Elsevier's Integrated
Histology

Elsevier's Integrated
Histology

Alvin G. Telser PhD

Northwestern University
Feinberg School of Medicine
Chicago, Illinois

with

John K. Young PhD

Department of Anatomy
Howard University College of Medicine
Washington, DC

Kate M. Baldwin PhD

Department of Anatomy
Howard University College of Medicine
Washington, DC

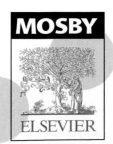

MOSBY

ELSEVIER

MOSBY
ELSEVIER

1600 John F. Kennedy Blvd
Suite 1800
Philadelphia, PA 19103-2899

ELSEVIER'S INTEGRATED HISTOLOGY   ISBN-13: 978-0-323-03388-6

Notice

Knowledge and best practice in this field are constantly changing. As new research and experience broaden our knowledge, changes in practice, treatment, and drug therapy may become necessary or appropriate. Readers are advised to check the most current information provided (i) on procedures featured or (ii) by the manufacturer of each product to be administered, to verify the recommended dose or formula, the method and duration of administration, and contraindications. It is the responsibility of the practitioner, relying on their own experience and knowledge of the patient, to make diagnoses, to determine dosages and the best treatment for each individual patient, and to take all appropriate safety precautions. To the fullest extent of the law, neither the Publisher nor the Authors assume any liability for any injury and/or damage to persons or property arising out or related to any use of the material contained in this book.

The Publisher

Library of Congress Cataloging-in-Publication Data

Telser, Alvin G.
    Elsevier's integrated histology / Alvin G. Telser, John K. Young,
Kate M. Baldwin.—1st ed.
        p. ; cm.—(Elsevier's integrated series)
    Includes index.
    ISBN 978-0-323-03388-6
    1. Histology. I. Young, John K. II. Baldwin, Kate M. III. Title.
IV. Title: Integrated histology. V. Series.
    [DNLM: 1. Histology. QS 504 T277e 2007]
QM551.T47 2007
611′018—dc22

                                2007002642

Acquisitions Editor: Kate Dimock
Developmental Editor: Andrew Hall

Printed in China

Last digit is the print number: 9   8   7   6   5   4   3   2   1

This book is dedicated to my loving wife, Karen, for her many years of unflagging support and encouragement.

I also wish to acknowledge the many excellent teachers I have had in my decades in higher education and learning. I learned from some in person and from many others by hearing them speak or by reading their excellent writings.

Alvin G. Telser, PhD

I would like to dedicate this book to the love of my life, my wife Paula.

John K. Young, PhD

Preface

The study and practice of medicine focuses on what goes wrong in the body and then how to restore it to a normal, healthy, functional state. For a physician to succeed in this endeavor, she or he needs considerable knowledge of both the normal and abnormal structures of the body's cells, tissues, and organs. Histology is that branch of medical science that describes the normal appearance and structure of cells, tissues, and organs at the microscopic level.

The molecular composition, biochemical composition, and functional aspects of these body components flow directly from the details of their structures. The ability to look at a structure and know what it comprises and to discern what its appearance and composition indicate about its ability to function properly is an invaluable skill for a physician—one that requires keen powers of observation and the application of detailed information. Histology is one of the few basic medical science disciplines that help the budding physician develop his or her observational skills.

This book assumes that the student has already taken a basic course in histology. It presents many light and electron micrographs of the cells, tissues, and organs of the body and seeks to place these structural features in a functional context. In many cases, only some of the structural features in an image are labeled, allowing the learner to locate and identify unlabeled examples of the same features. Diagrams are used to help connect structural features with their functional roles. Study them with a curious eye and mind; your diagnostic and clinical abilities will improve accordingly.

Alvin G. Telser, PhD
John K. Young, PhD
Kate M. Baldwin, PhD

Editorial Review Board

Chief Series Advisor
J. Hurley Myers, PhD
Professor Emeritus of Physiology and Medicine
Southern Illinois University School of Medicine
and
President and CEO
DxR Development Group, Inc.
Carbondale, Illinois

Anatomy and Embryology
Thomas R. Gest, PhD
University of Michigan Medical School
Division of Anatomical Sciences
Office of Medical Education
Ann Arbor, Michigan

Biochemistry
John W. Baynes, MS, PhD
Graduate Science Research Center
University of South Carolina
Columbia, South Carolina

Marek Dominiczak, MD, PhD, FRCPath, FRCP(Glas)
Clinical Biochemistry Service
NHS Greater Glasgow and Clyde
Gartnavel General Hospital
Glasgow, United Kingdom

Clinical Medicine
Ted O'Connell, MD
Clinical Instructor
David Geffen School of Medicine
UCLA
Program Director
Woodland Hills Family Medicine Residency Program
Woodland Hills, California

Genetics
Neil E. Lamb, PhD
Director of Educational Outreach
Hudson Alpha Institute for Biotechnology
Huntsville, Alabama
Adjunct Professor
Department of Human Genetics
Emory University
Atlanta, Georgia

Histology
Leslie P. Gartner, PhD
Professor of Anatomy
Department of Biomedical Sciences
Baltimore College of Dental Surgery
Dental School
University of Maryland at Baltimore
Baltimore, Maryland

James L. Hiatt, PhD
Professor Emeritus
Department of Biomedical Sciences
Baltimore College of Dental Surgery
Dental School
University of Maryland at Baltimore
Baltimore, Maryland

Immunology
Darren G. Woodside, PhD
Principal Scientist
Drug Discovery
Encysive Pharmaceuticals Inc.
Houston, Texas

Microbiology
Richard C. Hunt, MA, PhD
Professor of Pathology, Microbiology, and Immunology
Director of the Biomedical Sciences Graduate Program
Department of Pathology and Microbiology
University of South Carolina School of Medicine
Columbia, South Carolina

Neuroscience
Cristian Stefan, MD
Associate Professor
Department of Cell Biology
University of Massachusetts Medical School
Worcester, Massachusetts

Pharmacology
Michael M. White, PhD
Professor
Department of Pharmacology and Physiology
Drexel University College of Medicine
Philadelphia, Pennsylvania

Physiology
Joel Michael, PhD
Department of Molecular Biophysics and Physiology
Rush Medical College
Chicago, Illinois

Pathology
Peter G. Anderson, DVM, PhD
Professor and Director of Pathology Undergraduate Education
Department of Pathology
University of Alabama at Birmingham
Birmingham, Alabama

Contents

Series Preface

How to Use This Book

The idea for Elsevier's Integrated Series came about at a seminar on the USMLE Step 1 exam at an American Medical Student Association (AMSA) meeting. We noticed that the discussion between faculty and students focused on how the exams were becoming increasingly integrated—with case scenarios and questions often combining two or three science disciplines. The students were clearly concerned about how they could best integrate their basic science knowledge.

One faculty member gave some interesting advice: "read through your textbook in, say, biochemistry, and every time you come across a section that mentions a concept or piece of information relating to another basic science—for example, immunology—highlight that section in the book. Then go to your immunology textbook and look up this information, and make sure you have a good understanding of it. When you have, go back to your biochemistry textbook and carry on reading."

This was a great suggestion—if only students had the time, and all of the books necessary at hand, to do it! At Elsevier we thought long and hard about a way of simplifying this process, and eventually the idea for Elsevier's Integrated Series was born.

The series centers on the concept of the *integration box*. These boxes occur throughout the text whenever a link to another basic science is relevant. They're easy to spot in the text—with their color-coded headings and logos. Each box contains a title for the integration topic and then a brief summary of the topic. The information is complete in itself— you probably won't have to go to any other sources—and you have the basic knowledge to use as a foundation if you want to expand your knowledge of the topic.

You can use this book in two ways. First, as a review book . . . When you are using the book for review, the integration boxes will jog your memory on topics you have already covered. You'll be able to reassure yourself that you can identify the link, and you can quickly compare your knowledge of the topic with the summary in the box. The integration boxes might highlight gaps in your knowledge, and then you can use them to determine what topics you need to cover in more detail.

Second, the book can be used as a short text to have at hand while you are taking your course . . . You may come across an integration box that deals with a topic you haven't covered yet, and this will ensure that you're one step ahead in identifying the links to other subjects (especially useful if you're working on a PBL exercise). On a simpler level, the links in the boxes to other sciences and to clinical medicine will help you see clearly the relevance of the basic science topic you are studying. You may already be

confident in the subject matter of many of the integration boxes, so they will serve as helpful reminders.

At the back of the book we have included case study questions relating to each chapter so that you can test yourself as you work your way through the book.

Online Version

An online version of the book is available on our Student Consult site. Use of this site is free to anyone who has bought the printed book. Please see the inside front cover for full details on the Student Consult and how to access the electronic version of this book.

In addition to containing USMLE test questions, fully searchable text, and an image bank, the Student Consult site offers additional integration links, both to the other books in Elsevier's Integrated Series and to other key Elsevier textbooks.

Books in Elsevier's Integrated Series

The nine books in the series cover all of the basic sciences. The more books you buy in the series, the more links that are made accessible across the series, both in print and online.

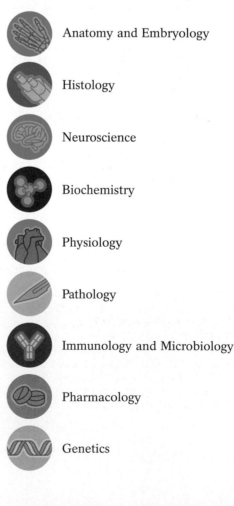

Anatomy and Embryology

Histology

Neuroscience

Biochemistry

Physiology

Pathology

Immunology and Microbiology

Pharmacology

Genetics

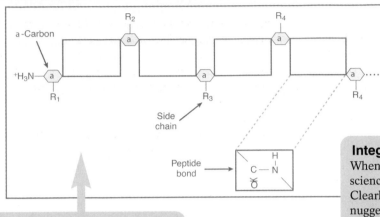

Figure 3-1. The peptide bond linking α-carbons and their side chains together into a polypeptide. The *trans* conformation is favored, producing a rigid structure that restricts freedom of movement except for rotation around bonds that join to the α-carbons.

Artwork:
The books are packed with 4-color illustrations and photographs. When a concept can be better explained with a picture, we've drawn one. Where possible, the pictures tell a dynamic story that will help you remember the information far more effectively than a paragraph of text.

Integration boxes:
Whenever the subject matter can be related to another science discipline, we've put in an Integration Box. Clearly labeled and color-coded, these boxes include nuggets of information on topics that require an integrated knowledge of the sciences to be fully understood. The material in these boxes is complete in itself, and you can use them as a way of reminding yourself of information you already know and reinforcing key links between the sciences. Or the boxes may contain information you have not come across before, in which case you can use them as a springboard for further research or simply to appreciate the relevance of the subject matter of the book to the study of medicine.

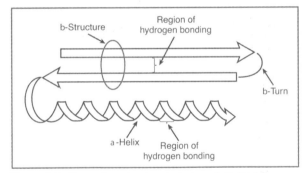

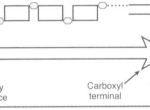

MICROBIOLOGY

Prion Diseases

Prions (PrP^Sc) are formed from otherwise normal neurologic proteins (PrP) and are responsible for encephalopathies in humans (Creutzfeldt Jakob disease, kuru), scrapie in sheep, and bovine spongiform encephalopathy. Contact between the normal PrP and PrP^Sc results in conversion of the secondary structure of PrP from predominantly α-helical to predominantly β-pleated sheet. The altered structure of the protein forms long, filamentous aggregates that gradually damage neuronal tissue. The harmful PrP^Sc form is highly resistant to heat, UV irradiation, and protease enzymes.

Figure 3-3. Secondary structure includes α-helix and β-pleated sheet (β-sheet).

Since proline has no free hydrogen to contribute to helix stability, it is referred to as a "helix breaker." The α-helix is found in most globular proteins and in some fibrous proteins (e.g., α-keratin).

Text:
Succinct, clearly written text, focusing on the core information you need to know and no more. It's the same level as a carefully prepared course syllabus or lecture notes.

rmation
-structure) consists of
tabilized by hydrogen f adjacent sequences.
(parallel) or opposite (antiparallel) direction. β-Structures are found in 80% of all globular proteins and in silk fibroin.

Supersecondary Structure and Domains

Supersecondary structures, or *motifs*, are characteristic combinations of secondary structure 10–40 residues in length that recur in different proteins. They bridge the gap between the less specific regularity of secondary structure and the highly specific folding of tertiary structure. The same motif can perform similar functions in different proteins.

- The four-helix bundle motif provides a cavity for enzymes to bind prosthetic groups or cofactors.
- The β-barrel motif can bind hydrophobic molecules such as retinol in the interior of the barrel.
- Motifs may also be mixtures of both α and β conformations.

Discovering and Describing Cell Structure

1

TECHNIQUES FOR STUDYING THE CELL

Virtually all living organisms, whether single-celled protists or multicellular metazoans, are compartmentalized to protect themselves from the environment and to control and regulate the myriad functions, processes, behaviors, and homeostatic mechanisms that are the essence of life. The compartments range in scale from protein-protein associations (e.g., a transcription complex); to structures (e.g., ribosomes); to cell organelles (e.g., mitochondria); to individual cells (e.g., lympho-cytes); to groups of similar cells, called tissues (e.g., muscle); to organs (e.g., parotid gland). Histology is a science devoted to a detailed study of the microscopic organization, appearance, and function of these cells, tissues, and organs, as well as the fluids and extracellular macromolecules found in the human body.

A major emphasis of modern histology is to provide an accurate description of the appearance, organization, and composition of the cells, tissues, and organs of a typical normal adult individual to provide a basis for understanding their function as well as understanding abnormal changes that may occur.

The main tool used in histology is a microscope; most routine histology is done by examining thin sections of material on glass slides with a light microscope viewed with transmitted light in the bright-field mode. Electron microscopy, both transmission and scanning, has also been a powerful tool in modern histology research because of the greater resolution the instruments afford. Specimens have to be prepared in special ways to be studied with any of these instruments. For the study of normal histology, a typical specimen is about one cubic centimeter or smaller. In a clinical setting, biopsy specimens are typically much smaller, perhaps a few cubic millimeters; they may be collected with a large-bore needle or sometimes as tissue scrapings. Typical specimen preparation entails fixation of the specimen with chemical agents. Specimens are then embedded in paraffin or plastic and sliced into very thin sections—on the order of a few micrometers thick for light microscopy to fractions of a micron thick for electron microscopy.

After sectioning, a stain is applied to make the specimen visible in the microscope. In the case of light microscopy, the stain (usually colored chemical dyes) imparts optical contrast to the specimen. In electron microscopy, the stains are heavy metal salts that absorb some of the electrons in the beam such that the specimen acquires contrast owing to the varying degrees to which the electrons penetrate the specimen.

A major challenge confronts the student in histology—how to interpret and understand the three-dimensional structure and organization of tissues and organs by looking at (apparently) random two-dimensional slices of these structures. Figure 1-1 illustrates how a number of section planes through

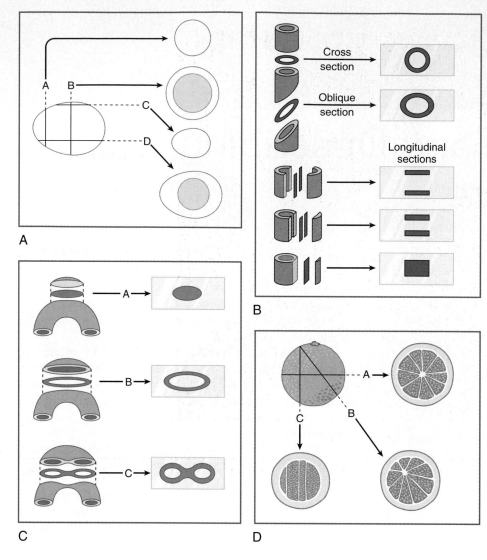

Figure 1-1. A, A hard-boiled egg sectioned in four planes. **B,** A cylinder sectioned transversely, obliquely, and in several vertical planes. Thin slices cut through a straight tube as at the left of this figure appear as on the right when mounted on glass slides. **C,** A curved cylinder sectioned in several planes. **D,** An orange cut to show transverse, oblique, and longitudinal sections.

common objects are interpreted relative to the structure of the whole, which then can provide a useful impression of the three-dimensional appearance of the object.

●●● LIGHT MICROSCOPY

Bright Field

Transmitted light bright-field microscopy is the most common and widely used technique in histology. A section in a thickness range of 1.5 to 20 μm is mounted on a glass slide and covered with a thin glass coverslip. It is illuminated from below with a bright light, and the image is seen in the eyepieces (or on a monitor) after passing through a substage condenser, the microscope objective, and the eyepieces. Specimens are viewed in a magnification range of about 25× to 1000×. Optical resolution increases significantly from the lower magnification ranges to the higher ones owing to the increased resolving power of high-power objectives (40× or greater). The optical resolution of this type of microscopy is on the order of 0.2 μm. This means it is possible to see

(resolve) objects that are 0.2 μm apart but no closer or those that are 0.2 μm in diameter but no smaller. Figure 1-2 shows a high magnification image of a white blood cell with some small cytoplasmic granules the smaller of which are about 0.1 μm in diameter and the larger about 0.3 to 0.4 μm in diameter.

Immunofluorescence

Immunofluorescence microscopy is used extensively in modern cell biology, molecular biology, immunology, and pathology research. It is also widely used in clinical laboratories to assist in the diagnosis of many diseases. Specimen preparation for immunofluorescence microscopy is different from that for transmitted light microscopy. Most immunofluorescence microscopy is done with illumination from above (epi-illumination) rather than from below. Figure 1-3 illustrates the use of immunofluorescence to label a major component of the cytoskeleton, vimentin intermediate filaments, in a normal interphase cell grown in tissue culture. Figure 1-4 illustrates the same technique used to localize a

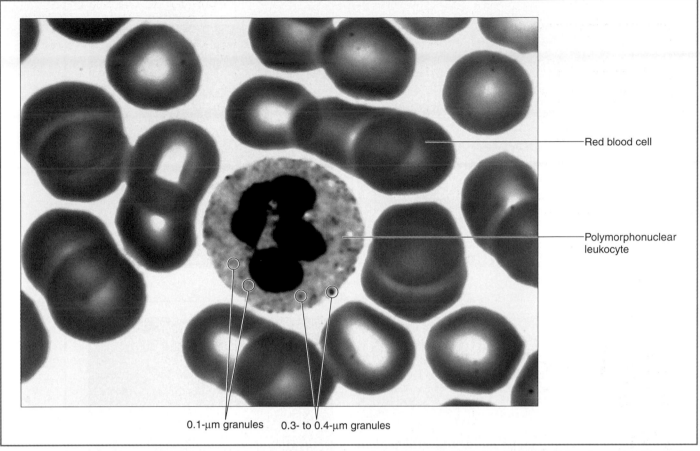

Red blood cell

Polymorphonuclear leukocyte

0.1-μm granules   0.3- to 0.4-μm granules

Figure 1-2. A white blood cell (polymorphonuclear leukocyte) from the peripheral circulation (1600×). This micrograph illustrates the limit of resolution of the light microscope.

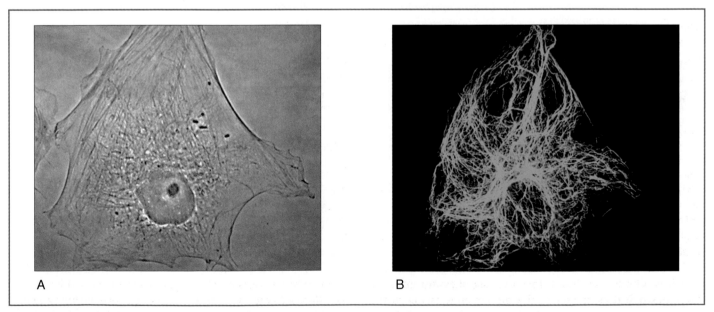

A   B

Figure 1-3. A, Phase-contrast image of an epithelial cell from a rat kangaroo (PtK2 cell) grown in tissue culture. **B,** The same cell as seen in an immunofluorescence microscope after the cell was stained with an antibody to the intermediate filament protein vimentin. (Courtesy of L. Chang and R. D. Goldman.)

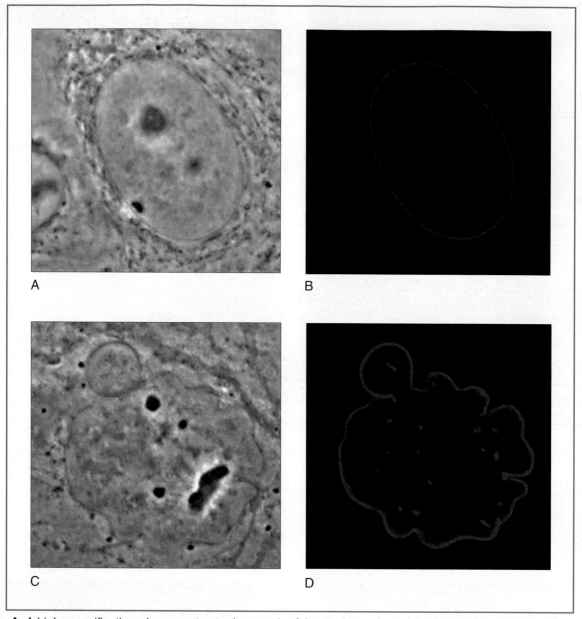

A

B

C

D

Figure 1-4. A, A high-magnification phase-contrast micrograph of the nucleus of a normal human fibroblast. **B,** The same nucleus as seen in an immunofluorescence microscope after the cell was stained with an antibody to lamins A and C. **C,** High-magnification phase-contrast micrograph of the nucleus of a human fibroblast obtained from a patient with progeria. **D,** The same nucleus as seen in an immunofluorescence microscope after the cell was stained with an antibody to lamins A and C. (Courtesy of S. Khuon and R. D. Goldman.)

different intermediate filament protein, lamin (a specific component associated with the inner surface of the nuclear envelope), in a normal fibroblast nucleus (see Figs. 1-4A and 1-4B) and a fibroblast nucleus (see Figs. 1-4C and 1-4D) from a patient with progeria—a disease that causes premature aging in affected individuals. Lamins are an important determinant of nuclear shape and are involved in gene transcription. Patients with progeria have a mutation in the lamin A gene that results in a profound alteration in nuclear shape.

●●● PHASE-CONTRAST MICROSCOPY

Phase-contrast microscopy is a technique most commonly used to examine living, unstained cells growing in laboratory tissue culture plates (see Figs. 1-3A, 1-4A, and 1-4C). Considerable cellular detail can be seen in such cells grown in culture. However, the organization of unstained tissues and organs as seen in sectioned material are too "phase-similar" and too complex to be interpreted with phase-contrast microscopy.

PATHOLOGY

Use of Immunofluorescence Microscopy in Disease Diagnosis

For more than a century pathologists have used light microscopy to great advantage to understand and diagnose diseases.

In the ensuing years, more and more information regarding the normal biochemical composition and organization of tissues and organs has become available. Furthermore, specific antibodies have been produced against many of these molecules. Since it is possible to localize these molecules by indirect immunofluorescence microscopy, a much larger number of diseases can be identified and with greater certainty.

BIOCHEMISTRY

Synthesis of Thyroglobulin and the Thyroid Hormone Thyroxine

The thyroid hormone thyroxine (tetraiodothyronine) is synthesized and secreted by the follicular cells of the thyroid gland. Hormone synthesis is a multistep process that involves most of the basic steps of cell function. The gene for thyroglobulin, a 660-kDa glycoprotein, is transcribed in the nucleus.

Thyroglobulin is translated in the rER, glycosylated in the Golgi apparatus, and constitutively secreted by exocytosis at the apical surface of the thyroid follicular cell into follicular lumen. Thus, thyroglobulin is stored extracellularly in the follicles in a gel-like mass called colloid.

Iodide ions are taken up from the bloodstream at the basal surface of the cell in an energy-dependent process, then transported to the apical surface of the cell, where the iodide is oxidized to iodine and released into the colloid. Many of the 120 tyrosine residues in thyroglobulin are iodinated and oxidatively coupled to generate triiodothyronine (T_3) and tetraiodothyronine (T_4). Iodinated thyroglobulin is taken up from the colloid by endocytosis and degraded in lysosomes to produce T_3 and T_4, which are released into the bloodstream at the basal surface of the follicular cells.

BIOCHEMISTRY

Ribosome Biogenesis and Export from the Nucleus

Ribosomal subunits are synthesized and assembled in the nucleolus and exported from the nucleus to the cytoplasm via nuclear pores.

Ribosomal (rRNA) genes, which reside in the nucleolus, are transcribed and assembled into small (40S) and large (60S) ribosomal subunits in the nucleolus. Ribosomal proteins, which have a nuclear import signal, are synthesized in the cytoplasm and imported to the nucleus by specific nuclear importins. Subunit assembly requires all the ribosomal proteins and low-molecular-weight rRNAs whose genes reside on non-nucleolar chromosomal loci. The 40S and 60S subunits are then transported to the cytoplasm via the nuclear pores. They assemble into 80S ribosomes in the cytoplasm or on the rER.

●●● ELECTRON MICROSCOPY

Specimens are prepared for electron microscopy (EM) using techniques similar to those used for light microscopy except that they are thought to preserve tissue appearance and structure in a more faithful reflection of the living state than those used in light microscopy. Small pieces of tissue are fixed in a different set of reagents than those used in light microscopy, embedded in plastic, and sectioned with a very sharp glass or a diamond knife, stained with heavy metal stains (uranyl, lead, or osmic acid salts) and examined in the transmission electron microscope (TEM). Optimal section thickness is 60 to 90 nm. A major advantage of EM is that the electron microscope has a much higher resolution than the light microscope (i.e., about 1 to 2 nm vs 0.2 μm [200 nm]). Figures 1-5A to 1-5C illustrate a section of the follicular cells of the thyroid gland in two light micrographs at medium (A) and high magnification (B) and a relatively low magnification electron micrograph (C). While the main features of these cuboidal epithelial cells are evident in all three micrographs, it is only in the electron micrograph that many subcellular details can be resolved. For example, the apical filopodia, chromatin, mitochondria, components of the endoplasmic reticulum and secretory vesicles (the secretory pathway), as well as pinocytotic vesicles and lysosomes (the endocytic pathway), are visible only in the electron micrograph (D).

Several special techniques in electron microscopy are particularly well suited to the examination of certain subcellular structures (e.g., nuclear pore complexes, components of the cytoskeleton) and certain components of the extracellular matrix (e.g., collagen fibers, proteoglycan aggregates). One of these techniques is negative staining. For negative staining, the material of interest is placed on a small, plastic-coated metal grid and flooded with stains containing heavy metal salts (e.g., uranyl acetate). The grid is examined in the electron microscope where the specimen is seen as a less electron-dense structure surrounded by the heavy metal stain (i.e., as a "negatively stained" or "negatively contrasted" structure) (Fig. 1-6).

Using another technique, a specimen may be metal-coated by vaporizing a heavy metal on it (often platinum), thus enabling detailed surface features to be examined at high resolution in the electron microscope (Fig. 1-7). Freeze-fracture etching is yet another technique in which tissue is frozen, etched, and coated with heavy metals under high vacuum, permitting internal and external membrane surfaces to be examined. In this technique, a fresh specimen is frozen under special conditions, the specimen is fractured while frozen, some of the frozen water is sublimed away (etched)

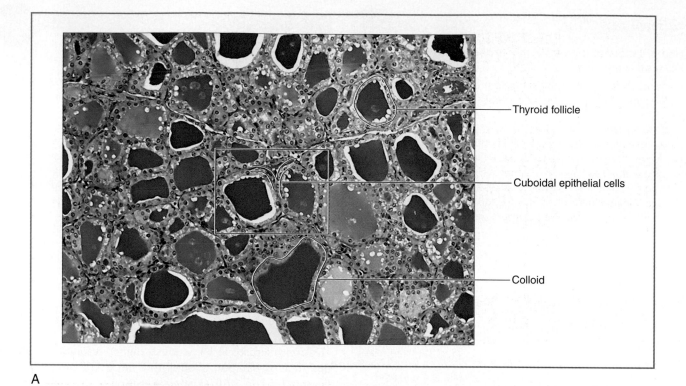

A

B

Figure 1-5. Light and electron micrographs of thyroid follicles illustrating the appearance of the cuboidal epithelial cells that comprise the cellular surface of the follicles at increasing magnification and resolution. **A,** A 1.5-μm section of the thyroid gland stained with H&E (125×). **B,** The same section at 500×.

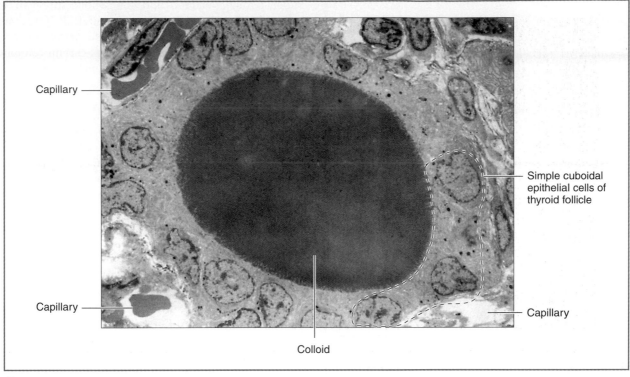

C

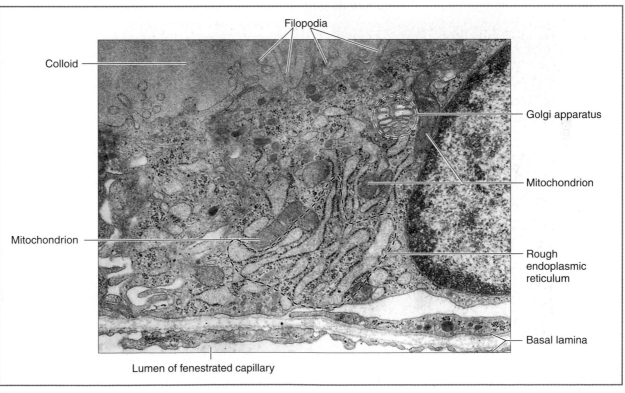

D

Figure 1-5 cont'd. C, A similar section of a thyroid follicle as seen in an electron micrograph (1800×). **D,** A higher magnification electron micrograph of a thyroid follicular cell showing several cell organelles (10,000×). (**C** and **D,** Courtesy of Judith Taggert Rhodin.)

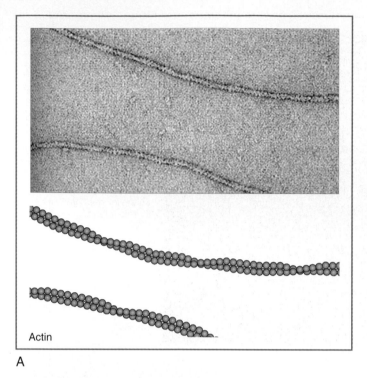

Actin

A

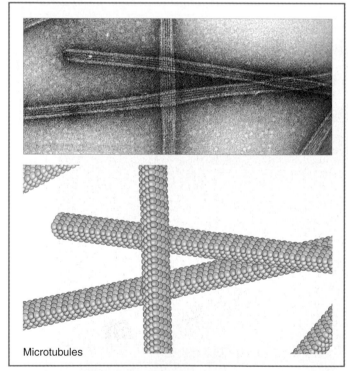

Microtubules

B

Figure 1-6. A, Electron micrograph of two actin filaments as seen by the negative stain technique. **B,** Electron micrograph of negatively stained microtubules. Below each micrograph is an interpretive drawing of the polymers.

under a high vacuum, and the whole specimen is subsequently coated with a heavy metal. This technique is especially useful for seeing very fine details of structures embedded in plasma membranes (e.g., certain cell junctions, the cytoskeleton, or in this example, nuclear pores) (Fig. 1-8).

A somewhat newer kind of electron microscope, the scanning electron microscope (SEM), provides still another way to study cell, tissue, and organ fine structure. This instrument operates in a resolution range that falls between the resolution of the light microscope and the transmission electron microscope, namely, about 20 nm. Cells, tissues, and whole organs can easily be studied with the SEM after they are coated with a metal. Specimen preparation for the SEM does not require cutting thin sections although specimens are first frozen and then dried in a special way (called critical point drying) before they are coated with vaporized metal. Some specimens are fractured before critical point drying and coating with a heavy metal. The distinctive three-dimensional appearance of many structures in the SEM can be more informative than the way they are seen in either the light microscope or the TEM (Fig. 1-9).

●●● STAINS

The extremely thin slices of tissue examined in a light or electron microscope are essentially invisible in the beam that illuminates them unless a stain is applied to the tissue. While some stains used in light microscopy provide information about the substance that takes up the stain, for the most part, the stain should be thought of primarily as an agent that provides contrast to a specimen that otherwise has little or no intrinsic contrast. The most commonly used stain is hematoxylin and eosin (H&E); with this stain, nuclei are a dark blue to black color, and cytoplasm and most extracellular materials stain a light to intense pink color. A variety of stains comprise three (or more) different stains to help reveal different components of a cell's cytoplasm or to help differentiate various components of the extracellular matrix; these are called trichrome stains and often carry the name of the person who developed them (Fig. 1-10). Many other stains are used in light microscopy; these will be introduced in the context of the tissues or other structural features where they are most frequently used.

Generally speaking, it is not necessary or even useful to learn what different cellular or matrix features (or components of either) are stained what specific color by the many stains used. It may be most useful to imagine all stains as if you were seeing in black and white—much the way a movie or television show is just as understandable in black and white as in color—albeit perhaps not as appealing.

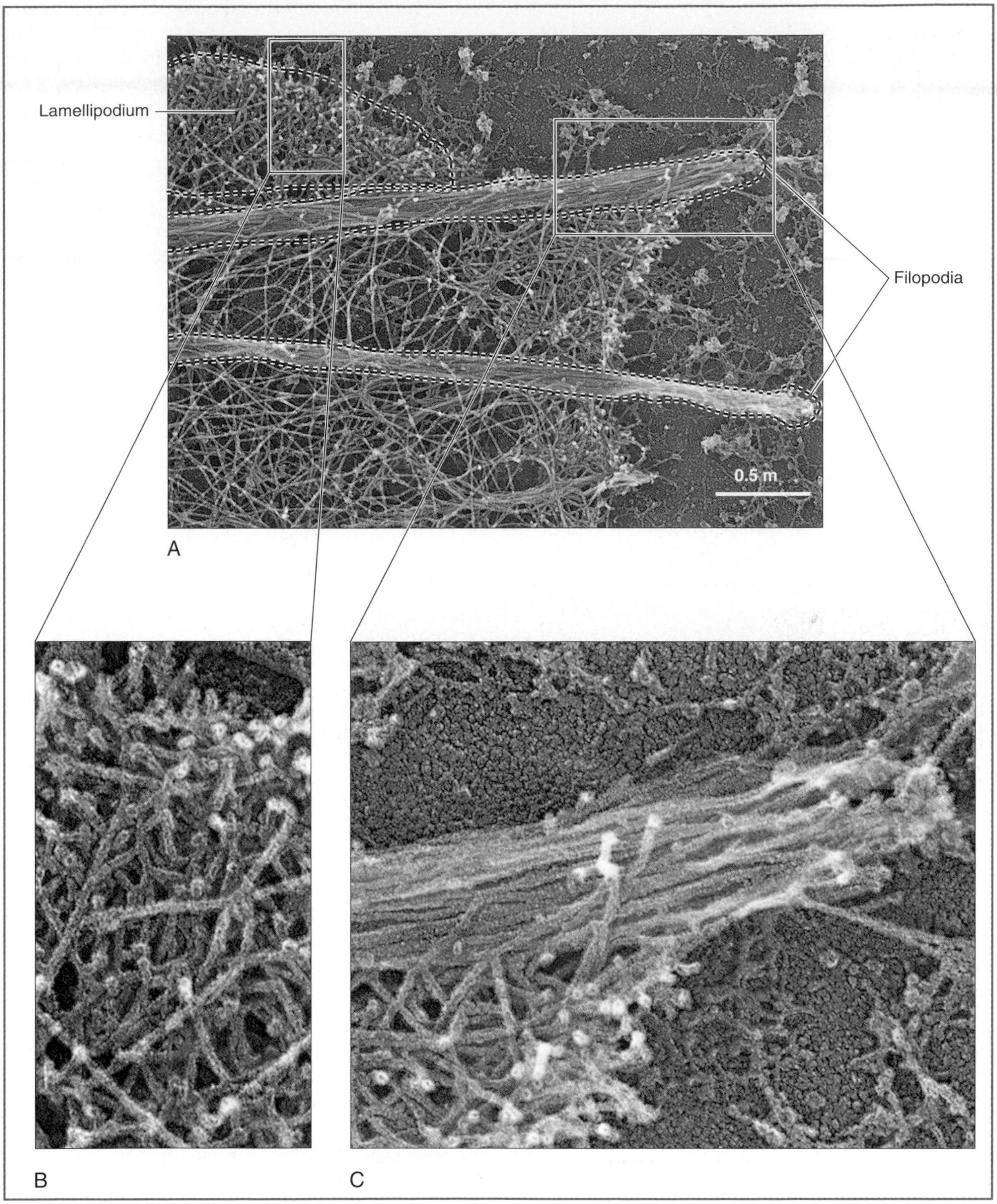

Figure 1-7. A, Electron micrograph of a migrating, cultured, frozen, deep-etched, platinum-coated fish keratocyte. In the lower magnification view, part of the migratory edge of the cell can be seen; the region in the box at the upper left is seen at higher magnification in part B, and the region at the upper right is seen in part C. The extensive meshwork of actin filaments (**B**) and the large bundle of actin filaments (**C**) are seen in the higher magnification image. (Courtesy of T. Svitkina and G. G. Borisy.)

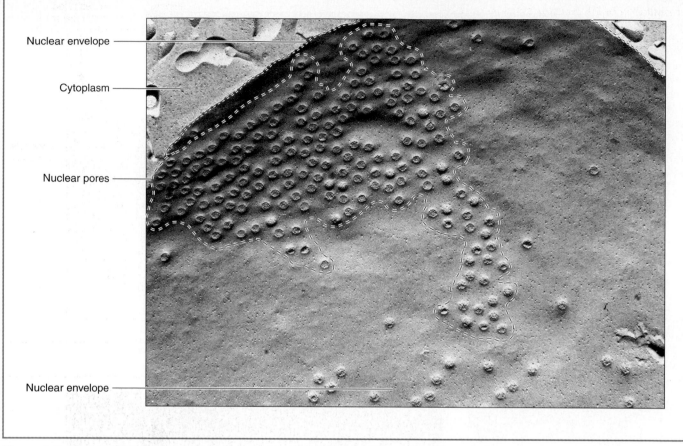

Figure 1-8. Freeze-fracture-etch preparation of a nuclear envelope. (Courtesy of Don W. Fawcett.)

Figure 1-9. A, Diagrammatic representation of the complex structure appearing in the lower part of part B. (Redrawn from Gartner LP, Hiatt JL. *Color Textbook of Histology,* 2nd ed. Philadelphia, WB Saunders, 2001, pp 441–442.) **B,** A scanning electron micrograph of the cells (podocytes) that envelop the capillaries of the glomerular capillary tuft in the renal corpuscle. (Courtesy of Don W. Fawcett.)

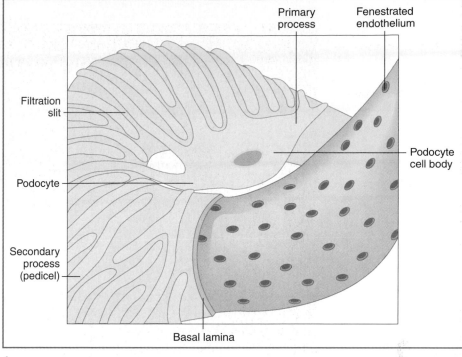

A

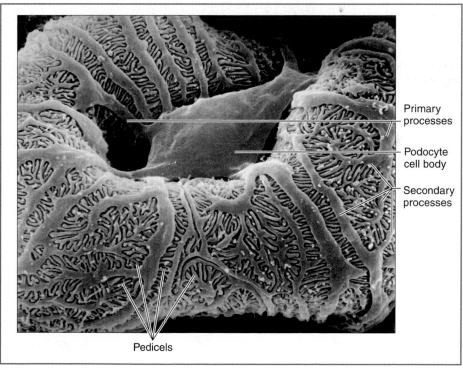

B

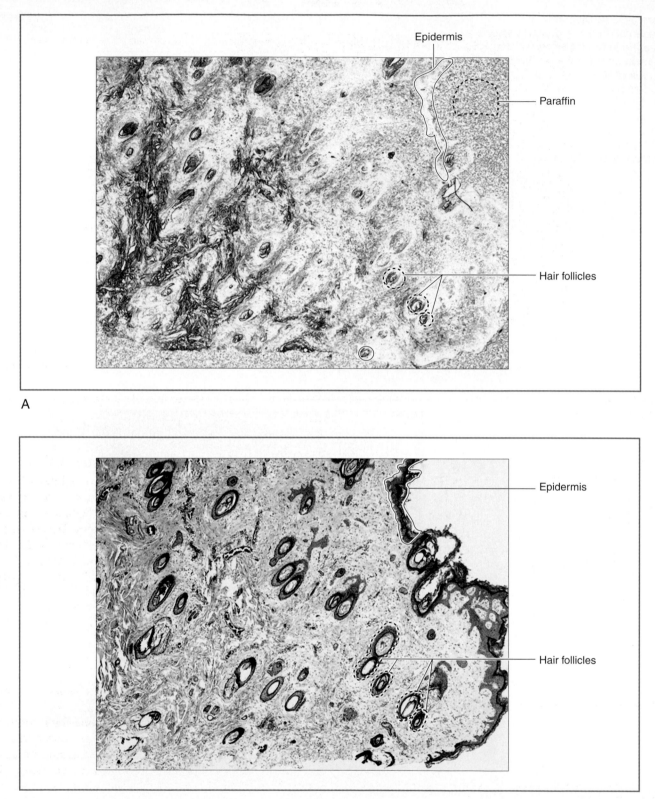

A

B

Figure 1-10. A, Section of scalp fixed, embedded in paraffin, and mounted on a slide without being stained. **B,** Nearby section from the same block stained with H&E.

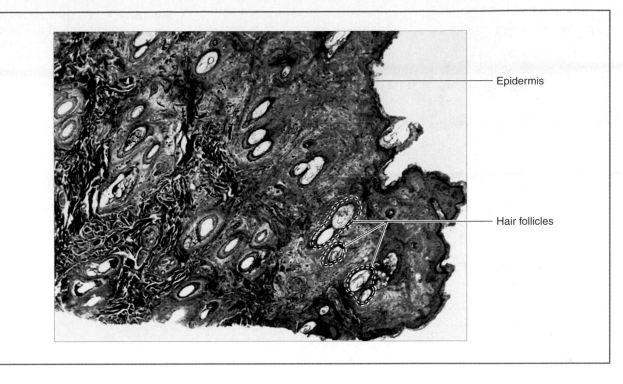

C

Figure 1-10 cont'd. C, Another nearby section from the same block stained with a trichrome stain. (All three images photographed at 20×.)

KEY POINTS ABOUT HISTOLOGY

- All cells are compartmentalized.
- Histology is the study of cells, tissues, and organs by light microscopy (transmitted, immunofluorescence, or other types), transmission electron microscopy, and scanning electron microscopy.
- A major difference among these types of microscopy is their resolving power (resolution).
- Each technique can be used to advantage to study specific features of normal cells, tissues, and organs.
- Most of these techniques are routinely used in the study of pathologic specimens and in many diagnostic methods.

CELL STRUCTURE AND FUNCTION

The cell is the fundamental unit of life; every structural and functional unit of the human body consists of cells and the extracellular products they produce. The precise composition of the fluids in which the internal environment of the organism is bathed is also created and maintained by the cells of the body. Since the invention of the light microscope over three centuries ago, scientists have studied and described the cells of living organisms. In the past 50 years or so, a far more detailed description of cell structure has been made possible by the use of biological electron microscopy. Described here are the major structural features of "generic" cells, their composition, and a brief description of what they do. Later chapters will describe and discuss specific cells in greater detail.

●●● PLASMA MEMBRANE

Structure

All cells are surrounded by a semipermeable membrane called the plasma membrane. Most (ca. 75%) of the membrane consists of lipids (phospholipids, cholesterol, and glycolipids); the balance is proteins, glycoproteins, and some lipoproteins. The components are arranged into a lipid bilayer: the phospholipids are positioned so that their hydrophilic "heads" are in contact with the internal cytoplasm or the external environment, and the hydrophilic "tails" are in contact with one another. Dispersed among the phospholipids are numerous cholesterol molecules and many proteins. This arrangement leads to the characteristic appearance of the plasma membrane in electron micrographs that is described as a trilaminar unit membrane. The term that describes our current understanding of the plasma membrane is the modified fluid mosaic model (Fig. 1-11).

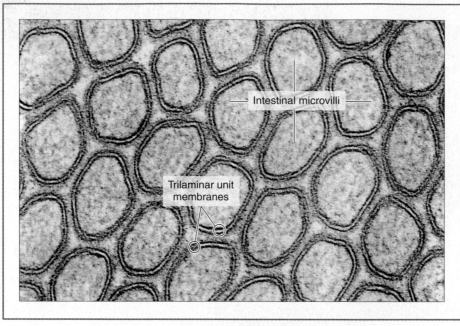

A

Figure 1-11. A, High-magnification electron micrograph of the brush border of intestinal absorptive cells showing the trilaminar structure of the lipid bilayer of the plasma membrane (Courtesy of Don W. Fawcett.) **B,** Diagram depicting the current understanding of the disposition of proteins and lipids in the plasma membrane.

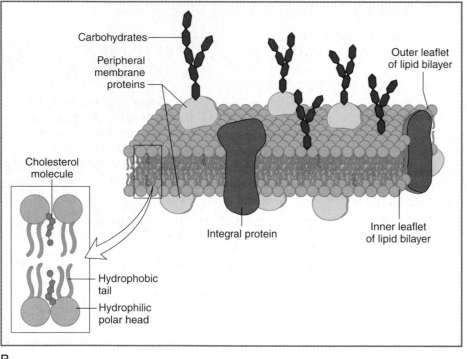

B

Composition and Organization

The protein components of the membrane are associated with it in a variety of ways. Some are embedded in the lipid bilayer, or span it with a portion in the extracellular or intracellular space, or are in both spaces; these proteins are called *integral membrane proteins*. Some are associated only with the cytoplasmic or the extracellular leaflet of the lipid bilayer. Most of the proteins that are in contact with the extracellular space are glycosylated. Many of the proteins have a small lipid molecule (myristate) covalently attached to them which helps anchor the protein to the lipid bilayer. A large number of proteins are associated with the cytoplasmic face of the membrane, either interacting with the hydrophilic heads of the lipids or with proteins embedded in the bilayer. Many of the proteins embedded in the membrane have hydrophobic regions that span the bilayer 1 to as many as 12 times.

Function

The plasma membrane serves as a semipermeable barrier between the cytoplasm and the extracellular environment of the cell. It is freely permeable to gases (e.g., O_2 and CO_2) and a number of small, uncharged molecules (e.g., urea). It is responsible for maintaining the correct intercellular ionic composition and pH and for transporting nutrients into the cell and waste products out. There are many membrane transporters, some general and some specific. There are many terms for the transporters (symports, antiports, etc); some require the expenditure of energy to function, and others exchange internal components with external ones. The plasma membrane even has specific water channel proteins (aquaporins).

The plasma membrane controls the ingress and egress of virtually everything (except for the few things to which it is freely permeable) that enters or leaves the cell. Molecules such as ions, amino acids, monosaccharides, and other nutrients enter the cell via specific transporters. Many integral plasma membrane proteins and membrane-associated proteins are involved in taking material into the cell by a process called *endocytosis*. When cells take up solutes (e.g., growth factors, immunoglobulins), the process is called *pinocytosis* (cell drinking); when they take up particulate materials (e.g., bacteria, yeast, carbon particles [smoke]), it is called *phagocytosis* (cell eating).

Pinocytosis and phagocytosis do not usually involve membrane receptors and are considered *unregulated* cell uptake processes. Endocytosis typically does involve specific plasma membrane receptors for each molecule (or class of molecules) taken into the cell. Many plasma membrane proteins involved in endocytosis are receptors for hormones or other biologically active molecules. Endocytosis proceeding via this *regulated* pathway is called receptor-mediated endocytosis (RCME), and the vesicles that result are called coated vesicles. Furthermore, other proteins are associated with the inner surface of the plasma membrane that are critical for the proper formation and internalization of the vesicles. A molecule central to this part of the endocytosis process is clathrin, which is a major component of the coat. Many other signaling molecules, such as cytokines, growth factors, and lymphokines, also interact with plasma membrane receptors but are not internalized. The signaling molecules and their receptors are key components of signal transduction mechanisms.

Another very important function of the plasma membrane is its role in the immune system. Bacteria, yeast, other pathogens, even fragments of foreign materials, can activate the immune system after they are phagocytosed by certain cells, called antigen-processing cells. This is a very complex process that involves a number of plasma membrane proteins, in particular, the major histocompatibility complex.

When cells release materials into the extracellular space, the process is called *exocytosis*. In general, exocytosis involves the fusion of intracellular vesicles with the plasma membrane.

Proteins and lipids in the vesicular membrane bind to cognate molecules in the plasma membrane; the membranes fuse so that the contents of the vesicle are released from the cell. Most macromolecules are exocytosed via a regulated or a constitutive pathway. Figure 1-12 shows several of these events in a schematic diagram.

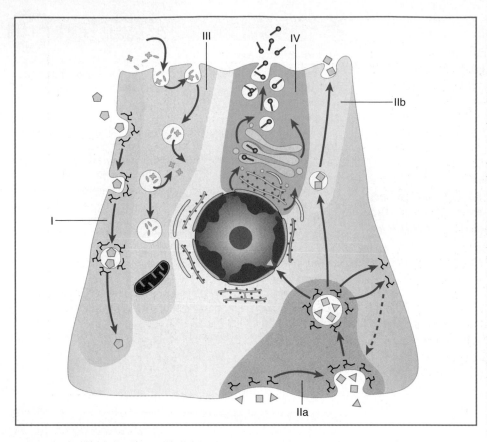

Figure 1-12. Diagram of a cell illustrating several types of endocytosis and exocytosis. On the left and bottom of the cell, RCME of materials from the external environment (I, pale orange) or the internal environment (IIa, deep orange) are illustrated. Some molecules taken up by RMCE (IIa, green squares) are transported to the apical surface of the cell and released, a process called transcytosis (IIb, yellow). Others taken up this way may travel to the nucleus (green triangles). The triskelions (purple) involved in RMCE are recycled as indicated near IIa and the lower right part of the cell. Unregulated pinocytosis and phagocytosis are shown at the upper left apical surface of the cell (III, pink). Some materials taken up this way may be released into the cytoplasm or may end up in lysosomes (small yellow ovals). The synthesis and secretion of proteins by exocytosis is indicated in the green area (IV). In highly polarized cells (those with distinct "tops," "sides," and "bottoms"), the different activities tend to be compartmentalized to the different surfaces. However, all cells carry out all these activities, often side by side. In this diagram, the symbols of materials taken up into the cell or secreted from it are not intended to convey any information about their structure; similarly, internal regions of the cell are colored to aid in following each of the several activities in the diagram.

●●● NUCLEUS

The nucleus is the most structurally prominent organelle of the eukaryotic cell (Fig. 1-13). While it contains roughly equal amounts of DNA, RNA and protein, it is the genetic material, (i.e., DNA) and its functional implications that makes the nucleus such an important organelle. Cells may either be dividing (mitotically or meiotically)—a state they are in for a very small proportion of their lifetime—or not dividing (interphase). What follows is a description of the interphase nucleus.

BIOCHEMISTRY

DNA Structure and Replication

Nuclear DNA is a double helix consisting of a linear polymer of the four deoxynucleoside bases—adenine (A), thymine (T), guanine (G), and cytosine (C). Chromatin contains double-stranded DNA and many proteins, some of which are structural, others enzymes, and still others regulatory.

The double-stranded helix results from A pairing with T, and G with C, via hydrogen bonds. The DNA is organized into several higher orders of structure to produce the chromatin seen in the light or electron microscope. Each linear strand is replicated by enzymes, which generates a complementary strand. DNA has a significant ability to repair replication errors and damage to individual bases or small groups of bases following chemical, radiation, oxidative, or other types of injury. In genetic terms, unrepaired errors are mutations.

Nuclear structure appears to be relatively simple, but its molecular organization is very complex. It is bounded by the nuclear envelope, composed of two concentric membranes and perforated by a few thousand nuclear pore complexes (see Figs. 1-7 and 1-13). The number of nuclear pore complexes is thought to be functionally related to the transcriptional activity of the nucleus (Fig. 1-14).

A distinct class of intermediate filaments (the nuclear lamins—lamin A and lamin B) is associated with the inner membrane of the nuclear envelope (see Fig. 1-4). The lamins help maintain nuclear shape, participate in anchoring chromatin to the nuclear envelope, are involved in gene transcription, and participate in nuclear assembly-disassembly during cell division.

Associated with the outer membrane of the nuclear envelope are many ribosomes. The outer membrane itself is continuous with the rough endoplasmic reticulum (rER).

Chromatin

Two terms are used to describe the major contents of the nucleus—those visible in the light and electron microscopes. The general term used to describe nuclear contents is chromatin, a complex consisting of DNA, histones, and other proteins. *Euchromatin* is the portion of chromatin that is or has recently been transcriptionally active. *Heterochromatin* is the transcriptionally inactive portion of chromatin.

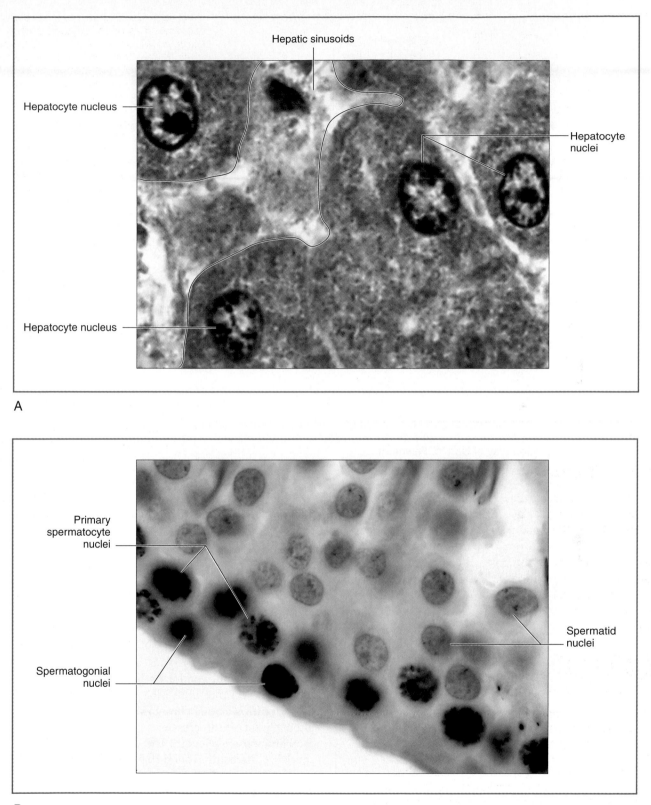

Hepatic sinusoids

Hepatocyte nucleus

Hepatocyte nuclei

Hepatocyte nucleus

A

Primary
spermatocyte
nuclei

Spermatid
nuclei

Spermatogonial
nuclei

B

Figure 1-13. A, Hepatocyte nuclei at high magnification (H&E, 1250×). **B,** Nuclei of spermatogenic cells in a seminiferous tubule of the testis (Feulgen stain, 1250×) (compare with the phase-contrast images of the nuclei in Figures 1-3A and 1-4A). *Continued*

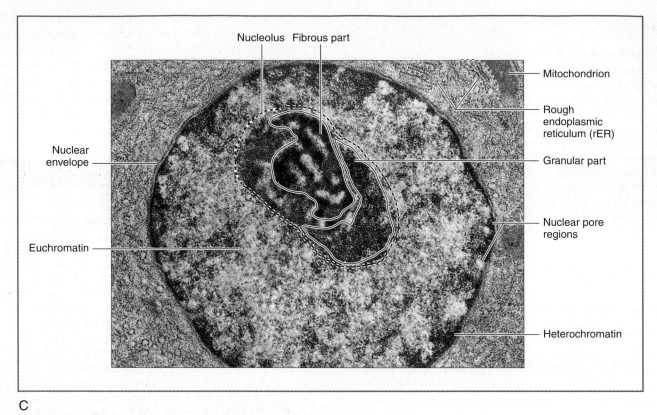

C

Figure 1-13 cont'd. C, Electron micrograph of a nucleus; note the nuclear envelope, euchromatin, heterochromatin, and nucleolus. The cytoplasm surrounding the nucleus has two mitochondria and many profiles of cytoplasmic and membrane-bound ribosomes (rER). (Courtesy of Don W. Fawcett.)

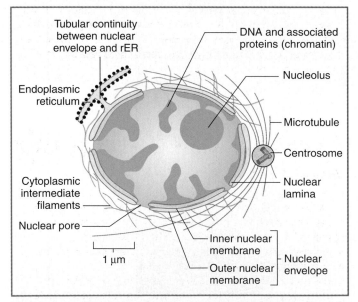

Figure 1-14. Diagram of a typical eukaryotic nucleus. Note the location of the centrosome with its paired centrioles and associated microtubules. Many cells have a "cage" of intermediate filaments surrounding the nucleus, as shown here. The lumen of the rough endoplasmic reticulum (rER) is continuous with the space between the two nuclear membranes.

Nucleolus

The nucleolus is the locus of the ribosomal DNA genes, ribosomal RNA synthesis, and the intranuclear assembly of ribosome subunits.

Chromosomes

During interphase, the chromosomes are not visible as distinct structural entities, although their chromatin is highly organized at the level of the DNA double helix and its many associated structural proteins and enzymes. As cells enter mitosis, chromatin condenses into more compact structures (chromosomes) that are visible in the light microscope. The characteristic shape of chromosomes is an X-shaped structure, although not all the crossover points are at the mid-point of the chromosome's length. The crossover point of the X is a specialized structure called the centromere. The centromere, together with specific associated proteins, is referred to as the kinetochore. The very ends of the chromosomes also contain structures called telomeres, which consist of many repeats of short, identical DNA sequences. Their function is thought to be related to cellular senescence and possibly to molecular events that may be related to the etiology of cancer. The chromosomes themselves are composed of highly coiled and super-coiled molecules of DNA, histones, and many other proteins.

DNA, Genes, and Chromosomes

DNA (both nuclear and mitochondrial) encodes all the genetic information in the cell. The mechanism of DNA replication assures that a faithful copy is passed from one generation of cells (and organisms) to the next.

Human DNA is organized into 23 pairs of chromosomes. Each chromosome contains one long strand of double-stranded DNA and many proteins. Only a very small proportion of the DNA in each chromosome consists of genes (sequences that code for proteins or for RNA). Mutations in DNA, or alterations in gene expression, or regulation of gene expression, are the main molecular events that underlie genetics.

●●● CYTOPLASM

Membranous Organelles

Mitochondria

Nearly all cells except red blood cells and the outermost layers of the skin contain mitochondria; mitochondrial number in a specific cell type may range from 10 or 20 to thousands. The main function of mitochondria is to provide energy, in the form of ATP, to drive the metabolic reactions of the cell. Mitochondria have evolved from aerobic micro-organisms that were phagocytosed by primitive cells eons ago and have been incorporated into the overall structure and metabolism of the cell. As such, they contain a small amount of mitochondrial DNA, mitochondrial ribosomes, and mitochondrial transfer RNAs. Mitochondrial DNA codes for 13 mitochondrial proteins; the remaining mitochondrial proteins (about 85) are coded for in the nuclear genome. A complex set of regulatory factors have evolved ensuring that a correct balance of mitochondrial proteins is transcribed and translated from each genome. Mitochondrial DNA also contains two ribosomal RNA and 22 transfer RNA genes. Although a significant number of proteins and RNAs are encoded in the mitochondrial DNA, the overwhelming majority of mitochondrial proteins are encoded in the nucleus.

The shape of a *typical* mitochondrion is an elongated oval (Fig. 1-15), but mitochondria may also be spherical, branched, coiled, or filamentous. When living cells are observed in tissue culture, mitochondria are highly dynamic—they are in constant motion and undergo fission and fusion. Specific cell types (e.g., hepatocytes, steroid-synthesizing cells, spermatozoa) contain mitochondria that are metabolically and structurally characteristic of that cell type. Like the nucleus, the mitochondrion is bounded by two concentric membranes. Mitochondrial membranes contain a much higher proportion of protein than other cellular membranes. The outer membrane of the mitochondrion is in contact with the cytoplasm of the cell; next is an intermembrane space; then an inner mitochondrial membrane; and finally the mitochondrial matrix. The inner membrane is usually arranged into many long folds called cristae. Associated with the inner membrane and the cristae are the enzymes of cellular respiration. The innermost compartment, the mitochondrial matrix, contains the mitochondrial DNA, mitochondrial ribosomes, and enzymes of the tricarboxylic acid cycle and of fatty acid metabolism. Therefore, it is helpful to think of the mitochondrion as having four functional domains: outer membrane, intermembrane space, inner membrane, and matrix.

Mitochondrial Structure and Function

Mitochondria are complex organelles that convert the main fuel of the cell, glucose (and all other cell fuels), into a form of energy the cell can use by accepting electrons from reduced nucleotides generated during metabolism. ATP is a major form of energy that the cell uses for nearly all its metabolic work. Mitochondria are also responsible for generating the heat that maintains body temperature. The outer mitochondrial membrane is freely permeable to many of the smaller molecules, and many proteins, that are found in the cytoplasm. The inner membrane is impermeable to many anions and cations, a characteristic that enables the chemiosmotic gradient of H^+ that drives the synthesis of ATP within the mitochondrial matrix. The segregation of enzymes into the intermembrane space and the mitochondrial matrix by the double membrane system as well as the permeability characteristics of each of the two membranes are the key mechanisms that underlie mitochondrial function. The enzymes of the citric acid cycle (Krebs' cycle) and other metabolic enzymes are located in the matrix. The folding of the inner membrane into cristae, which contain the enzymes of the respiratory chain (oxidative phosphorylation), greatly facilitates the production of ATP owing to the spatial organization conferred by cristae.

Mitochondrial Diseases

Mutations in many mitochondrial enzymes have been described in recent years, a substantial number of which lead to disease. Most of these mitochondrial disorders are due to mutations in the nuclear DNA-encoded proteins of the mitochondrion, although a significant portion occur when the mitochondrial DNA is mutated.

The number of diseases due to mitochondrial dysfunction grows yearly, but the following list includes some of the better known and better characterized. Each of the diseases referred to below reflects defects in different mitochondrial enzymes.

- There are skeletal muscle myopathies and cardiac muscle myopathies.
- Some of the diseases affect the nervous system such as optic atrophy, seizures, neuropathy, and hearing loss.
- Some mitochondrial mutations are suspected of playing a role in the etiology of diseases of aging such as Parkinson's and Alzheimer's diseases.

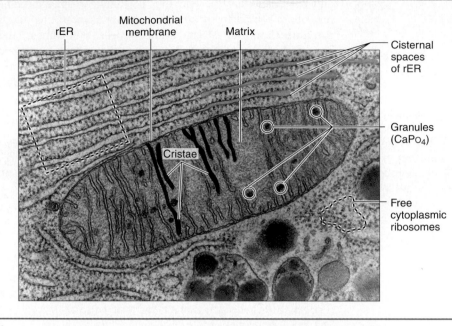

A

Figure 1-15. A, Electron micrograph of a mitochondrion. (Courtesy of Keith R. Porter and Don W. Fawcett.) **B,** Diagram of a typical eukaryotic mitochondrion.

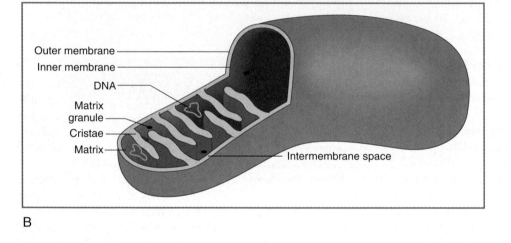

B

Endoplasmic Reticulum

The endoplasmic reticulum (ER) is an extensive network of intracellular membranes that play a central role in managing the biosynthesis and distribution of many proteins of the cell. Proteins whose functional destiny is to become part of the plasma membrane, of the extracellular environment, or of certain intracellular organelles are synthesized by the endoplasmic reticulum. The ER is classified into two major functional and morphologic categories: the rER and the smooth endoplasmic reticulum (sER). The rER is so-named because its cytoplasmic surface is studded with many ribosomes and the sER because its membranes lack ribosomes and are smooth. A significant number of ribosomes in cells are not associated with the ER; these are called free, or cytoplasmic, ribosomes (see Fig. 1-15). Many proteins that function in the cytoplasm are synthesized on cytoplasmic ribosomes (e.g., hemoglobin).

Although the structural relationship between the nuclear envelope and the rER is not obvious in electron micrographs, they are in fact continuous via small, short, tubular or funnel-shaped connections. Because of this spatial relationship, it follows that the rER and sER create a topologically separate compartment in the cytoplasm, the ER lumen or ER cisternal space. The rER generally appears as flattened, stacked membranes enclosing a cisternal space. In some cells, the total area of the rER and sER is several times greater than that of the plasma membrane (Figs. 1-16 and 1-17).

A third intracellular membrane compartment is seen in nearly all cells—the *Golgi apparatus*; many cells (particularly neurons) have multiple Golgi apparatuses. The Golgi is seen as a light-staining or unstained area in the light microscope, usually near the nucleus. In the electron microscope, it is seen to consist of a series of stacked, flattened cisternae with dilated edges, not unlike a stack of flattened paper cups. The

Figure 1-16. The relationship of the nuclear envelope to the rER is demonstrated in this diagram. The process by which the cisternal space of the rER is established from the nuclear envelope is depicted. Also shown is the subsequent establishment of the sER, Golgi apparatus, and secretory vesicles.

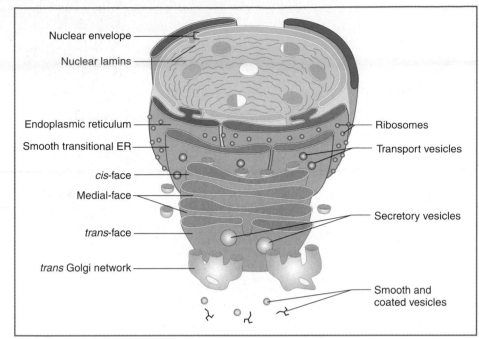

Nuclear envelope

Nuclear lamins

Endoplasmic reticulum

Smooth transitional ER

cis-face

Medial-face

trans-face

trans Golgi network

Ribosomes

Transport vesicles

Secretory vesicles

Smooth and coated vesicles

BIOCHEMISTRY

Protein Synthesis and the Signal Hypothesis

Biosynthesis of cellular proteins destined for export from the cell, or those which will become membrane proteins, takes place in association with the rER; these proteins have a short N-terminal extension called the signal sequence. The cell has a specific mechanism for translocating these proteins into the lumen of the rER. The proposed mechanism is called the signal hypothesis.

Immediately after a messenger RNA binds to the small subunit of a ribosome, the complex binds the large subunit of the ribosome and translation begins. The signal sequence binds to a signal recognition particle (SRP), which consists of proteins and RNA. Once bound, protein translation pauses until the SRP binds to an SRP receptor on the rER. The nascent peptide is translocated across an aqueous channel in the rER membrane using energy from the hydrolysis of GTP to GDP. Once translocation occurs, translation of the nascent protein resumes.

part of the Golgi apparatus closest to the rER or the sER is called the *cis*-Golgi and that farthest from the rER is the *trans*-Golgi. The *cis*-Golgi is often in a juxtanuclear location. As the biosynthesis of proteins or glycoproteins is completed, vesicles bud off from the dilated edges of the cisternae and finally from the *trans*-Golgi until they reach their final destination.

The lumens of all three compartments—rER, sER and Golgi apparatus—are in a dynamic functionally interrelated

state owing to a highly regulated series of vesicle budding and fusion events. Furthermore, the three compartments of the Golgi apparatus (*cis*-, stacks, and *trans*-) are morphologically and biochemically highly specialized. The *trans*-Golgi region is a major site for the sorting and final targeting of proteins to their ultimate cellular destinations; for this reason, it has been called the *trans*-Golgi network (TGN) (Fig. 1-18).

Once in the lumen of the ER, proteins are targeted to their various specific final destinations by a complex series of modifications; e.g., specific proteolytic events, specific glycosylation (and deglycosylation) reactions at particular amino acid residues, the covalent attachment of lipids, and complexing with other proteins that assist in proper folding of the protein or with still other proteins that help target the newly synthesized proteins to their intended location. Collectively, these are called posttranslational modifications.

Lysosomes

Lysosomes are small, membrane-bounded vesicles that are filled with about 40 hydrolytic enzymes; these hydrolases are active only at an acidic pH (between pH 4.5 and 5.0). The main function of lysosomes is to carry out the controlled hydrolysis of nearly every macromolecule in the cell—whether endogenous or exogenous. Their membranes contain a set of specific proteins, some of which are proton pumps, that generate the acidic internal environment of the lysosome.

Lysosomal enzymes (in the form of prohydrolyases) are synthesized and sequentially processed in the ER and Golgi apparatus. The signal that targets the prohydrolyases to nascent lysosomes is mannose-6-PO$_4$ (man-6-P); this sugar phosphate is produced by a series of glycosylation steps and

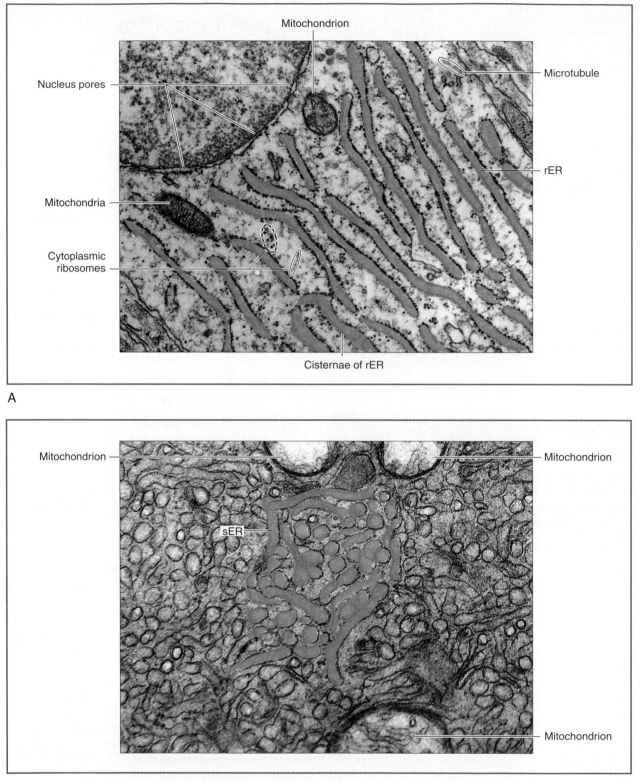

Figure 1-17. A, Electron micrograph of the rER in a hepatocyte. The cisternae are colored pale blue. A nucleus with several nuclear pores is also seen. The cytoplasm has two mitochondria. **B,** Electron micrograph of sER in a steroid-secreting cell. Cisternal spaces are colored pale blue. Profiles of the sER are seen throughout the figure. Several mitochondria and lipid droplets typical of steroid-secreting cells are also present. (Courtesy of Don W. Fawcett.)

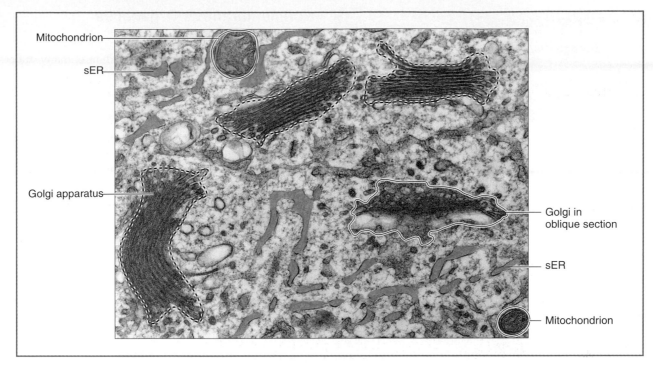

A

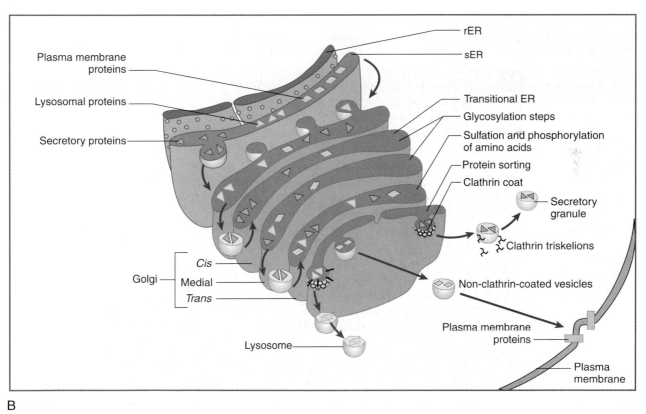

B

Figure 1-18. A, Electron micrograph of the Golgi apparatus. Profiles of four Golgi apparatuses are shown. The upper right-hand-most is sectioned in a plane perpendicular to the membrane stacks, and the one below it is more obliquely sectioned; the *cis* (upper side) and *trans* (lower side) faces of the Golgi are seen in the latter case. **B,** Diagram of the Golgi apparatus. (Modified from Gartner LP, Hiatt JL. *Color Textbook of Histology,* 2nd ed. Philadelphia, WB Saunders, 2001, p. 28.)

Lysosomal Storage Diseases

Many diseases are caused by defects in one or more of the lysosomal hydrolases. The consequence of these enzyme defects is that the lysosomes of the cell become engorged with partially degraded macromolecules and the cells ultimately die. Many of the lysosomal storage diseases affect individuals early in life; they usually have characteristic phenotypes, and most of the diseases lead to premature death. A partial list of lysosomal storage diseases follows:

- In several diseases called gangliosidoses, the degradation of the carbohydrate portion of cerebral gangliosides is defective (e.g., Tay-Sachs disease, Sandhoff's disease, Niemann-Pick disease).
- Another group of diseases is caused by defects in enzymes that degrade glycoproteins.
- A third category of diseases results in the accumulation of partially degraded glycosaminoglycans (called mucopolysaccharidoses in an older nomenclature system). Among these disorders, enzyme replacement strategies have achieved some therapeutic success, leading to a marked reduction in symptoms.

processing of the glycosyl group in the TGN. Certain regions of the TGN have transmembrane man-6-P receptors and a distinct set of membrane components compared to other intracellular membranes; these are the nascent lysosome membranes. Thus, the lysosomal prohydrolases are targeted to specific regions of the TGN, where they bud off into the cytoplasm to form primary lysosomes. The budding is accomplished by specific lysosomal membrane proteins and clathrin, which facilitate the formation of lysosomes. The lysosomes fuse with endosomes to form late endosomes. Following these steps, the clathrin and man-6-P receptors are recycled, clathrin to any of several cellular sites and man-6-P to the TGN. These events are summarized in Figure 1-19.

Peroxisomes

Peroxisomes are another group of vesicular organelles found in the cytoplasm of all cells. They are specialized to carry out oxidative reactions via a group of oxidative enzymes (oxidases) that utilize molecular O_2 to produce H_2O_2. Excess H_2O_2 is removed by catalase, of which peroxisomes contain considerable quantities. The catalase (and general protein) concentration of the peroxisome is so high that it is often seen as a crystalline inclusion in the peroxisome, which can serve as a useful marker to recognize this organelle in electron micrographs. The lipid membrane of peroxisomes is thought to be derived from components of the ER. The oxidases are synthesized on cytoplasmic ribosomes and are imported into peroxisomes owing to a three-amino-acid signal sequence near the carboxyl terminus of the protein; there may be other import signals on some peroxisome-bound proteins. Peroxisomes contain no DNA or RNA and are self-replicating; new organelles arise by fission of preexisting organelles.

Nonmembranous Organelles

Cytoskeleton

The cytoplasm of cells is organized into many functional domains created and maintained by the cytoskeleton. The term cytoskeleton collectively refers to three separate classes of proteins seen as fine cytoplasmic filaments. In filament diameter, the smallest class is the actin filaments; they are about 6 nm in diameter. The next largest class is the intermediate filaments; they are about 8 to 10 nm in diameter. The third and largest class is the microtubules, which are about 25 nm in diameter. One or more of these classes of filaments are present in all human cells. Although they are quite distinct in appearance, composition, and function, these filaments share many properties. In situ, all three can be many micrometers long; they are all capable of self-assembly (in vivo and in vitro) from globular protein subunits, are in a state of dynamic equilibrium in vivo, have many specific associated (or accessory) proteins that control or modulate their behavior, and in almost all cases interact with one another in a functionally coordinated manner.

Actin Filaments

Actin filaments are found in great abundance in muscle cells, where they function as a major component of the contractile machinery (they make up about 60% of the protein in these cells). They are found as a major protein (ca. 10% to 15%) in essentially all nonmuscle cells as well, where they play a central role in cell locomotion, maintenance of cell shape, translocation of cell organelles, formation and function of the contractile ring in mitosis, and numerous other activities. Humans have six genes encoding actin, and there are three major isoforms of actin: α, β, and γ. α-Actin is found in muscle cells, and β and γ are found together in all nonmuscle cells. The cytoplasmic actin filament is a 6-nm wide, very long polymer of a globular actin monomer; it is a homopolymer in that all its protein subunits are the same. The filament has an inherent helical structure and polarity (Fig. 1-20). The polarity is revealed by "decoration" of actin filaments with the actin-binding fragment of myosin; when visualized this way, the filaments appear to have a barbed end and a pointed end, and the barbed end is the faster-growing one. More than 50 proteins interact with actin (the globular subunits or the filaments); one of the most common of these proteins is myosin, a so-called motor protein (see Chapter 4). The organization of actin filaments in cells varies by cell type, specific location in the cell, and functional state of the cell. The actin filaments in a cell are in a constant state of assembly and disassembly; typically, there is net assembly at one end (plus end) and net disassembly at the other end (minus end).

Intermediate Filaments

This type of filament is also found in nearly all human cells; it is particularly abundant in stratified squamous epithelial cells, such as those found in the outer layer of the skin (epidermis). Intermediate filaments have a similar diameter

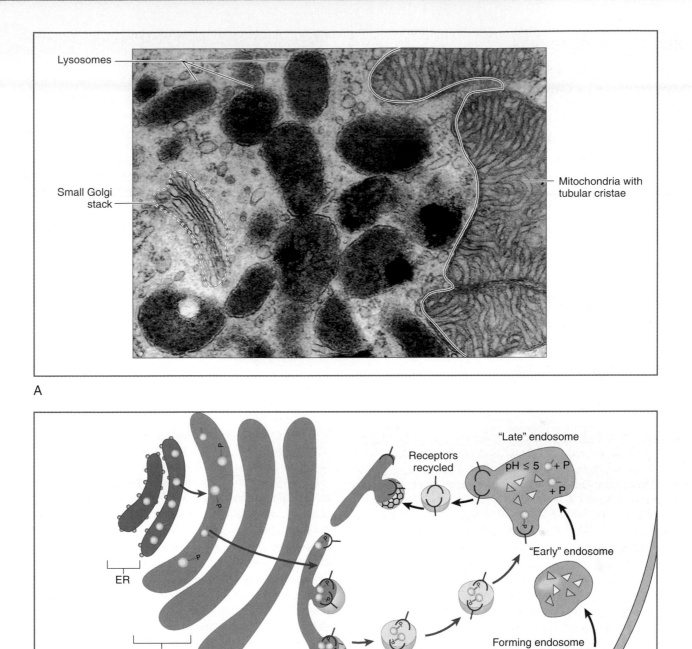

A

B

Figure 1-19. A, Electron micrograph of several lysosomes and mitochondria from a mammalian cell; a Golgi profile is seen at left. (Courtesy of Don W. Fawcett.) **B,** Diagram of lysosome formation from the rER, through the Golgi apparatus, and budding of lysosomes from the *trans*-Golgi network (TGN), where they fuse with late endosomes.

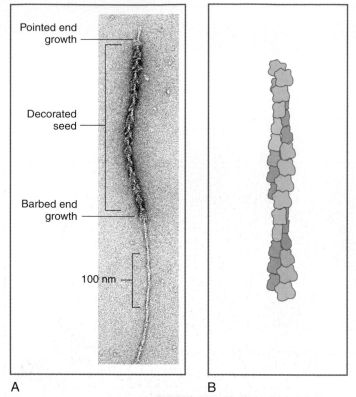

A   B

Figure 1-20. Electron micrograph of a negatively stained actin filament polymerized in vitro. **A,** In the upper part of the image, an actin filament seed was decorated with myosin heads to demonstrate its polarity. The seed served as a site for further polymerization, which occurs much faster at the barbed end than at the pointed end. **B,** Diagram of an actin filament illustrates its double helical nature. (From Pollard TD, Earnshaw WC. *Cell Biology.* Philadelphia, WB Saunders, 2002, p 563.)

and morphology in the EM. There are more than 50 genes for intermediate filaments in humans, and they share several protein structural motifs. Their assembly is less well understood than that of actin filaments or microtubules, but like the others, they are assembled from protein subunits. There are six major classes of intermediate filaments that are somewhat, but not exclusively, tissue specific. Furthermore, each class contains several isoforms some of which are developmentally expressed. Figure 1-3 illustrates the pattern of the intermediate filament vimentin in a cultured epithelial cell. Figure 1-4 illustrates the organization of the nuclear intermediate filament lamin in cultured fibroblasts. Although the exact function of intermediate filaments is not known, mutations in their structure, and the consequent pathology, clearly indicate a key role in the function of normal cells.

Microtubules

Microtubule filaments are composed of two globular protein subunits: α-tubulin and β-tubulin. Dimers of these two proteins assemble into cylindrical structures with an outer diameter of about 25 nm and a hollow core of about 10 nm.

The polymerized microtubule has a distinct helical pitch; the circumference of the microtubule has 13 parallel protofilaments in which α- and β-tubulin alternate. A third isoform of tubulin, γ-tubulin, is found in all human (and just about all other eukaryotic) cells, albeit in much lower concentrations than α- or β-tubulin. γ-Tubulin is involved in nucleating microtubules from specialized structures called *microtubule organizing centers* (MTOCs). Like actin, tubulin is highly conserved across the phylogenetic tree. Humans have six genes encoding α-tubulin and six for β-tubulin. Microtubules have a number of important functions in cells; they comprise the mitotic spindle, play a major role in maintaining cell shape, are critical to the intracellular movement of organelles and nonorganelle-associated "cargo," are important in cell migration during development, and in adult cells, are the major structural proteins in cilia and flagella. Figure 1-21 shows electron micrographs and diagrams of microtubules. (See also Fig. 1-6B for an electron micrograph of negative-stained microtubules polymerized in vitro.)

Cells contain substantial amounts of the three types of cytoskeletal filaments. An understanding of their distribution and organization has elucidated many important aspects of cell structure and function. Because of the large cellular content of filaments and their intermingled cellular distribution, it is difficult to appreciate how they look in situ. One technique that is well suited to studying their distribution in whole cells is immunofluorescence microscopy. Figure 1-3B shows the vimentin intermediate filament distribution in a cultured epithelial cell. Figure 1-22 shows a migrating melanoma cell stained with antibodies to two cytoskeletal filaments—microtubules (green) and actin filaments (cyan). The bright red spots at the leading edge of this migrating cell

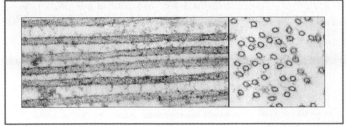

A

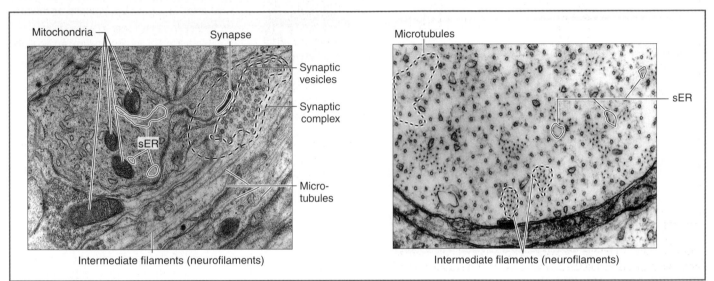

B

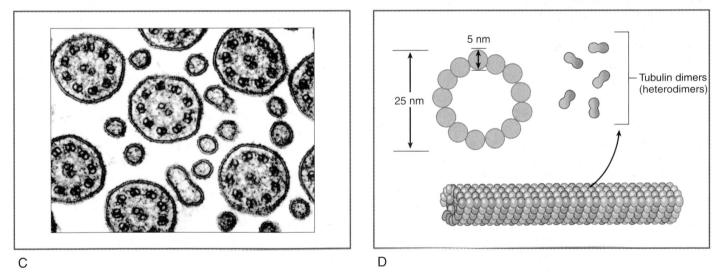

C   D

Figure 1-21. A, Transmission electron micrographs (TEMs) of microtubules polymerized in vitro, embedded, and sectioned in longitudinal and transverse planes. (From Pollard TD, Earnshaw WC. *Cell Biology.* Philadelphia, WB Saunders, 2002, p 589.) **B,** Electron micrograph of a cerebellar dendrite sectioned longitudinally *(left)* and a different dendrite sectioned transversely *(right).* The dendrite in the image on the left shows a number of microtubules and neuronal intermediate filaments (neurofilaments). The transversely sectioned dendrite in the image on the right shows cross-sections of many microtubules and neurofilaments as well as numerous profiles of the smooth endoplasmic reticulum. (Courtesy of Enrico Mugnani *[left]* and Don W. Fawcett *[right].*) **C,** Electron micrograph of several cilia, sectioned transversely, found on epithelial cells in the respiratory tract. Note the ciliary axoneme with its array of nine radially arranged pairs of microtubules and a central pair of microtubules. These epithelial cells also have numerous microvilli. (Courtesy of Don W. Fawcett.) **D,** Diagram of microtubules that shows the arrangement of subunits in a microtubule.

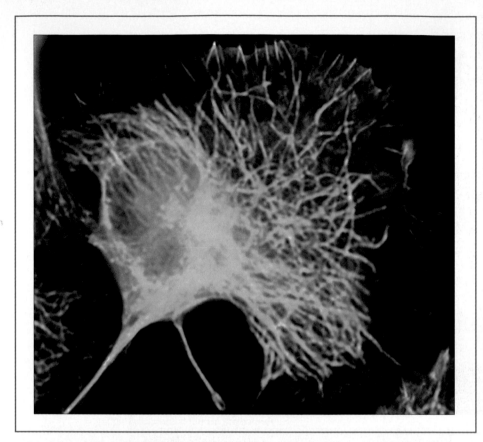

Figure 1-22. Melanoma cell grown in tissue culture. At the time of fixation and staining, it was migrating from the lower left to the upper right corner of the field of view. It was stained with three different immunofluorescent labels—tubulin with an antibody with a green fluorescent label, actin with phalloidin labeled with a cyan fluorescent label, and phosphotyrosine with an antibody with a red fluorescent label. (Courtesy of Kristiana Kandere-Grzybowska and Gary G. Borisy.)

represent phosphotyrosine, a posttranslational modification of many proteins that are found in high concentration at focal adhesion contact sites in cells.

It is possible to see all three cytoskeletal filaments in specially prepared cells grown in tissue culture. Figure 1-23 shows two versions of the same electron micrograph, one unlabeled and the other labeled. Each of the three filaments is colored in the lower micrograph; one of the many proteins that bind to both actin and intermediate filaments, plectin (also present in hemidesmosomes; see Chapter 9), is colored green.

Most human cells have MTOCs except some terminally differentiated cells such as red blood cells, platelets, and the outermost layer of the epidermis. In those cells that have an MTOC (which is commonly called the *centrosome* in animal cells), a distinctive organelle—the paired centrioles—are seen near its center. They are structures oriented at 90 degrees to each other. The centriole is made of many proteins, a major one of which is tubulin. To date, centrioles in all cells throughout the phylogenetic tree look essentially the same; furthermore, they all contain relatively high concentrations of γ-tubulin. They consist of nine triplet microtubules arranged in a precise, blade-like geometric pattern (Fig. 1-24). Apart from their role in nucleating microtubules, centrioles play two other important roles in cells. At the beginning of the

PHARMACOLOGY

Antitubulin Drugs

Similarly to the situation with actin, there are drugs that stabilize or destabilize microtubules. Their primary effect is to inhibit cell division, since a major component of the mitotic apparatus is spindle fibers that are largely made of microtubules. Cells treated with these agents are typically blocked at the metaphase stage of mitosis; thus, these agents are said to be "mitotic blockers." They are widely used in treating cancer and certain other diseases in which disruption of microtubule structure is effective.

Paclitaxel is a drug isolated from a genus of yew trees that prevents the dynamic turnover of microtubules. It freezes cells at the metaphase stage of mitosis, with an intact spindle apparatus, thereby preventing the progression of mitosis and inhibiting cell growth.

There are two drugs that interfere with the polymerization of tubulin dimers into microtubules—colchicine and nocodazole. They increase the rate of microtubule depolymerization and block cells at metaphase. Colchicine is widely used as an anticancer drug and to treat gout. In the latter case, it inhibits the phagocytic uptake of uric acid crystals by polymorphonuclear neutrophils by depolymerizing cytoplasmic microtubules.

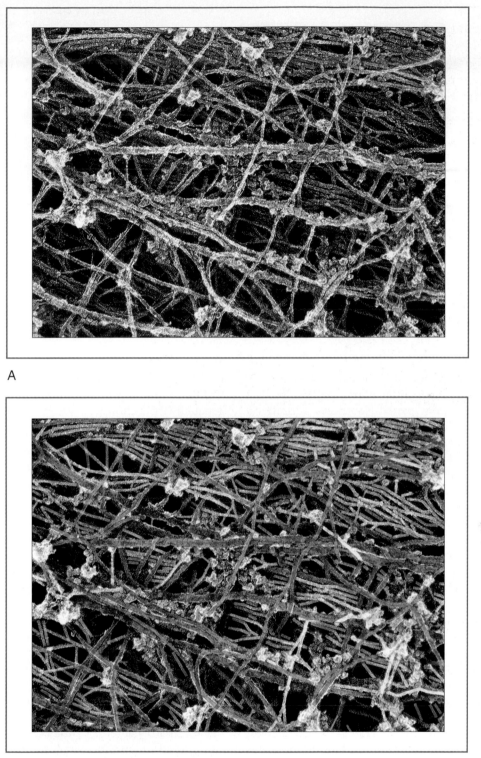

A

B

Figure 1-23. Electron micrograph of a tissue culture cell prepared and examined by the technique of platinum replica electron microscopy. **A,** A region of the cell with all three cytoskeletal filaments. All three of the filaments are coated with a variety of associated proteins. **B,** The same micrograph with transparent colored overlays of the three filaments; microtubules are red, actin filaments are yellow, intermediate filaments are blue. The cross-linking protein plectin is colored green. (Courtesy of Tatyana Svitkina.)

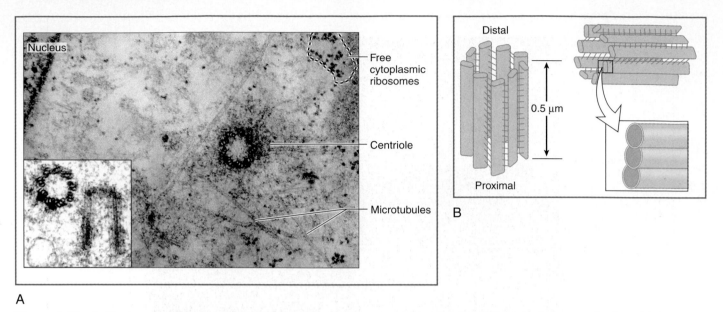

A

Figure 1-24. A, Electron micrograph of a centriole in the centrosome region of a cell. The inset shows a pair of centrioles oriented at right angles to each other. (Courtesy of Guenter Albrecht-Buehler.) **B,** Diagram of a centriole.

S phase of the cell cycle (see Cell Cycle), the two centrioles separate from each other and replicate to produce two identical paired structures. The new paired centrioles migrate to opposite poles of the cell and nucleate the astral microtubule arrays of the mitotic apparatus. In cells that produce cilia or flagella, they replicate and give rise to the basal bodies that are found at the base of each cilium or flagellum. Based on numerous studies in tissue culture cells, centrioles have been shown to serve as a high-level cellular integration center (the "brain" of the cell?) in that they regulate cell locomotion, the spatial organization of cellular microtubules, the response of the cell to light in the infrared range of the spectrum, and other functions.

Cytoplasmic Inclusions

There are several distinct morphologic features in the cytoplasm of many cells that are not surrounded by membranes. Two of the more important are glycogen and lipid droplets. Glycogen is the major storage form of glucose; in the electron microscope, glycogen particles are seen as irregular, somewhat stellate, electron-dense clusters (Fig. 1-25). The amount of glycogen in a cell is related to the overall nutritional status of the individual or to the type of cell it is. Parenchymal cells of the liver, skeletal muscle, and chondrocytes may have substantial glycogen deposits in their cytoplasm.

Lipid droplets are a common cytoplasmic feature of many cells. The liver has a central role in lipid metabolism; therefore, hepatocytes usually have numerous lipid droplets. Cells that synthesize steroid hormones also typically have numerous lipid droplets. Special stains and staining procedures are required to visualize lipid droplets in the light microscope, but they have a characteristic appearance in

electron micrographs, since they are well preserved with the fixatives used in electron microscopy (glutaraldehyde and osmium) (Fig. 1-26).

●●● CELL DYNAMICS

Cell Renewal

From the moment of fertilization, a hallmark of the life cycle of humans, at the cellular level, is cell growth, cell division, cell renewal, and cell death. As body size and mass increase in embryonic, fetal, childhood, and adult life, there is a concomitant increase in cell number until a steady state is attained by the late teens or early twenties. However, different populations of cells can be placed in different groups in terms of their growth behavior. Some cell or tissue types divide rarely or not at all in the adult; others may undergo cell renewal or cell replacement via activation of undifferentiated "reserve" cells or satellite cells by specific signals, and still others are constantly undergoing cell renewal at a characteristic rate, depending on the specific cell or tissue type. Cells in the blood are renewed at a rather high rate throughout life (see Chapter 7). Although there are many cell and tissue renewal populations in the body, epithelial tissues tend to be among the most active. For example, the basal layer of the epidermis (see Chapter 9) and essentially all the epithelial lining of the digestive system (see Chapter 11) undergo constant cell renewal; each is discussed in more detail later.

Cell Cycle

Cells are in one of two general states in terms of the cell cycle: interphase or mitosis. The interphase state is simply defined as the state between the events of mitosis even

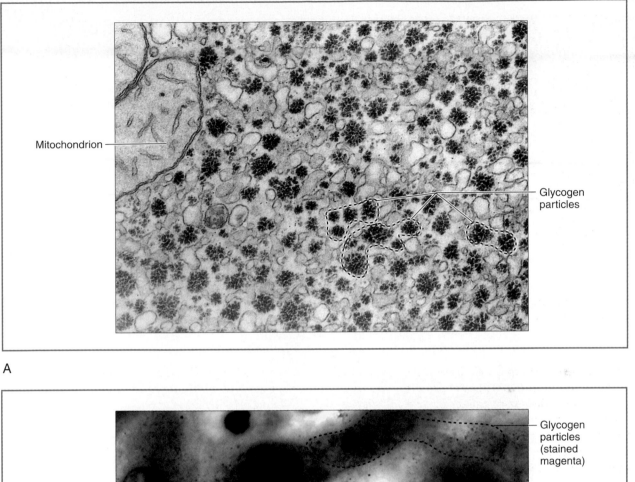

Mitochondrion

Glycogen particles

Glycogen particles (stained magenta)

Liver cell nuclei

A

B

Figure 1-25. A, Electron micrograph of a liver cell showing glycogen particles associated with the sER. (Courtesy of Don W. Fawcett.) **B,** Light micrograph of liver fixed and stained to preserve the glycogen content of the hepatocytes.

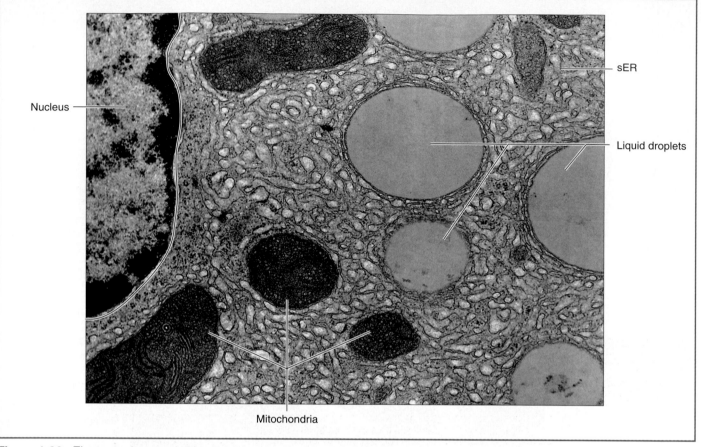

Nucleus

sER

Liquid droplets

Mitochondria

Figure 1-26. Electron micrograph of a steroid-synthesizing cell showing several lipid droplets, mitochondria, and extensive smooth endoplasmic reticulum. (Courtesy of Don W. Fawcett.)

though it consists of three distinct phases of its own. The four cell cycle phases are called G_1 (first gap phase), S (DNA synthesis phase), G_2 (second gap phase), and M (mitosis). A diagrammatic representation of the cell cycle is shown in Figure 1-27. The major characteristic of the G_1 phase is growth of the cell in mass and volume; it is typically the longest and most variable phase of the cycle. The S phase is characterized by DNA synthesis (replication) of nuclear chromosomes. Each chromosome has many specific sites of replication, termed *origins of replication*. As DNA replication proceeds, the regions of replicated DNA are called *replicons*. In higher eukaryotes, the unit of chromosome replication is a cluster of replicons. The replicated chromosomes have two sister chromatids each of which retains the constriction (kinetochore) of the parent chromosome. Generally, euchromatin replicates early in S phase and heterochromatin replicates late in S. Cells "proofread" the replicated DNA and prepare for mitosis during G_2. Cells then enter M phase, during which they undergo karyokinesis (nuclear division) and cytokinesis (cell division), giving rise to two essentially identical sibling cells.

Understanding of the cell cycle and how it is controlled has increased dramatically in recent years. Like many events in the cell, a major mode of regulation is the phosphorylation or dephosphorylation of a protein, whether or not it is an enzyme. A group of enzymes called *cyclins* are key in regulating progress through the cell cycle. They interact with specific kinases (protein-phosphorylating enzymes) to form cyclin-dependent kinases (Cdks), which control progression of a cell through the cycle. There are a number of checkpoints that determine whether a cell will successfully complete its progress through the cycle, be delayed, or even be triggered into a suicidal pathway (programmed cell death). Four of the checkpoints have been particularly well studied: (1) the restriction point in the G_1 phase checks for cell size and certain environmental parameters; (2) the DNA damage checkpoint in G_1 monitors the integrity of DNA before the cell enters S phase; (3) a separate DNA damage checkpoint also functions in G_2 to ensure that the DNA has been fully replicated and there is little or no damaged DNA; and (4) the metaphase checkpoint restrains the cell in metaphase until all the chromosomes are properly attached to the mitotic spindle. One of the major ways the checkpoints exert their controlling functions is via Cdks, which work by a number of mechanisms specific to each Cdk.

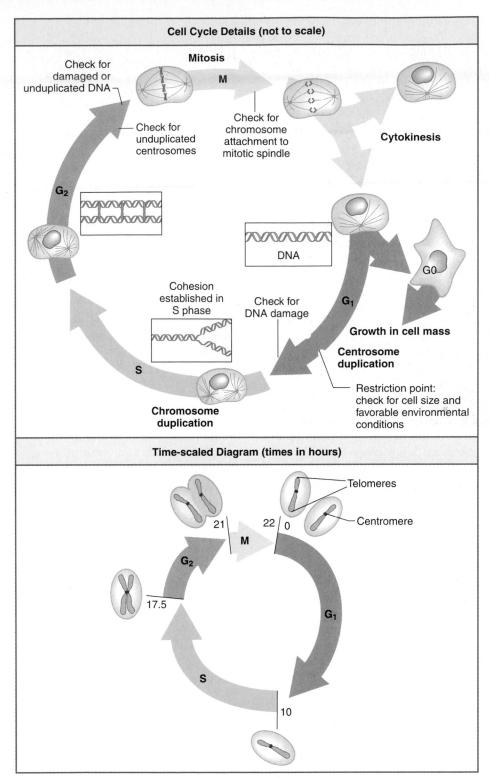

Figure 1-27. The cell cycle based on a human cell grown in tissue culture. The four phases and four main checkpoints are labeled. The approximate time this cell spends in each phase of the cycle is indicated on the diagram; these times are based on a 22-hour cycle. The behavior of a single chromosome is shown at its relevant points in the cycle. (From Pollard TD, Earnshaw WC. *Cell Biology*. Philadelphia, WB Saunders, 2002, p 674.)

Cell Division

The details of cell division, both mitosis and meiosis, have been observed and studied for over 150 years. The process of mitosis consists of the following six steps (Fig. 1-28). *Prophase* (step 1) is the time when nuclear DNA begins to condense into strands readily visible in the light microscope. Toward the end of prophase, the centrioles and associated pericentriolar material (i.e., the centrosome) duplicate and migrate to opposite poles of the cell. They each nucleate one pole of the mitotic spindle. At about this time, the nuclear envelope breaks down into hundreds of vesicles and the chromosomes randomly attach to microtubules arising from the poles of the mitotic spindle; this is called *prometaphase* (step 2). The chromosomes, attached to spindle microtubules, align along the equator of the cell. It is worth noting that the chromosome pairs do *not* align near each other during mitosis, as they do in meiosis. This is the step monitored by the metaphase checkpoint; all the chromosomes must be properly aligned at the metaphase plate, and the kinetochores of both sister chromatids must be attached to a spindle microtubule. This step is called *metaphase* (step 3). Next, the sister chromatids separate rapidly in *anaphase* (step 4). Anaphase has two distinct parts: anaphase A, when the sister chromatids rapidly separate from each other, and anaphase B, when the chromatids and the poles to which they have migrated separate from one another. The new nuclear envelopes begin to reassemble during anaphase B. The cell is now in *telophase* (step 5). Collectively, these five steps are referred to as *karyokinesis*. During telophase, a contractile ring, consisting largely of actin and myosin, assembles midway between the spindle poles and constricts to separate the sibling cells from one another. These last events of mitosis are called *cytokinesis* (step 6). The overall result is that two genetically identical, diploid, sibling cells are produced.

Meiosis, discussed in greater detail in Chapter 14, follows two sequential steps that are morphologically similar to those seen in mitosis. They are known as *meiosis I* and *meiosis II*; the chromosomal events of meiosis I are unique to meiosis, whereas the steps in meiosis II are essentially the same as mitosis. The major difference between the two is that in meiosis the end result is four genetically nonidentical, haploid cells (spermatozoa in males; however, in females a single haploid ovum is produced). Meiosis is often called a "reductive" process, since the cells (gametes) that are the end result have half the DNA and half the number of chromosomes of the parental cell from which they are derived. It is the production of gametes that is the basis for sexual reproduction in eukaryotes.

Programmed Cell Death (Apoptosis)

It is currently thought that the ability to undergo programmed cell death is a latent capacity of virtually all cells of multicellular organisms. Programmed cell death (sometimes referred to as cellular suicide) occurs among many groups of adult cells as well as many cells during development. Specific

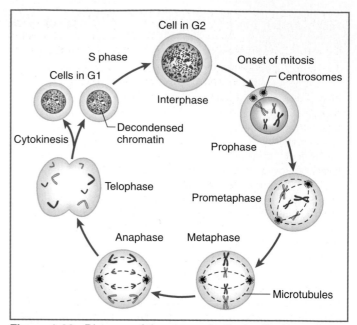

Figure 1-28. Diagram of the steps of mitosis. (Redrawn from Nussbaum RL, McInnes RR, Willard HF. *Genetics in Medicine,* 6th ed. Philadelphia, WB Saunders, 2001, p. 5.)

cell death events that occur in the epiphyseal plate of endochondral bone formation (see Chapter 5) are one example of programmed cell death. Cells may be programmed for death if they become infected with certain viruses, are exposed to certain drugs, or fail to meet the correct checkpoint criteria during the cell cycle.

Although, strictly speaking, apoptosis is a specific subset of programmed cell death, the terms are often used interchangeably. A distinct series of morphologic steps characterize the apoptotic pathway that is not seen in all cells undergoing programmed cell death. The intracellular program that leads to cell death is mediated by a large number of signals and enzymes. A group of enzymes called *caspases* are key players in programmed cell death. There are two major classes of caspases; one class is found in a precursor form and the other is not. The former may be autoactivated by its own proteolytic activity. Caspases participate in the destruction of cytoplasmic proteins and degradation of nuclear DNA in characteristic patterns.

Two major pathways lead to cell suicide. One is called the death receptor pathway; it is initiated by the binding of certain ligands to specific receptors. The other apoptotic pathway involves mitochondria, in particular, a key enzyme of respiration—cytochrome *c*. An ever-lengthening list of diseases involving defects in programmed cell death is being compiled. Among these are neurodegenerative diseases such as Alzheimer's disease, many autoimmune diseases, and several kinds of cancer.

Cells may also die as a result of damage or cellular trauma. When this happens, the process is termed *necrosis* (or

GENETICS

General Genetic Mechanisms of Human Diseases

As a result of the large number of complex steps involved in producing gametes and the amount of time it takes to produce them, many defective gametes are formed. A significant number of defective gametes are not viable, but some are. As a result, children are born with a genetic defect. Errors also can occur in somatic cells during mitosis. The errors can be at the level of mutations in a single base in the DNA up to the level of chromosome structure and "handling."

Single-base changes can result in the synthesis of a completely or partially defective protein (e.g., sickle cell anemia, cystic fibrosis) or one with a novel function or pattern of expression. Microdeletions or translocations can result in the synthesis of truncated proteins or of extra long, fused proteins. There can be mutations or chromosome translocations in proteins that regulate gene expression (e.g., the translocation in chronic myelogenous leukemia [CML], which leads to a loss in regulation of cell proliferation of certain bone marrow cells). Chromosomes may translocate or exchange whole parts of their structure, as in the case of CML, which is characterized by the appearance of the so-called Philadelphia chromosome—a shortened form of chromosome 22 due to a translocation with chromosome 9 during mitosis. These are called structural anomalies of chromosomes. There are a number of syndromes in which chromosome numbers are abnormal (aneuploidies) because of errors in chromosome handling during meiosis I. These can produce mild to severe phenotypes that begin during fetal life and are evident in the adult. Examples of aneuploidy diseases are Down syndrome (trisomy 21), the most common chromsomal anomaly. Children with Down syndrome have 47 chromosomes. Turner's syndrome is a condition in which females only have one X chromosome and therefore have a total of 45 chromosomes.

ANATOMY & EMBRYOLOGY

Programmed Cell Death and Fetal Development

Embryologic and fetal life are times of considerable cell growth and differentiation as well as development of the whole organism. In addition to the net increase in cell number and size of the developing infant, in specific locations and at specific times, many cells undergo programmed cell death. Some well-characterized examples follow.

The upper and lower limbs make their first appearance at about 5 weeks of life. Initially, they are buds on the lateral aspects of the embryo. Within the next few days, the hands and feet form as webbed flipper-like structures, and by the end of the sixth week, the general location of the fingers and toes is evident. The loss of webbing between the primordial digits is due to programmed death of the cells that comprise the webbing.

At about 7 to 8 weeks of development, the left and right palatal shelves (lateral palatine processes) fuse to form the secondary palate. The epithelial cells that cover the two fusing surfaces die as the result of programmed cell death.

Many of the neurons in embryonic ganglia die as a result of programmed cell death.

Immature T cells in the fetal thymus gland undergo massive programmed cell death (about 95% of the cells die) in the process of growth and maturation of the gland in utero.

---

accidental cell death). Cells that die by necrosis usually induce an inflammatory process. Necrosis often begins following damage to the plasma membrane; too much water enters the cell, causing swelling of organelles, release of lytic enzymes into the damaged cytoplasm, and digestion of many cellular organelles and macromolecules.

It should be evident from the preceding brief discussions that every aspect of cell growth, division, renewal, and death is under exquisite regulation by many complex pathways. Cells pay attention—so should you!

Types and Classification of Tissues and Organs

2

CONTENTS

It is useful to think about the overall organization of the body, from atoms to the whole organism, to position histology in its appropriate biologic hierarchy. Figure 2-1 represents such a hierarchy; the lower left corner of the figure includes those parts typically included as the domain of histology. Histology is a descriptive science. The study of tissues and organs at the microscopic level has led to the declaration of a few simple and useful principles. Namely, there are four, and *only* four, basic tissue types; organs comprise at least two to all four of these tissue types; organs are either solid or hollow and each kind has a recognizable set of structural characteristics. These principles of tissue and organ organization have made a significant contribution to the understanding of normal function and of most pathologic disorders.

●●● MEANING AND CONCEPT OF TISSUES

It is often said that the basic unit of life is the cell. This generalization applies to essentially all members of the plant and animal kingdoms as well as to archi- and eubacteria and to fungi. In Chapter 1, cells were discussed in terms of their general structure and organization, discrete organelles, and other ultrastructural features, all without regard for the many different types of cells often used to illustrate the characteristics and components of cells. Although it is difficult to be precise, examination and enumeration of the cells in the human body would reveal many hundreds, if not a few thousand, different cell types. However, after careful study of

all these cell types, it is clear they can be grouped into only four different categories. These categories are *tissue* types.

The value of the concept of tissues became apparent early in the study of the histology of human specimens at the light microscopic level. For years, scientists and physicians had recognized certain characteristics of living or postmortem specimens at the gross anatomic level based on their appearance, texture, patterns of location in the body, functions, common pathologic presentations, and other aspects. The microscopic appearance of human specimens reinforced these observations, since it was noted that cells occurred in clusters or in layers such that many cells in a specific location had a similar appearance to each other and to cells seen in analogous locations elsewhere in the body. Embryologic studies helped us understand the early differentiation and development of tissues into the four basic or fundamental types now recognized: epithelial tissue, connective tissue, muscle tissue, and nerve tissue. Bear in mind the use of one or more of the following criteria for assigning any cell (or groups of cells) to one of these basic tissue types: embryologic origin, appearance and texture, and functional properties. As will be pointed

ANATOMY & EMBRYOLOGY

Tissue Development

The four basic tissue types of the body characteristically develop from one of the three embryonic layers: ectoderm, mesoderm, or endoderm. Since the four tissues originate from three embryonic layers, it is obvious that their development is not a simple precursor-product relationship. The process of tissue development is called histogenesis.

Epithelial tissues arise from both ectoderm and endoderm (i.e., the epidermis of the skin arises from ectoderm, and the epithelia of the gut or the lungs arise from endoderm). Connective tissues arise from mesoderm, but some connective tissues of the cranium (including cranial bones) arise from ectoderm. Muscle tissues also arise from mesoderm. Nerve tissue arises from ectoderm after first differentiating into neuroectoderm in the form of either the neural tube or the neural crest.

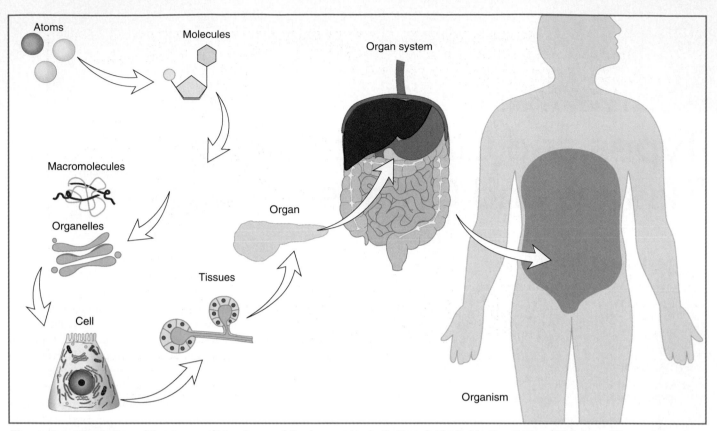

Figure 2-1. Illustration of the range of structures of the human body that are included in the study of histology. The main criterion for including these structures is that they can be seen by an electron or light microscope (or even a low-power magnifying glass) with sufficient resolution to interpret the structure. Thus, many macromolecules and all organelles, cells, tissues, organs, or parts of organs are visible. The organ used to illustrate this principle is the pancreas and many of its smaller components.

out in later chapters, *all cells* of the human body can be assigned to one, and only one, of these four basic tissue types.

Epithelial Tissue

The external and internal surfaces of the body are covered or lined with epithelial tissue; in other words, the outer and inner free surfaces of the body are composed of epithelia. These epithelia are avascular. Most epithelial tissues are derived from embryonic ectoderm or endoderm. All the glands of the body, including exocrine and endocrine glands, are also derived from these same two layers of the embryo. Nonetheless, some epithelia, such as those lining the vascular system and parts of the urinary system, are of mesodermal origin. Epithelial tissues are subclassified into several groups based on their morphologic appearance and organization in situ (see Chapter 3).

The subclassifications are based on the shape of the most superficial cells in the epithelium and on the number of cells in the layer. Many epithelia consist of only a single layer of cells; these are called simple epithelia. When there are two or more layers of cells in the epithelium, it is called a stratified epithelium. A special case, pseudostratified epithelium, is composed of a single layer of cells that has the appearance of being stratified. However, all the cells of pseudostratified epithelium are in contact with the basal lamina.

All covering and lining epithelial cells and all exocrine gland secretory cells are in close apposition to one another. Specialized cell-to-cell junctions are found in these regions of apposition; the junctional specializations consist of four distinct structures that are seen at the ultrastructural level. The junctions are discussed in detail in the next chapter, but it is important to note that they serve three important roles: (1) they hold adjacent cells together, (2) they prevent the unregulated movement of materials from entering or leaving tissue spaces by sealing "outside" from "inside," and (3) one of the junctions is specialized for intercellular communication. Epithelia have very little space between them, and the small amount that is found is filled with interstitial fluid. Figure 2-2A illustrates an epithelium with a single layer of flattened cells (a simple squamous epithelium), and Figure 2-2B shows an epithelium consisting of many layers of cells, the most superficial of which are also flattened; hence this is a stratified squamous epithelium.

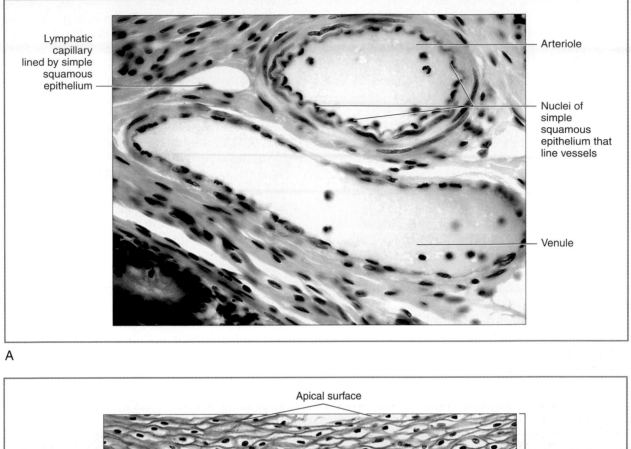

Lymphatic capillary lined by simple squamous epithelium

Arteriole

Nuclei of simple squamous epithelium that line vessels

Venule

A

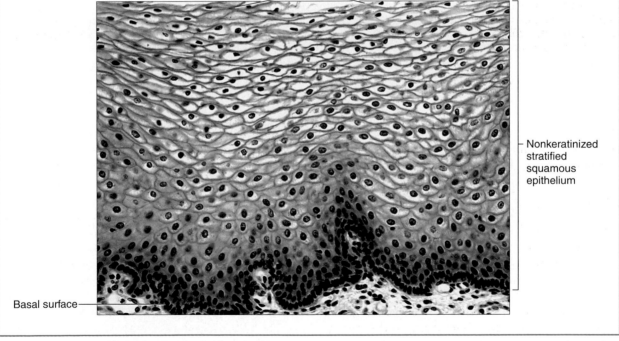

Apical surface

Nonkeratinized stratified squamous epithelium

Basal surface

B

Figure 2-2. **A,** Micrograph of a small arteriole and venule from the small intestine. A small lymphatic capillary is also seen just above and to the left of the blood vessels. All three of these vessels are lined with a simple squamous epithelium. H&E stain (280×). **B,** Micrograph of the nonkeratinized stratified squamous epithelium of the esophagus. The cells at the basal surface of the epithelium are more or less cuboidal while those at the free surface are flattened (squamous) cells. H&E stain (160×).

In virtually all locations, epithelia have a thin, mesh-like layer between the epithelial cells and the adjacent connective tissue—the basal lamina; the basal lamina is synthesized by the epithelial cells.

Connective Tissue

A defining characteristic of connective tissue (CT) is that it consists of relatively few cells embedded in a large volume of extracellular matrix. Most CT is derived from mesoderm. The connective tissues are classified into two main categories: CT proper and supporting CT. The supporting CTs are cartilage and bone.

There are several subclasses of CT proper, each of which has a characteristic appearance, feel, and composition. In some of the more common examples, a number of different connective cells are found within any given type of CT; this is in contrast to epithelia in which all the cells in any one epithelial tissue type are essentially the same. Each CT type has its own characteristic matrix composition; some are very loose, appear disorganized, and have a high water content; others are very homogenous, dense, highly ordered, and tough. One common kind of connective tissue, loose CT, is found subjacent to many epithelia, as illustrated in Figure 2-3, where a trichrome stain of human skin can be seen. The keratinized, stratified squamous epithelium is seen (incompletely) to the right. To the left of the epithelium is a layer of loose CT, a layer of dense irregular CT, and still another layer of loose CT with many adipose cells. Major components of connective tissue matrix are the fibrous proteins, collagen and elastin. These two fibrous proteins are seen in this micrograph; collagen fibers are stained aqua blue and elastin fibers are the thicker, reddish purple fibers seen particularly well in the region of dense connective tissue.

Loose CT, in particular, is a compartment with many blood vessels and nerves. This type of CT is relatively cellular compared with other types. The outer covering of blood vessels (see Fig. 2-2A) and nerves consists of a connective tissue sheath, which holds them in place and blends imperceptibly into the surrounding CT. Connective tissues and individual CT cells do not have a basal lamina associated with them with one exception—adipose cells. Consequently, it could be stated that in addition to its function of literally connecting the cells and tissues of the body to each other, CT provides a compartment, or "highway," in the body in which cells and many macromolecules can travel (in principle) throughout the body without having to cross a basal lamina.

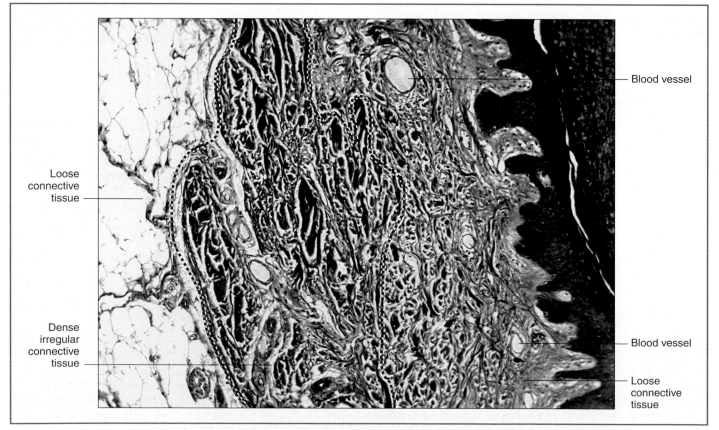

Figure 2-3. Section of skin showing two different kinds of loose connective tissue and dense irregular connective tissue. The keratinized stratified squamous epithelium is seen to the right, although the free surface is not included in this micrograph. The loose CT just under the epithelium is rich in collagen fibers (light blue), cells, and small blood vessels, although good examples of the latter two are difficult to see at this magnification. The dark magenta–staining fibers seen in abundance in the dense CT layer are elastin fibers. Mallory's trichrome stain (160×).

Determinants of Protein Structure

Some proteins are globular and some are fibrous. Many proteins form functional associations with other proteins to form higher order structures. The structure of a protein and where in the cell it is synthesized determine whether it will remain in the cytoplasm, become part of a membrane—an intercellular membrane or the plasma membrane of the cell—or be exported and function in the extracellular space (e.g., proteins of the extracellular matrix) or at some other location in the body (e.g., hormones or cytokines).

- The primary structure of a protein refers to its linear amino acid sequence.
- The secondary structure of a protein refers to a number of structural domains including α-helices, β-pleated sheets, and membrane-spanning domains.
- The tertiary structure of a protein refers to the manner in which the protein folds to form its native structure.
- The quaternary structure of a protein refers to other proteins with which it associates to form a functional unit.

Globular proteins tend to be soluble in physiologic salt solutions. Some proteins are fibrous owing to their amino acid sequence and form macroscopic fibers in the extracellular space (e.g., triple helical collagen and elastin).

Proteins synthesized on free cytoplasmic ribosomes are destined to remain in the cell. In general, proteins synthesized on the rough endoplasmic reticulum are destined to reside in membrane-bound organelles, such as lysosomes, or to be packaged into vesicles to be released from the cell by exocytosis.

Muscle Tissue

Contractility is the defining characteristic of muscle tissue. Most muscle is derived from mesoderm. Histologically, muscle tissue is described as being smooth or striated; striated muscle is further subdivided into skeletal and cardiac muscle. For historical reasons, muscle cells (of all three types) are called fibers rather than cells; this is an appropriate nomenclature, since muscle fibers are elongated compared with most other cell types. Each individual muscle cell is invested with a delicate lamina externa, which in terms of appearance and composition is similar to the basal lamina. All three types of muscle are vascular; each is endowed with a considerable number of capillaries.

The contractility of all three muscle types is regulated by the intracellular concentration of Ca^{++}. The principal contractile proteins of muscle are actin and myosin, yet each of the three muscle types has a substantial number of "muscle-specific" proteins associated with the actin-myosin. These muscle-associated proteins are critical for the normal structure and function of muscle fibers and for whole anatomic muscles. Actin and myosin, as well as many specific associated proteins, are found in all cells of the body, albeit in much smaller concentrations than in muscle fibers.

Examples of all three types of muscle are shown in Figure 2-4.

Muscle Types

Smooth Muscle

Smooth muscle is widely distributed in many organs, where it may have contractile or supporting functions, or both. Smooth muscle is also found in the walls of all blood vessels larger than capillaries. It is generally referred to as involuntary muscle, since its contraction is regulated by the autonomic nervous system. Smooth muscle fibers exhibit an intrinsic contractility, so they may contract in the absence of external or nervous stimuli; the peristaltic waves of contraction of the intestine are an example of this intrinsic contraction.

Skeletal Muscle

This type of tissue comprises the major muscle mass of the body and its contraction is under voluntary control. An entire skeletal muscle is surrounded by a connective tissue sheath called the *epimysium* (equivalent to deep fascia). Skeletal muscles are organized further into fascicles and individual fibers by connective tissue sheaths called the *perimysium* and the *endomysium*.

Cardiac Muscle

Cardiac muscle is found only in the heart. The contraction rate of the heart is under the control of sympathetic (accelerates heart rate) and parasympathetic fibers (decelerates heart rate) of the autonomic nervous system. Compared with smooth and skeletal muscle, cardiac muscle fibers have significantly more interstitial CT.

Nerve Tissue

The fourth basic tissue type is nerve tissue. Nerve cells (neurons) and their processes are found throughout the body. Based on the location of the neurons (and their associated structures and supporting cells), the central nervous system (CNS) can be described as consisting of the brain and spinal cord and the peripheral nervous system (PNS) as consisting of all the neurons and associated cells and structures in the rest of the body. Figure 2-5 shows examples of neurons in the brain and the spinal cord. Nerve tissue is derived from the neural tube, which is an early developmental derivative of ectoderm. In the simplest terms, the PNS consists of clusters of cell bodies, the ganglia, and their long processes, and the nerves seen at the gross anatomic level. It is these latter structures that comprise the named anatomic nerves. Figure 2-6 shows a ganglion and a peripheral nerve. Peripheral nerves are invested with connective tissue sheaths, in a manner analogous to skeletal muscle. An entire nerve is surrounded by a sheath of connective tissue called *epineurium*. Within the nerve there are fascicles surrounded by a distinctive CT sheath called *perineurium*; each individual nerve process has a delicate CT sheath called *endoneurium*.

The CNS is responsible for regulating all the higher functions of humans and other animals. The entire nervous system integrates, coordinates, and regulates the functions of

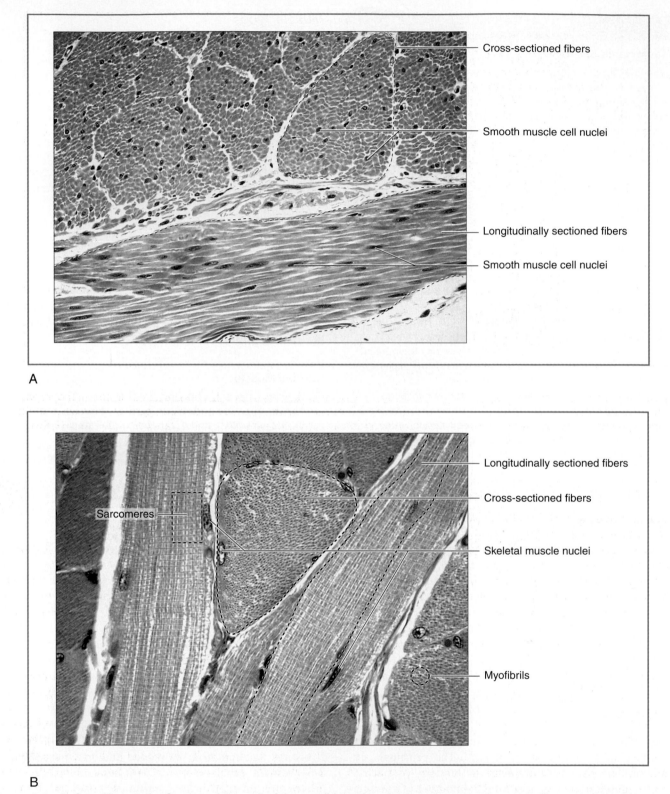

A

B

Figure 2-4. A, Smooth muscle. Section of the wall of the small intestine shows many smooth muscle fibers sectioned in transverse and oblique-longitudinal planes. Nuclei of smooth muscle fibers are cigar-shaped, so when seen in transverse section, they appear circular such that the circles exhibit a small range of different diameters. In longitudinal planes, the tapered oval shape of the nucleus can be seen. H&E stain (200×). **B,** Skeletal muscle. In this section of the tongue, the skeletal muscle fibers in transverse and longitudinal planes of the section are visible. Skeletal muscle nuclei are flattened oval structures located at the periphery of the muscle fiber. The hundreds of small dots seen in the transversely sectioned fibers are myofibrils. In the longitudinal planes of the section, many sarcomeres are seen. Iron hematoxylin stain (440×).

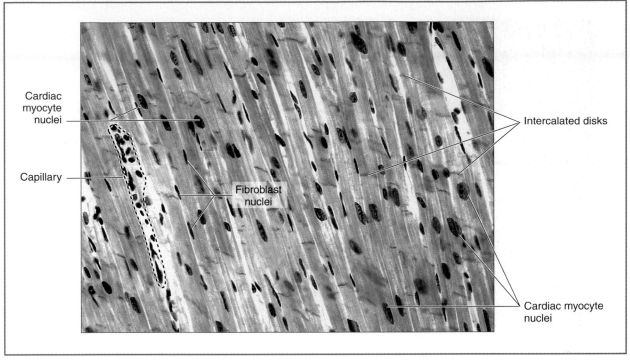

Cardiac myocyte nuclei

Capillary

Fibroblast nuclei

Intercalated disks

Cardiac myocyte nuclei

C

Figure 2-4 cont'd. **C,** Cardiac muscle. Two of the distinctive features of cardiac muscle fibers are seen in this micrograph: (1) the centrally placed oval nuclei of the fibers and (2) the intercalated disks. It is also possible to gain an impression of the branching nature of the cardiac myocytes, especially in comparison with the other two kinds of muscle. H&E stain (250×).

ANATOMY & EMBRYOLOGY

Embryonic Development of the Heart and Cardiovascular System

The heart and cardiovascular system form the first organ system to develop and function in the embryo. The system first functions at day 22 of development when the heart is a primitive tube and the first set of blood vessels carries blood to and from the developing embryo and placenta.

- The primitive heart tube begins to beat at about this time, since cardiac myocytes exhibit an intrinsic or spontaneous contractility.
- The four chambers of the heart appear at about 4 to 5 weeks of development.
- The heart valves are complete by about 8 weeks of development.

PHYSIOLOGY

Regulation of Heart Rate

There are at least two levels of heart rate regulation:
- One level is the intrinsic rate of firing of specialized cardiac myocytes, called pacemaker cells, which are in the sinoatrial (SA) node.
- Overall regulation of heart rate is mediated by the autonomic nervous system acting on SA node cells.

---

organs of the body. Neurons are also responsible for receiving and processing sensory input from the environment.

Neurons are specialized to receive, integrate, and send electrical signals within the body—to and from the body organs as well as to and from each other. All cells of the body exhibit electrical properties, but neurons have special capabilities in this regard. The specializations are seen in the structure of the neurons and their elaborate and extensive processes. Each neuron has a single, usually long, axon, which carries information away from the cell body (soma), and

usually many other processes, dendrites, that convey information toward the soma. The processes can be very long (many micrometers to many centimeters), so they are virtually impossible to see in their entirety in the light microscope; even when one is seen, the two types of processes look very similar, so it is practically impossible to distinguish axons from dendrites by conventional light microscopy. The fine structure of neurons seen with the electron microscope reveals the structural complexity of these cells (Fig. 2-7). In addition to the structural specializations of neurons, they are highly specialized in biochemical terms to synthesize and secrete many different chemicals, called neurotransmitters, which initiate or facilitate the propagation of nerve impulses from one neuron to another. The neurotransmitters are released at specialized regions near the end of an axon or a dendrite. These regions are called *synapses* (Fig. 2-8). Synapses may

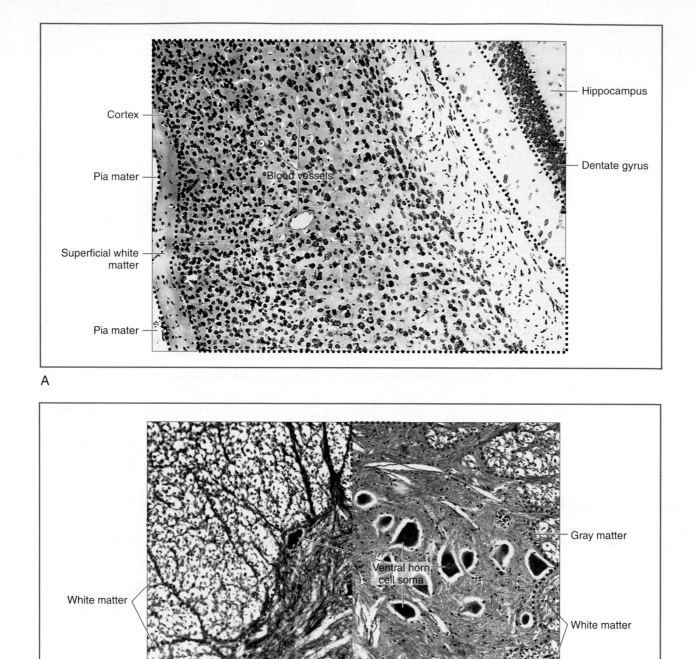

A

B

Figure 2-5. A, Section of brain stained with the Nissl stain, which has a high affinity for ribonuclear protein, both nuclear and cytoplasmic. Part of the hippocampus is seen in the upper right part of the section, alongside the dentate gyrus. The rest of the section shows part of the cortex, its superficial white matter, and the pia mater. Cresyl violet stain (70×). **B,** The spinal cord stained with two different stains. Many of the same features can be seen with both stains: spinal motor neurons, gray and white matter, nuclei of glial cells in the gray matter, the neuropil that makes up the rest of the material that stains in the gray matter, and cross-sections of the myelinated axons in the white matter. Several large neurons and their processes are seen against a background of glial cells. Silver stain *(left),* H&E stain *(right)* (80×).

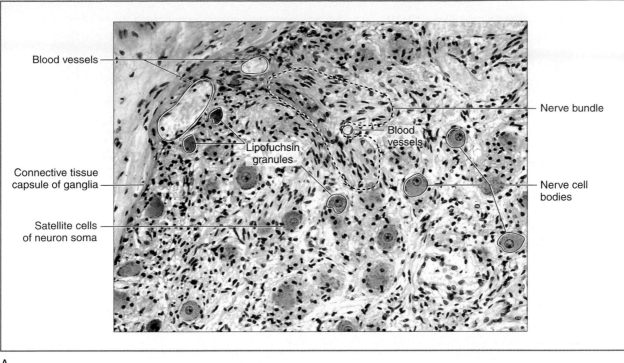

A

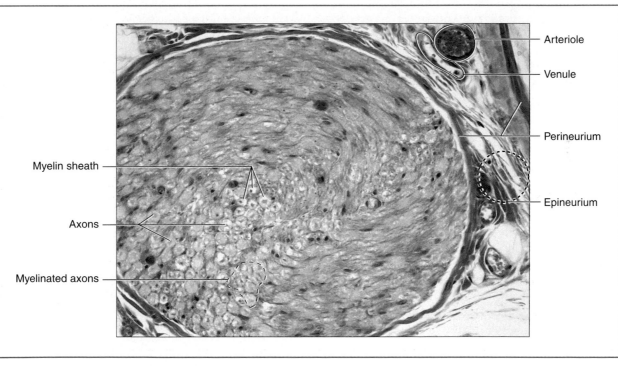

B

Figure 2-6. A, A typical sensory ganglion is seen in this micrograph. Numerous cell bodies are seen (many with yellowish-brown lipofuchsin granules), as are the satellite cells that surround the neuronal soma, myelinated axons, and the CT capsule of the ganglion. H&E stain (150×). **B,** An entire small nerve bundle is seen in this micrograph. In those axons sectioned transversely, it is possible to see individual axons and their myelin sheaths. The axons in nerve bundles such as these travel in curving, tortuous paths, which accounts for the large number of curved, swirling profiles seen in about 60% of this section. The bundle is surrounded by a dark-staining CT sheath, the perineurium; a small part of the perineurium of another nerve bundle can be seen in this preparation. The moderately loose to dense irregular CT that is seen between the bundles is the epineurium. H&E stain (140×).

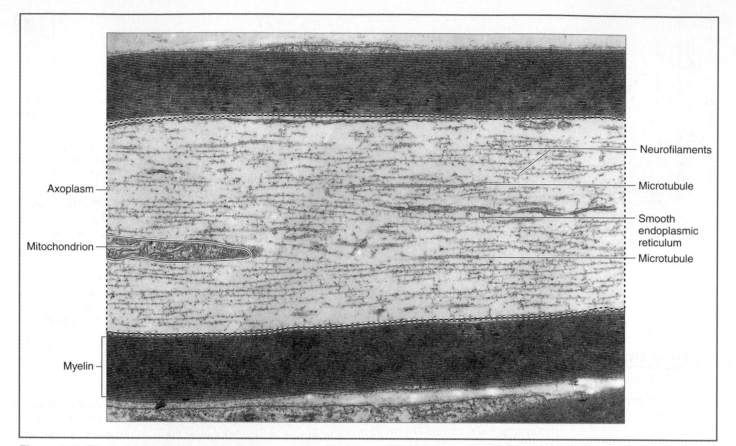

Figure 2-7. Electron micrograph of a myelinated axon sectioned longitudinally. The electron dense myelin sheath is seen on each side of the axoplasm. Many neuronal intermediate filaments (neurofilaments) are seen in the axoplasm, as are several microtubules and a mitochondrion. (Courtesy of Enrico Mugnani.)

release their neurotransmitters in proximity to another axon, a dendrite, or a neuronal cell body.

Nerve tissue has little if any supporting connective tissue, but there is a large and diverse population of supporting cells in the nervous system. In the CNS, these cells are called the *neuroglia* of which there are three major types: oligodendrocytes, astrocytes, and microglia. There are hundreds of billions of cells in the CNS; estimates tell us that more than 90% of them are neuroglia. The supporting cells in the PNS are called Schwann cells, which are analogous to the oligodendrocytes in the CNS, and the satellite or capsule cells of ganglia. Neurons, like muscle fibers, have a delicate basal lamina surrounding them.

●●● BASAL LAMINA

In defining each of the basic tissue types above, reference has been made to the presence or absence of an extracellular structure called the basal lamina. The specific functions of the basal lamina have not been precisely defined. It has been described as a supporting layer for epithelia, a structural-biochemical barrier to the movement of cells from the connective tissue compartment to the epithelial (or muscle or neuronal) compartment, a path to guide migrating cells

ANATOMY & EMBRYOLOGY

Development of the Central Nervous System

The precursors of the brain and nerve tissue appear early and throughout development. A general characteristic of neural development is extensive migration of neuroblast cells to specific locations where they further proliferate and differentiate into more mature forms.

- Neurulation begins during the first week of embryonic life when the early stages of development of the fore-, mid-, and hindbrain are seen.
- Spinal nerves grow into the body wall, and autonomic nerves grow into the viscera within the forming body cavities.
- The brain develops throughout prenatal and postnatal life up to and including the teenage years.

during embryonic development, and so on. However, as a structural and biochemical entity, much is known about the basal lamina. Histologists had described an amorphous layer underlying many, but not all, epithelia for decades; certain epithelia (e.g., the trachea and the glomerular capillaries in the kidney) have an easily recognized basement membrane. They called this layer the *basement membrane* because of its

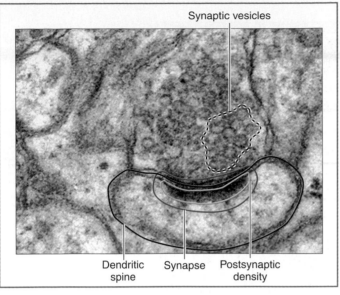

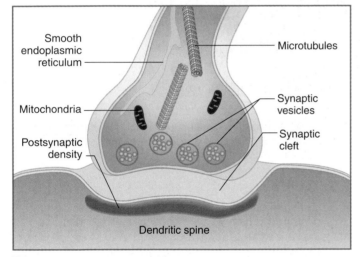

B

Figure 2-8. A, High-magnification electron micrograph of a synapse. The pre- and postsynaptic densities and the cleft between them are seen; the axonal ending (bouton) has many small, round synaptic vesicles. This is a synapse between an axon and a dendritic spine. (Courtesy of Yuri Geinisman.) **B,** A similar synapse is diagrammed in this part of the figure.

location. When tissue sections were stained with the periodic acid–Schiff method (PAS is a stain that reacts with carbohydrates and results in an intense magenta color [Fig. 2-9]), this same layer stained intensely. In addition, a greater range of epithelia and some of the other basic tissue types (e.g., smooth muscle) were PAS-positive, suggesting a more widespread distribution of basement membrane than had been thought.

As histologists and cell biologists began to study the ultrastructure of tissues, they noted a thin, moderately electron dense, amorphous, mesh-like layer where the basement membrane was seen in the light microscope. More significant

PATHOLOGY

Tumor Metastasis and the Basal Lamina

The growth of tumors (neoplasms) in the body is an unfortunately common occurrence. In simple terms, tumors can be classified into two categories: benign (noninvasive) and malignant (invasive). The growth of all tumors reflects a loss in the regulation of cell division. Unregulated cell division (growth) can result from mutations in growth-regulating proteins, from chromosomal translocations, or from other causes. Several factors determine whether a tumor becomes malignant:

- It may become malignant if it grows beyond a certain size.
- It may become malignant if it is locally invasive.
- It may become malignant if it synthesizes and secretes proteases, especially those that degrade the matrix and the basal lamina.
- When tumor cell proteases degrade the basal lamina of the microvasculature in proximity to the primary tumor, the tumor cells enter the circulation and are dispersed to distant regions of the body, where they seed the growth of new tumors.

was the fact that they saw such a structure associated with all epithelia, with individual epithelial cells in glands, with all three types of muscle fibers, and with neurons and the supporting Schwann cells. None of the connective tissue cells, except adipose cells, had a basal lamina. Depending on the type of tissue with which the layer was associated, they called it the basal lamina, or lamina externa. Coupled with biochemical studies of certain basement membranes, especially those in the kidney, it quickly became clear that one biochemical component was found ubiquitously in the basal lamina/basement membrane, namely, type IV collagen. It is now known that there are many more "universal" components of the basal lamina. In this text, the term basal lamina usually refers to this layer, since the term applies to both light and electron microscope images; when basement membrane is used, it should be understood that light microscopy is implied. Table 2-1 summarizes the general characteristics of the basic tissue types.

●●● ORGAN CLASSIFICATION

Solid Organs

The solid body organs are described in terms of a general structural "plan" (Fig. 2-10). Those cells in the organ that are responsible for its main functions are called *parenchymal* (Greek, "anything poured in beside") cells. These cells are supported by a connective tissue called *stroma* (Greek, "bed"). A solid organ has a CT capsule and is subdivided into lobes and lobules by CT septae (Greek, "walls") that radiate inward from the capsule to deeper parts of the organ. Emanating from the capsule or the septae may be found smaller, thinner CT structures called *trabeculae* (Greek,

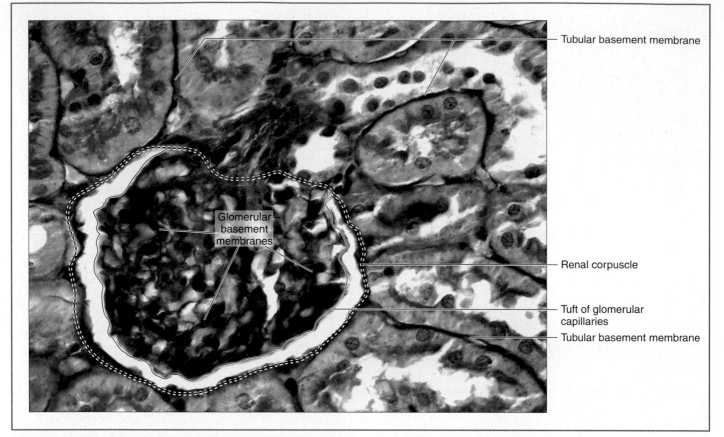

Figure 2-9. Micrograph of the renal cortex, stained with periodic acid–Schiff, which stains carbohydrate-rich molecules, shows the basement membranes that are so abundant in the kidney. The wall of the renal corpuscle and the tuft of glomerular capillaries it contains show prominent basement membranes, as do the tubular parts of the nephron. PAS stain (400×).

"spike"). Finally, the parenchymal cells are often supported by fine CT fibers.

A common shape for a solid organ is that of a bean; at the indented part of the circumference (which is called the *hilum*), an artery and a vein carrying blood to and from the organ are visible. Solid organs are innervated, so the nerve and an efferent lymphatic vessel carrying lymph produced by the organ at the hilum may be seen. Since most exocrine glands are solid organs, they have a large secretory duct, exiting the gland at the hilum. The secretory duct is the largest-diameter part of a series of smaller ducts that originate in the parenchyma of the organ. A number of solid organs (e.g., the liver, the salivary glands) are not bean shaped, but they have the same general organization, including a hilum and its associated structures.

Many, but not all, solid organs have a distinct outer region called the *cortex* and a distinct inner region called the *medulla*. The cortex lies under the capsule, and the medulla occupies the space between the cortex and the hilum.

Hollow Organs

Hollow organs have four layers: (1) the innermost is called the *mucosa*, (2) the second is a connective tissue layer called the *submucosa*, (3) the third is a layer of smooth muscle called the *muscularis externa*, and (4) the outermost is called the *adventitia* or *serosa* (see below). Figure 2-11 presents a diagram of a typical hollow organ.

Glands and glandular secretions are a characteristic feature of hollow organs. In many cases, the mucosal epithelium itself is a secretory epithelium. There are also numerous examples in which glands are external to the hollow organ; they empty their contents into the lumen of the organ via a duct.

Mucosa

The mucosa is further subdivided into an epithelial layer (*mucosal epithelium*) and its basal lamina, a connective tissue layer (*lamina propria*), and a thin muscular layer (*lamina muscularis mucosae*, or *muscularis mucosae*). The specific kind of mucosal epithelium depends on the organ and the specific part of the organ or organ system. The lamina propria is typically a loose CT layer with many blood vessels, nerves, and nerve endings; furthermore, it is where the system of lymphatic capillaries in each organ originates. The lamina propria typically contains many lymphocytes and macrophages, which are part of the front line of the body's immune defense system. In certain locations, the lamina propria may have small exocrine glands; these are called *mucosal glands*. In nearly all cases, the muscularis mucosae is a thin layer of smooth muscle.

TABLE 2-1. General Characteristics of the Basic Tissue Types*

Tissue Type	Major Categories	Relative Cell: Matrix Ratio	Cellular Hetero-geneity	Vascularity	Basal Lamina	Cell-Cell Communication	Special Features
Epithelia	Covering/lining Simple	99:1	1+	0	Yes, at interface with CT	Yes, via gap junctions and local growth factors	Individual cells or whole epithelium is polarized
	Stratified/ pseudostratified	99:1	2+	0	Yes, at interface with CT	Yes, via gap junctions and local growth factors	Apical cells touch a free/ external surface Cells are held together at or near apical surface by junctional complexes
	Glands Exocrine	95:5	2+	2+	Yes, at basal surface each cell	Yes, via gap junctions	Usually is a single cell layer thick Cells are polarized and have junctional complexes Secretory products are deposited on a free surface
	Endocrine	98:2	4+	5+	Yes, each surrounding cell		Cells typically occur in groups large enough to be called anatomic glands Secretory products are released into extensive capillary bed
Connec-tive tissue	Proper CT Loose, high water content	5:95	5+	5+	No	Responsive to locally secreted growth factors or growth inhibitors, activators of cell function, etc	Cellular population may be very heterogeneous and relatively cell rich Low content of extracellular fibers Extremely vascular and the major compartment to find nerve fibers and sensory endings
	Adipose	95:5	1+	4+	Yes, each cell		Very cellular and vascular
	Dense, low water content	2:98	2+	1+	No		Small number of cells, mostly fibroblasts, very fibrous, relatively avascular
	Supporting CT Cartilage	5:95	1+	0	No		Homogenous cell population Dense, gel-like, rubbery matrix with high water content
	Bone	5:95	1+	3+	No	Yes, via gap junctions	Homogeneous cell population Dense, ossified matrix

*This summary of the major features of the four basic tissue types provides a convenient basis for comparison.

Table continued on following page

TABLE 2-1. General Characteristics of the Basic Tissue Types*—*cont'd*

Tissue Type	Major Categories	Relative Cell: Matrix Ratio	Cellular Hetero-geneity	Vascularity	Basal Lamina	Cell-Cell Communication	Special Features
Muscle	Smooth	98:2	1+	2+	Yes	Yes, via gap junctions	Individual, mononucleate, fusiform fibers (cells)
	Striated Skeletal	98:2	1+	3+	Yes		Very long, cylindrical, multinucleated fibers (cells)
	Cardiac	90:10	1+	5+	Yes	Yes, via gap junctions	Individual, branching, mono- or binucleated fibers held together end-to-end by specialized cell junctions
Nerve	CNS Neurons	98:2	5+	5+	Yes	Yes, via gap junctions and through many types of synaptic mechanisms	Many types of cells Soma are specialized to synthesize large quantities of protein Cellular processes (axons and dendrites) are long and contain large amounts of intermediate filaments and microtubules
	Glia	98:2	3+	4+			Three major cell types in CNS Carry out important supporting roles for neurons
	PNS Neurons	95:5	2+	3+	Yes	Yes, via gap junctions and synaptic mechanisms	Soma are specialized to synthesize large quantities of protein Cellular processes (axons and dendrites) are long and contain large amounts of intermediate filaments and microtubules
	Ganglia	98:2	2+	2+			Two major cell types
	Supporting cells	90:10	2+	2+	Yes		Two major cell types that support axons and two major types that support neuronal cell bodies in ganglia

*This summary of the major features of the four basic tissue types provides a convenient basis for comparison.

Submucosa

The submucosa can be a relatively thick layer of loose to moderately dense CT. It has larger blood vessels, larger nerve fibers, neuronal soma in certain locations, and larger lymphatic vessels (than those seen in the lamina propria). In certain locations, the submucosa may have exocrine glands; these are called *submucosal glands*.

Muscularis Externa

Although there is considerable variation in the organization of the muscularis externa, the most common pattern is that of an inner circular and outer longitudinal layer of smooth muscle fibers. The muscularis externa in the small and large intestines has neuronal soma (as individual cells and as small ganglia) throughout its length.

Figure 2-10. Schematic diagram of a solid organ with all main parts labeled. The left half of the diagram shows the general appearance of a solid organ (such as a lymph node) that is not subdivided into lobes and lobules. The right side of the diagram illustrates the general appearance of a solid organ that is subdivided into lobes and lobules; this architecture would be seen in the salivary glands. The hilum of a solid organ is the area where arteries enter and veins leave. Nerves enter and lymph (via a lymphatic vessel) leaves the organ at the hilum; if this were a secretory organ, the excretory duct would be seen.

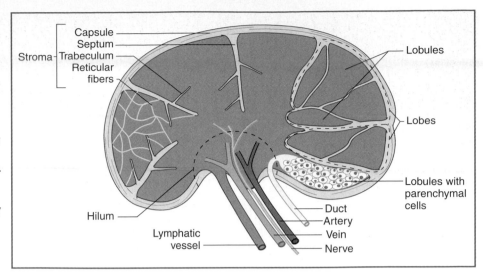

Figure 2-11. Schematic diagram of a typical hollow organ, even though it is based largely on the intestine. The four layers of the organ are indicated by Roman numerals. Different specializations in the inner three layers are indicated in three of the quadrants. Epithelial *(blue)*, connective *(green)*, muscle *(red)*, and nerve *(yellow)* tissues are depicted.

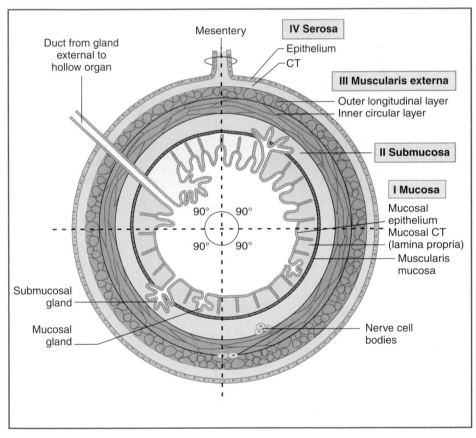

Adventitia or Serosa

In places where a hollow organ is in contact with the body wall or other internal organs, the outermost layer (adventitia) is an irregular layer of moderately dense CT. When the hollow organ faces a body cavity (e.g., the peritoneum), it is covered with serosa, which is a very thin layer of wet, simple squamous epithelium.

Epithelial Tissues and Exocrine Glands

3

●●● CHARACTERISTICS AND CLASSIFICATION OF EPITHELIAL TISSUES

General Characteristics of Epithelia

Epithelial tissues cover all the external and line all the internal surfaces of the body; it is helpful to think of these epithelia as sheets of cells that follow the contour of their anatomic location. All these epithelia are *avascular*. Covering and lining epithelia "sit" on a basal lamina, which is synthesized and secreted by the epithelial cells; there always is a layer of loose connective tissue under the basal lamina in these kinds of epithelia. The parenchymal cells of exocrine glands and their ducts, as well as the parenchymal cells of endocrine glands, are composed of epithelial cells; both kinds of glands are highly vascular. Parenchymal cells in exocrine glands have a delicate basal lamina at their basal surface while endocrine glands are surrounded by a delicate basal lamina.

The cells that line the blood and lymphatic vascular systems are epithelial cells, as are the cells that make up the thin, wet membranes of internal body cavities, such as the pleural, pericardial, and abdominal cavities; epithelial cells in all these locations also have a basal lamina. The presence of these epithelial linings and their function play a major physiologic role in local and systemic homeostasis.

Essentially all epithelial cells are held together by a set of specializations of the plasma membrane called *cell junctions*. There are five types of junctions, which are described in greater detail below, but it is worth noting now that the junctions are seen in characteristic locations of the cell. Three of the junctions are usually seen as a group very close to the apical margins of the cell—the *zonula occludens* (the tight or occluding junction), the *zonula adherens* (the adhering zone), and the *macula adherens* (the adhering spot) or *desmosome*. Two terms are used to describe this group of junctions, the *terminal bar* (a term used in light microscopy) and the *junctional complex* (a term used in electron microscopy). While a major role of the junctions is to hold the cells in close proximity to one another, a second critical role is in regulating the movement of solvents and solutes across the epithelium. The desmosome is also seen as a solitary junction distributed in many locations on the lateral surfaces of the cell. The other two junctions are the *communicating junction* (gap junction or nexus) and the *hemidesmosome*. The nexus can be found in many places on the lateral surfaces of the cell, and the hemidesmosome is always found on the basal surface of the cell, where it interacts with the basal lamina and the underlying connective tissue.

Although epithelial cells carry out many functions, two of the most common are *synthesis* and *secretion* of proteins, glycoproteins, enzymes, hormones, etc, and the *absorption* or *resorption* of fluids, salts, nutrients, proteins, etc, in a number of organs.

Generally speaking, epithelia, or at least some of the cells that make up an epithelium, divide throughout life (i.e., they are in a life-long state of cell renewal). Cells found in the skin, intestinal lining, hair, virtually all glands, and so on, remain active in the cell cycle throughout life.

Classification of Epithelia

The primary criteria for naming epithelia are the *number of cells in the full thickness of the epithelium* and the *shape of the cells at the free or apical surface*. When the epithelium is a single cell layer thick, it is a simple epithelium. When the epithelium is two or more cell layers thick, it is a stratified epithelium; only the basal cell layer is in contact with the basal lamina in a stratified epithelium. Particularly in lining epithelia, the apical surface of the cell has a number of specializations such as microvilli, cilia, flagella, filopodia, and others; each of these surface modifications has one or more specific functions. The whole epithelium is named according to the shape of the cells at the free surface using the following three terms: squamous, cuboidal, or columnar epithelium.

A *squamous epithelial* cell is wide and flat but not very high—you can think of such a cell as looking like a fried egg, where the yolk is the cell nucleus and the white is the cytoplasm; in most sections, the cytoplasm of a squamous epithelium is hard to see, so the most identifiable feature is the cell nucleus. Like the yolk of a fried egg, the nucleus of a squamous epithelial cell is a flattened disk. These cells are usually sectioned perpendicular to their large, flat surface. If you look down at the surface of a *simple squamous epithelium*, you see cells that are more or less hexagonally close-packed. Figure 3-1 shows two such preparations. Figure 3-1A shows a whole mount of frog epidermis stained with a silver stain and hematoxylin. The silver stains the cell boundaries of the surface layer of cells while the nuclei stain with hematoxylin. Since this thin sheet of tissue is a few cell layers thick (i.e., it is not a simple squamous epithelium), some cells appear to have more than one nucleus. Nonetheless, the edges of only the surface cells are stained, providing an accurate impression of a simple squamous epithelium. Figure 3-1B shows a whole mount of squamous epithelial cells scraped from the inner surface of the cheek.

Figure 3-2 shows simple squamous epithelia in sectioned specimens of the lymphatic and blood vascular system. Figure 3-2A is a section of a large lymphatic vessel in the soft palate. Many of the epithelial cells that line the inner surface of this vessel are sectioned perpendicular to their flat surface, and some are sectioned tangentially. Figure 3-2B is an electron micrograph of a capillary that consists of only a single squamous epithelial cell. The cytoplasm of this cell is seen to contain many organelles and a nucleus with a significant proportion of euchromatin.

There are two widely distributed kinds of stratified squamous epithelium: *nonkeratinized stratified squamous epithelium* and *keratinized stratified squamous epithelium*. These two kinds of epithelia illustrate the principle of naming epithelia on the basis of the free surface morphology. Figure 3-3 shows a nonkeratinized stratified squamous epithelium and a keratinized stratified squamous epithelium. In both cases, the basal cells are more or less cuboidal, the cells in the intermediate layers are cuboidal or stellate, and the superficial cells are squamous—either nonkeratinized or keratinized.

A cuboidal epithelial cell has a height, width, and depth that are approximately the same. The nucleus of a cuboidal epithelial cell is usually spherical and centrally placed in the cell. The most widely distributed kind of cuboidal epithelium is a *simple cuboidal epithelium*. Figure 3-4 shows two examples of cuboidal epithelial cells. Rare examples of *stratified cuboidal epithelia* are found in the larger ducts of exocrine glands (see Fig. 3-4C).

A columnar epithelial cell is about two to four times taller than it is wide. The nucleus of a columnar epithelial cell is usually oval and is in the lower third of the cell. The surface specializations mentioned above are commonly found on columnar epithelial cells, so that if the columnar epithelial cells had cilia, we would call it a ciliated columnar epithelium. As for cuboidal epithelia, most columnar epithelia are *simple columnar epithelia*. Figure 3-5 shows an example of columnar epithelial cells from the stomach. Very rare examples of *stratified columnar epithelium* are found in the largest ducts of exocrine glands.

In actual tissue or organ specimens, intermediate forms of the "standard" cells types mentioned above (e.g., a high—or thick—squamous epithelium or a low columnar epithelium) are often seen. The standard practice is to use the shape closest to one of these three cell morphologies and expand the description to describe the epithelium more completely if necessary.

In a few locations, modified versions of the epithelia named above are found. In the upper parts of the respiratory system and in certain regions of the male reproductive tract are *pseudostratified columnar epithelia*. The distinguishing characteristic is that *all the cells in the epithelium are in contact with the basal lamina* even though this can only be verified definitively by electron microscopy. Another modification is found in the lower urinary tract, where the epithelium found from the minor calyces of the kidney to the proximal part of the urethra is called *transitional epithelium* or *urothelium*. It appears to be a stratified cuboidal epithelium in most tissue sections, but when the bladder is first distended and then fixed, it can appear to be a simple squamous epithelium or at most about two to three cell layers thick (Fig. 3-6).

●●● CELL POLARITY

Polarity is a characteristic of epithelia. In simple epithelia, each individual cell is polarized because the apical, lateral,

Text continued on page 61

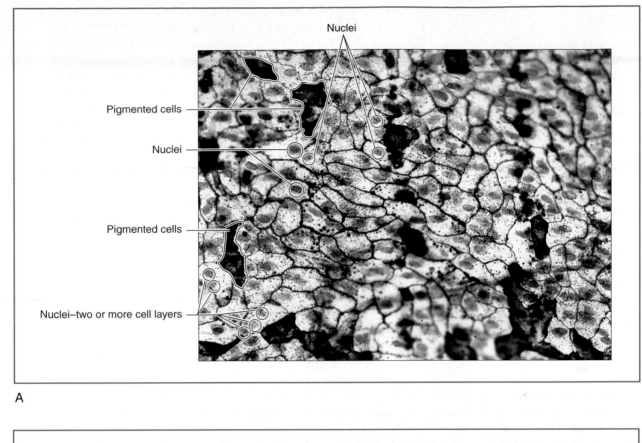

Nuclei

Pigmented cells

Nuclei

Pigmented cells

Nuclei—two or more cell layers

A

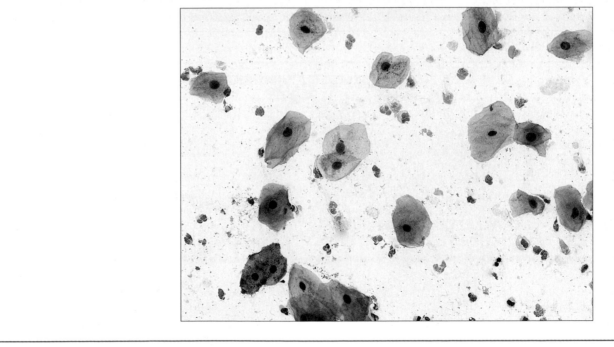

B

Figure 3-1. A, A small piece of frog epidermis mounted flat on a slide—a whole mount—stained with silver and hematoxylin (200×). Since the specimen does not lie perfectly flat on the slide, parts are out of the focal plane. The hexagonal packing of the surface cells and their nuclei are seen clearly. Some nuclei from underlying cells are visible. The very dark staining cells are pigmented cells. **B,** H&E stain of cells scraped from the inner surface of the cheek (180×). The same features of individual simple squamous epithelial cells are seen here. The many other small cells in the field of view are polymorphonuclear neutrophils.

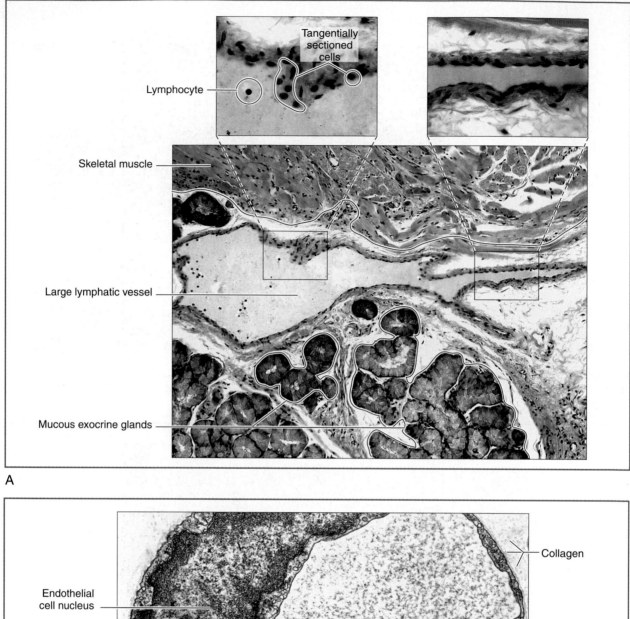

Tangentially
sectioned
cells

Lymphocyte

Skeletal muscle

Large lymphatic vessel

Mucous exocrine glands

A

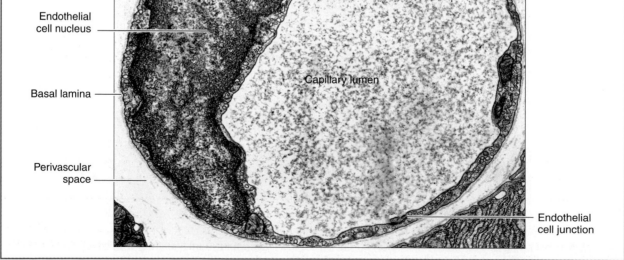

Collagen

Endothelial
cell nucleus

Capillary lumen

Basal lamina

Perivascular
space

Endothelial
cell junction

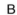

B

Figure 3-2. A, H&E stain from the soft palate with a large lymphatic vessel in the middle of the field (75×). The darker staining groups of cells are mucous exocrine glands. A number of skeletal muscle fibers are seen in the upper part of the field. Only the nuclei of the simple squamous epithelial cells on the right part of the vessel are visible *(right inset)* and others are sectioned tangentially *(left inset)* so the whole nucleus and part of the cell can be seen. **B,** Electron micrograph of a blood capillary. The capillary is made entirely of a single cell wrapped around to make a tiny cylindrical structure.

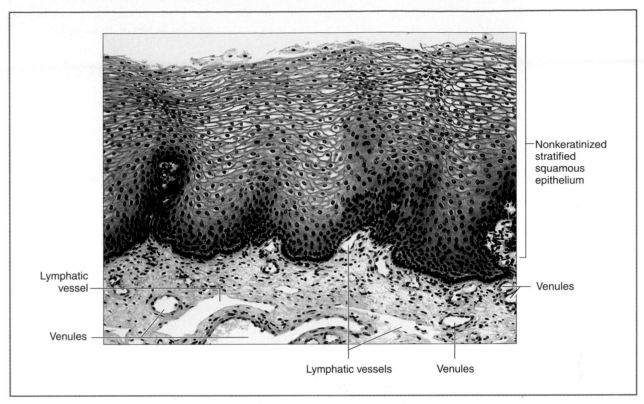

A

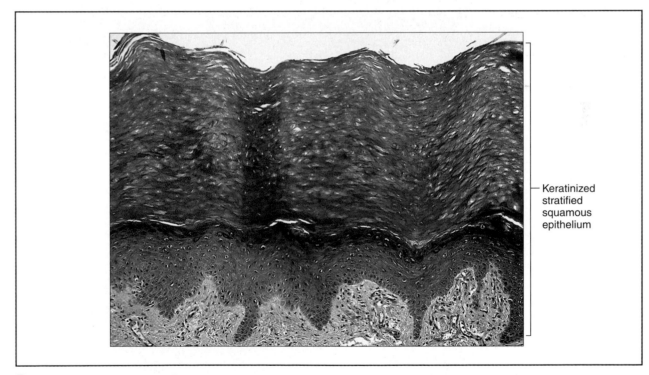

B

Figure 3-3. A, Section of the epithelial lining of the vagina (100×). This is a nonkeratinized stratified squamous epithelium. Note that the lymphatic vessels and venules are lined with simple squamous epithelium. **B,** Section of skin that is a keratinized stratified squamous epithelium. Both specimens are stained with H&E (70×).

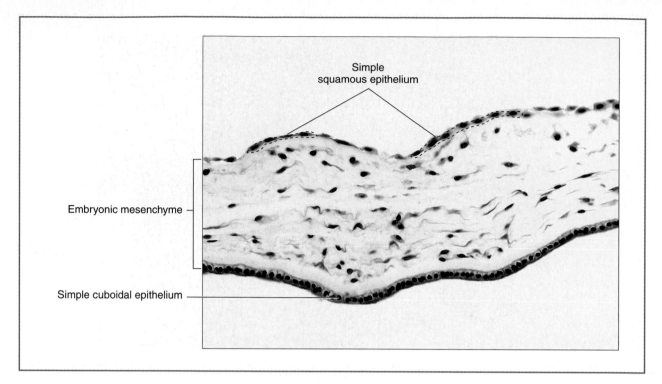

A

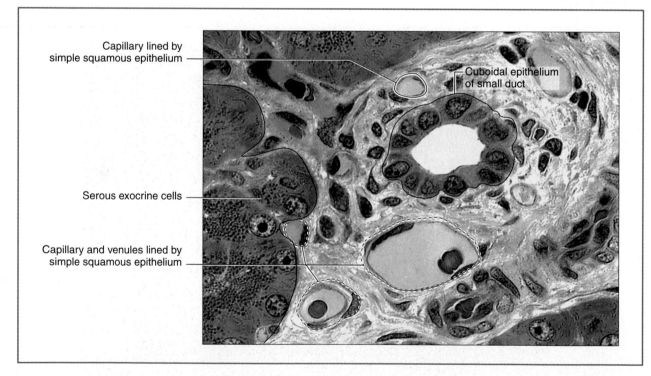

B

Figure 3-4. A, H&E stained section of amnion (200×). This membrane enclosing the developing embryo has simple squamous epithelium on one surface and simple cuboidal epithelium on the other. Embryonic mesenchyme is found between the two epithelial layers. **B,** H&E stained semi-thin (1.5 μm) section of the pancreas in a region where a small duct and several small blood vessels are seen (700×). The duct is lined by simple cuboidal epithelial cells and the blood vessels by simple squamous epithelial cells.

Continued

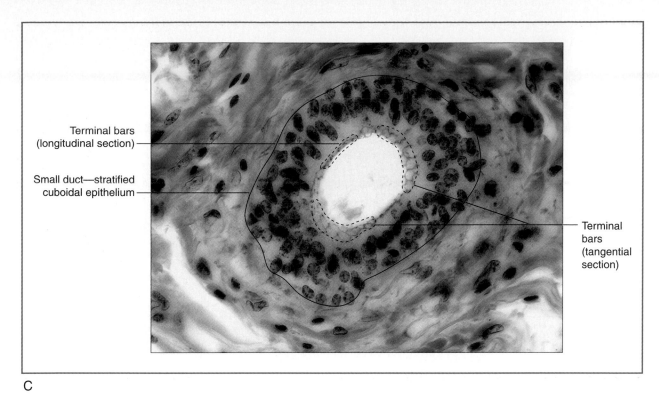

Terminal bars
(longitudinal section)

Small duct—stratified
cuboidal epithelium

Terminal
bars
(tangential
section)

C

Figure 3-4 cont'd. C, A region of the submandibular gland that shows a duct lined with stratified cuboidal epithelial cells. (Mallory-Azan trichrome stain, 440×).

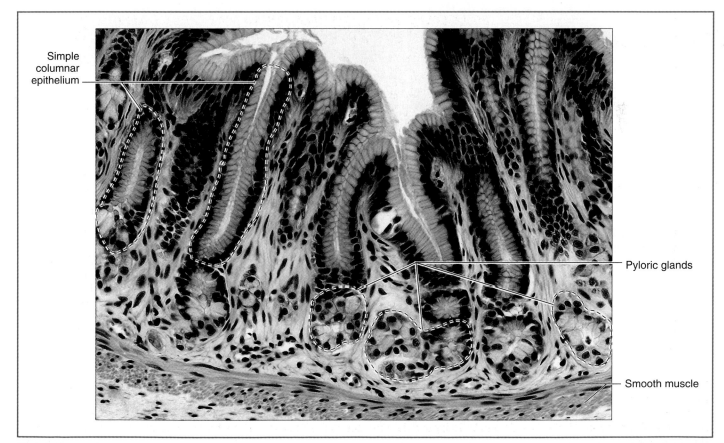

Simple
columnar
epithelium

Pyloric glands

Smooth muscle

Figure 3-5. H&E section of the pyloric region of the stomach (150×). The majority of the epithelial cells in this section are simple columnar epithelium. Owing to the highly folded surface of the stomach, the cells are sectioned in many planes, which can make it difficult to recognize their true morphology. Two areas where their nature is clearly seen are indicated. The thin layer of smooth muscle near the bottom of the specimen is the muscularis mucosae; in this location, the smooth muscle fibers are shown in longitudinal section and cross-section.

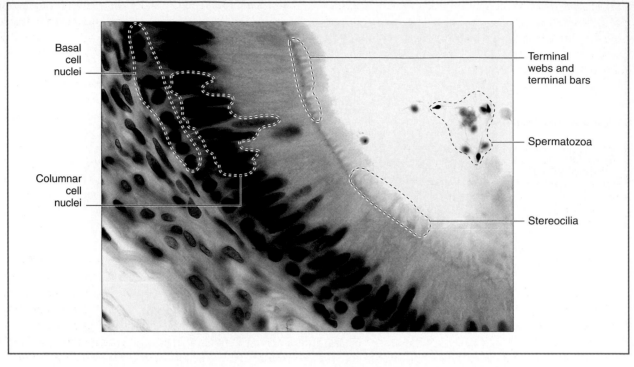

Basal cell nuclei

Columnar cell nuclei

Terminal webs and terminal bars

Spermatozoa

Stereocilia

A

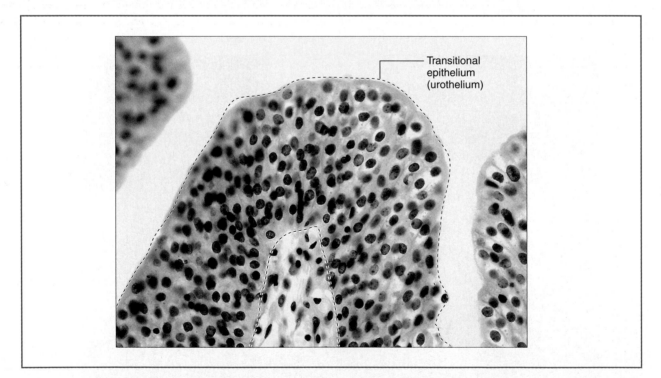

Transitional epithelium (urothelium)

B

Figure 3-6. A, A section of epididymis stained with H&E showing a part of the wall of this long convoluted tube (500×). The locations of basal cell and columnar cell nuclei of this pseudostratified epithelium are indicted. A few spermatozoa are indicated in the lumen. **B,** An H&E stained section of urothelium (310×). In this specimen, the epithelium has the appearance of a thick stratified cuboidal epithelium, but the cells become more flattened when the bladder is distended.

and basal surfaces of the cell have different biochemical, molecular, structural, and functional components and characteristics. Stratified and pseudostratified epithelia also are polarized because the cells at the free surface exhibit significant structural and functional differences compared with the cells at intermediate and basal levels.

Apical Specializations

Many epithelia have one or more apical specializations; these may be distinct structural features, or they may be biochemical or molecular in nature. In every case, the specializations carry out functions specific to the cell or the whole epithelium. The structural specializations are *filopodia*, *microvilli*, *stereocilia*, *cilia*, and *flagella*.

The biochemical specializations are reflected in functions, such as *endocytosis*, *pinocytosis*, and *receptor-mediated endocytosis* (functional features also found in other basic tissue types), or locations such as the substantially thickened inner leaflet and complex membrane plaques seen in the apical plasma membrane of the superficial cells of uro-thelium, or the keratin-filled, membrane cross-linked plasma membranes of the superficial cells of the epidermis. All cells have glycoproteins in or associated with their plasma membranes. Absorptive epithelia such as those found in the gastrointestinal tract, renal nephrons, and parts of the

reproductive tract have a more elaborate set of glycoproteins associated with the apical plasma membrane; this display of glycoproteins is called the *glycocalyx*. Figure 3-7 is an electron micrograph of the glycocalyx and the tips of the microvilli found on the absorptive cells of the intestine; the glycocalyx contains many enzymes that are critical to the absorptive functions of these epithelial cells.

Furthermore, most sensory organs in humans have highly specialized epithelia, intermixed with sensory neuron endings, each having unique apical specializations. These specializations are discussed in more detail in later chapters, but the olfactory epithelium (sense of smell), the retinal pigmented epithelium (visual system), the taste buds (sense of taste), and the cochlear epithelium of the inner ear (sense of hearing) are where these specialized sensory epithelia are located.

Actin-containing Structural Specializations

Three of the five structural specializations involve protrusions of the apical plasma membrane that are supported internally by bundles of actin filaments. *Filopodia* are short ($\leq$0.1 µm), irregularly spaced surface features of many epithelia; they are more or less perpendicular to the membrane surface and are of irregular lengths. *Microvilli* are prominent in the absorptive epithelia of the small intestines and the proximal convoluted tubule of the renal nephron. They are of uniform length (ca. 1–2 µm long, 0.1 µm in diameter) and densely

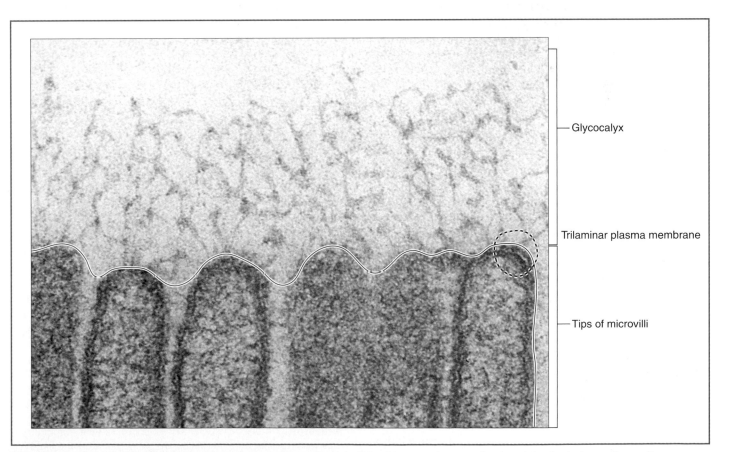

Glycocalyx

Trilaminar plasma membrane

Tips of microvilli

Figure 3-7. The glycocalyx and the tips of microvilli are seen in this electron micrograph of an intestinal absorptive cell. (Courtesy of Don W. Fawcett.)

packed on the apical surface of the cell. In both the light and electron microscope they have the appearance of a brush; thus, this arrangement is called a *brush border*. Within each microvillus, the actin filaments are anchored to the apical tip of the plasma membrane by one of many actin-binding proteins (ABPs)—villin in this case. The actin filaments within the microvillus are cross-linked to each other at regular intervals by two other ABPs (fimbrin and fascin) and to the plasma membrane of the microvillus by yet another ABP. The bundle of actin filaments project from the microvilli down into the apical part of the cytoplasm of the cell, where they are associated with another spectrum of fine filamentous proteins, oriented orthogonally, that include actin filaments, intermediate filaments, and a nonmuscle isoform of myosin. This region, called the *terminal web*, spans the entire apical region of cytoplasm. It is as though the microvilli are held in a felt-like pad that sits atop the apical cell cytoplasm (Fig. 3-8).

The third type of actin filament–containing specialization is the *sterocilia*, which are unusually long apical protrusions of variable length and thickness. Sterocilia is something of a misnomer, since they are unrelated to cilia (see next section) and are a variant of the microvilli class of apical cell membrane specializations. They are found in only a few locations: the epididymis and ductus deferens of the male reproductive tract, and the sensory (hair) cells of the inner ear. In the former case, they are part of an active absorptive epithelium, and in the latter a sensory epithelium. Their actin filament bundles are anchored to the plasma membrane by an ABP (ezrin) and to each other by a different ABP (fimbrin). They are much thicker at their base (or stem) than at their tips, and they may form anastomoses along their length; in the region of the thick stems and anastomoses is yet another ABP (α-actinin; see Fig. 3-6A).

Microtubule-containing Structural Specializations

Many of the columnar epithelial cells that line the upper (conducting) parts of the respiratory system and the uterine tubes (oviducts) of the female reproductive tract have several hundred thin, motile projections of uniform length on their free surface (5–10 μm long, 0.2 μm in diameter). These are *cilia*, apical specializations that contain a distinctive set of microtubules arranged in a circular array such that there are nine pairs of outer doublet microtubules surrounding a central pair of microtubules; the entire structure at the core of the cilium is called the *axoneme*. Each of the outer doublet pairs consists of a 13-protofilament "complete" microtubule, the A tubule, and a 10-protofilament "incomplete" B tubule (Fig. 3-9). At the base of each cilium is a *basal body*, which is a structure similar to a centriole. The basal body has an important role in the growth of the cilium from the cell body and in anchoring it to the cell. Cilia contain a large number of proteins many of which are involved in generating the motile activity and others that are thought to be purely structural. Ciliated epithelial cells beat in a characteristic coordinated pattern called a metachronal wave. The prominent arms on the outer doublet pairs of microtubules consist of a complex of proteins, including one group called ciliary dynein. Ciliary dynein is a motor protein that utilizes ATP to generate motility; it is associated with the A microtubule of each outer doublet pair. In cilia it is responsible for the sliding of an outer doublet pair of microtubules relative to the adjacent pair. Ciliary structure and motility are both complex, yet the basic structure of a cilium, the motile mechanism, and the associated proteins are highly conserved throughout evolution.

In humans, we find one other axoneme-containing motile structure, the *flagellum*. It is the long, thin tail of the male germ cell, the spermatozoon. Structurally, the central part of the flagellum, the axoneme, is similar to the ciliary axoneme, although the flagellum is about 90 μm long and has an additional group of major accessory structures associated with it. The detailed structure of the mature spermatozoan is discussed in Chapter 14.

Sensory neuroepithelial cells in the olfactory, auditory, and visual systems have nonmotile cilia; these cilia have a typical (9 + 2) or modified (9 + 0) axonemal microtubule structure. Certain epithelial cells in liver bile ductules, renal parietal epithelium, and renal collecting tubules have a single, nonmotile cilium. These are called *primary cilia*; they are thought to have chemosensory capabilities. Primary cilia are also found on epithelial and nonepithelial cells grown in tissue culture. Recent studies have shown that primary cilia are found on certain cells in early embryonic development. These cilia are motile and have been shown to play a role in establishing the correct left-right orientation of certain organs in early organogenesis.

Cell Junctions

Junctional Complex

The terminal bar (light microscopy term) or junctional complex (electron microscopy term) consists of a set of membrane specializations at the apical regions of the lateral margins of adjacent cuboidal or columnar epithelial cells (see Fig. 3-8). Examine the lumen of the duct shown in Figure 3-4C; the terminal bars of the apical cells are sectioned to advantage in this specimen. Figure 3-10 shows a diagram of the junctional complex and a high-magnification electron micrograph of a junctional complex (a similar one is seen at lower magnifica-

---

ANATOMY & EMBRYOLOGY

Kartagener's Syndrome

Kartagener's syndrome is an inherited disease that affects embryonic development. In this disorder, cilia and flagella lack dynein arms and are therefore nonmotile. Individuals with this syndrome may have their heart on the right side of the body—a condition called situs inversus. Affected individuals have serious respiratory problems, since the cilia of their respiratory epithelium are nonmotile. Males are sterile because the flagella of their spermatozoa are nonmotile.

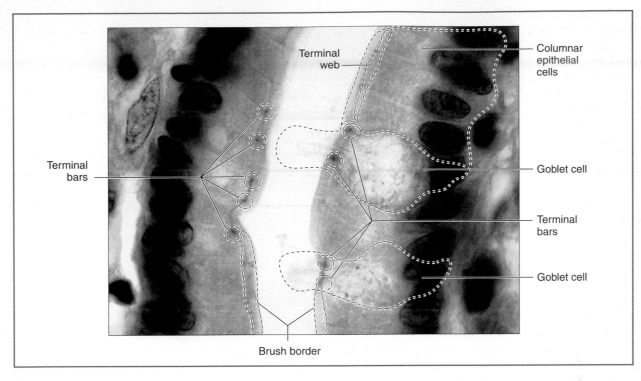

Terminal
web

Columnar
epithelial
cells

Terminal
bars

Goblet cell

Terminal
bars

Goblet cell

Brush border

A

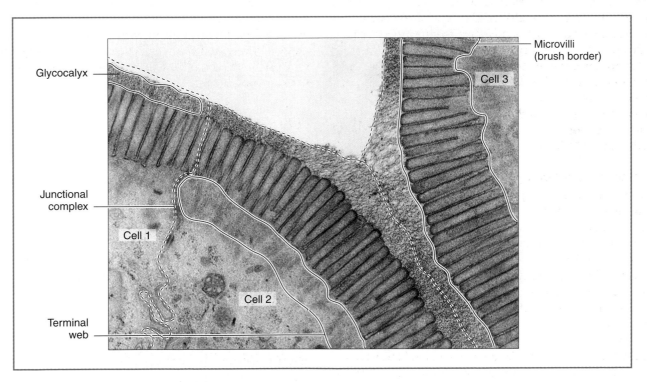

Glycocalyx

Microvilli
(brush border)

Cell 3

Junctional
complex

Cell 1

Cell 2

Terminal
web

B

Figure 3-8. A, Cross-section of a villus from the jejunum stained with Milligan's trichrome stain (1000×). A number of intestinal absorptive cells are seen in this micrograph; there are also two goblet cells (unicellular glands) with some of their mucous secretions in the right-center of the micrograph. The brush border, terminal web, and terminal bars are labeled. **B,** Electron micrograph of the apical portions of three similar cells showing the microvilli (brush border) at the ultrastructural level. The uniform appearance of the microvilli (with their associated glycocalyx) is seen. The terminal web is seen as a slightly more electron dense area just under the microvilli. Two adjacent cells are seen in the lower left. A junctional complex (terminal bar in light microscopy terminology) is indicated at the apical region of the cells. (Courtesy of Don W. Fawcett.)

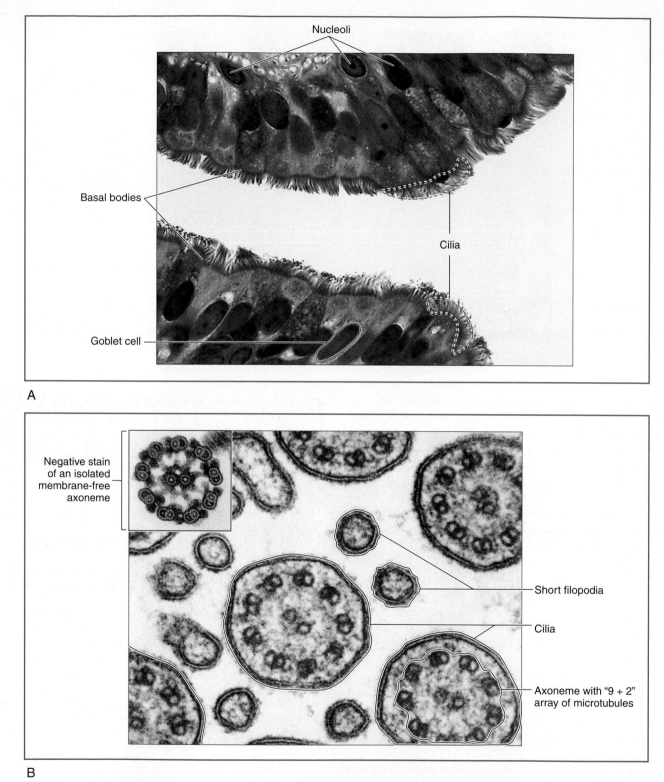

Figure 3-9. A, Section of a plastic-embedded bronchus stained with toluidine blue (900×) showing a pseudostratified ciliated columnar epithelium. The ciliated cells are indicated in the micrograph; a dark line just at the base of the cilia, consisting of basal bodies, is also seen. This row of basal bodies should not be confused with the terminal web seen in Figure 3-8. **B,** Electron micrograph of several cilia cut in cross-section. The organelle is enclosed by the plasma membrane of the cell and contains an array of microtubules, with nine doublet pairs arranged in a circle surrounding a central pair; this array is called an axoneme. The inset is a ciliary outer doublet negatively stained with tannic acid to reveal the individual protofilaments of the microtubules.

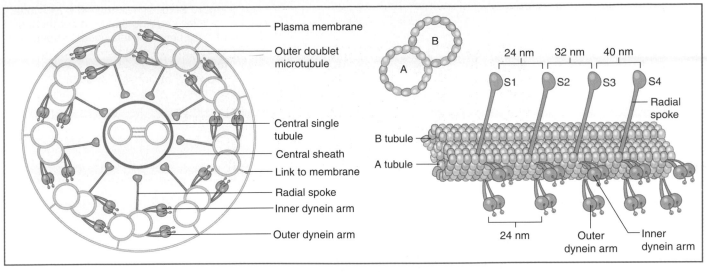

C

Figure 3-9 cont'd. C, Diagram of a cross-sectioned axoneme naming its major structural features. The lower part of this diagram is a three-dimensional representation of a single outer doublet pair of microtubules; note that the α-subunits of the α-β tubulin dimers are a darker red/orange shade than the yellower β-subunits. (Modified from Pollard TD, Earnshaw WC. *Cell Biology*. Philadelphia, WB Saunders, 2004, p. 641.)

tion in Fig. 3-8B). When this region is examined at even higher magnification in the electron microscope, it is shown to consist of three distinct structures: the *occluding junction*, the *adhering* or *intermediate junction*, and the *spot desmosome*. In tissues, the junctions are usually seen in the order named. A number of specific proteins are associated with each of these junctions; some are extracellular, some are membrane proteins, and some are cytoplasmic proteins. The specific proteins are numerous and their interactions are complex and are not discussed in detail here.

The occluding (tight) junction (*zonula occludens*) derives its name from its major function, which is to prevent (occlude) the movement of ions and small molecules from tissue spaces to the external environment and vice versa. Of the three components of a junctional complex, the occluding junction is closest to the apical end of a cuboidal or columnar epithelial cell; it encircles the cell much as a purse string does a purse. Occluding junctions consist of an anastomosing set of membrane proteins that form a series of linear contacts between adjacent cells (Fig. 3-11). Depending on the specific epithelium under study, the number of tiers of anastomosing contacts can vary considerably, as well as the extent to which the contact lines are more or less complete. The physiologic consequence of these variations is that some occluding junctions are very tight (impermeable) or relatively leaky (permeable). The cytoplasmic face of occluding junctions is associated with a small number of short actin filaments.

Because of its structural characteristics and location, the occluding junction also serves to hold adjacent cells to one another and to restrict the movement of molecular components of the plasma membrane from the apical domain to the basolateral domain and vice versa. Hence, the occluding junction plays a key role in maintaining the polarity of

MICROBIOLOGY

Cause of Gastric Ulcers

One of the most common causes of chronic gastritis and gastric ulcers is infection by the bacterium *Helicobacter pylori*. The bacteria disrupt proteins of the tight junction, which can lead to inflammation or ulcers.

- *H. pylori* is a curved, gram-negative rod that does not form spores.
- Many people carry this bacterial infection in their gastric mucosa for decades with no pathology.
- In addition to its causal role in chronic gastritis and gastric ulcers, there is a strong association between infection with *H. pylori* and gastric carcinoma.
- *H. pylori* disrupts the zonula occludens (occluding junction, or tight junction) by associating with the proteins of the junction and compromising their barrier function.
- It is thought that survival of *H. pylori* in the acidic mucous environment of the stomach is aided by the production of ammonia by the bacterial enzyme urease.
- *H. pylori* can be eliminated by treatment with antibiotics and proton pump inhibitors.

epithelial cells and facilitating the transport functions of these cells.

Occluding junctions are also found at the margins of adjacent simple squamous epithelial cells wherever these cells are found, such as mesothelial cells and the endothelial cells that line blood vessels.

The adhering junction is located just basal to the occluding junction (see Figs. 3-10A and 3-10B). It is characterized by a uniform, electron-lucent, 20-nm space between the adjacent

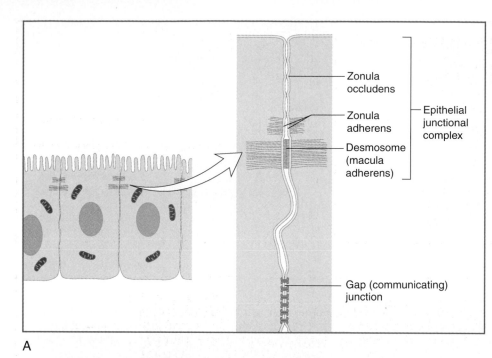

A

Figure 3-10. A, Diagram of a junctional complex showing the three components of the junction as they would appear in an electron micrograph. **B,** Electron micrograph of a junctional complex. (Courtesy of Don W. Fawcett.)

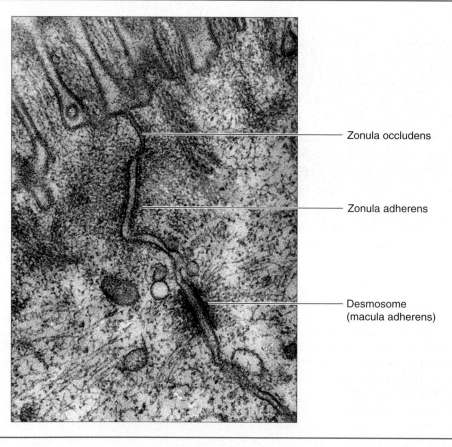

B

cells, a "fuzzy plaque" on the cytoplasmic face, and a band of actin filaments that circles the cell, in a belt-like fashion, very close to the fuzzy plaque. The structure called the terminal bar at the light microscopic level is thought to reflect the presence of the fuzzy plaque and the associated actin

filaments. In certain columnar cells, e.g., intestinal absorptive cells, there is a felt-like network of cytoplasmic actin filaments, cytoplasmic myosin filaments, and a smaller amount of intermediate filaments that span the entire cytoplasm at the level of the adhering junction. The terminal

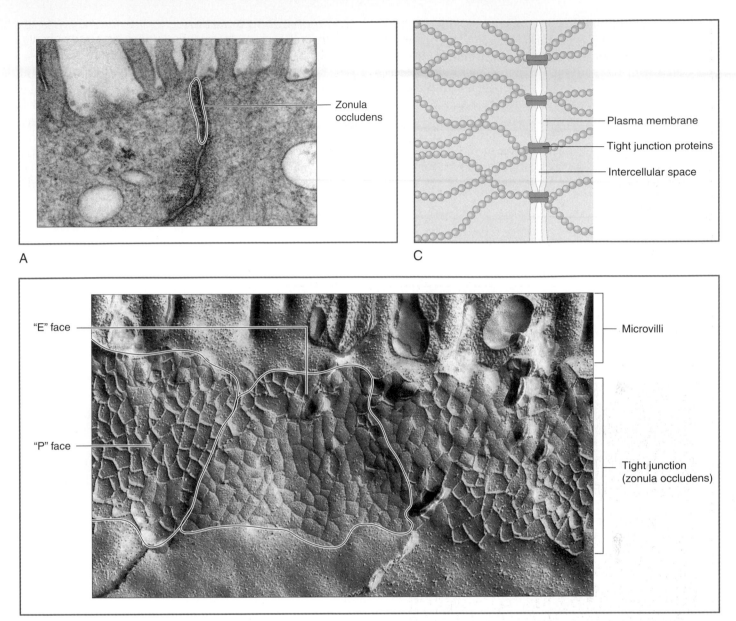

A

C

Zonula
occludens

Plasma membrane

Tight junction proteins

Intercellular space

"E" face

"P" face

Microvilli

Tight junction
(zonula occludens)

B

Figure 3-11. High-magnification electron micrograph of a typical occluding junction (**A**) and the same in a freeze-fracture etching (ffe) preparation (**B**). (**A,** Courtesy of Patricia C. Cross, PhD, Stanford University School of Medicine; **B,** Courtesy of Don W. Fawcett.) The detailed structure of the junction shown in part A is difficult to appreciate in sectioned material, but several membrane-to-membrane contact points can be seen in the labeled zonula occludens. The ffe preparation permits a view of the junction in the plane of the membrane and reveals more detail. The anastomosing network of the membrane proteins that make up the contact lines (points) of the junction are clearly seen. The ffe technique cleaves the trilaminar membrane through its hydrophobic plane. When the specimen is "etched" (ice is sublimed away in a high vacuum), two membrane surfaces may be seen. One is the "P" (protoplasmic) face of the membrane, and the other is the "E" (ectoplasmic) face of the membrane. Both faces are shown. **C,** Diagrammatic representation of this junction.

web seen in many epithelial cells, particularly those with a brush border, probably reflects this network of filaments. The membrane specialization itself encircles the cell like a belt. Its main functions are to contribute to the adhesive force between adjacent cells and to provide support to the apical region of the cell.

The third component of the junctional complex is the desmosome (macula adherens, or adhering spot). This junction serves as a strong anchoring structure. It is disk-shaped when viewed from within the cytoplasm of either of the two cells it holds together. It has an electron-dense cytoplasmic attachment plaque that contains several desmosome-specific proteins; a large number of intermediate filaments loop into and out of the plaque. The extracellular space between the two adjacent cells is filled with a large number of highly ordered proteins that serve to strengthen the adhering forces at the site of the junction. The degree of order of these extracellular proteins generates a distinctive appearance to the entire desmosome (Fig. 3-12). In addition to being associated with the junctional complex, many desmosomes are seen on the lateral surfaces of columnar and cuboidal epithelial cells. Keratinized and nonkeratinized stratified squamous epithelia are particularly rich in these junctions; in fact, the desmosome was first characterized in these two kinds of epithelia. A modified version of the desmosome is seen in cardiac muscle, the fascia adherens. Desmosomes may even be seen in nerve tissue occasionally.

Communicating Junction

One type of cell junction, the communicating junction (gap junction, or nexus) may be found in all four basic tissue types (Fig. 3-13). It is found in nearly all epithelial cells; in smooth and cardiac muscle fibers; in many neuronal cell types; and in osteocytes, the specialized connective tissue cells found in bone. As its name suggests, this junction serves as a communicating channel between adjacent cells. This communication is achieved via a large number of closely (hexagonally) packed transmembrane channels in the plasma membranes of each of two adjacent cells. Each transmembrane channel is called a

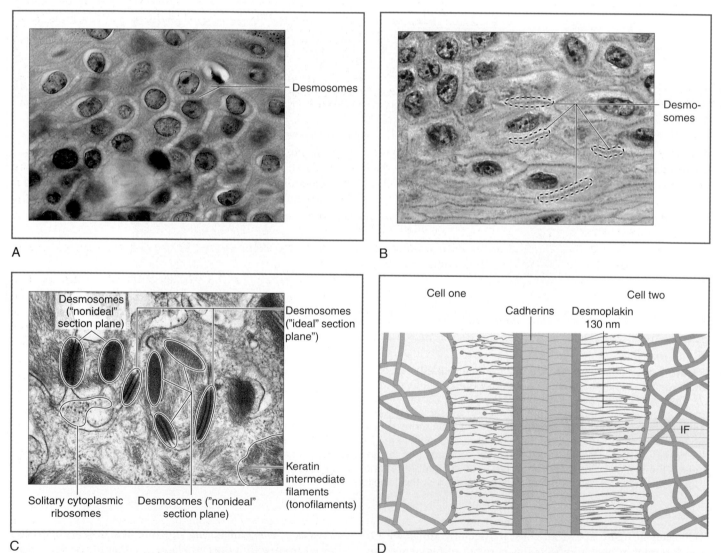

Figure 3-12. A, H&E stain of a layer of the epidermis (stratum spinosum) that is especially rich in desmosomes (1000×). **B,** Semi-thin (1.5 μm) section of nonkeratinized stratified squamous epithelium of the tongue stained with iron hematoxylin (1000×). Groups of desmosomes are seen as short dark bars in a zigzag pattern along the margins of the cells. **C,** Electron micrograph of similar cells from the esophagus. Two of the desmosomes are sectioned perpendicular to the plane of disk-shaped desmosomes; even at this medium-power magnification, many details of the substructure of the desmosome can be seen. (Courtesy of Kathleen Green.) **D,** Diagram of a desmosome with some of the structural components labeled. IF, intermediate filament.

Figure 3-13. Freeze-fracture etch preparation of a plaque of connexons in the plasma membrane of an ovarian granulosa cell. The connexons are randomly packed together into a loose approximation of hexagonal arrays. The inset on the lower right shows negatively stained purified connexons in the open configuration. The dark central dot in each connexon is the water channel through which ions and other small molecules diffuse from cell to cell. The hexagonal packing of the connexons is more evident in the negatively stained micrograph. The inset on the lower left is a diagrammatic representation of a few connexons in the open configuration. (Courtesy of Don W. Fawcett; inset from the work of N. B. Gilula.)

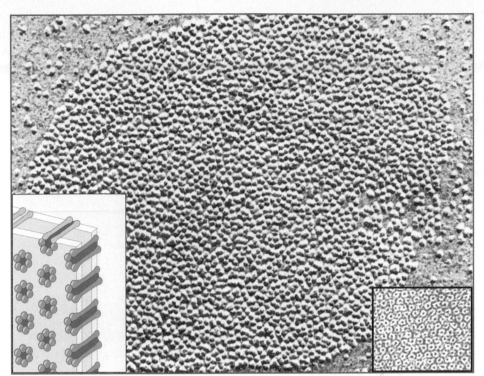

connexon, and the integral membrane proteins that comprise it are *connexins*. The connexons are aligned to allow the movement of ions and small molecules between cells. The largest molecule that can be passed between cells is about 1 kDa, but it is thought that the main function of connexons is to permit the passage of ions and small signaling molecules between cells. The channels can fluctuate rapidly between an open or a closed state owing to reversible conformational changes in the connexins.

Hemidesmosome

Epithelial cells are tightly anchored to their basal lamina and the underlying connective tissue by a junction called the hemidesmosome. Morphologically, the hemidesmosome resembles a half-desmosome, but its molecular constituents are quite different. The morphologic appearance is due to the presence of a cytoplasmic plaque with associated intermediate filaments. However, the plaque is attached to the basal lamina through the involvement of a specific integrin, fibronectin, other proteins, and one of the minor collagen types. There are also specific structures deeper in the connective tissue that stabilize the anchoring of the hemidesmosome to the connective tissue (Fig. 3-14).

●●● EXOCRINE GLANDS

The two major types of glands or glandular tissue throughout the body are exocrine glands—epithelia derived from ectoderm or endoderm—and endocrine glands—epithelia derived from the same two embryonic tissue layers plus neuroectoderm. The simple distinction between these two

types of glands is that the secretions of exocrine glands are carried to a body surface by a duct or system of ducts, whereas the secretions of endocrine glands are delivered directly to the bloodstream via an extensive system of fenestrated capillaries found in these glands. Endocrine glands are discussed in greater detail in Chapter 10.

Exocrine glands may be classified on the basis of several criteria:

- One criterion is the physicochemical nature of the secretion—thin and watery or thick and sticky (mucus). Cells or glands that secrete the former are called *serous cells/glands*, and cells or glands that secrete the latter are called *mucous cells/glands*. This criterion emphasizes *what* the cell is secreting. The simplest gland is a unicellular gland that secretes mucus; it is called a goblet cell because of its resemblance to a wine goblet. Two goblet cells are shown in Figure 3-8A, and others can be seen in Figure 3-9A. Examples of serous, mucous, and mixed exocrine glands are seen in Figures 3-15 to 3-17.
- Another criterion describes *how* the cell actually secretes the products it has synthesized (i.e., secretion mechanisms).
  - In *merocrine* secretion, the secretory product arrives at the cytoplasmic surface of the plasma membrane in a vesicle that fuses with the cell membrane, releasing the secretory products into the extracellular space. The membrane components are recycled back into the cell to participate in another round of secretion. This is the most common form of secretion and is seen in both exocrine and endocrine glands.
  - In *apocrine* secretion, the secretory product arrives at the cytoplasmic surface of the plasma membrane in a

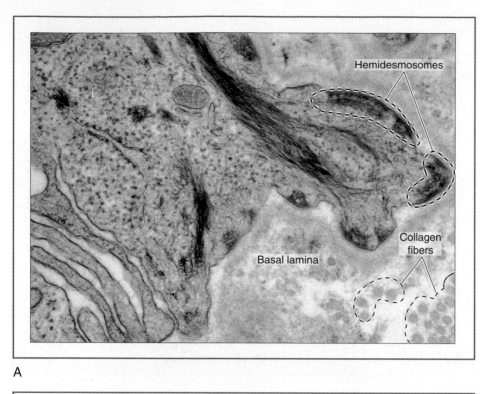

A

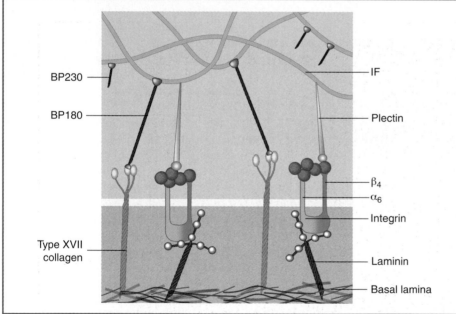

B

Figure 3-14. **A,** Medium-power electron micrograph of several hemidesmosomes as seen in the epidermal-dermal interface. (Courtesy of Jonathan Jones.) **B,** Diagram of a hemidesmosome. It shows looping intermediate filaments inside the cell and the many proteins that interact to anchor the cell to the basal lamina and the underlying connective tissue. BP180 and BP230 are glycoproteins of molecular weight 180 KDa 230 KDa, respectively. The BP indicates that they were identified on the basis of their immunoreactivity to autoantibodies found in the serum of patients with bullous pemphigoid, an autoimmune blistering disease of skin. IF, intermediate filament.

vesicle. The whole vesicle and a thin rim of apical cytoplasm and apical plasma membrane are released into the extracellular space. It is seen in only a few types of exocrine glands (e.g., mammary epithelial cells).

- In *holocrine* secretion, the secretory product is an entire terminally differentiated cell that has undergone apoptosis. This type of secretion is seen in sebaceous glands.
- *Cytocrine* secretion is seen in the glands of the male and female reproductive systems—the testes, which produce spermatozoa, and the ovaries, which produce oocytes. In this case, the secretory "product" is an entire viable cell.
- A third criterion is based on the *structural or architectural organization* of the gland. Some glands are a simple, or coiled, or branched tube; hence, they are called simple tubular, simple coiled tubular, or branched tubular glands. The secretory cells of these two types of glands may be serous, mucous, or both; hence, there are simple coiled tubular serous glands (e.g., sweat glands) or branched, mixed seromucous glands (e.g., minor salivary glands in the tongue).

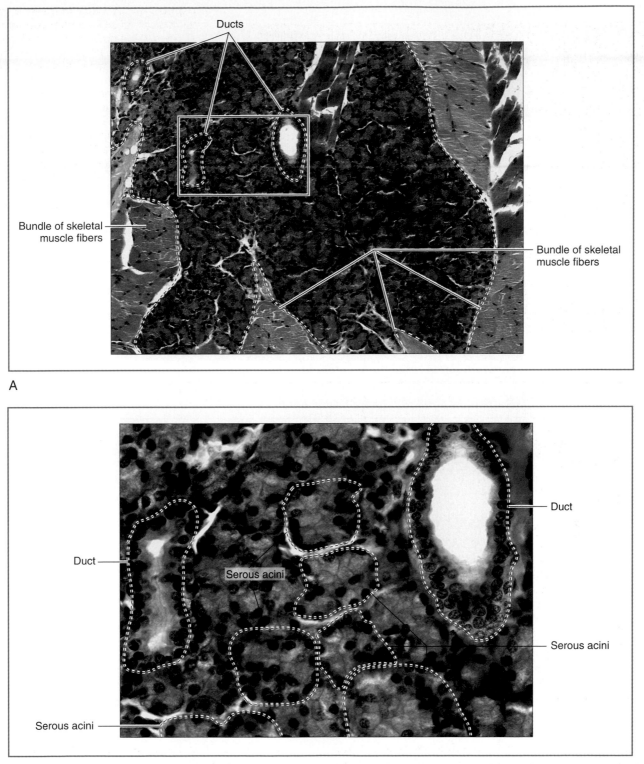

A

B

Figure 3-15. A, H&E stained section of a small serous gland within the body of the tongue (120×). **B,** Higher magnification image (400×) of the same specimen showing two small ducts and several serous acini. Note the spherical nuclei in the basal one-third of the cells and the cuboidal to pyramidal shape of the secretory cells. The cytoplasm of serous cells usually stains a rather uniform dark color with most stains.

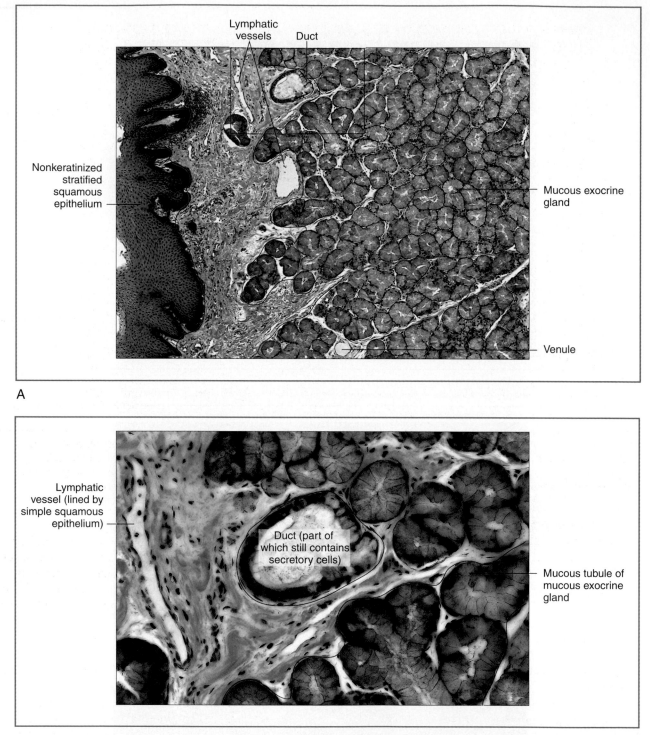

A

B

Figure 3-16. A, H&E stained section of a small mucous gland within the body of the soft palate (60×). **B,** Higher magnification image (120×) of the same specimen showing several mucous tubules and a duct that shows the transition from secretory to duct cells along part of its circumference. Note the flattened nuclei and cytoplasm filled with secretory material. Because of the fixative used for this specimen, the cytoplasm of the secretory cells is well stained instead of its more usual appearance, as seen in the next figure.

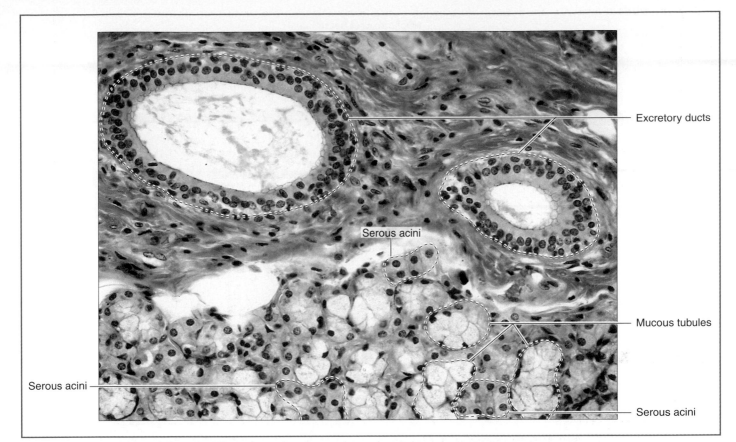

Excretory ducts

Serous acini

Mucous tubules

Serous acini

Serous acini

Figure 3-17. Submandibular gland (Mallory-Azan stain, 200×). This gland contains a mixture of serous acinar and mucous tubular cells. The more typical darker-staining serous and lighter-staining mucous cells are seen. Note the characteristic morphology and location of the nucleus in each type of secretory cell. The upper part of the figure shows two large ducts (surrounded by connective tissue) lined by stratified cuboidal to columnar cells.

- A further structural criterion recognizes the *shapes of the terminal secretory units* plus the branching pattern of the whole gland. The terminal secretory units may be tubular, acinar (shaped like a small grape cluster), or alveolar (flask shaped).
- Yet another criterion addresses *where the secretion goes* or *what it does* once it leaves the cell.
  - When cells secrete by the *exocrine mechanism*, their secretory product is delivered to an external or internal body surface.
  - Cells that secrete by the *endocrine mechanism* release their secretory product directly into the bloodstream.
  - In the case of *paracrine* secretion, the secretory product of a single cell affects the function or behavior of a small group of neighboring cells. The secretory product is secreted into the paracellular space (i.e., the small volume of tissue fluid that surrounds all cells).
  - In *autocrine* secretion, the product of the secretory cell affects its own function. As in the case of paracrine secretion, the secretory product is secreted into the paracellular space.

Figure 3-18 illustrates the secretion mechanisms and cellular arrangements of exocrine glands by means of several diagrams. Note that the mechanisms and organization of the glands are presented but no specific examples are given regarding where these types of glands are found, although examples follow later in this book.

The structure of exocrine glands ranges from the unicellular goblet cell to more complex exocrine glands such as the submandibular gland (a compound, branched, tubuloacinar, seromucous exocrine gland), and even glands that produce secretions by both exocrine and endocrine mechanisms, such as the pancreas (a compound acinar exocrine gland with clusters [islets] of endocrine cells) and the liver (a branched lobar/lobular gland in which the parenchymal cells [hepatocytes] secrete an exocrine product—bile—into a system of ducts and endocrine products [e.g., serum proteins] into the bloodstream).

The ability to understand the type and organization of an exocrine gland takes practice and relies on the ability to recognize and recall the characteristics of exocrine cells and the principles and details of their organization.

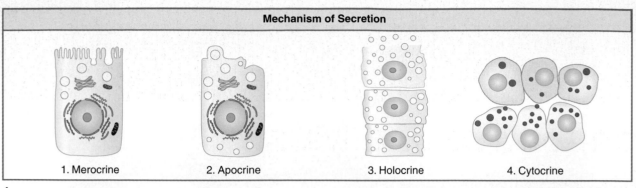

Mechanism of Secretion

1. Merocrine   2. Apocrine   3. Holocrine   4. Cytocrine

A

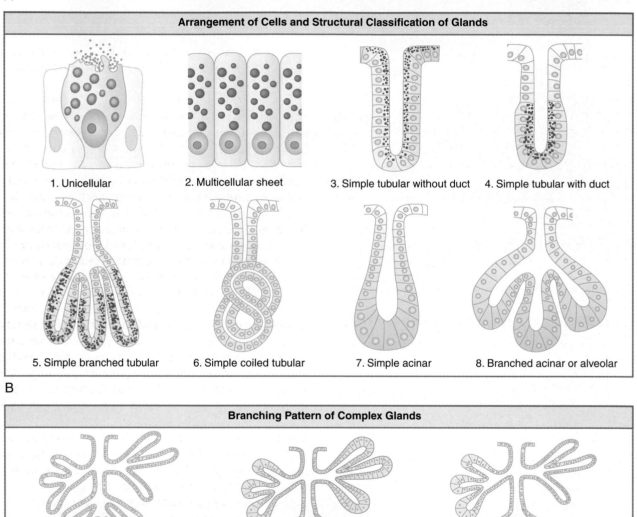

Arrangement of Cells and Structural Classification of Glands

1. Unicellular   2. Multicellular sheet   3. Simple tubular without duct   4. Simple tubular with duct

5. Simple branched tubular   6. Simple coiled tubular   7. Simple acinar   8. Branched acinar or alveolar

B

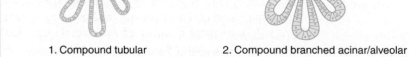

Branching Pattern of Complex Glands

1. Compound tubular   2. Compound branched acinar/alveolar   3. Compound branched tubulo-acinar

C

Figure 3-18. A, The four secretion mechanisms. **A1,** Merocrine secretion: the contents of secretory vesicles are released into the extracellular space after fusion of the vesicular membrane with the plasma membrane. **A2,** Apocrine secretion: the entire secretory vesicle and a small rim of apical cytoplasm, and its plasma membrane, are released into the extracellular space. **A3,** Holocrine secretion: an entire cell and its remaining contents after undergoing programmed cell death are secreted into the extracellular space. **A4,** Cytocrine secretion: an entire viable cell is secreted into the extracellular space after a period of differentiation or maturation. **B,** A set of idealized diagrams of the different architectural patterns of exocrine glands from a unicellular gland to a branched acinar gland. **C,** Three major variations of the patterns shown in part B that reflect the organization of many of the larger glands in the body. In these cases, the secretory parts are branched in complex ways and entire secretory units may contain serous and mucous secretory cells.

Connective and Muscle Tissues

4

CONNECTIVE TISSUE

●●● CHARACTERISTICS AND CLASSIFICATION OF CONNECTIVE TISSUE

General Characteristics of Connective Tissue

Embryonic connective tissue, connective tissue proper, and one of the specialized connective tissues, adipose tissue, are discussed in the first part of this chapter. Subsequent chapters deal with the specialized connective tissues cartilage and bone (Chapter 5), blood (Chapter 7), and the lymphoid tissue (Chapter 8).

In the broadest sense, connective tissue proper does just what its name says—it connects and holds the structures of the body to one another. Connective tissues are classified into a number of different types based on their appearance, texture, matrix composition, matrix organization, and "density," in addition to the specific cells or the spectrum of cells found in a given kind of connective tissue. In many connective tissue locations, different types of connective tissue blend imperceptibly into one another; in other locations, the tissue is of a consistent, distinct, and easily recognized type.

It is worth noting that the prototypical cell of connective tissue proper is the fibroblast. This cell synthesizes and secretes all the matrix components of the tissue in which it is found. Connective tissue matrices have characteristic metabolic turnover rates (half-lives) that differ significantly from one specific kind of tissue to another and from one matrix component to another. It is important to realize that connective tissue matrix components are degraded and replaced throughout life. The metabolic turnover is the result of a delicate interplay between extracellular proteases and protease inhibitors. The fibroblast plays a central role in this process although some other cells in the tissue (or adjacent to it; e.g., epithelial tissue) also participate in degradation of matrix components. However, replacement of matrix components is the sole task of the fibroblast.

Connective tissues differ from the other basic tissue types in several important ways. The first and most striking difference is that compared with the other basic tissue types, connective tissues are relatively cell-poor and matrix-rich. The matrix contains an array of fibers (collagen, elastin, and reticular) and an amorphous ground substance (proteoglycan aggregates and glycoproteins) whose composition varies widely from one specific type of connective tissue to another.

A second important difference is that the cell types found in certain of the most common connective tissues are quite diverse although in certain types of connective tissue only a single connective tissue cell (fibroblast, chondrocyte, osteocyte) is found.

Thirdly, since connective tissues do not produce a basal

Protein Degradation and Biological Half-Life

Intracellular and extracellular proteins are subject to degradation by specific pathways at several time points following their synthesis. If protein degradation were not a carefully regulated process, cells—and the whole organism—would suffer disastrous consequences. Some of the degradation pathways deal with errors in biosynthesis and others with the normal turnover of proteins. A useful concept in considering protein turnover is biological half-life ($t_{1/2}$). It is a measure of the amount of time it takes for half of a newly synthesized protein to be degraded.

One of two major pathways of intracellular protein degradation is dependent on lysosomes. Proteins degraded by this mechanism are typically those with longer $t_{1/2}$—days to weeks. The second major pathway of protein degradation is the proteosome, a cylindrical structure found in the nucleoplasm and cytoplasm that is composed of multiple protein subunits. Proteins typically degraded in the proteosome are abnormal owing to translational or posttranslational errors or have experienced folding errors; in fact, as many as 20% to 30% of newly synthesized proteins are degraded by cellular quality-control mechanisms. In addition, proteins with a short $t_{1/2}$ (minutes to a few hours) are degraded in proteosomes. Many defective intracellular proteins are marked for degradation by the covalent attachment of a distinctive small protein, ubiquitin (mol. wt. ca. 8 kDa). Extracellular proteins, collagen, elastin, and other structural components of the extracellular matrix are degraded by a carefully coordinated series of proteolytic enzymes that are synthesized by most connective tissue and epithelial cells. Although the $t_{1/2}$ of proteins (and glycosaminoglycans) of the extracellular matrix is on the order of weeks to many months, these macromolecules are degraded and replaced on a regular basis by the cells that normally synthesize them.

lamina (with the exception of adipose cells), the cells and the soluble components of connective tissue can, in principle, travel to all connective tissue compartments of the body without having to cross a basal lamina; hence, the connective tissue compartment of the body can be thought of as an organism-wide thoroughfare. Furthermore, it is the compartment through which the larger blood vessels, nerves, and lymphatic vessels travel.

Cells of Connective Tissue

Many different cell types are found in adult connective tissue. They can be classified into two sets each with two categories of cells. One set considers an important aspect of cell behavior—cell motility. Certain connective tissue cells are, or can be, motile, and others are not. The second set refers to the permanent or transient presence of connective tissue cells in a given kind of adult connective tissue. Some connective tissue cells are full-time residents of a tissue, and others are visitors (i.e., they migrate into the tissue from the vascular system in response to tissue injury, infection, or other stimuli). Table 4-1 presents a list of connective tissue cells in each of these sets and categories.

Embryonic Connective Tissues

Most connective tissues develop from the middle embryonic tissue layer, the mesoderm. Two different kinds of embryonic connective tissue, mesenchymal connective tissue and mucous connective tissue, are described in the following sections.

Mesenchymal Connective Tissue

As mesoderm develops and differentiates, there are large volumes of mesenchymal connective tissue, the embryologic precursor of most adult connective tissues. The connective

Biological Aging

Normal biological aging is a reflection of many changes at the molecular, subcellular, cellular, extracellular matrix, and organ levels. Proteins and nucleic acids may be subject to damage by free radicals. Over time, the number of stem cells in different populations declines or their proliferative capacity is diminished, resulting in a slower or absent ability to renew the tissues or organs they normally maintain. Mutations may accumulate in nuclear and mitochondrial DNA, leading to the biosynthesis of defective gene products or to the lack of their synthesis altogether. This can lead to defective metabolic or biosynthetic pathways or to significant rate reductions in these pathways. The components of the extracellular matrix of skin are maintained by a delicate balance of synthesis and degradation. Imbalances in these events, usually due to a reduced rate of biosynthesis, lead to a gradual deterioration in the integrity of the matrix and the appearance of the skin.

TABLE 4-1. Cells of Connective Tissue Proper	
Cells	**Tissues**
Motile Cells	*Permanent Residents of Connective Tissue*
Mesenchymal cells, fibroblasts, monocytes, macrophages, polymorphonuclear leukocytes, eosinophilic leukocytes, lymphocytes, basophilic leukocytes, mast cells	Fibroblasts, mesenchymal cells (pericytes and other connective tissue "stem" cells), adipose cells, plasma cells, macrophages, mast cells
Nonmotile Cells	*Visitors to Connective Tissue*
Adipose cells, plasma cells	Monocytes, polymorphonuclear leukocytes, eosinophilic leukocytes, basophilic leukocytes, lymphocytes

tissues found in the head also develop from mesenchyme, but most of this tissue is derived from embryonic neuroectoderm rather than mesoderm. Mesodermal and neuroectodermal mesenchyme are indistinguishable in morphologic terms although they have some molecular and biochemical differences. Mesenchymal cells exhibit many different shapes and have a high nuclear to cytoplasmic ratio. Their large nuclei are nearly completely euchromatic and have one or two prominent nucleoli; these morphologic features indicate that they are transcriptionally and translationally active. The mesenchymal cells are separated from one another by large amounts of a delicate, highly hydrated matrix with a scant fibrous appearance. It is not uncommon to find mesenchymal cells that are in contact with each other via thin cytoplasmic processes. Gap junctions may be seen in these regions of contact, suggesting that the cells are in electrical and other kinds of signaling communication with each other. Mesenchyme is found in many locations throughout fetal development.

Mucous Connective Tissue

Mucous connective tissue is found in several locations in the embryo but is most abundant in the umbilical cord and just deep to the epidermis. The mesenchymal cells in mucous connective tissue are sparse and stellate in shape; the connective tissue matrix has a thick, gel-like consistency owing to its rich content of a high-molecular-weight glycosaminoglycan called hyaluronic acid (see discussion on pp 93–94 and Fig. 4-9). There are few fibers in mucous connective tissue (Fig. 4-1); those present are delicate and best visualized in the electron microscope.

Connective Tissue Proper

Loose Connective Tissue

Loose connective tissue is distributed widely in the body; in particular, it is found beneath those epithelia that cover or line the body. Its overall organization is that of a three-dimensional meshwork. It encompasses a range of tissue appearances, textures, and cellular and matrix composition. Not only is it more cellular than most other kinds of connective tissue, but the cells found in loose connective tissue are more diverse than those found in other kinds of connective tissue. Figure 4-2 illustrates six different kinds of connective tissue all of which are called loose, or areolar, connective tissue. General characteristics of loose connective tissue are the following: (1) many cell types may be seen in a

---

ANATOMY & EMBRYOLOGY

Embryologic Origin of Connective Tissue

The connective tissues primarily develop from mesoderm, but some develop from ectoderm. The mesenchyme in most of the body originates from mesoderm. Much of the mesenchyme in the cranium originates from ectoderm. In the adult, there is no histologic difference in the connective tissues that develop from either of these two different embryologic origins.

---

given volume of loose connective tissue; (2) the fibrous component of the matrix contains relatively few fibers compared with the dense connective tissues, and those present are thin and delicate; (3) it has a relatively higher content of ground substance; (4) individual or small clusters of adipose cells are found in some varieties of loose connective tissue; and (5) it contains many arterioles, capillaries, and venules as well as nerve fibers and lymphatics.

It is not surprising that a tissue with these characteristics is the locus of many biochemical and physiologic activities. Because of its vascularity, especially its rich content of capillaries, it is the site where O_2 and other nutrients are delivered to other tissues and where CO_2 and metabolic waste materials are returned to the vasculature to be carried to organs that are responsible for their ultimate removal from the body. It is also a major site of inflammatory and immune reactions owing to its proximity to covering or lining epithelia.

Dense Irregular Connective Tissue

Dense irregular connective tissue is a kind of connective tissue essentially made entirely of fibers. The fibers exhibit a wide range of length, orientation, composition, and diameter, hence the name. The fibers commonly appear to be branched and wavy. A small amount of ground substance is associated with dense irregular connective tissue. This tissue is found as a distinct layer, the submucosa, in the walls of hollow organs. It also makes up the deep layer of the dermis of the skin as well as surrounds the nests of epithelial cells in the mammary gland. It is found in numerous other locations. The predominant cell found in dense irregular connective tissue is the fibroblast. Capillaries, larger blood vessels, and nerves often pass through regions of dense irregular connective tissue. Collagen comprises the majority of the fibrous mass of the submucosal and mammary gland dense irregular connective tissue, but the dermis contains a substantial content of elastin fibers in addition to the collagen fibers. The capsules and trabeculae of solid organs display the characteristics of dense irregular connective tissue; the larger solid organs of the body have significant amounts of elastin fibers intermingled with the collagen fibers (Fig. 4-3).

Dense Regular Connective Tissue

The fibers in dense regular connective tissue tend to have a uniform length and a large and uniform diameter, are packed in tight parallel arrays, and are notably unbranched. This arrangement of fibers provides a strong "connector" and is found in tendons, the structures that hold muscles to bone; aponeuroses, which hold muscle to each other; and ligaments, which hold bones to each other. Tendons are surrounded by a thin, cellular connective tissue sheath, the *epitendineum*, in which the collagen fibers are not so thick, dense, or ordered as the body of the tendon itself. Extensions of the epitendineum into the body of the tendon divide it into fascicles. The only cell found in dense regular connective tissue is the fibroblast; all that can be seen of this cell in the light microscope is its nucleus, which is tightly squeezed between

Text continued on page 84

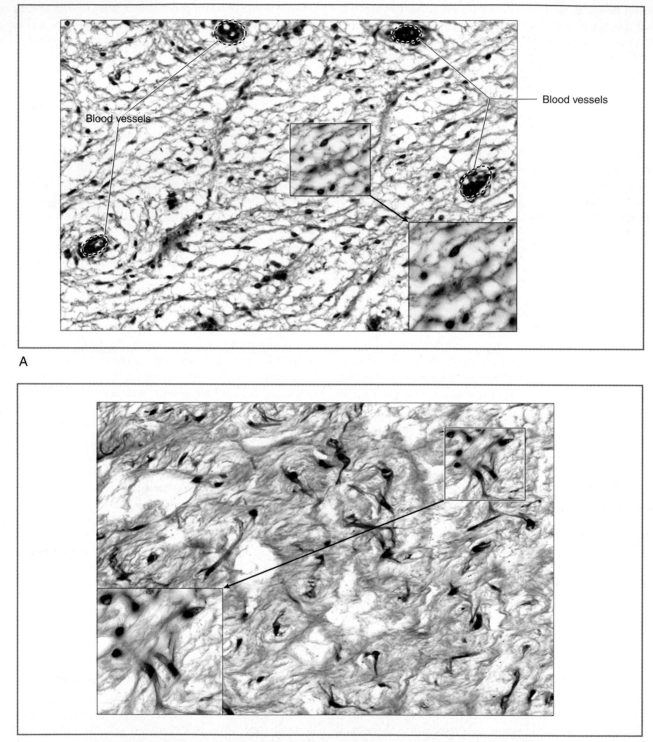

A

B

Figure 4-1. A, Light micrograph of mesenchyme near the spinal cord of a developing pig fetus stained with H&E (200×). Note the delicate fibers, large areas of unstained material (ground substance), and numerous cells with two or three long cytoplasmic extensions. Four growing blood vessels are circled. The inset at right is at a higher magnification (950×). **B,** A trichrome stain of a full-term umbilical cord (160×). The morphology of the mesenchymal cells is similar to that in the adjacent panel, but the extensive matrix shows little evidence of fibers and there are fewer cells in the field of view. The inset at left is at a higher magnification (1000×).

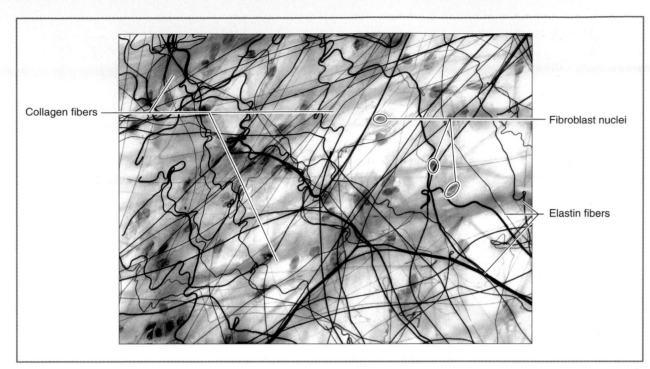

Collagen fibers

Fibroblast nuclei

Elastin fibers

A

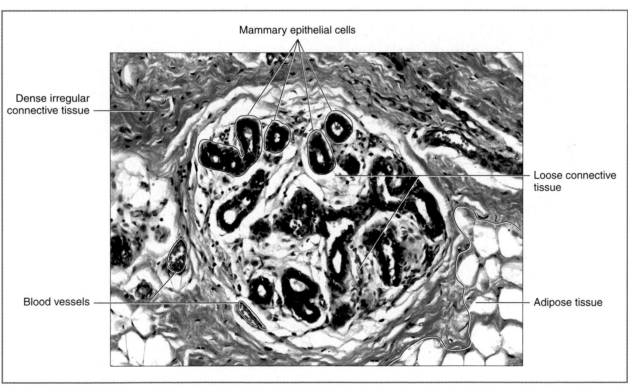

Mammary epithelial cells

Dense irregular connective tissue

Loose connective tissue

Blood vessels

Adipose tissue

B

Figure 4-2. Six different kinds of loose connective tissue. **A,** A spread, whole-mount preparation of loose (areolar) connective tissue (H&E plus an elastin stain, 200×). The most prominent features are the many black, thin, branched elastin fibers; some are straight; others, which have been cut, are wavy. The collagen fibers are the thick pink (eosinophilic) cables that appear to be in the background. There are many nuclei in this field of view; most are fibroblasts, some may be macrophages, but it is difficult to identify any of the cells with certainty. **B,** A section of inactive mammary gland (H&E, 125×). The dark-staining nuclei of the inactive mammary epithelial cells are seen clustered as acini and ducts. The epithelial cells are surrounded by a very sparse, somewhat cellular (mostly fibroblasts) bed of loose connective tissue. Also in the field of view are several blood vessels, areas of adipose cell-rich loose connective tissue, and some regions of dense irregular connective tissue.

Continued

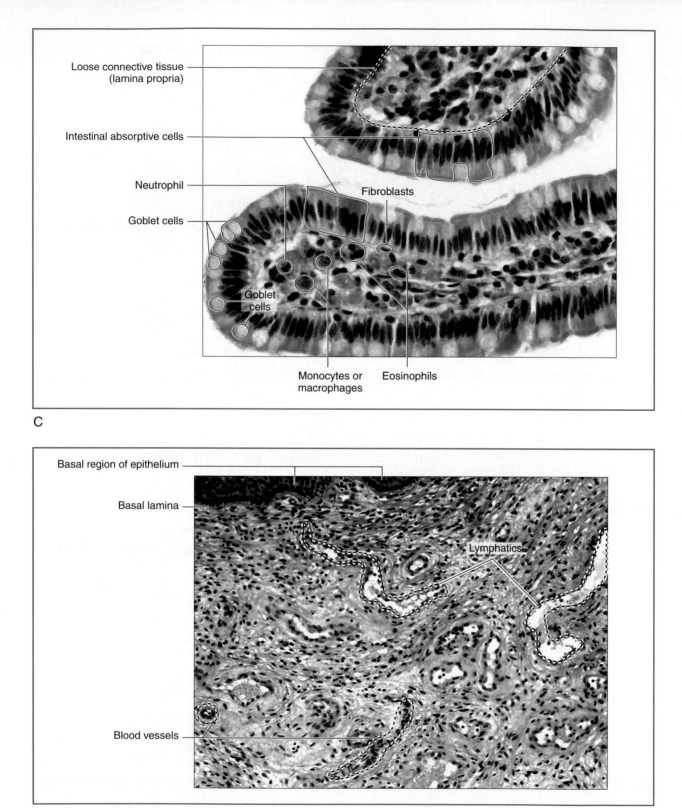

C

Loose connective tissue (lamina propria)

Intestinal absorptive cells

Neutrophil

Goblet cells

Fibroblasts

Goblet cells

Monocytes or macrophages

Eosinophils

D

Basal region of epithelium

Basal lamina

Lymphatics

Blood vessels

Figure 4-2 cont'd. C, A section of the tips of two intestinal villi from the jejunum (H&E, 320×). The epithelium is simple columnar and is made up of intestinal absorptive cells and mucus-secreting goblet cells. The central part of each villus is filled with loose connective tissue; in this location, the term lamina propria is given to this connective tissue in accordance with the nomenclature used for hollow organs. It is difficult to identify most of the individual cells, but several can be identified—eosinophils, fibroblasts, a neutrophil, and several large cells that could be macrophages. The lamina propria also has blood and lymphatic capillaries and several isolated smooth muscle cells that are extensions of another structural feature of hollow organs—the muscularis mucosae. **D,** A section of vagina just below the epithelium (H&E, 100×). The connective tissue here is highly cellular (mostly fibroblasts) and filled with many small-diameter collagen fibers. Many lymphatic vessels and a few blood vessels are interspersed throughout the connective tissue.

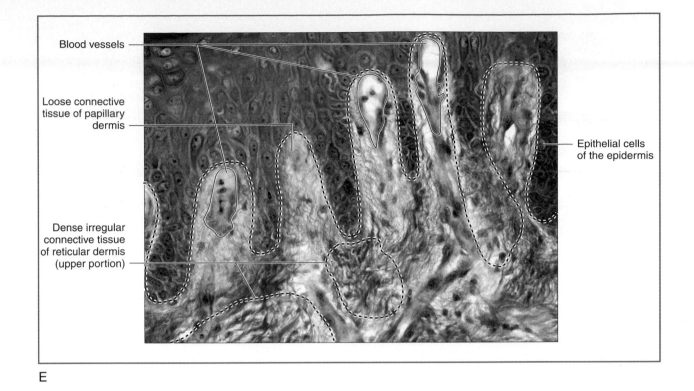

Blood vessels

Loose connective tissue of papillary dermis

Dense irregular connective tissue of reticular dermis (upper portion)

Epithelial cells of the epidermis

E

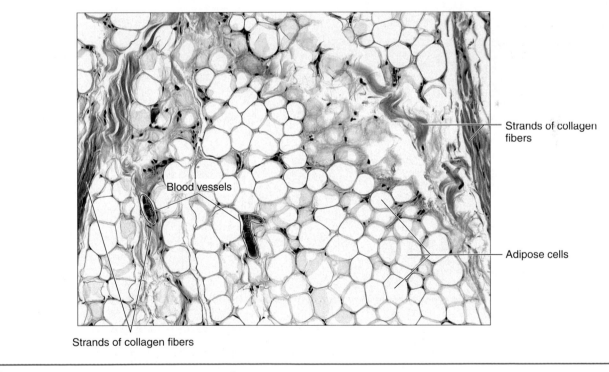

Strands of collagen fibers

Blood vessels

Adipose cells

Strands of collagen fibers

F

Figure 4-2 cont'd. E, A section of skin showing the region just below the epidermis (H&E, 250×). The loose connective tissue that is just under the epidermis is called the papillary dermis. It is filled with delicate fibers, blood vessels, and often the nerve fibers that innervate the epidermis. The lower part of the field in this image shows some of the collagen fibers that are part of the dense regular connective tissue of the reticular dermis that lies under the papillary dermis. **F,** A section of the hypodermis, the fatty, loose connective tissue that is the deepest layer of skin (H&E, 75×). In gross anatomy terminology, this layer is the superficial fascia. This type of loose connective tissue is mostly made up of adipose cells and is supported by widely spaced strands of collagen fibers.

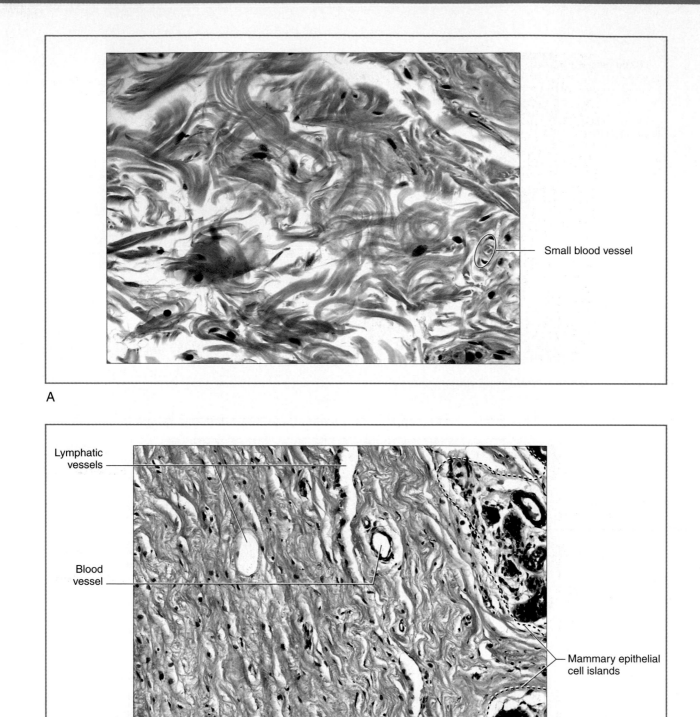

A

Lymphatic
vessels

Small blood vessel

Blood
vessel

Mammary epithelial
cell islands

B

Figure 4-3. Examples of dense irregular connective tissue. **A,** A section of the submucosa of the intestine (H&E, 250×). The dense irregular arrangement of the collagen fibers is evident; note the significant space between the fibers. **B,** A different field of view (H&E, 125×) of the same section of inactive mammary gland seen in Figure 4-2B. The irregularly arranged collagen fibers are closely packed and have many more fibroblasts per unit area than the example in Figure 4-3A. On the right side of the field are a few groups of mammary epithelial cells surrounded by loose connective tissue.

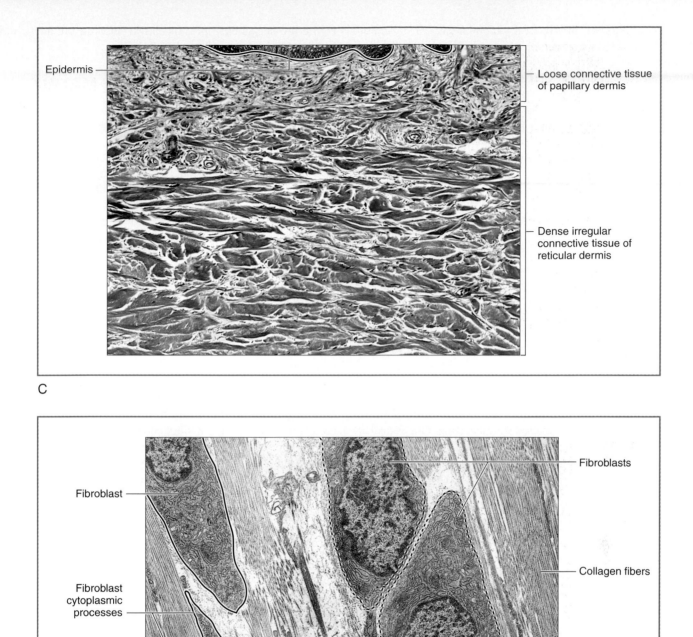

Epidermis

Loose connective tissue
of papillary dermis

Dense irregular
connective tissue of
reticular dermis

C

Fibroblasts

Fibroblast

Collagen fibers

Fibroblast
cytoplasmic
processes

D

Figure 4-3 cont'd. C, Low-magnification image of skin (Mallory's trichrome stain, 80×). A bit of the epidermis is seen in the upper part of the field with a band of loose connective tissue of the papillary dermis just under it. The lower 70% or so of the field is filled with the dense irregular connective tissue of the reticular dermis. At this magnification, very few fibroblasts can be seen. **D,** Electron micrograph of dense irregular connective tissue. Parts of four fibroblasts are seen in this micrograph. The nuclei of all four have large amounts of euchromatin; the cell nucleus in the lower right center has a prominent nucleolus. The cytoplasm of all four cells (and the cytoplasmic processes below them) is nearly completely filled with rER and other organelles; note that many of the rER cisternae are dilated. All these cellular features are indicative of a high rate of protein (mostly collagen) synthesis and secretion. The extracellular space is filled with many bundles of collagen fibers the cross-banded structure of which can be seen. (Courtesy of Jeffrey B. Kerr.)

the thick fibers of the tendon, aponeurosis, or ligament (Fig. 4-4). Electron micrographs of a tendon reveal that the fibroblast has a full complement of cytoplasmic organelles. There are occasional small blood vessels or capillaries in tendons.

Dense regular connective tissue is also found in the cornea of the eye, an avascular tissue. It consists of layers of bundles of collagen fibers of a uniform diameter. The bundles of collagen fibers in each adjacent layer are deposited at an approximately 90-degree angle to each other by the corneal fibroblasts (see Fig. 4-4B). This highly organized *orthogonal arrangement* is thought to be responsible for the transparency of the cornea. This organization of collagen fibers is called an *aponeurosis* although the term is used more commonly to describe broad, flat tendons. It is noteworthy that the collagen fiber diameter and the fiber-to-fiber spacing in the corneas in all five orders of vertebrates (fish, amphibians, reptiles, birds, and mammals) are the same.

Reticular Connective Tissue

The supporting framework *(stroma)* of several organs—lymph nodes, spleen, adrenal gland, and liver—are seen to consist of a network *(reticulum)* of delicate collagen fibers especially when stained with certain stains (periodic acid–Schiff [PAS] or silver-containing stains). Both of these stains react with sugar aldehydes, suggesting that reticular fibers contain a relatively high content of carbohydrate moieties. It is known that the specific type of collagen (type III) in reticular fibers is relatively highly glycosylated and that the fibers have a number of glycoproteins associated with them, making them even more reactive to these stains. Reticular fibers are synthesized by fibroblasts ("reticular cells" according to some authors), which are more intimately associated with the delicate fibrous reticulum than is usually the case in other types of connective tissue. Examples of reticular fibers from a lymph node and fetal adrenal gland are visible in Figure 4-5.

Elastic Connective Tissue

Some authors describe elastic connective tissue as a distinct kind of tissue. This may lead to some confusion, since there are several places where an abundance of elastin fibers is found as part of a tissue or organ region and where a different tissue designation than elastic connective tissue is used. For example, the muscular layer of the largest blood vessels (tunica media) contains abundant elastin fibers even though the cells that synthesize them and which are embedded in them are smooth muscle cells. The reticular layer of the dermis of the skin contains a large number of coarse and fine elastin fibers, yet this layer of skin is more properly called dense irregular connective tissue. And finally, certain ligaments of the spinal cord (the ligamenta flava) contain many elastin fibers, which leads to their being called elastic ligaments. However, as a specific connective tissue type, these ligaments are examples of dense regular connective tissue. Nonetheless, they are connective tissue types that have a higher content of elastin fibers than other connective tissues.

Figure 4-6 shows examples of elastin fibers in the aorta and in the reticular layer of the dermis.

●●● CONNECTIVE TISSUE MATRIX COMPOSITION

Fibrous Components

Collagen

Collagens are abundant, widely distributed, diverse, and centrally important to the development, structure, and function of humans.

Collagen is the most abundant connective tissue protein. The collagen fibers seen in tissue sections are long with no discernable ends. In some locations, they have thin diameters and in others thick. They may form thick, straight bundles, or be wavy in appearance; they assume many morphologies and sometimes appear to branch. Many types of collagen have been described. The first one characterized, and the most abundant by far, is *type I collagen.*

Collagen fibers in any of the specific tissues described above are flexible; however, they have high tensile strength; i.e., they cannot be stretched without breaking. These properties contribute significantly to the physiologic function of collagen-rich structures such as tendons, with respect to muscle movement; skin, a tough, nontearable, flexible covering for the body; and in the submucosa of hollow organs, a collagen fiber–rich layer of the intestine.

The collagen fibers seen in tissue sections at the light microscope or electron microscope level are huge multimeric assemblies of subunits called *tropocollagen.* An understanding of the structure of collagen fibers best begins with a description of these subunits.

Tropocollagen is a trimeric protein synthesized and assembled intracellularly from three α-chains. These three α-chains wind around each other to form a triple helical protein that is stabilized by hydrogen bonds; its conformation is that of a coiled-coil. The trimer is called tropocollagen and has a molecular weight of about 3×10^5 Daltons (Da). It is a long, thin asymmetric molecule, 1.5 nm wide $\times$ 300 nm long. Visible collagen fibers are built from these long, thin, fibrous tropocollagen molecules.

The α-chains have some unusual and distinctive characteristics. The initial translated polypeptide has a signal peptide that is cleaved as the chain enters the lumen of the endoplasmic reticulum. The intracellular form of each α-chain has a molecular weight over 140,000 Da, but in the final tropocollagen molecule it has a molecular weight of about 100,000 Da. Glycine (the smallest of the amino acids) comprises approximately 33% of all its amino acids and proline plus hydroxyproline another 30%. Furthermore, glycine occurs in every third position of each α-chain and is usually followed in sequence by proline or hydroxyproline. Collagen contains another hydoxylated amino acid, hydroxylysine. These two hydroxylated amino acids are found in small amounts in only a few other noncollagenous proteins. A generalized sequence of collagen α-chains can be

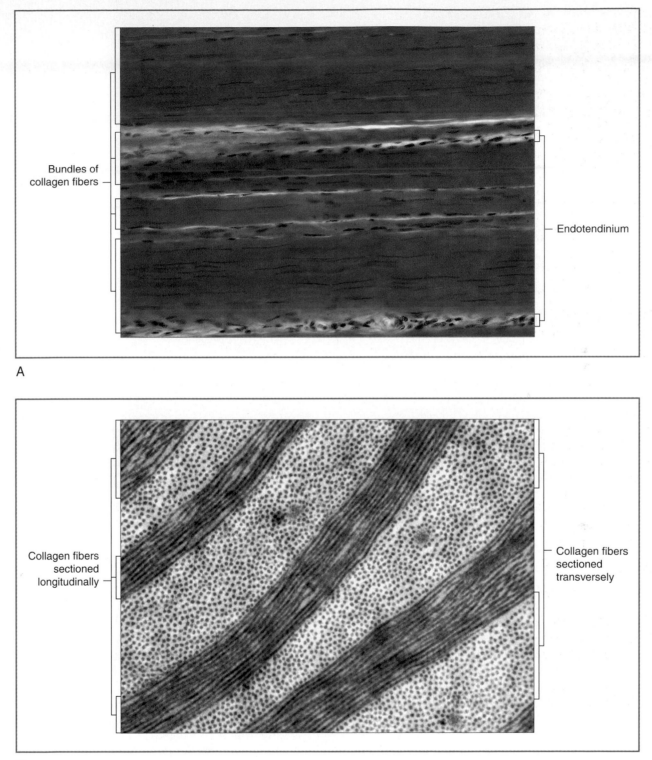

Bundles of collagen fibers

Endotendinium

A

Collagen fibers sectioned longitudinally

Collagen fibers sectioned transversely

B

Figure 4-4. A, Light micrograph of a longitudinal section of a tendon (H&E, 200×). Note the long, straight cables of collagen fibers with only long, thin fibroblast nuclei visible squeezed between the fibers. There are three or four extensions of the more cellular epitendineum (called endotendineum when inside the substance of the tendon), which divide the collagen fibers into fascicles. **B,** Electron micrograph of the cornea (35,000×). Note the uniform diameter of all the collagen fibers, the absence of any fibroblasts or their cell processes, and the orthogonal arrangement of the nearly uniform lamellae of fiber bundles. (Courtesy of Don W. Fawcett and M. Jakus.)

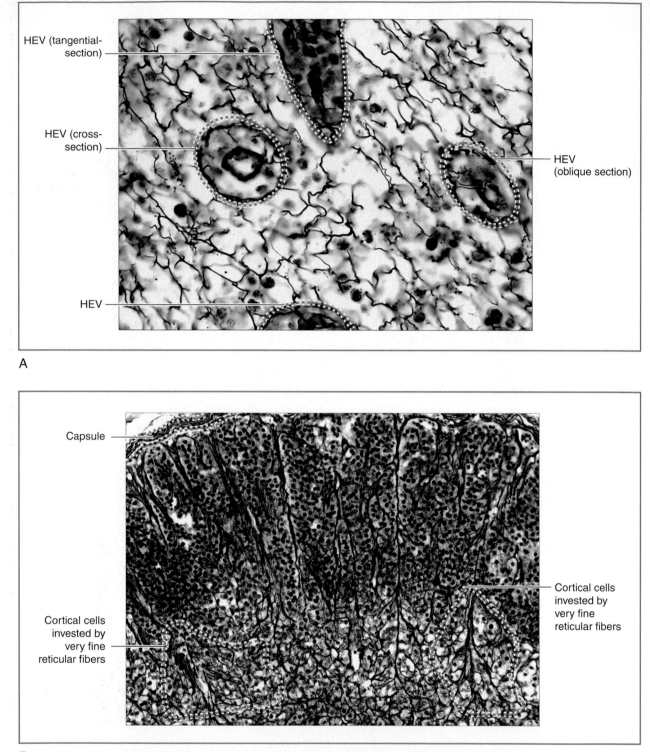

Figure 4-5. A, Silver stain of a lymph node (400×). The thin, highly branched network of reticular fibers that comprises the stroma of the lymph node is seen throughout the field. Some of the fibers are above the focal plane and others are below it—the greenish and reddish out-of-focus fibers. Most of the black dots are lymphocyte nuclei; there are also four sections of special lymph node venules (high endothelial venules [HEVs]) in the field. **B,** A silver stain of the cortex of a fetal adrenal gland (140×). There are many thin to very thin black fibers in this image; some are in the capsule, some divide clusters of adrenal parenchymal cells into columnar groups, and the finest are associated with cell clusters in the lower third of the image.

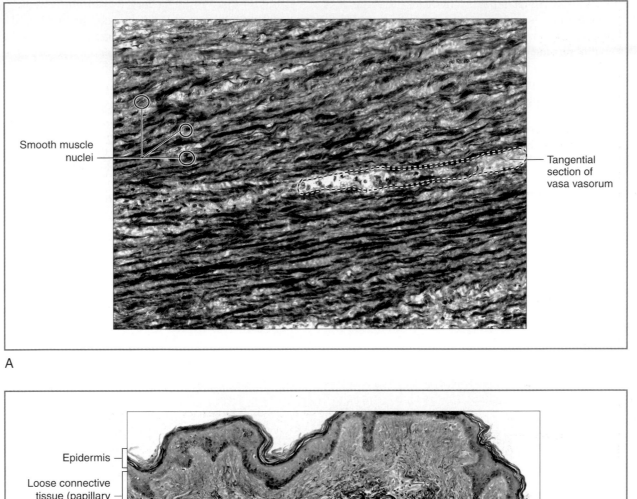

Smooth muscle nuclei —

Tangential section of vasa vasorum

A

Epidermis —

Loose connective tissue (papillary dermis) —

Nerve fiber bundle

Dense irregular connective tissue (reticular dermis) —

Nerve fiber bundle

B

Figure 4-6. A, Section of aorta (iron hematoxylin, azure blue, 160×). The elastin fibers are dark reddish-brown, and collagen fibers are azure blue. Some of the elastin fibers are thin and wavy, others are thick and wavy, and still others are straight. This illustrates the variable structure of these fibers as well as some "plane of section" factors that make some fibers appear to be more different than they actually are. It is difficult to discern any smooth muscle cells in the wall of this vessel, since they are relatively unstained; however, some smooth muscle nuclei are labeled in the upper left part of the field. **B,** Section of skin showing the epidermis and dermis (Mallory's trichrome stain, 100×). The lower three-quarters of the field is the dense irregular connective tissue of the reticular dermis, which in this specimen demonstrates the intermingled nature of the blue collagen fibers and reddish-brown elastin fibers particularly well. Note that the elastin fibers closer to the papillary dermis are thinner than those in the lower part of the field. The loose connective tissue of the papillary dermis has very little elastin, but some short, thin fibers can be seen. The basal layer of the epidermis is highly pigmented owing to the presence of melanin granules.

represented by the triplet repeat, $(Gly-X-Y)_{333}$, where X is usually proline and Y is hydroxyproline or hydroxylysine or any of the other 20 common amino acids.

Hydroxyproline and hydroxylysine are posttranslational modifications of the nascent collagen α-chains that occur in the lumen of the endoplasmic reticulum. Other changes that occur in this compartment (and in the Golgi apparatus) are glycosylation of some of the hydroxylysine residues, winding of the three α-chains to form the triple helical cable, covalent cross-linking of the α-chains, and packaging of tropocollagen into secretory vesicles.

The collagen molecules secreted into the extracellular space are actually precursors of the molecules that will be used to build mature collagen fibers (Table 4-2). The secreted form is called procollagen and contains carboxyterminal ("heads") and amino-terminal ("tails") propeptides that are globular in nature (i.e., they do not become part of the triple helical cable although they participate in the intracellular formation of tropocollagen). The long triplet repeat part of the molecule contains few, if any, cysteine residues, but the carboxyl and amino-terminal peptides have a number of cysteines that form several disulfide bonds. As the procollagen is secreted from the cell, the heads and tails are cleaved by specific procollagen peptidases associated with the plasma membrane of the cell prior to the assembly of the newly formed tropocollagen into fibrils.

GENETICS

Collagen Gene Mutations

Several mutations in collagen genes result in serious defects in connective tissues:

- Ehlers-Danlos syndrome is a group of diseases in which defects in collagen type I or III result in significant structural defects in dense irregular connective tissue. At least 10 mutations of these types of collagen are classified as Ehlers-Danlos syndrome.
- Osteogenesis imperfecta is another disease caused by a mutation in type I collagen (the α_1-chain gene). (See Chapter 5.)

TABLE 4-2. Collagen Biosynthesis: From the Cytoplasm to the Matrix

Biochemical Steps	Locus
Cellular Loci	
1. Uptake and synthesis of amino acids needed for collagen biosynthesis	Plasma membrane and cytoplasm
2. Transcription of collagen genes and processing of collagen mRNA—a high-molecular-weight RNA with 42 exons	Nucleus
3. Translation begins, producing preprocollagen, which docks on cytoplasmic surface of rER	Cytoplasm and cytoplasmic surface of rER
4. Preprocollagen translocates to rER lumen to produce procollagen	Cytoplasmic surface of rER and rER lumen
5. Specific procollagen proline and lysine residues are hydoxylated to form hydroxyproline and hydroxylysine	rER lumen
6. Some of the ∂-amino groups of lysine are glycosylated with Gal-Glu or Gal	rER lumen and sER lumen
7. The globular ends of the C-terminal propeptides become cross-linked by a specific enzyme, disulfide isomerase, to produce inter-α-chain cysteines	sER lumen and *cis*-Golgi lumen
8. This brings the three α-chains into register and initiates the process of triple helical procollagen formation	Golgi lumen
9. The triple helical procollagen molecules "zip up" from the carboxyl terminus and are secreted from the cell	Golgi lumen, secretory vesicles, and in some fibroblasts via specialized secretory structures
Extracellular Loci	
10. Specific proteases (procollagen proteases) cleave the propeptides to form the mature tropocollagen	Pericellular and extracellular spaces
11. The tropocollagen assembles into fibrils (a process inhibited in procollagen by the presence of propeptides	Pericellular and extracellular spaces
12. Selected lysine residues form covalent cross-links with lysine residues in nearby α-chains to stabilize the fibrils	Extracellular space
13. Fibrils assemble into mature collagen fibers	Extracellular space

When collagen fibers are studied in situ under the electron microscope, they have a regular repeating cross-banded pattern with a periodicity of 68 nm (Fig. 4-7). The banding pattern is the result of the specific way tropocollagen molecules pack together—first into fibrils and ultimately into fibers. Adjacent tropocollagen molecules align with all their carboxyl and amino-terminal ends oriented in the same direction to produce a *unit fibril*. A key feature of this packing is that each tropocollagen molecule is displaced by 68 nm (a little less than 25% of its length) with respect to adjacent tropocollagens and there is a small gap (ca. 35 nm) from the head of one to the tail of the next molecule; this is called the *quarter-stagger* model. Hundreds of unit fibrils assemble into larger and larger structures, which can be seen in the light or electron microscope. As an individual ages, the tropocollagen molecules in the dense irregular and dense regular types of connective tissue become progressively more and more cross-

linked by covalent bonds. Thus, collagen from these tissue types is essentially insoluble, whereas tropocollagen molecules from the same tissue types in young individuals can be readily solubilized.

Collagen Types

Many different types of collagen have been described in humans and other animals. The primary basis for stating that one kind of collagen is a different type from another is the length and specific amino acid sequence of its α-chains. The types have been assigned Roman numerals in order of their discovery, and this nomenclature has no relationship to their function or tissue location. More than 25 different types of collagen have been described in humans, and since the α-chains are primary gene products, we also know there are over 40 different collagen genes in the human genome. Some have as few as 600 amino acids and others as many as 3000;

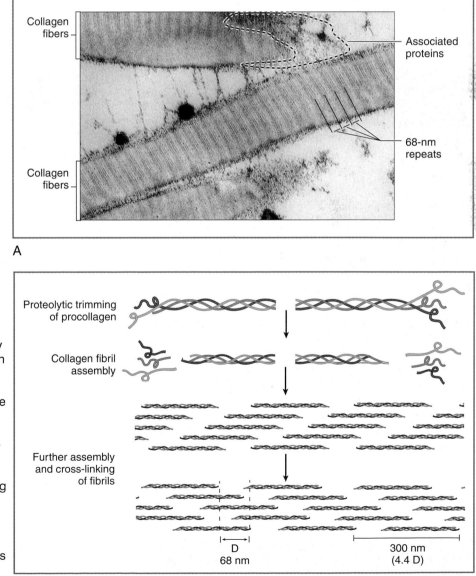

Figure 4-7. A, Electron micrograph of collagen showing the distinctive 68-nm cross-banded pattern of the collagen fibers and associated proteins. (Courtesy of Jeffery B. Kerr.) **B,** Diagram of collagen fiber assembly showing most of the extracellular steps. The non–triple helical portions of the procollagen molecules are cleaved by specific proteases; the triple-helical tropocollagen molecules assemble into small fibrils that are cross-linked and assemble further to form collagen fibers (see steps 10 through 13 in Table 4-2). The cross-banded repeating pattern shown is that for type I collagen; other collagen types have similar cross-banded patterns, but the spacing and details of the patterns are slightly different. The repeating pattern spacing is referred to as the "D" period.

however, most α-chains have about 1000 amino acids. Major defining characteristics of a protein as a collagen α-chain are that (1) one third of its amino acids are glycine in a repeating Gly-X-Y sequence, (2) they form a triple-helical fibrous cable, and (3) they are extracellular matrix proteins.

Type I collagen (the prototype) has two different α-chains in its triple-helical tropocollagen cable; one is called alpha 1, type I [α1(I)], and the other is called alpha 2, type I [α2(I)]. The type I tropocollagen cable has the formula [α1(I)$_2$ α2 (I)]. Since there are two different type I α-chains in a single triple helical cable, type I collagen is called a *heterotrimer*. Type II collagen, which is found in cartilage and the vitreous humor of the eye, is a *homotrimer*, since its molecular formula is α1(II)$_3$. Collagen types I to V are considered the major collagens, since they comprise a substantial percentage (ca. 25% to 100%) of the protein in their native locations. All the others are considered minor collagens, since they make up 2% or less of the total connective tissue protein. Table 4-3 presents a list of the collagens, their tropocollagen molecular formulas, whether they form fibers or some other structure, and their principal location.

So far collagen has been presented as a fibrous protein; with regard to the triple-helical tropocollagen cable, this is true for nearly all of the collagens. Many of these collagen cables assemble into fibers, but not all do so. Some form a sheet-like meshwork, others are associated with plasma membranes, and still others serve to anchor or connect cells to the matrix or one matrix component to another. The majority of the fiber-forming cables make fibers with diameters in the range of 15 to 300 nm. However, some tropocollagen cables, type IV in particular, assemble into mesh-like sheets. Type IV collagen is a major component of the basal lamina of all cells and tissues that have a basal lamina. Others function in a number of different ways (see Table 4-3). Furthermore, collagens are synthesized by cells representing all four basic tissue types. Epithelia synthesize type IV collagen; the basal lamina associated with smooth, skeletal, and cardiac muscle fibers is synthesized by the muscle cells themselves; smooth muscle cells in the walls of blood vessels synthesize types I and V collagen; and in the nervous system, Schwann cells synthesize type IV collagen.

Some collagens are developmentally expressed, i.e., the collagen is expressed only at a specific stage of development, degraded, and never again expressed during the lifetime of the individual. Many of the collagen fibers we see in the light or electron microscope contain more than one type of collagen (e.g., the dense irregular connective tissue in the dermis of skin has collagen fibers containing types I and III collagen as well as several minor collagens). The walls of blood vessels contain mixed collagen fibers of types I and V.

To date, seven transmembrane collagens have been described, two of which are listed in Table 4-3 (types XII and XVII). Of the other five, types XXIII and XXV have been assigned Roman numerals, and the remaining three have not. All seven have wide tissue distributions and are synthesized by many different cell types. All have the amino terminus in the cytoplasm of the cell that synthesized them, a short transmembrane segment, a noncollagenous domain on the ectoplasmic face of the cell, and a large ectoplasmic domain that is either all collagenous or that has collagen-like domains interrupted by noncollagenous domains. They are, or can be, cleaved by specific proteases to produce a matrix tropocollagen cable that may or may not have flexible hinges along its length depending on the presence or absence of noncollagenous domains.

Elastin Fibers

Elastin (or elastic fibers) is the other main fibrous component of the connective tissue matrix. In order to be seen clearly in its native tissue locations (deep layer of the dermis, loose connective tissue, walls of blood vessels, elastic cartilage, the delicate connective tissue layers in the lung) in the light microscope, the tissue needs to be secured with certain fixatives or stained with specific dyes, such as orcein or resorcin-fuchsin (see Fig. 4-6). In all tissue locations, elastin fibers exhibit a wide range of fiber diameters and branch extensively. The appearance of elastin fibers in the electron microscope reveals they are amorphous; in tissue locations other than the walls of blood vessels, the large elastin fibers are associated with a number of microfibrillar components called fibrillin (Fig. 4-8). In physicochemical terms, elastin fibers exhibit the same properties as rubber bands—they can be stretched to 150% of their length without breaking and when the tension is released, they snap back to their original length.

Elastin fibers are synthesized by fibroblasts in connective tissue and by smooth muscle cells in the walls of blood vessels. Their biosynthetic pathway is similar to that of collagen: (1) they are synthesized as a proelastin precursor that is cleaved by specific proteases at the cell membrane upon secretion into the extracellular space; (2) the cleaved product is a fibrous protein called tropoelastin; (3) they contain large amounts of glycine and proline as well as more alanine, valine, and lysine than do collagen and other proteins; (4) they assemble into fibrils and larger fibers in the extracellular space; and (5) they are cross-linked in the extracellular space (more extensively than is collagen) by a series of steps involving four lysine residues. The cross-linking produces two cyclic amino acids called desmosine and isodesmosine; these amino acids are diagnostic for the presence of elastin. It is the high alanine and valine content as well as the desmosine and isodesmosine cross-links that gives elastin its stretchable properties.

As the tropoelastin molecules form the large, thick extracellular fibers seen in the light and electron microscopes, a group of acidic proteins, the fibrillins, becomes associated with the surface of the elastin fibers. It is fibrillins that make up the microfibrils seen in electron micrographs of elastin fibers.

Elastic fibers in situ have an extremely low metabolic turnover rate (i.e., a very long half-life). This means that the elastic fibers made in an individual's earliest years—more or less through puberty—last for a lifetime. The aging of skin, particularly wrinkling, is largely due to damage to the elastin content of the dermis of skin by exposure to direct sunlight.

TABLE 4-3. Collagen Types and Distribution

Type	Tropocollagen Composition	Assembled Form of Tropocollagen	Synthesized by	Distribution
I	$[\alpha 1(I)_2\ a2\ (I)]$	Fibers	Fibroblasts, osteoblasts/ osteocytes, smooth muscle cells, odontoblasts	Dense regular connective tissue, dense irregular connective tissue, loose connective tissue, bone, blood vessel walls, dentin
II	$[\alpha 1(II)_3]$	Fibers	Chondroblasts/chondrocytes	Cartilage, vitreous body
III	$[\alpha 1(III)_3]$	Fibers, reticular fibers	Fibroblasts	Dense irregular connective tissue, loose connective tissue, reticular connective tissue
IV	$[\alpha 1(IV)_2\ a2\ (IV)]$	Meshwork sheets	Epithelial cells, muscle cells, Schwann cells	Basal lamina
V	$[\alpha 1(V)_2\ a2\ (V)]$ or $[\alpha 1(V)\ a2\ (V)\ [a3(V)]$	Fibers	Fibroblasts, smooth muscle cells	Dense irregular connective tissue, placenta, blood vessel walls
VI	$[\alpha 1(VI)_2\ a2\ (VI)]$ or $[\alpha 1(VI)\ a2\ (VI)\ [a3(VI)]$	Beaded fibrils	Fibroblasts	
VII	$[\alpha 1(VII)_3]$	Anchoring fibrils	Fibroblasts	Epidermal-dermal interface
VIII	$[\alpha 1(VIII)_2\ a2\ (VIII)]$	Meshwork sheets	Endothelial cells	Descemet's membrane (of the cornea)
IX	$[\alpha 1(IX)\ a2\ (IX)\ [a3(IX)]$	Fibrils	Chondrocytes	Cartilage—interacts with type II collagen at chondrocyte lacunar boundaries
X	$[\alpha 1(X)_3]$	Fibrils	Hypertrophic chondrocytes	Hypertrophic zone of epiphyseal plate
XI	$[\alpha 1(XI)_2\ a2\ (XI)]$ or $[\alpha 1(XI)\ a2\ (XI)\ [a1(II)]$	Fibrils	Chondrocytes	Cartilage matrix
XII	$[\alpha 1(XII)_3]$	Fibrils	Fibroblasts	Fetal connective tissues, loose connective tissue, dense irregular connective tissue
XIII	$[\alpha 1(XIII)_3]$	Cables with noncollagenous flexible hinges	All four basic tissues	Transmembrane—associated with several components of basal lamina
XIV	$[\alpha 1(XIV)_3]$	Fibrils	Fibroblasts	Fetal connective tissues, placenta, skin, bone marrow
XV	$[\alpha 1(XV)_3]$	Fibrils	Fibroblasts	Associated with basal lamina
XVI	$[\alpha 1(XVI)_3]$	Fibrils	Fibroblasts, smooth muscle	Loose connective tissue, dense irregular connective tissue, blood vessel walls
XVII	$[\alpha 1(XVII)_3]$	Cables with noncollagenous flexible hinges	Keratinocytes in basal layer of the epidermis	Transmembrane—component of hemidesmosomes, interacts with integrins and other basal lamina components
XVIII	$[\alpha 1(XVIII)_3]$	Fibrils	Epithelial cells, fibroblasts	Epidermal-dermal interface, interacts with basal lamina and proteoglycans

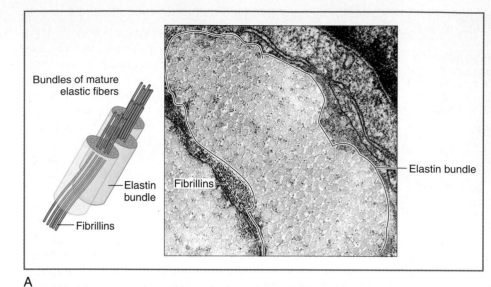

Bundles of mature elastic fibers

Elastin bundle

Fibrillins

Fibrillins

Elastin bundle

A

Figure 4-8. A, Electron micrograph of a large group of elastin fibers, in cross-section, next to a fibroblast. Large clusters of fibrillin fibers can be seen at the edge of the elastin bundles as well as a few in their midst. (From Kierszenbaum A. *Histology and Cell Biology.* Philadelphia, Mosby, 2002, p 102. **B** and **C,** Electron micrographs of a smaller bundle of elastin fibers (stained black) that illustrate the number and relationship of the fibrillin fibers to the elastin fibers. Part B is a longitudinal section, and part C is a cross-section of a similar bundle. (From Pollard TD, Earnshaw WC. *Cell Biology.* Philadelphia, WB Saunders, 2004, p 481.)

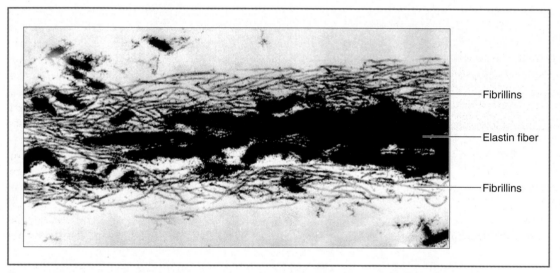

Fibrillins

Elastin fiber

Fibrillins

B

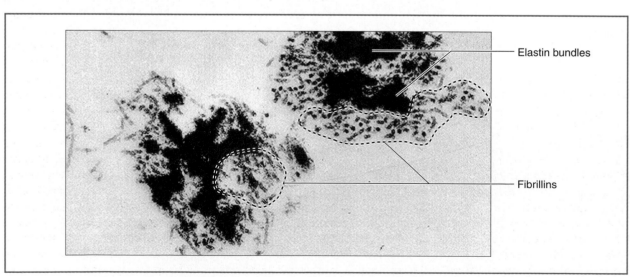

Elastin bundles

Fibrillins

C

GENETICS & PATHOLOGY

Marfan Syndrome

A disease known as Marfan syndrome is caused by a mutation in the fibrillin-1 gene. There are several different fibrillins, and mutations have been described in many of them. Marfan syndrome is particularly interesting in that the phenotype demonstrates variable expressivity.

- Marfan syndrome is an autosomal dominant disease.
- It is commonly associated with bone overgrowth.
- About 10% of affected individuals develop emphysema.
- Many individuals with Marfan syndrome have aneurysms of the aorta as well as heart valve defects.
- It has long been thought that the defect in fibrillin-1 caused structural abnormalities in the structure and hence the function of elastin fibers, which have a "coating" of fibrillins.
- Recent evidence strongly suggests the underlying cause of the connective tissue defect is that normal fibrillin-1 binds the transforming growth factor–β (TGF-β) family of cytokines, down-regulating their activities.
- Mutant fibrillin-1 does not bind TGF-β, which leads to its overactivity, particularly during development. This results in gross abnormalities in the structure of elastin- and fibrillin-rich connective tissues.

Other Fibrous Proteins of Connective Tissue

Fibronectin and *laminin* are the two main fibrous proteins of connective tissue other than collagen and elastin. Their abundance is much lower than that of the major fibrous structural proteins, and they are not visible in any routine light or electron microscopic sections. Nonetheless, they each play central roles in anchoring cells to the matrix that surrounds them or underlies them (in the case of epithelial cells).

Ground Substance

Structure

Ground substance represents the majority of the balance of connective tissue matrix that is not occupied by fibrous proteins. Because of its chemical composition and physical characteristics, ground substance—acidic proteoglycans—is not well fixed or visualized by the most common chemical fixatives or stains used for light or electron microscopy. Even when appropriate fixatives and stains are used to preserve and visualize ground substance, it has an amorphous appearance in light or electron microscopy. Polysaccharides bind five to six times their weight of water; furthermore, ground substance has a high net negative charge at physiologic pH, so it also binds (chelates) a substantial amount of cations; these characteristics make ground substance highly water soluble.

Ground substance is a complex mixture of high-molecular-weight polymers of acidic carbohydrates (*glycosaminoglycans*, or *GAGs*) all but one of which is covalently attached to a core protein. Those and the core proteins to which they are covalently bound are called proteoglycans. Glycosaminoglycans may have a relatively simple or highly complex structure. In general, GAGs consist of repeating disaccharides with the formula [hexose uronic acid–hexosamine]$_n$. The GAG with the simplest structure is *hyaluronan* (formerly, hyaluronic acid), which is a very high molecular weight linear polymer of the disaccharide [D-glucuronic acid–N-acetyl D-glucosamine]. A single molecule of hyaluronan may have up to 2500 repeats of this disaccharide and a molecular weight of $\geq 10^6$ Da; such a molecule is more than 20 μm long—greater than the diameter of many cells.

Composition

Most GAGs in tissue occur as proteoglycans whose general structure can be thought of as being similar to a bottle brush—the wire stem of the brush is the core protein and the bristles are the GAG chains. Although the structure of proteoglycans in a given tissue displays a degree of uniformity with respect to core protein molecular weight, number, type, and length of GAG chains, within any one category the structures are much more heterogeneous than those of many other biological macromolecules. Like the collagens, proteoglycans have characteristic half-lives, with some as short as 30 days. Also like the collagens, some protoglycans are components of the plasma membrane of the cell that synthesized them; they participate as coreceptors for specific ligands. A few collagens (IX, XII, and XVII) have GAG chains covalently attached to them; these collagens, therefore, are proteoglycans. Although they are synthesized by connective tissue cells, certain specific proteoglycans are also synthesized by epithelial cells, muscle cells, and nerve cells. Table 4-4 lists the composition and characteristics of the major GAGs.

In many native tissue locations, the proteoglycans listed in Table 4-4 occur as huge aggregates of hyaluronan, a large number of proteoglycans, and two specific link proteins per proteoglycan. The type found in cartilage, aggrecan, may have as many as 100 chondroitin sulfate proteoglycans noncovalently bound, via the link proteins, to hyaluronan, resulting in an aggregate with a molecular weight in excess of 10^8 Da. Cartilage aggrecan interacts with type II collagen fibers in the tissue to produce a stable, compression-resistant, gel-like substance that occupies many cubic centimeters of volume. Similar types of aggregates of hyaluronan and proteoglycans are found in loose connective tissue and dense irregular connective tissue, albeit of lower molecular weight. Since the aggregates are so large and are held together by covalent and noncovalent bonds, they are susceptible to degradation following only a few proteolytic or glycosidic cleavages as well as exposure to ultraviolet irradiation or other agents (e.g., free radicals) that may disrupt the noncovalent interactions holding the aggregates together. In fact, it is the gradual reduction in size of these aggregates in the dermis of skin over a lifetime that contributes to the aging (wrinkling) of skin. The structure of aggrecan and other typical proteoglycans is diagrammed in Figure 4-9.

TABLE 4-4. Glycosaminoglycans (GAGs) and Proteoglycans

Type of GAG	Repeating Disaccharide	GAG Molecular Weight Range (Da)	Covalently Linked to Protein and Nature of Linkage
Hyaluronan	GlcUA–GlcNAc	$0.8–1.2 \times 10^6$	No
Chondroitin 4-sulfate	GlcUA–GalNAc-4-SO$_4$	$1.5–2.5 \times 10^3$	Yes: GlcUA-Gal-Gal-Xyl to serine
Chondroitin 6-sulfate	GlcUA–GalNAc-6-SO$_4$	$1.5–2.5 \times 10^3$	Yes: GlcUA-Gal-Gal-Xyl to serine
Dermatan sulfate	IdUA–GalNAc-4-SO$_4$	$2.5–3.0 \times 10^3$	Yes: GlcUA-Gal-Gal-Xyl to serine
Keratan sulfate	Gal–GlcNAc-4-SO$_4$	$1.0–1.5 \times 10^3$	Yes: branched linkage containing Man, Fuc, and GlcNAc to aspartic acid
Heparan sulfate/heparin	GlcUA (or IdUA-2-SO$_4$)– GlcNAc (or N-sulfamyl GlcN)	$1.2–4.0 \times 10^3$	Yes: GlcUA-Gal-Gal-Xyl to serine

GlcNAc, N-acetyl D-glucosamine; GalNAc, N-acetyl D-galactosamine; GlcUA, D-glucuronic acid; IdUA, L-iduronic acid; Xyl, D-xylose; Gal, D-galactose; Fuc, fucose; Man, D-mannose.

Biosynthesis

The biosynthesis of proteoglycans follows the same general steps as for any other glycoprotein destined for secretion from the cell (i.e., by a series of posttranslational modifications of the core protein): (1) the core protein is translated from its mRNA and translocated into the lumen of the rough endoplasmic reticulum (rER) by its signal peptide sequence; (2) the serine residues are glycosylated by UDP-xylose in the rER and smooth endoplasmic reticulum (sER); (3) further glycosylation by UDP-galactose, UDP-glucuronic acid, and UDP-*N*-acetylgalactosamine occurs in the sER and the Golgi apparatus; (4) galactosamine (or other carbohydrate) residues of the nascent GAG chains are sulfated in the Golgi apparatus; (5) the completed proteoglycans are packaged into secretory vesicles by the Golgi apparatus; (6) the proteoglycans are secreted into the extracellular space by exocytosis of the vesicles.

The biosynthesis of hyaluronan differs significantly from that of proteoglycans, since its repeating disaccharides are added sequentially to the growing chain by enzymes associated with the plasma membrane. It is as though this very long molecule "spins" off the surface of the plasma membrane. Furthermore, hyaluronan is not bound to protein and is not modified postsynthetically as are proteoglycans.

Once in the extracellular space, the proteoglycans and hyaluronan interact to generate the large aggregates characteristic to each specific tissue type.

●●● CELLS OF CONNECTIVE TISSUE

Fibroblasts

The cell that synthesizes and secretes the matrix components of connective tissue proper is the fibroblast. It is an elongated, spindle shaped (fusiform) cell with a prominent nucleus and scant cytoplasm, particularly when seen in the light microscope. Unlike many other cells having the suffix "blast" (e.g., myoblast, neuroblast, lipoblast), the fibroblast is not considered to be an immature form of a more mature cell— the fibrocyte. It is called a fibroblast because of its capacity to

GENETICS

Mucopolysaccharidoses

There is a group of genetic diseases in which the degradation of glycosaminoglycans (GAGs) is defective owing to mutations in the lysosomal enzymes that normally degrade them. Collectively, these diseases are called mucopolysaccharidoses (based on earlier nomenclature for GAGs). In some of these diseases, the partially degraded GAG chains are stored in lysosomes. In others, the partially degraded GAG chains are excreted in the urine. All mucopolysaccharidoses exhibit pleiotropic phenotypes that commonly involve the skeletal system and liver, with significant mental retardation and a shortened life span in the absence of treatment.

synthesize and secrete connective tissue fibers, as well as connective tissue ground substance and glycoproteins. In embryonic development, fibroblasts differentiate from mesenchymal cells. Fibroblasts of adults may divide and may undergo periods of active matrix synthesis and secretion and periods of quiescence, but they maintain a basal level production of matrix. In most locations where loose or dense irregular connective tissue is found, fibroblasts remain in the cell cycle and undergo mitosis throughout life. Fibroblasts in dense regular connective tissue divide infrequently or not at all.

When fibroblasts are examined in the transmission electron microscope, their cytoplasm is seen to be richly endowed with dilated rER, sER, one or more Golgi apparatuses, secretory vesicles, a full complement of cytoskeletal filaments, and all the other cellular organelles. A useful indicator of the matrix synthesis activity of a fibroblast (in both light and electron microscopy) is the appearance of the nucleus; those having one or more nucleoli and about 80% or more euchromatin are in an active phase of matrix synthesis at the time of their fixation.

Fibroblasts can be readily grown in tissue culture and have been used for important cellular and biochemical studies of

Figure 4-9. A, Diagram of aggrecan, the prototypical proteoglycan. About 100 of the large aggrecan subunits *(top)* form a noncovalent complex with hyaluronan stabilized by two "link" proteins. This complex interacts with type II collagen fibers to produce the firm gel characteristic of cartilage *(bottom).* **B,** Schematic diagrams of five other proteoglycans. Decorin binds to collagen fibrils and modulates their assembly; serglycin binds histamine (a basic molecule) in leukocyte secretory granules; perlecan is part of basal lamina structure. Syndecan and glypican are membrane-associated proteoglycans and associate with several components of the pericellular matrix.

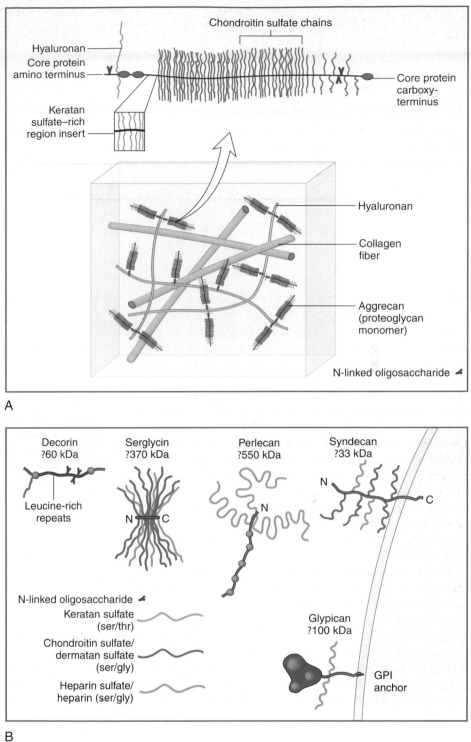

collagen synthesis, cell motility, receptor mediated endocytosis, and many other fundamental cellular activities. Figure 4-10 shows three examples of fibroblasts.

Adipose Cells

Like fibroblasts, adipose cells differentiate from mesenchymal cells. In the human embryo, fat first appears as a distinct cell type about midway through fetal development. The fetus has two forms of fat—white and brown—based on the appearance of the tissue in the living state.

The cells of brown fat have many small fat droplets, a centrally placed nucleus, and a large number of mitochondria; the high cytochrome content of mitochondria gives these cells their brown color. Because the fat droplets of these cells are dissolved by the solvents used in typical histologic preparation techniques, brown fat cells appear to have many holes and are called multilocular adipocytes. The main

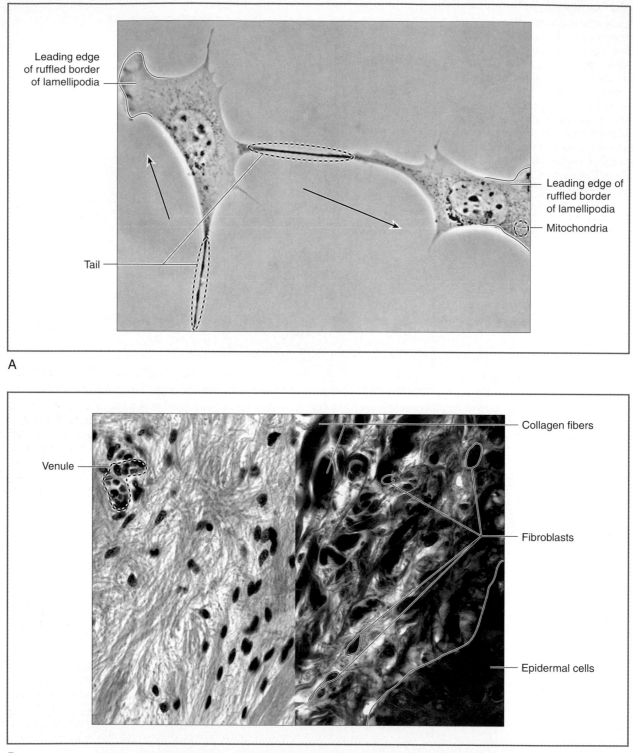

A

B

Figure 4-10. A, Phase-contrast image of two fibroblasts (3T3 cells) in tissue culture. These are two sibling cells that are moving away from each other *(arrows)*. Note the large oval nuclei each with several phase dark nucleoli, the thread-like mitochondria (particularly clear near the leading edge of the cell at right), and the numerous phase light and dark cell organelles. (Courtesy of Guenter Albrecht-Buehler.) **B,** A composite of two light micrographs of fibroblasts in the papillary layer *(left,* H&E, 400×) and the reticular layer *(right,* Mallory's trichrome, 1000×) of the dermis of skin. In the micrograph at left, nearly all the nuclei in the field of view are fibroblast nuclei, but hardly any cytoplasm can be seen, since it stains the same color as the surrounding collagen fibers. Note the spindle (fusiform) shape of the cells in the micrograph at right and the large nuclear to cytoplasmic ratio (also see Fig. 4-12B). It is noteworthy that the collagen fibers in the micrograph at left are finer than those in the one at right, even though the latter is at a higher magnification. However, few other cellular details can be seen in either image.

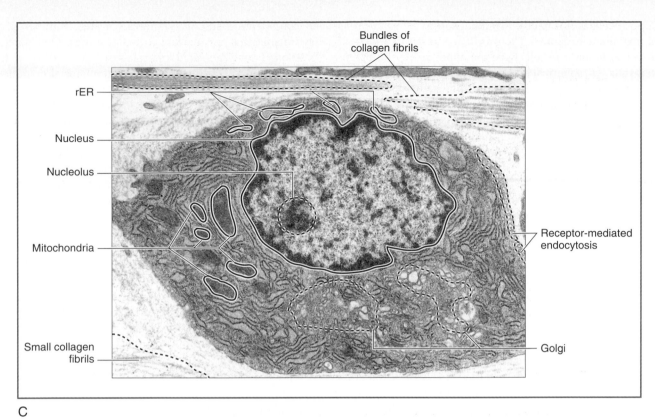

Bundles of
collagen fibrils

rER

Nucleus

Nucleolus

Mitochondria

Receptor-mediated
endocytosis

Small collagen
fibrils

Golgi

C

Figure 4-10 cont'd. C, Electron micrograph of a fibroblast sectioned transversely (an interpretation based on the shape of the cell profile and the location of its nucleus, and by comparison to the general fusiform shape of fibroblasts as seen in Fig. 4-10B). There are two small bundles of collagen fibrils above the cell and numerous individual fibrils in other locations around the cell. This fibroblast shows many characteristics of a cell engaged in a high rate of protein synthesis and secretion: the nucleus has a large proportion of euchromatin; there is a prominent nucleolus; the plasma membrane has many coated (pinocytotic) vesicles; there are many mitochondria; there is a large and extensive Golgi complex; and the cytoplasm is filled with many profiles of rER, many of which are dilated. All six of these cytologic features are labeled on the image. Some profiles of rER are labeled only at upper left even though they are seen throughout the cell. (Courtesy of Jeffery B. Kerr.)

metabolic role of brown fat is to produce heat. It is rather abundant in newborns, and its content in the body gradually declines in the first decade of life although small amounts may be found in the adult.

White adipose cells (adipocytes, lipocytes, fat cells) are large, spherical cells (some may be as large as 100 μm in diameter) found in many locations. In loose connective tissues, they are often seen as individual cells or in small groups. The hypodermis typically contains large amounts of adipose cells, which are visible as a layer of subcutaneous fat (see Fig. 4-2F); women have a slightly thicker layer of subcutaneous fat than men. More internally, larger muscles may have a thick covering of adipose cells, so much in fact that this accumulation of fat cells is called adipose tissue. Substantial masses of adipose tissue also are associated with the visceral pericardium, with the superior poles of the kidneys—near the adrenal glands, the greater omentum, and other places. The cells of white fat have a flattened nucleus and scant cytoplasm. In typical preparations, the fat content

BIOCHEMISTRY

Energy Storage

Within cells, energy may be stored as glycogen or in the form of triglycerides, which are stored mostly in adipose cells. When cells need chemical energy, the triglycerides in white adipose tissue are degraded and the fatty acids are metabolized in mitochondria to produce ATP. When the body needs energy in the form of heat, special mechanisms in brown fat allow for the catabolism of triglycerides to produce heat—the nonshivering thermogenic response. The thermogenic response is mediated by a group of proteins called thermogenins that are distributed in a tissue-specific manner. The thermogenins are uncouplers of oxidative phosphorylation. They work by allowing the passage of protons from the intramembranous space into the inner mitochondrial matrix, which diminishes the electrochemical gradient between these two compartments and partially uncouples ATP synthesis. Thus, the energy produced by metabolism is released as heat.

of adipose cells is not fixed or stained, so the cells appear as large, unstained structures. There is little stroma in a mass of adipose tissue, and the cells have the appearance of a tightly packed mass of spherical to polygonal cells. Adipose tissue has a rich supply of capillaries. When adipose tissue is stained with a silver stain, a number of delicate reticular fibers (type III collagen) are seen in the stroma.

As white adipose cells differentiate, they accumulate more and more fat droplets in their cytoplasm. Early in their development, numerous fat droplets can be seen in the cytoplasm of the lipoblasts; such cells are called multilocular lipoblasts or mid-stage lipoblasts. As the cells mature, all the droplets coalesce into a single large fat droplet; at this time the cells are called unilocular adipocytes.

The ultrastructure of white adipose tissue reveals several interesting and distinctive features. Despite the scant cytoplasm and flattened nucleus, the adipocyte has all the organelles of any metabolically active cell—mitochondria, lysosomes, and cytoskeletal components throughout the cytoplasm as well as small amounts of rER, a Golgi apparatus, and free ribosomes in the perinuclear region. The large lipid droplet that occupies the majority of the cytoplasm is not membrane bounded but is anchored to the surrounding cytoplasm by an array of short, parallel-oriented intermediate filaments of the vimentin type. Figure 4-11 shows two examples of adipose tissue—a light micrograph and an electron micrograph of a single adipocyte.

Free Cells of Connective Tissue

Free cells of connective tissue originate in the bone marrow, circulate in the bloodstream, and are known collectively as leukocytes, or white blood cells. Some of the leukocytes found in connective tissue are morphologically mature in the peripheral blood: the polymorphonuclear neutrophil, the eosinophil, the lymphocyte, and the basophil. Others are derived from a peripheral blood cell called the monocyte. Although the monocyte is described as a single leukocyte species found in the circulation, in fact it is an immature precursor (a stem cell) that can differentiate into a number of different mature cells when it leaves the circulation. In the case of connective tissue, these cells are macrophages and mast cells.

Macrophages

The macrophages found in loose connective tissue are derived from a cell in the circulating blood, the monocyte. Monocytes leave the circulation by a process called diapedesis; following an appropriate tissue signal, the monocyte is capable of inducing a pore to open in the cytoplasmic "wall" of an endothelial cell and entering the surrounding connective tissue space, where it undergoes postmitotic cellular differentiation to become a mature macrophage (sometimes called a histiocyte). The primary function of the macrophage is phagocytosis. It engulfs and degrades damaged tissue, foreign bodies, and microbes that may be present as the result of a wound or an infection. During the course of its differentiation

in connective tissue, it synthesizes a large number of acid hydrolases that are packaged in lysosomes. One particular lysosomal enzyme, acid phosphatase, is used as a histochemical marker for macrophages. The material degraded by the macrophage is secreted (or excreted) into the extracellular space and returned to the circulation. The macrophage has a prominent Golgi apparatus, rER, and sER and a full complement of actin filaments and associated proteins, which equips the cell for active cell motility and phagocytosis. In certain locations (e.g., the loose connective tissue of the gut), occasional monocytes persist in the connective tissue for a brief period of time, likely less than a day, before they differentiate into macrophages.

Unless special techniques are used to stimulate the phagocytic activity of a macrophage before histologic preparation, they can be difficult to identify in the light microscope; however, the ultrastructural appearance of a macrophage is distinctive. They have a large, eccentrically placed nucleus, numerous lysosomes, and a large surface area owing to the presence of hundreds of thin, curved filopodia. These surface elaborations play an active role in the phagocytic activity of the cell as well as being a central component in macrophage motility. Figure 4-12 shows light and electron micrographs of macrophages.

In addition to their general distribution in connective tissue, macrophages are found in many other locations around the body. For example, they are found in the liver, where they are called Küpffer cells; dispersed in the lymphoid parenchyma; on the luminal surface of pulmonary alveolar cells; and as the microglia in the central nervous system.

In addition to their primary role as phagocytes, they play an important role in the immune system by virtue of a class of cell surface molecules known as the major histocompatibility complex II (MHC II) molecules. Macrophages ingest and degrade foreign cells and biological macromolecules. The peptide degradation products interact with the MHC II complex and "present" the peptides to T lymphocytes as an important early step in the immune response. When functioning in this capacity, macrophages are referred to as antigen-presenting cells (APCs).

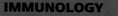

IMMUNOLOGY

Macrophages as Antigen-Presenting Cells (APCs)

The degradation products produced by macrophages from foreign cells and proteins are short polypeptides, which are usually about 7 to 10 amino acids long. These polypeptides typically serve as antigens. Because of their important role in the immune response, the macrophages are described as APCs. The peptides are displayed on the surface of the macrophage in association with the MHC II complex. The peptide-MHC complexes activate T lymphocytes, which stimulates the cell-mediated immune system. They also stimulate the humoral immune system through similar mechanisms involving B lymphocytes.

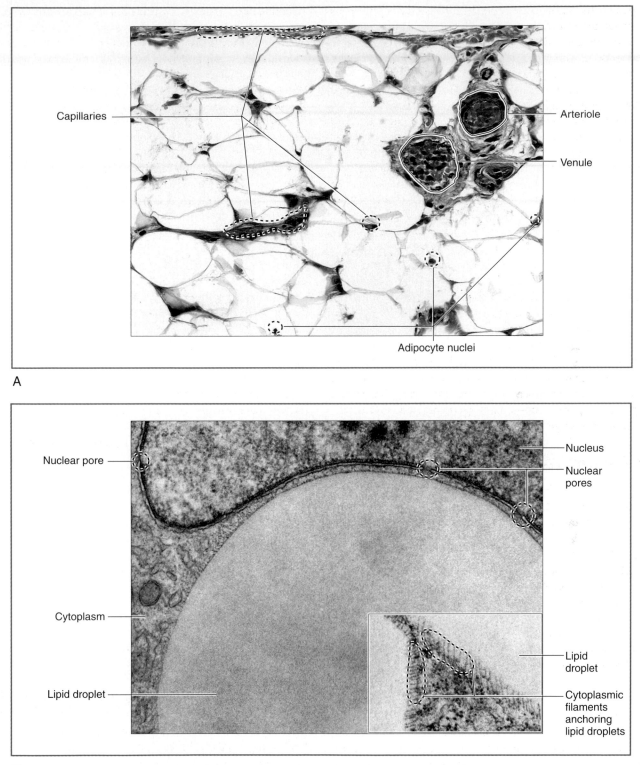

A

B

Figure 4-11. A, Light micrograph of adipose tissue. In this example, the adipocytes are unstained and only a hint of a nucleus can be seen in 5 to 7 of the cells (H&E, 180×). **B,** Electron micrograph of an adipose cell (34,000×). Part of the nucleus is seen in the upper part of the field; a large lipid droplet occupies the majority of the central part of the field, and some of the cytoplasm surrounding the lipid droplet is seen. Note that the lipid droplet is not membrane bound. The inset is a higher magnification of the cytoplasm-lipid interface (87,000×) illustrating two important features: the absence of a membrane surrounding the lipid is more evident; and there are fine cytoplasmic filaments (of the vimentin intermediate filament type) at the interface that anchor the lipid droplets in place. (Courtesy of Don W. Fawcett.)

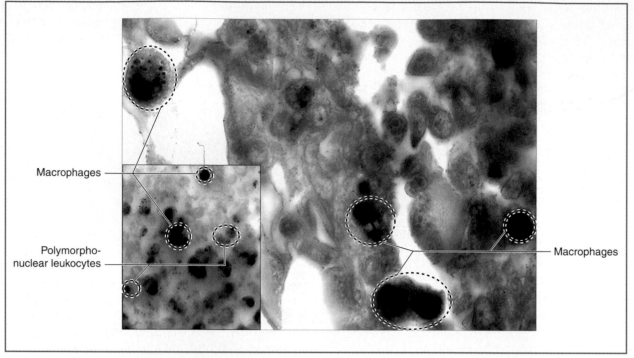

A

Macrophages

Polymorpho-
nuclear leukocytes

Macrophages

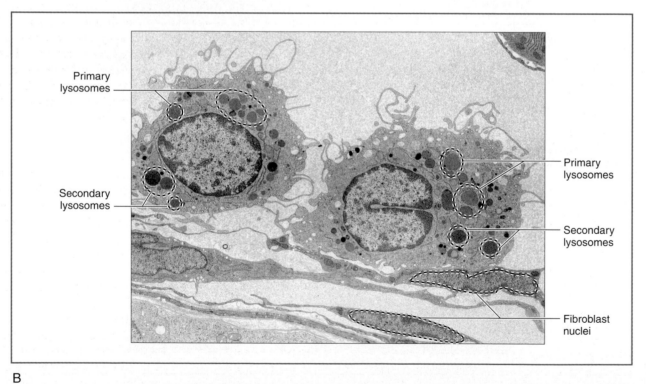

B

Primary
lysosomes

Secondary
lysosomes

Primary
lysosomes

Secondary
lysosomes

Fibroblast
nuclei

Figure 4-12. A, Light micrograph of loose connective tissue (eosin stain, 800×) taken from an animal that had been injected with trypan blue a few hours before it was sacrificed. Trypan blue is a "vital" dye, since it can be taken up—phagocytosed—by living cells. Most of the blue-stained cells are macrophages; the smaller ones are polymorphonuclear neutrophils. Although little cellular detail can be seen in these phagocytes, this staining technique gives a good impression of their abundance (*inset*, 400×). **B,** Electron micrograph of two macrophages. The cytoplasm is filled with many primary and secondary lysosomes, and the plasma membrane has numerous filopodia. Portions of three fibroblasts are seen below the macrophages. (Courtesy of Jeffery B. Kerr.)

Nongranular Cells Derived from the Circulation

As part of the body's immune response, lymphocytes are recruited to compartments of loose connective tissue via diapedesis. Lymphocytes are small cells with a spherical nucleus and relatively little cytoplasm. They may differentiate into plasma cells (as described in the next paragraph), or they may interact with other cells of the immune system to participate in the immune response. A more complete discussion of lymphocytes is found in Chapter 8.

Under appropriate stimuli, some of the lymphocytes in connective tissue will differentiate into an antibody-secreting cell, the plasma cell (Fig. 4-13). Each plasma cell is highly specialized to synthesize and secrete a single specific class of antibody molecules (immunoglobulins of the A, D, E, G, or M types). A plasma cell is usually elliptical in shape, with an eccentrically placed nucleus containing a "cartwheel" pattern of chromatin and a cytoplasm filled with rER. Immunoglobulins are secreted from plasma cells via the constitutive pathway. During times when the cells are especially active in immunoglobulin synthesis and secretion, numerous profiles of dilated rER and a well-developed Golgi apparatus can be seen by electron microscopy, but secretory vesicles, as such, are not a feature of plasma cells.

Granular Cells Derived from the Circulation

Polymorphonuclear leukocytes (PMNs, polys, neutrophils) are phagocytic cells found in loose connective tissue near sites of tissue injury, inflammation, or infection. They are recruited to these locations by cytokines and chemokines produced locally by other connective tissue cells following injury or infection; as such, they are found only rarely in normal connective tissue. The most distinctive feature of the polymorphonuclear leukocyte is its nucleus, which is highly lobulated (it may have from two to five lobes); the specific lobulation pattern differs from one PMN to another—hence the term polymorphonuclear. The cell has many granules, but they tend not to stain well with nearly all commonly used stains, which is why these cells are often called neutrophils. The primary function of PMNs is to serve as a phagocyte; a particular target of their phagocytic activity is bacteria, giving rise to the description of their function as bactericidal. With respect to their phagocytic activity, they are similar to macrophages, and in fact, PMNs were first described as "microphages" to distinguish them as cells smaller than macrophages but apparently carrying out the same functions. PMNs also play an important role in the immune response.

Eosinophils

Eosinophils are found in the loose connective tissue adjacent to mucosal surfaces, particularly in the gut, where they play an important role in the immune response. Eosinophils have a bilobed nucleus and a cytoplasm filled with granules containing basic proteins that stain intensely with eosin (an acidic stain). Though they exhibit phagocytic activity, phagocytosis is not considered one of their main functions. They release histamine-degrading enzymes at sites of high histamine concentration. For this reason, they are considered to play a role in allergic reactions. Eosinophils interact with immune system cytokines and with immunoglobulins. They are also involved with the late-phase reaction of the hypersensitivity response. In the case of parasitic infections, their numbers in the circulation and in connective tissue increase substantially. The protease contents of their granules are effective in killing a number of parasites, but the proteases also cause tissue destruction.

Mast Cells

Mast cells (MCs) are found in most loose connective tissue compartments. Mast cell precursors originate in the bone marrow and enter the circulation. Once their precursor leaves the circulation and enters a connective tissue compartment, it proliferates and differentiates into mature mast cells. They are the largest mononuclear cells of connective tissue; MCs are large, oval cells with a round to oval nucleus and a cytoplasm filled with darkly staining granules. The granules have high concentrations of glycosaminoglycans, particularly heparin (see previous discussion), as well as several proteases; consequently, the granules stain with basic dyes. Certain of these dyes undergo a color shift when they bind to the GAGs and hence are called *metachromatic* dyes. Mast cells are widely distributed in subepithelial connective tissues and loose (areolar) connective tissue. They are frequently found in association with blood vessels and nerves (Fig. 4-14).

Mast cells play an important role in allergic reactions, the immune response, and particularly in the *immediate reaction of hypersensitivity*. They are found in abundance in the stroma of the lung. They release a number of bioactive compounds and are therefore thought to play a significant role in bronchiolar asthma. They are also abundant in the lamina propria of the small intestines, other mucosal

---

IMMUNOLOGY

Plasma Cells and the Humoral Immune System

Plasma cells secrete different classes (or isotypes) of immunoglobulins depending on the different signals and mechanisms by which they are programmed in the immune system. Immunoglobulin G (IgG) is the prototypical molecule, since it was the first whose structure and functions were known; it is also the most abundant, being found in serum at a concentration of about 13.5 mg/dL. IgG might be regarded as the central structural and functional theme of the humoral immune system and the other isotypes as variations on this theme.

There are five classes of immunoglobulins: IgA, IgD, IgE, IgG, and IgM, each having a characteristic structure and physiologic function. Three are secreted (IgA, IgE, and IgG), and two are bound to the plasma cell membrane (IgD and IgM). There are complex genetic and molecular mechanisms that give rise to antibody diversity. These mechanisms are responsible for the programming and proliferation of antigen-specific B cells.

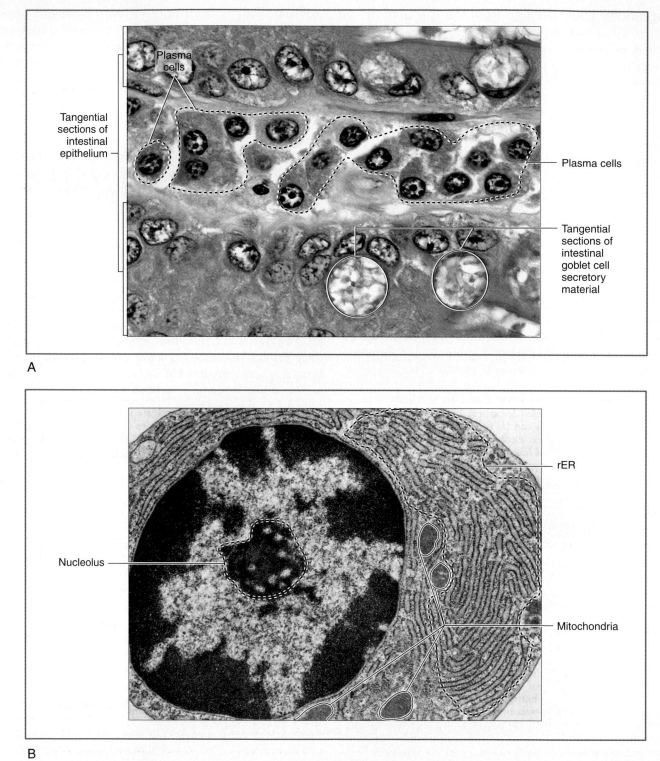

Figure 4-13. A, Light micrograph of plasma cells from the lamina propria of the intestines (H&E, 1500×). There are about 15 plasma cells in this field of view. Note the distinctive cartwheel pattern of chromatin in the nuclei—the light euchromatin, the dark heterochromatin, and a prominent nucleolus in the center of nearly every nucleus. **B,** Electron micrograph of a plasma cell. The nucleus shows the characteristic cartwheel distribution of chromatin and a prominent nucleolus. The cytoplasm is filled with many moderately dilated profiles of rER and several mitochondria. This section does not show the Golgi apparatus. (Courtesy of Don W. Fawcett.)

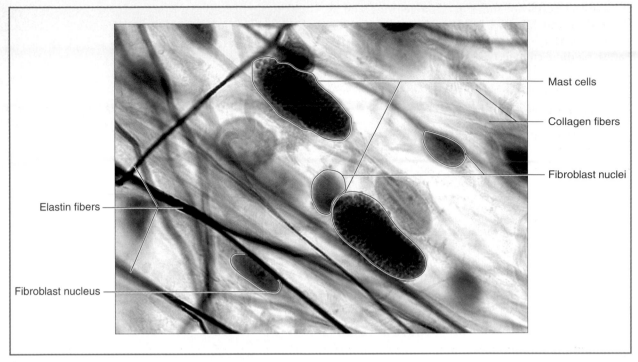

A

Mast cells

Collagen fibers

Fibroblast nuclei

Elastin fibers

Fibroblast nucleus

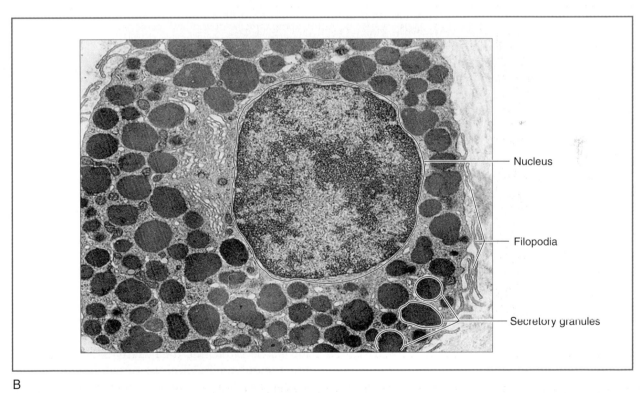

B

Nucleus

Filopodia

Secretory granules

Figure 4-14. **A,** Light micrograph of a spread of loose connective tissue with two prominent mast cells filled with refractile eosinophilic granules. **B,** Electron micrograph of a mast cell. The cytoplasm of the cell is filled with many electron-dense secretory granules; the plasma membrane has many filopodia. (From Abbas AK, Lichtman AH. *Cellular and Molecular Immunology*, 5th ed. Philadelphia, WB Saunders, 2005, p 438.)

locations, and the dermis of the skin. Mast cells (as well as basophils and eosinophils) are stimulated to release their granules when surface receptors (Fc receptors) are cross-linked after binding to IgE or to specific components of complement. Upon such activation, mast cells also secrete a number of lipid mediators of inflammation, which are synthesized de novo at the time of activation.

The degranulation of MCs occurs in an unusual manner. After receiving a degranulation signal, cytoplasmic secretory granules fuse with one another and then fuse with the plasma membrane, opening a large membrane-bounded secretory channel; this process is called *compound exocytosis*. After they degranulate, MCs are able to synthesize and accumulate new cytoplasmic granules. The mature cells have a prolif-erative capacity in the connective tissue. MCs persist for weeks to months in the loose connective tissues.

There are two subtypes of MCs. The two types are morphologically identical but differ in several ways. Human MC granules have high levels of heparin (a powerful anti-coagulant) and chondroitin sulfate proteoglycans, histamine (a potent vasodilator), more than 15 cytokines, plus a number of neutral proteases including tryptase and chymase. A major difference between the two types is that one type expresses both tryptase and chymase (MCTCs) and the other expresses only tryptase (MTCs). In rodents, in which mast cell (and basophil) biology have been studied extensively, mast cells display the same differences, plus others; one type is called a connective tissue mast cell (CTMC) and the other a mucosal mast cell (MMC). Mast cells have many important functions including a significant role in acquired immunity through the IgE-associated immune response.

Basophils

Basophils are the rarest of the circulating leukocytes, comprising less than 1% of all white cells. They are even rarer in connective tissue and are only found there after recruit-ment to the tissue in the case of inflammation. Their function and morphology are similar to those of mast cells, but they are not so widely distributed or so numerous. The granules of basophils contain chondroitin sulfate proteoglycans but not heparin. Basophils have proteases and a more limited number of cytokines than mast cells.

MUSCLE TISSUE

●●● GENERAL CHARACTERISTICS OF MUSCLE TISSUE

Muscle is the biological motor that provides humans with the power to move about, pump the blood around the body, support and control the movement of all the internal organs, and regulate blood pressure in the blood vessels. The molecular basis for all this movement resides in the two major muscle proteins, actin and myosin, which are organized into precisely structured filaments within muscle cells. These

---

IMMUNOLOGY

Hypersensitivity and the Immune Response

The granular leucocytes of connective tissue have a variety of functions, but each of them plays a role in the immune system:

- Mast cells have an important role in the immediate hypersensitivity response, since they rapidly release stored granule contents and newly synthesized lipid mediators of this response.
- Eosinophils and basophils, to the extent the latter are involved at all, are more part of the late-phase response.
- Mast cells exhibit a phenomenon called mast cell heterogeneity, which refers to their variable content of proteoglycans, proteases, various phenotypes, and varied tissue distribution. Nonetheless, their degranulation is an important part of the hypersensitivity response.

PATHOLOGY

Inflammation and Tissue Repair

The free cells of connective tissues (visitors) play an important role in inflammation and in tissue repair. Macrophages and PMNs are recruited from the circulation into connective tissue compartments during both acute and chronic phases of inflammation. Tissue repair is a complex process that begins with removal and degradation of foreign materials and of injured cells and tissue matrix. The above two visiting cells and the resident fibroblasts are central to the process of removal. The fibroblasts alone are then responsible for rebuilding the tissue matrix.

---

two proteins, in concert with many associated proteins, are responsible for the contraction of muscle cells.

Structurally there are two major types of muscle: striated and smooth. Striated muscle has two subtypes: skeletal and cardiac.

All three types of muscle cells are elongated and arranged in parallel arrays, or bundles. As such, they have a fibrous appearance in the light and electron microscopes. The cytoplasmic protein components of muscle are collectively called sarcoplasm. In addition to this muscle-specific name for muscle cytoplasm, other parts of the muscle cell often begin with "sarco"; these terms will be introduced as they arise. Owing to the parallel orientation of muscle cells, their length, and their physical properties, they are usually referred to as muscle fibers (or *myofibers*) rather than as muscle cells.

Major Contractile Proteins

The actin and myosin filaments generate the contractile force in the cell (and consequently, a whole muscle, the heart, an organ, the body) by sliding relative to one another. The energy to drive the sliding comes from ATP, and in broad terms the process is regulated by Ca^{++}, although the detailed regulatory mechanism differs in the three types of muscle. Nevertheless, in all three cases, an increase in cytoplasmic Ca^{++} stimulates contraction. The molecular organization of the contractile machinery is much greater in striated muscle than it is in smooth muscle. In skeletal and cardiac muscle, the filaments are organized into a sarcomere, which is the fundamental contractile unit.

Sarcomeres are made of thin (actin) filaments and thick (myosin) filaments. There are many other proteins in the sarcomere: some are structural, others participate in the contractile process, and still others are regulatory.

A sarcomere has three prominent striations oriented at right angles to the long axis of the myofiber:

The *A band* is rich in myosin thick filaments. It is a dark-staining part of the sarcomere in both light and electron microscopy. It is called the A band because when viewed with polarized light, it appears light or dark when the polarizers are crossed or uncrossed (i.e., it is *anisotropic*).

The *I band* is rich in actin thin filaments. It is the lightest staining part of the sarcomere in both light and electron microscopy. It is called the I band because its appearance does not change when viewed in polarized light with crossed or uncrossed polarizers (i.e., it is *isotropic*).

The *Z disk* or *Z line* is rich in α-actinin. It is the darkest staining part of the sarcomere in both light and electron microscopy. It bisects the A band; its name comes from the German word *Zwischenscheibe* meaning "between disks."

I Band Actin Thin Filaments

The I band thin filaments are about 6 nm in diameter and can be more than 1 μm long. The filaments are made of globular actin protein monomers (G-actin) that self-assemble into double helical actin filaments (F-actin); each filament contains thousands of actin monomers. The F-actin filaments have polarity (with a pointed end and a barbed end) because the G-actin molecules are all oriented in the same configuration in the F-actin filament. The barbed end is the rapidly growing end of the filament. The F-actin in a sarcomere is complexed with tropomyosin and a trimeric complex of troponins—troponin C (TnC), troponin I (TnI), and troponin T (TnT). In striated muscle, the pointed end of the filament is capped by a protein dimer called tropomodulin. A diagram of an actin thin filament is seen in Figure 4-15.

A Band Myosin Thick Filaments

The A band thick filaments are about 15 nm thick and 1.5 μm long. They are assembled from protein subunits into bipolar thick filaments. Thick filament subunits are hexameric proteins that have a long tail and a globular head. The hexamer has a molecular weight of 510 kD and contains two heavy chains (222 kD each) and four regulatory light chains (two 18 kD and two 22 kD). The two heavy chain tails form a coiled-coil α-helix that self-associates with other myosin tails to produce the bipolar myosin thick filament. Each myosin globular head has an ATP and an actin-binding site; each also binds two regulatory light chains.

Diagrams of a myosin thick filament and its assembly into bipolar filaments are seen in Figure 4-16. The myosin tails associate with one another such that the large globular actin-binding and ATP-binding heads are directed toward the opposite ends of the bipolar filament.

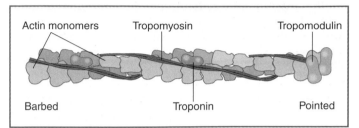

Figure 4-15. Diagram of an actin filament. The G-actin molecules assemble into a double helical filament. The thin filament is complexed with tropomyosin, a long fibrous molecule, and the troponin complex at about every seven dimer pairs of G-actin. The end of the filament is capped by tropomodulin.

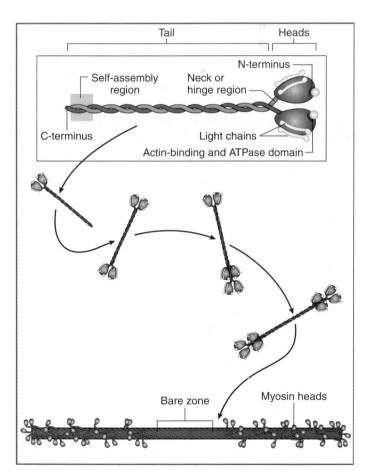

Figure 4-16. A myosin subunit is seen at the top of this diagram. The tails of the two heavy chains associate with each other to produce a double "lollypop-like" structure. The globular heads of each heavy chain bind an 18-kD and a 22-kD regulatory light chain. The fibrous tails self-assemble (in the middle part of the figure) to produce the bipolar thick filament (bottom of the figure). The central part of the bipolar filament (the bare zone) is free of globular heads; this is where the H band and M line are located.

●●● SKELETAL MUSCLE

The vast majority of skeletal muscle is connected to the skeleton, is under voluntary control, and is responsible for movement of the body. Skeletal muscle fibers are very thin, long cylinders. They range in diameter from 10 to 100 μm and can be tens of centimeters long. An individual skeletal myofiber is a multinucleate *syncytium*; during fetal life mesodermal cells differentiate into cells called myoblasts, which fuse to form myofibers. Myofiber nuclei are flattened oval organelles that are pressed into the inner aspect of the plasma membrane (*sarcolemma*) of the myofibers (i.e., the nuclei are peripherally located). All skeletal myofibers have a delicate basal lamina (also called an external lamina).

A small percentage (ca. 3% to 5%) of the nuclei seen near myofibers belong to satellite cells. These are undifferentiated mesenchymal (or stem) cells located between the basal lamina and the sarcolemma that can be stimulated to proliferate and differentiate into myoblasts and ultimately into myofibers following injury to a skeletal muscle. Skeletal muscle has a rich blood supply; a cross-section of a bundle of myofibers reveals many capillaries. Skeletal muscle can undergo exercise-induced or hormone-induced hypertrophy.

Skeletal Muscle Structure

Connective Tissue Sheaths

Skeletal muscles are invested with a set of connective tissue sheaths: epimysium, perimysium, and endomysium. Epimysium surrounds an entire muscle such as the sartorius muscle of the lower limb; it is equivalent to the term *deep fascia* in gross anatomic nomenclature. The muscle is subdivided into fascicles by the perimysium, and each individual myofiber is surrounded by a delicate connective tissue sheath of endomysium. Epimysium and perimysium range in character from dense irregular to loose connective tissue, and endomysium is loose connective tissue. These connective tissue sheaths permit the whole muscle and each of its smaller subdivisions to slide with respect to adjacent myofibers, fascicles, tissues, or organs. An entire muscle is connected to bone via a tendon (dense regular connective tissue). These connective tissue components of skeletal muscle allow it to serve its mechanochemical functions in moving limbs and body. Figure 4-17 shows the hierarchy of organization of skeletal muscle from an entire muscle down to individual myofilaments.

Innervation

Motor neurons that originate in the brainstem or the spinal cord innervate skeletal myofibers. Each myofiber has a nerve fiber ending (a *motor end plate* or *neuromuscular junction*) that can stimulate the myofiber to contract. A single spinal nerve branches and innervates a group of myofibers to create a *motor unit* that contracts more or less simultaneously. A motor unit may consist of as few as six myofibers, in the case of ocular muscles, to hundreds of myofibers in the case of back muscles. Each myofiber has only a single motor end plate, no matter how long it is. The motor end plate is a specialized structure that has many synaptic vesicles in the

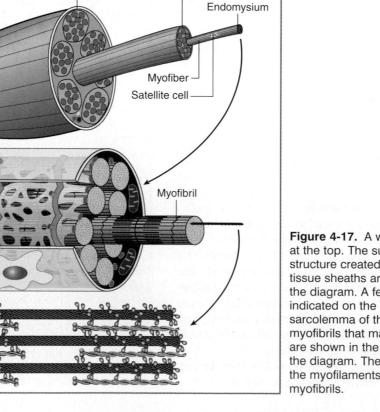

Figure 4-17. A whole muscle is shown at the top. The subdivisions of muscle structure created by the three connective tissue sheaths are shown in this part of the diagram. A few satellite cells are indicated on the surface of the sarcolemma of the myofiber. The myofibrils that make up each myofiber are shown in the middle part of the diagram. The lower part shows the myofilaments that comprise the myofibrils.

neuronal ending; the neurotransmitter in the vesicles is acetylcholine (ACh). The myofiber sarcolemma in close proximity to the motor end plate is highly folded (*junctional folds*) to increase surface area and hence the speed and efficiency of the stimulus. A delicate basal lamina is associated with the entire structure. A diagram of a motor end plate and light and electron micrographs of this structure are seen in Figure 4-18.

A specialized structure called a *muscle spindle* provides sensory innervation to the myofibers. These are complex structures containing several types of nerve fibers (Fig. 4-19).

Sections of skeletal muscle are seen in Figure 4-20. A cross-section of a portion of an entire small muscle is seen in Figure 4-20A. The three connective tissue sheaths and a number of myofibers are seen in this specimen. Figures 4-20B and 4-20C show myofibers from the tongue (one of the few locations in the body where skeletal muscle is not attached to bone) in both transverse and longitudinal section. Figure 4-20D shows longitudinal sections of a few skeletal myofibers stained with a trichrome stain. The cross-striations of the myofibers and details of sarcomere structure are evident in Figures 4-20B to 4-20D.

Sarcomere Structure

Cross-striations are part of the sarcomeres of striated muscle; a sarcomere is about 2.5 μm long. The fine details of the sarcomere are clearly seen in Figure 4-21. Here, a medium-power micrograph shows a large number of sarcomeres aligned into myofibrils; a single nucleus is seen at the periphery of a myofiber. Figure 4-21B, a high magnification of a sarcomere, shows many of its fine details. The sarcomere is bounded by two dark lines: the Z lines. Between and adjacent to the Z lines are two lighter staining regions, each is one-half of the I band—the thin actin filaments. The wide, dark-staining band in the middle of the sarcomere is the A band—the thick myosin filaments. The many profiles of membrane vesicles are visible in Figure 4-21A; these are the membranes of the *sarcoplasmic reticulum* (the sER of muscle cells), which store large amounts of calcium ions. These membranes occupy much of the space between and along myofibrils.

More details of the sarcomere are seen in diagrammatic form in Figure 4-22. This figure shows somewhat more than two sarcomeres to give a better impression of overall sarcomere structure as well as highlight the structure and function of some of the other proteins in the sarcomere. The sarcomere does its work in contracting muscles by coupling the hydrolysis of ATP with the sliding of I band actin filaments along and toward the bare zone of the A bands. This shortens each sarcomere by about one micron; the coordinated shortening of thousands of sarcomeres in many myofibers results in the contraction of an entire muscle. During contraction, the sarcomeres thicken somewhat, but the individual actin and myosin filaments (I bands and A bands) stay the same length.

The lateral boundaries of a sarcomere are the dark-staining Z lines (or Z disks—in three dimensions). The Z disk is a complex structure containing many proteins; a major one is α-actinin. The actin thin filaments of the half–I band are anchored to the Z disk and capped at their free ends with tropomodulin. A protein called nebulin is also anchored to the Z disk and is associated with the actin thin filaments; it is a nonelastic protein and is thought to help maintain actin filament attachment to the Z disk. The A band is made of myosin thick filaments; the central region of the A band is free of the globular heads, so it is somewhat narrower than the ends. A distinct substructure in this region is seen best in the electron microscope. A lighter staining region called the H band (German, *Hell*, "light") is bisected by a narrow line called the M line (German, *mitte*, "middle"). A number of proteins are associated with the H band and M line; these proteins help maintain A band structure by keeping the myosin molecules in register. One of them, titin, a very high molecular weight elastic protein (2500 kD), is connected to the Z disk and to the M line. Titin helps keep the A band centered in the sarcomere during contraction and also provides the passive resistance of relaxed muscle to stretching.

Calcium Regulation of Sarcoplasmic Contraction

The contraction process is regulated by the concentration of Ca^{++} in the sarcoplasm. The diagram in Figure 4-23 helps explain how this process works. The sarcoplasmic reticulum (SR) is extensive and is wrapped around each column of myofibrils. Near each of the A-I junctions, the cisternae of the SR are dilated. The sarcolemma is invaginated over its entire

Text continued on page 115

PATHOLOGY

Duchenne's Muscular Dystrophy

The most common form of muscular dystrophy is an X-linked type called Duchenne's muscular dystrophy. The defect involves a protein called dystrophin. One end of this protein binds to the actin thin filaments of the sarcomere near their attachments to the Z lines and the other end to two transmembrane glycoproteins of the sarcolemma—dystroglycan and sarcoglycan. Dystroglycan binds to an extracellular adhesion protein, α_2-laminin, which in turn binds to the basal lamina of the myofiber.

The disease occurs with a frequency of about one in 3500 live male births. It usually becomes evident at 4 to 5 years of age. It is manifested as a general muscle weakness. The defective dystrophin does not anchor the sarcomere to the sarcolemma and hence to the extracellular matrix. This deficient anchoring and consequent deficient interface between the contractile apparatus and the extracellular matrix leads to muscle atrophy. The myofibers become irregular in diameter and fewer in number and have increased endomysial connective tissue and many regenerating myofibers. In time, the rate of degeneration of the myofibers exceeds the replacement rate. More connective tissue and adipose tissue fill in the volume formerly occupied by the myofibers. As the respiratory muscles of the chest and the diaphragm weaken, the individual dies of respiratory failure.

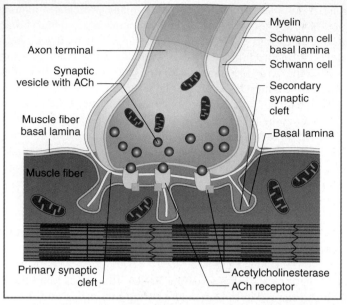

Myelin
Schwann cell basal lamina
Schwann cell
Axon terminal
Synaptic vesicle with ACh
Secondary synaptic cleft
Muscle fiber basal lamina
Basal lamina
Muscle fiber
Primary synaptic cleft
Acetylcholinesterase
ACh receptor

A

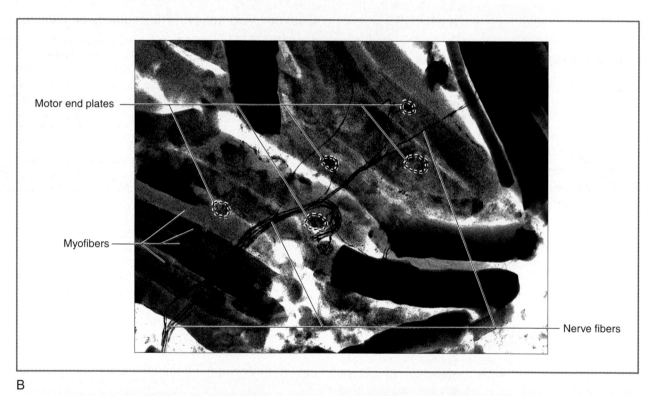

Motor end plates

Myofibers

Nerve fibers

B

Figure 4-18. A, A synaptic ending as it makes contact with a small depression of a myofiber in an area called a synaptic cleft. The surface of the sarcolemma is expanded owing to a large number of folds called junctional folds. A delicate basal lamina is associated with the synaptic ending and all the junctional folds. Many vesicles are present in the synaptic ending, which contains the neurotransmitter ACh. **B,** A motor unit at the light microscopic level (100×). Terminal branches of a nerve fiber are seen with their synaptic endings (six or more) touching individual myofibers.

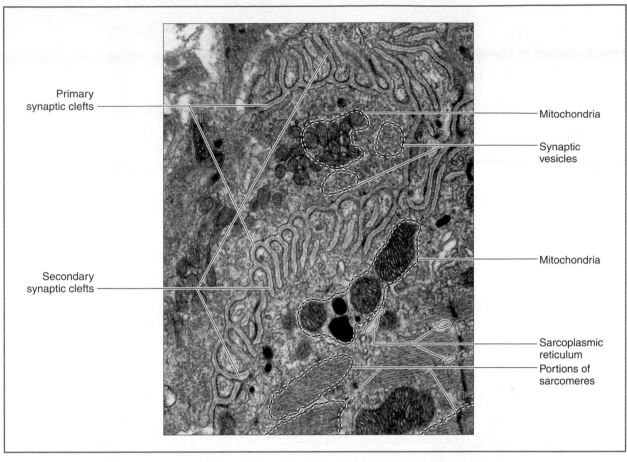

C

Figure 4-18 cont'd. C, Electron micrograph (51,000×) of a motor end plate. Several of the main features of a neuromuscular junction are labeled: the primary and secondary synaptic clefts, many (but not all) synaptic vesicles, much of the sarcoplasmic reticulum, and parts of a few sarcomeres; several mitochondria are seen in synaptic endings and myofibers. (Courtesy of Patricia Cross, Stanford University School of Medicine.)

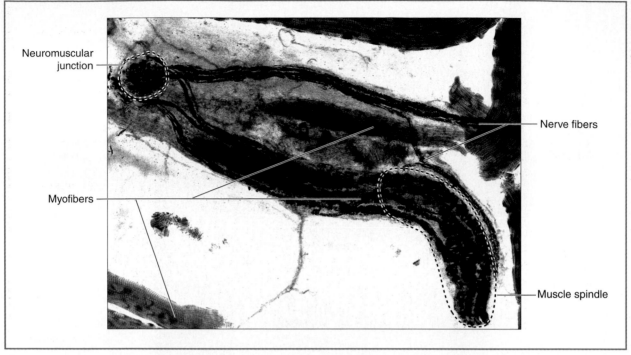

Neuromuscular junction

Nerve fibers

Myofibers

Muscle spindle

A

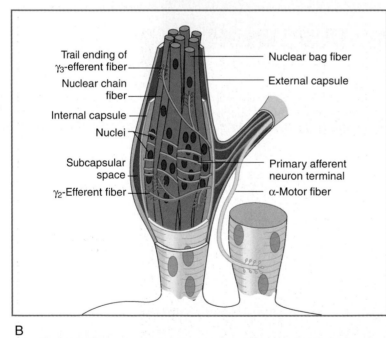

Trail ending of γ₃-efferent fiber

Nuclear chain fiber

Internal capsule

Nuclei

Subcapsular space

γ₂-Efferent fiber

Nuclear bag fiber

External capsule

Primary afferent neuron terminal

α-Motor fiber

B

Figure 4-19. A, Light micrograph of a muscle spindle (160×); the nerve fibers are stained dark brownish-black. **B,** Diagram of a muscle spindle as it would be seen in an electron micrograph; this complex structure is difficult to interpret in light or electron micrographs.

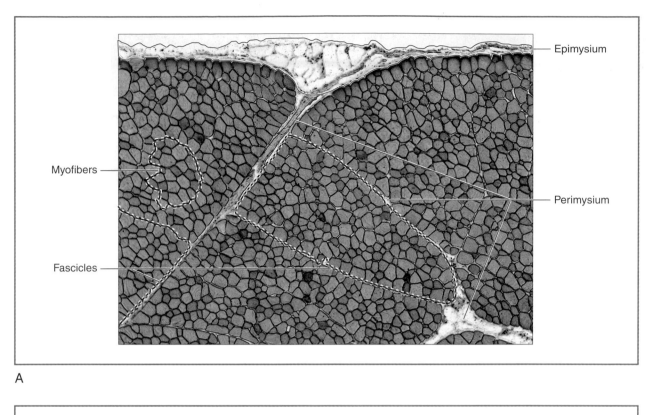

A

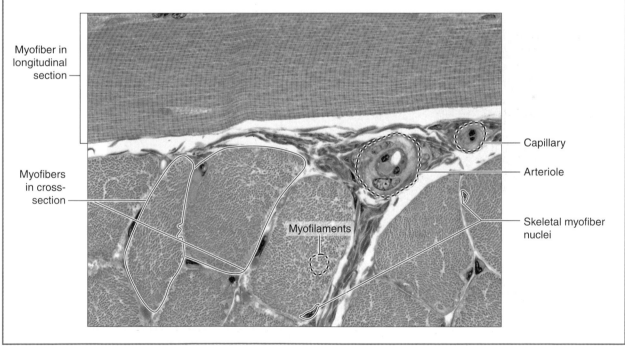

B

Figure 4-20. Sections of skeletal muscle. **A,** H&E stain of a portion of an entire small skeletal muscle (62.5×). The epimysium is seen only partially, but the other two connective tissue sheaths and many myofibers are seen; the myofibers are clearly grouped into fascicles by the perimysium. **B,** Iron hematoxylin stain of skeletal myofibers from the tongue (440×); this is a semi-thin section (1.5 µm) using modern fixatives, which minimizes tissue shrinkage. The sarcomeres, A bands, and I bands are seen in the longitudinally sectioned myofibers. The small dots in the transversely sectioned myofibers are individual myofibrils.

Continued

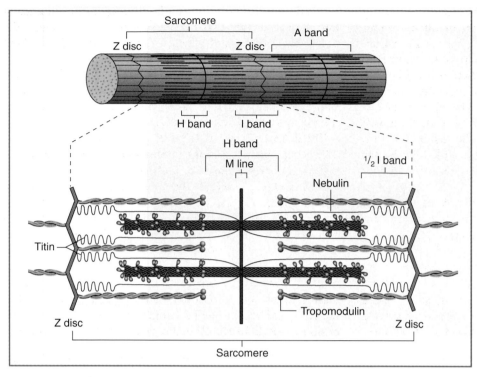

Figure 4-22. Diagram of a sarcomere.

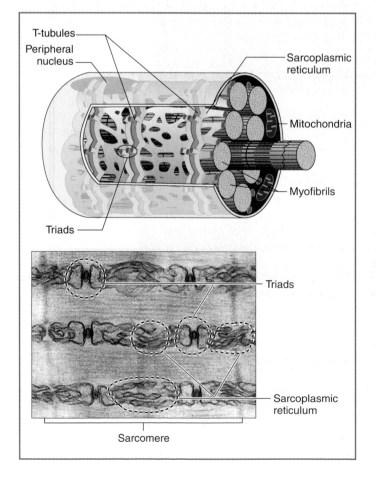

Figure 4-23. In this three-dimensional diagram of a single myofiber, a number of myofibrils are shown in association with the sarcoplasmic reticulum and T tubules of the sarcolemma. Note that the T tubules are seen at each A-I region of the sarcomere. The inset is an electron micrograph of T tubules from frog skeletal muscle, which clearly illustrates the appearance and position of the triads. (Inset courtesy of Don W. Fawcett.)

surface by small tubules that are oriented transversely along the length of the myofiber; they dip into the myofiber in close proximity to the myofibrils at the level of the A-I junction. The tubular invaginations are called *T tubules*; their lumen is extracellular. When the SR and T tubules are sectioned in an appropriate plane and examined in the electron microscope, these membranous structures appear as a triad (see inset in Fig. 4-23). The T tubule is in the center of the triad; the two outer parts of the triad are the dilated SR cisternae. Thus, each sarcomere has two sets of triads associated with it; this facilitates rapid and efficient contraction of the myofiber following neuronal stimulus.

When a myofiber is stimulated by the release of ACh at the motor end plate, the sarcolemma undergoes a rapid wave of depolarization along the length of the myofiber. The depolarization is delivered to the internal regions of the cylindrical myofiber by the T-tubule system. As the depolarization passes along the T tubules, Ca^{++}, stored in the SR, is released from the SR. This rapid increase in Ca^{++} in the sarcoplasm initiates a cascade of molecular events in which the actin filaments of the half–I band bind to the globular head of the myosin filaments of the A band; ATP is hydrolyzed by the myosin ATPase, and the actin filaments slide, ratchet fashion, toward the middle of the A band, shortening (contracting) the sarcomere as well as causing a slight increase in the diameter of the myofibrils. The Ca^{++} in the sarcoplasm is taken up quickly by the SR so that another contraction cycle can occur.

●●● CARDIAC MUSCLE STRUCTURE

Cardiac muscle is found only in the heart. Cardiac myofibers and skeletal myofibers look similar because they both have essentially the same sarcomeric organization of their contractile apparatus. Furthermore, it is not practically possible to distinguish atrial from ventricular cardiac myofibers at the microscopic level. Nonetheless, a number of features make distinguishing one from the other rather easy. Some of the features are evident in the light microscope while others can only be seen with the electron microscope.

The nuclei of cardiac muscle fibers are centrally located; there are one or two nuclei per fiber. About half of cardiac myofibers have two nuclei; this estimate is based on stereologic analysis of serial sections of cardiac muscle. Cardiac muscle has significantly more connective tissue per unit area than does skeletal muscle, but the connective tissue is not organized into layers of epimysium, perimysium, and endomysium. This difference in connective tissue content is most evident in trichrome stains of both muscle types. Because of the curving, almost helical, nature of cardiac myofiber bundles, it is common to see myofibers in many planes of section in a single field. Cardiac myocytes produce their own thin basal lamina.

Cardiac myofibers have a full complement of cell organelles; most are located in the perinuclear region. Cardiac myofibers have many more mitochondria and glycogen particles associated with their sarcomeres than do skeletal myofibers. The myofibers have a branching or step-like appearance; their

squared-off ends meet one another to give the appearance of longer muscle fibers. Where the squared-off ends meet, the cells have complex cell junctions that are visible in the light microscope; they are called *intercalated disks*.

Figure 4-24 shows two light micrographs of cardiac muscle. The branching structure of cardiac myocytes can be difficult to discern and can be better appreciated by comparing micrographs of skeletal and cardiac muscle.

The details of intercalated disk structure are seen in Figure 4-25. The appearance of the intercalated disk is similar to the zonula adherens of epithelial cells except the junction is more sheet-like; hence, it is called a fascia adherens. In addition to providing end-to-end cell adhesion, the fascia adherens serves as an attachment surface for actin thin filaments. As seen in Figure 4-25A, the intercalated disk extends to the lateral margins of the myofibers. The lateral parts of the intercalated disk are rich in gap junctions, which facilitate electrical communication between the cardiac myofibers. Desmosomes are also found along the intercalated disk interface and on the lateral margins near the gap junctions; desmosomes help stabilize the end-to-end and lateral cell adhesions.

The sarcoplasmic reticulum of cardiac myofibers is less extensive than that of skeletal myofibers. Cardiac myofibers also have a system of T tubules, but the tubular invaginations occur at the level of the Z line of the sarcomere. This results in a similar physiologic mechanism for carrying contraction signals to the interior of the myofiber as in skeletal muscle. Figure 4-26 shows a diagram of the organization of the T-tubule system of cardiac muscle as well as the other features of cardiac myocytes.

Contractile Properties of Cardiac Myocytes

Cardiac myocytes have an intrinsic ability to contract; this is evident from experiments in which dissociated cardiac myocytes are placed in tissue culture dishes. They proliferate and contract synchronously under appropriate culture conditions.

In the intact heart, the contractions are initiated, locally regulated, and coordinated by modified cardiac myocytes that are organized into specialized *pacemaker nodes* (the sinoatrial node, the atrioventricular node, and the bundle of His) and groups of other cells called Purkinje cells (Fig. 4-27). Physiologically, the rate of cardiac contraction is regulated by sympathetic and parasympathetic innervation that terminates in the nodes. Sympathetic stimulation accelerates heart rate, and parasympathetic stimulation slows heart rate.

●●● SMOOTH MUSCLE STRUCTURE

Smooth muscle myofibers are found in many parts of the body, sometimes as single myofibers but more often as clusters of a few dozen or larger masses of myofibers supporting the walls of many of the tubular or hollow organs of the body. Smooth muscle myofibers are responsible for

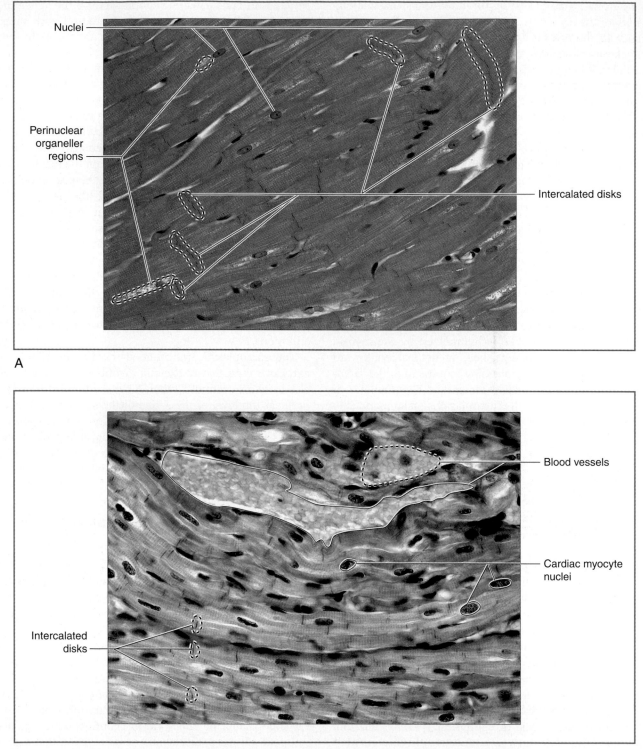

A

B

Figure 4-24. **A,** Several features of cardiac muscle are seen in this iron hematoxylin stain (210×); there are numerous intercalated disks, the striations of the myofibers are clearly evident, the centrally placed nuclei (with prominent nucleoli) are seen, and organelles are seen at the poles of the nuclei. **B,** Specimen of cardiac muscle stained with H&E (360×); many of the same features in part A can be seen in this micrograph. A small blood vessel, in oblique section, is seen in the upper center of the field.

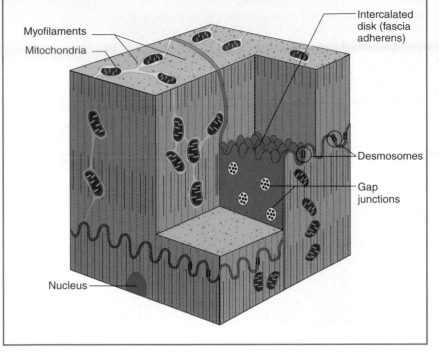

A

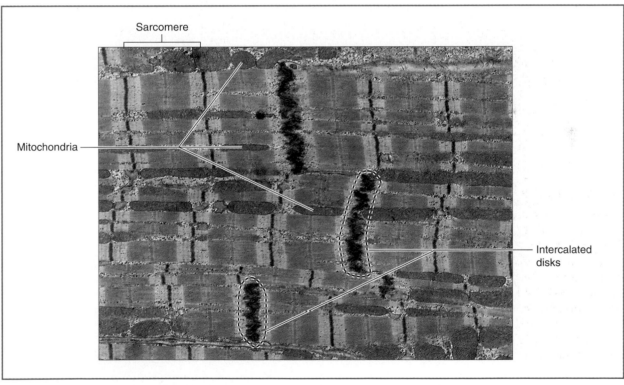

B

Figure 4-25. A, Diagram showing the centrally placed nucleus, abundance of mitochondria, end-to-end structure of the intercalated disks, and nonuniform diameter and shape of the myofibril bundles. **B** and **C,** These two electron micrographs of cardiac muscle show its main ultrastructural features. Part B is a medium-power micrograph of portions of several cardiac myocytes. Part C is a high-power magnification of an intercalated disk that shows the fine structure of the fascia adherens and the gap junctions of the lateral margins of the cell. Note that the I bands terminate in the fascia adherens. (Part C from Pollard TD, Earnshaw WC. *Cell Biology*. Philadelphia, WB Saunders, 2004, p 665.)

Continued

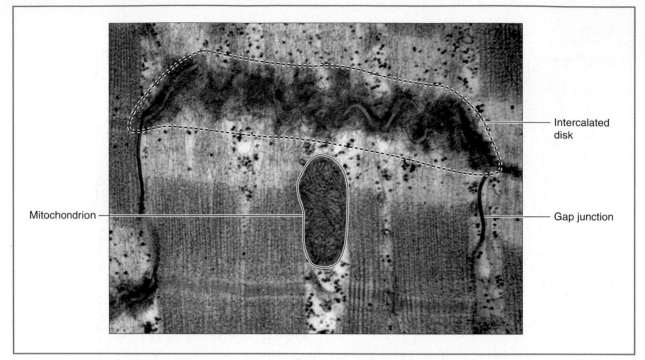

C

Figure 4-25 cont'd.

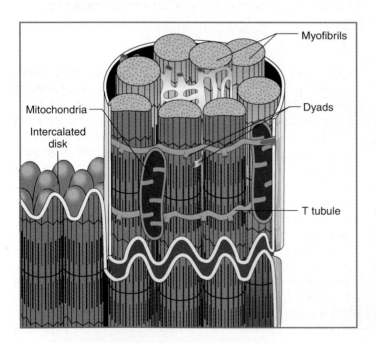

Figure 4-26. Diagram of part of a cardiac myocyte showing the organization of the sarcoplasmic reticulum with respect to the sarcomere and the T tubules of this cell. The T tubules of cardiac muscle have a larger diameter than those found in skeletal muscle and they are found at the level of the Z lines of the sarcomeres. Furthermore, the sarcoplasmic reticulum of cardiac myocytes is less extensive than is found in skeletal muscle. Therefore, the typical ultrastructural appearance of this membrane system is that of two membranous structures and is called a dyad. Other characteristics of cardiac myocytes seen in this diagram are an intercalated disk, mitochondria, and the nonuniform shapes of cardiac myocyte myofibrils. (Redrawn from Standring S. *Gray's Anatomy*, 39th ed. Philadelphia, Churchill-Livingstone, 2005, p 151.)

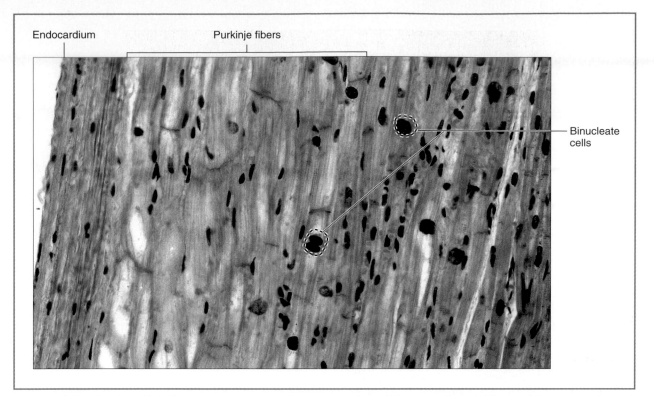

Endocardium   Purkinje fibers

Binucleate cells

Figure 4-27. H&E stain of Purkinje fibers close to the endocardial surface of the heart (180×). These cells are specialized cardiac myocytes and retain scant remnants of sarcomeres in their cytoplasm. Their cytoplasm appears empty in most micrographs, since it is rich in glycogen, a substance that does not fix well and is washed out of the cell during processing. There are two binucleate Purkinje fibers in this field of view.

relatively minor motile behavior such as hair "standing on end" and more major and physiologically significant motility such as the peristaltic movement of the hollow organs in the gastrointestinal system and male reproductive system, regulation of blood flow through much of the vascular system, the patency of a large proportion of the air-conducting system of the lung, and the expulsive actions of the urinary bladder, gallbladder, and the uterus during childbirth. Like striated muscle cells, smooth muscle cells synthesize and secrete a basal (external) lamina of type IV collagen and a small amount of delicate connective tissue and elastin fibers.

When viewed in the light microscope, smooth muscle cells are elongated, spindle-shaped cells with a single, centrally placed, cigar-shaped nucleus. Their cytoplasm is filled with high concentrations of actin and myosin that are not organized into arrays like the sarcomeres of skeletal or cardiac muscle; hence, the sarcoplasm has a uniform (or smooth) appearance when stained with most stains. Smooth muscle cells have a much higher ratio of actin to myosin than that found in the other two types of muscle. They have a small number of typical cell organelles located in the peri-nuclear region at the poles of the elongated nuclei. Figure 4-28 illustrates the appearance of smooth muscle sectioned transversely and longitudinally with three different stains.

The homogeneous character of smooth muscle cells is also evident in the electron microscope. The cytoplasm is packed with actin thin filaments and myosin II filaments. Dense plaques are seen along the sarcolemma and dense bodies in the cytoplasm. These electron-dense structures are rich in α-actinin; they serve as attachment sites for actin filaments and are therefore analogous to the Z disks of striated muscle. Myosin filaments are also oriented along these thin filaments, producing sarcomere-like cytoplasmic arrays of actomyosin complexes. It is common to find gap junctions between adjacent smooth muscle cells; these junctions serve to synchronize the contraction of the interconnected cells. However, not all smooth muscle cells are electrically coupled by gap junctions. The plasma membrane of a smooth muscle cell has a large number of vesicles called caveolae. These vesicles resemble pinocytotic vesicles and may have a role in increasing surface area to facilitate Ca^{++} entry into the cells. It is difficult to see the myosin chains of smooth muscle in the electron microscope unless the cells are extracted with mild detergents or labeled with appropriate antibodies. Smooth muscle myosin is a different isoform of myosin II than that found in striated muscle. Three electron micrographs and a diagram of smooth muscle are seen in Figure 4-29.

Contraction of Smooth Muscle and Its Regulation

Bundles of smooth muscle contract in waves. The waves are evident as curves of wavy cells and nuclei. In some cases, as

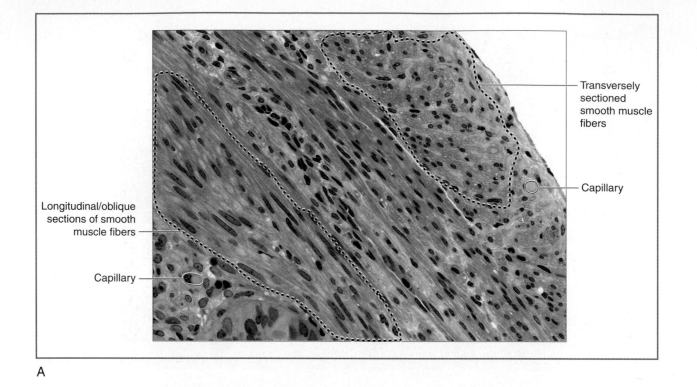

A

Transversely
sectioned
smooth muscle
fibers

Capillary

Longitudinal/oblique
sections of smooth
muscle fibers

Capillary

B

Figure 4-28. A, H&E stain of a semi-thin section of the muscular wall of a monkey oviduct (360×). The smooth muscle fibers in the outer layer of the wall are sectioned transversely, and the fibers in the inner layer are sectioned longitudinally or transversely. **B,** Milligan's trichrome stain of the muscular wall of the small intestine (250×). The plasma membrane and basal lamina of the fibers are seen to advantage in the transversely sectioned fibers. In these same fibers, the slight variation of the diameter of the nuclei is an indication of the cigar-shaped organelle—the smaller profiles are near the tapered ends of the organelle and the largest profiles are sections through the central part of the organelle. Many of the longitudinally sectioned nuclei have prominent nucleoli. The bright red material in this specimen is red blood cells.

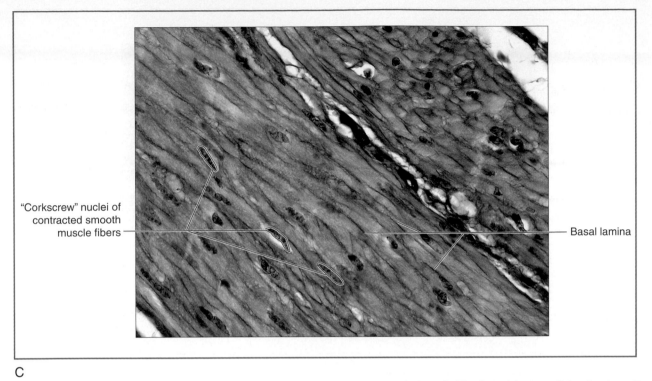

"Corkscrew" nuclei of contracted smooth muscle fibers

Basal lamina

C

Figure 4-28 cont'd. **C,** PAS-stained section of the muscular wall of the stomach (400×). The basal (external) lamina is well stained in this specimen. A number of nuclei of contracted smooth muscle fibers are clearly seen.

the contracted smooth muscle cell becomes shorter, thicker, and folded in accordion-like fashion, the nucleus acquires a twisted or corkscrew-like shape. Contracted cells are recognized by these characteristics. Figure 4-30 illustrates the appearance of a contracted smooth muscle cell in a diagram and in two sections of the wall of the stomach. Smooth muscle cells contract more slowly than striated muscle cells, yet they generate the same force as contracted striated muscle and can sustain the contracted state for prolonged periods.

Since smooth muscle cells do not have a sarcoplasmic reticulum or T-tubule system, the transient increases in cytoplasmic Ca^{++} concentration occur by a rapid uptake of extracellular Ca^{++} by the sarcolemma. The F-actin filaments of smooth muscle cells have tropomyosin bound to them, but instead of the troponin complex, they bind two other regulatory proteins—caldesmon and calponin—which interact with Ca^{++} to initiate contraction. The myosin II molecules of smooth muscle are much longer and thinner than the myosin II found in sarcomeres; this is thought to be a key feature of the sustained force generation in smooth muscle.

The physiologic factors that regulate smooth muscle contraction are more complex than those regulating skeletal and cardiac muscle contraction. Sympathetic and parasympathetic nerves of the autonomic nervous system usually initiate contraction of smooth muscle cells. Various hormones such as oxytocin, epinephrine, and norepinepherine also stimulate contraction. Smooth muscle plasma membranes have receptors for adrenergic or cholinergic ligands or one of the hormonal ligands; the kind and number of receptors differ in different anatomic locations, so the same ligand may or may not stimulate contraction depending on the type and location of the smooth muscle.

Smooth Muscle–like Cells

There are a number of locations where cells have characteristics of epithelial cells *and* smooth muscle cells, or of fibroblasts *and* smooth muscle cells. In the former case, the cells are called myoepithelial cells, and in the latter, myofibroblasts. The secretory cells of a number of glands (e.g., mammary glands, apocrine sweat glands, some of the salivary glands) have myoepithelial cells associated with them. The perineurium and certain cells in the aqueous outflow channel of the eye (the canal of Schlemm) are two locations that have myofibroblasts. These features will be identified as they arise in later chapters.

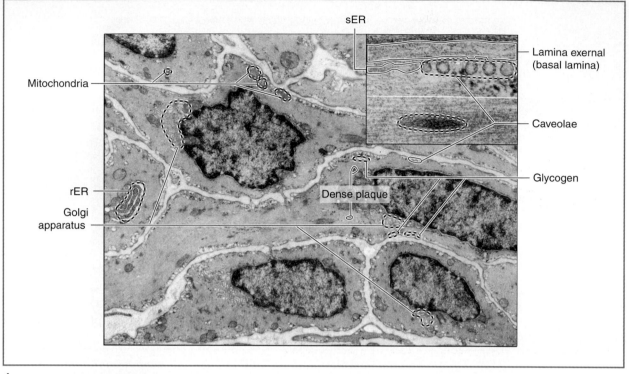

sER

Mitochondria

Lamina exernal (basal lamina)

Caveolae

Glycogen

rER

Golgi apparatus

Dense plaque

A

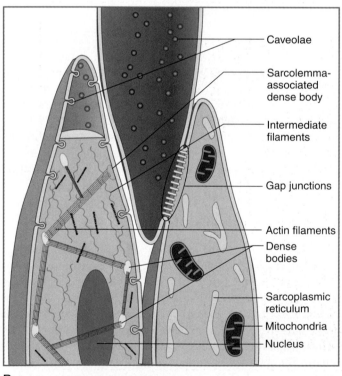

Caveolae

Sarcolemma-associated dense body

Intermediate filaments

Gap junctions

Actin filaments

Dense bodies

Sarcoplasmic reticulum

Mitochondria

Nucleus

B

Figure 4-29. **A,** Electron micrograph of smooth muscle cells in the wall of the ductus deferens (13,000×). Some of the myocytes are sectioned transversely and others in oblique-longitudinal section. Note the many labeled cell organelles (mitochondria, rER, sER, Golgi, mitochondria, glycogen granules) and the many caveolae (pinocytotic vesicles) that are found in abundance near the smooth muscle cell plasma membrane. The cytoplasm is filled with myofilaments, almost entirely actin-tropomyosin thin filaments; myosin thick filaments, which are not discernible in these micrographs; and a number of dense bodies or plasma membrane plaques, which serve as attachment sites for the contractile proteins. The insets (both 90,000×) show several features in greater detail. The upper one shows caveolae, a profile of sER, and some glycogen granules. The lower one shows a dense body and cytoplasmic myofilaments near it. (Courtesy of Judith Taggert Rhodin.) **B,** Major ultrastructural features of smooth muscle fibers. The part of the cell depicted at left shows the nucleus, the cytoplasmic dense bodies and sarcolemma-associated dense plaques, and the myofilaments that interconnect them. The parts of the two cells at right illustrate the caveolae in the sarcolemma, gap junctions between cells, and the scant sarcoplasmic reticulum in the cytoplasm.

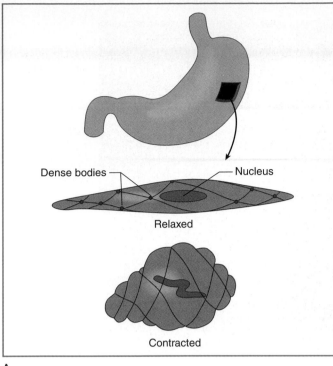

Dense bodies — Nucleus

Relaxed

Contracted

A

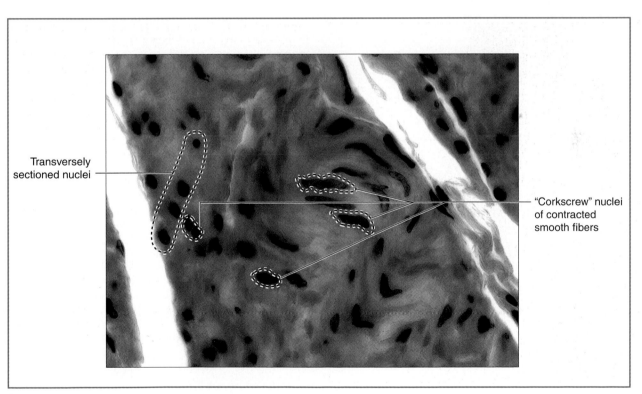

Transversely
sectioned nuclei

"Corkscrew" nuclei
of contracted
smooth fibers

B

Figure 4-30. A, Diagrammatic representation of a noncontracted and a contracted smooth muscle cell. The two insets show what contracted smooth muscle cells and their nuclei look like. **B,** High-magnification (H&E, 630×) section of a small bundle of smooth muscle fibers from the wall of the stomach. Although not much of the detail of the cytoplasm is visible, numerous corkscrew-shaped nuclei are seen as well as curved nuclei of cells in different states of contraction.

Continued

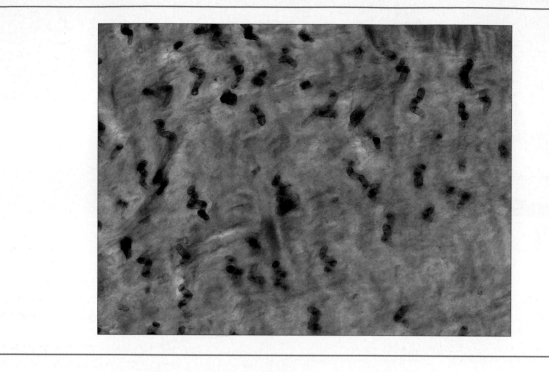

C

Figure 4-30 cont'd. C, Another group of contracted smooth muscle cells (H&E, 630×).

Cartilage and Bone 5

●●● GENERAL CHARACTERISTICS OF CARTILAGE

Cartilage is one of the two forms of connective tissue specialized to function as a supporting or weight-bearing tissue, bone being the other. There are three types of cartilage: hyaline, elastic, and fibrocartilage. Hyaline cartilage is the most abundant and has important roles during fetal development, postnatal growth and development, and in the adult. Because of this, most of our understanding of cartilage structure and function is based on hyaline cartilage. All three types of cartilage have many similarities but are differentiated by their matrix appearance and composition.

Hyaline cartilage has a matrix rich in proteoglycan aggregates and type II collagen. It is found in the fetus as the "models" from which most of the long bones of the body develop. In the adult, the articular surfaces of bone are covered with hyaline cartilage, the larger airway passages in the respiratory system are supported by rings and plates of hyaline cartilage, and the main supporting material of the nose is hyaline cartilage.

Elastic cartilage matrix also has proteoglycan aggregates and type II collagen plus significant quantities of elastin fibers. It is found in the epiglottis, parts of the auditory system (the external acoustic meatus and parts of the eustachian tubes), and in the pinnae of the ears.

Fibrocartilage is a mixture of dense regular connective tissue and small amounts of cartilage matrix. It is found in intervertebral disks and a number of specialized joints.

Cartilage has the properties of a firm, somewhat rubbery, resilient gel. In the living state, hyaline cartilage is bluish-white with a slight glassy translucence. In fixed and stained preparations, its matrix has an amorphous appearance. Cartilage is somewhat pliable, but when it is subjected to too much stress or to trauma, it will fracture. This can cause serious problems, since cartilage does not have the capacity to regenerate or "heal." Cracks fill in with fibrous connective tissue, much like a scar, and the mass of cartilage will malfunction for the remainder of life.

A distinctive characteristic of cartilage is that it is completely avascular, or more specifically, it lacks a microvascular (capillary) blood supply. This means that all nutrients have to diffuse through the matrix to the cartilage cells (chondrocytes), and waste materials have to diffuse out in order to sustain the vital functions of the chondrocytes. The physico-chemical properties of the firm cartilage matrix, with its high water content and high anionic charge, facilitate this diffusion. Like all components of connective tissue matrix, cartilage matrix undergoes metabolic turnover; the half-life of hyaline cartilage is on the order of 1 to 2 months.

The matrix of hyaline cartilage contains a high concentration of proteoglycan (aggrecan) molecules. Each aggrecan has a molecular weight of $3–5 \times 10^6$ Da, of which over 99% of the mass is the chondroitin sulfate and keratan sulfate chains. One hundred or more aggrecan molecules are noncovalently bound to very long molecules of hyaluronic acid to form enormous macromolecular complexes; a single complex

Degeneration of Articular Cartilage—Osteoarthritis

Many individuals experience degeneration of the hyaline cartilage on the epiphyseal surfaces of many bones. The degeneration can occur in the third decade of life or in later years. It may be due to a pathologic processes or to trauma. One of the pathologic changes that leads to osteoarthritis is loss of hyaline cartilage at the articular surface and death of chondrocytes. As a result of this erosion, the low-friction, protective surface of hyaline cartilage on the epiphyseal end of the bone will crack or erode. Since cartilage is a tissue that does not regenerate, the damaged areas fill in with type I collagen fibers, forming a kind of fibrocartilage scar or plug. Further erosion leads to exposed bone, local bone thickening, vascularization, and formation of new bone in place of the articular cartilage. Traumatic injury (a rather common situation in the knee joints of professional athletes) to articular surfaces may result in small pieces of hyaline cartilage breaking free and floating in the synovial space. Arthroscopic surgery may alleviate the immediate problems associated with this sort of injury, but ultimately the articular surface degenerates in a manner similar to that described above.

Biosynthesis of Proteoglycans

The proteoglycans of cartilage (aggrecans) are large molecules; an individual aggrecan has a molecular weight (MW) of about one million Daltons. It consists of a core protein (MW ca. 200 kD) to which are covalently attached a small number of keratan sulfate (KS) chains (MW of each is ca. 15 kD) and a larger number (50–100) of chondroitin sulfate (CS) chains (MW of each is ca. 20–50 kD). These molecules are synthesized on and within the cisternae of the endoplasmic reticulum as follows:

- The core protein is synthesized on the rER in the same manner as all proteins destined for secretion from the cell.
- The core protein has a high proportion of serine residues.
- As the protein passes through the rER cisternae, many of the serine residues are modified by posttranslational glycosylation.
- The sugars are added to the protein one at a time.
- Addition of the sugars begins in the rER, continues in the sER, and is completed in the Golgi apparatus.
- The first sugar added is the pentose xylose, followed by two galactose moieties, and then by alternating residues of D-glucuronic acid and N-acetylgalactosamine.
- The biosynthetic precursor of all the sugars in the KS and CS chains is UDP-sugars.
- Each of the UDP sugars is synthesized from UDP-glucose in the cytosol.
- As the KS and CS chains reach their full length, which occurs in the Golgi apparatus, they become sulfated.
- In the case of CS, it is the N-acetylgalactosamine that becomes sulfated in the C4 or the C6 position.
- If the carbon-4 atom becomes sulfated, chain growth is terminated.
- The completed aggrecan molecules are released into the extracellular space from large secretory vesicles that bud off the *trans* face of the Golgi apparatus.
- Many aggrecans bind to hyaluronic acid in the extracellular matrix to produce the full space-filling, hydrated proteoglycan aggregate.

of this type can be much larger (on the order of 40 μm) than most cells and can have a molecular weight of over 10^8 Da. The structure of an aggrecan molecule and the large aggregates it makes with hyaluronic acid are seen in Figure 5-1.

Cartilage matrix also has type II collagen fibers. Type II collagen is often called cartilage-specific collagen; however, it is found in a few other locations such as the vitreous body of the eye. Like other fiber-forming collagens, type II collagen fibers are cross-banded; the specific banding pattern is unique to type II fibers; their diameter is thinner than that of typical type I fibers; and the relative amount of proteoglycan aggregates to collagen fibers is much higher in cartilage than in other connective tissues. Other proteins are dispersed in the matrix of cartilage including some of the minor collagens, specifically types IX, X, and XI. Some of the staining characteristics of hyaline cartilage matrix reflect differential distribution of these minor cartilage collagens.

Hyaline Cartilage

Hyaline cartilage has many chondrocytes embedded in a large volume of cartilage matrix. The chondrocytes may occur as single cells or in groups of two, three, or four cells in close proximity. These groups (often called cell nests) are called isogenous groups for historical reasons—the presumption is that these close neighbors arose from a single precursor cell even though all the cells in the body arise from a single cell and have the same genome (i.e., all cells of the body are "isogenous"). The cartilage matrix is so firm that even if chondrocytes had the capacity to locomote, they would not be able to because of the rigidity of the matrix. In the living

state, the chondrocytes completely fill the space in which they are seen, but it is typical for the chondrocyte to shrink during fixation, which gives the impression that they reside in a small space or hole in the cartilage matrix. This small space is called a lacuna. The edges of the lacuna that are in contact with the chondrocyte often stain darker than the adjacent matrix, giving another impression, namely, that the chondrocyte has a "capsule." This is a reflection of the presence of another minor collagen, type VI, and therefore is not a capsule in any usual sense of the term.

While the matrix of hyaline cartilage is amorphous and glassy, it shows a variation in staining that depends on factors such as the distribution of minor collagens, the method of fixation, how close a given region of cartilage matrix is to chondrocytes, and which stain is used. The matrix may be relatively unstained, may be eosinophilic or basophilic, or

Figure 5-1. A, Diagram of an aggrecan molecule. The amino-terminal end of the core protein binds to hyaluronic acid (hyaluronan). A very long molecule of hyaluronan, the aggrecan, and two small "link" proteins form a stable, noncovalently linked structure. There is a short region of the core protein, closer to the amino-terminal end, to which are attached 15 to 20 keratan sulfate (KS) chains. CS, chondroitin sulfate. **B**, Diagrammatic representation of the structure described in A. **C**, Diagram of the matrix of hyaline cartilage emphasizing its major matrix components. The proteoglycan aggregates and collagen fibers form a large, space-filling complex that binds large amounts of water and anions. Since collagen molecules do not stretch and the matrix forms a rigid gel, a mass of cartilage resists compression very effectively.

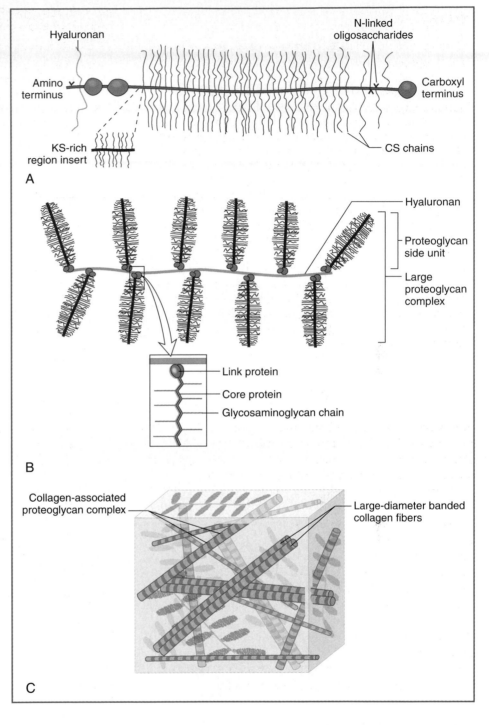

may show a shift in color (metachromasia) with certain stains such as alcian blue (Fig. 5-2).

Most cartilage is surrounded or enclosed by a fibrous connective tissue sheath—the perichondrium—with two notable exceptions, articular cartilage and fibrocartilage, neither of which have a perichondrium. The outer layers of the perichondrium consist of fibrous layers of type I collagen with a small number of fibroblasts embedded among them. The innermost layers of the perichondrium contain relatively undifferentiated mesenchymal cells, which can differentiate into new fibroblasts of the outer perichondrium or into chondroprogenitor cells that differentiate further into chondroblasts, the cells that actively synthesize and secrete cartilage matrix (Fig. 5-3).

Cartilage Development

Cartilage development begins when mesenchymal cells are stimulated to proliferate, differentiate, and secrete cartilage matrix molecules. This mass of mesenchymal tissue is called a blastema; it is often described as a condensation of cells, but more accurately, the increased cell density reflects cell proliferation, cell differentiation, and cell locomotion. The first

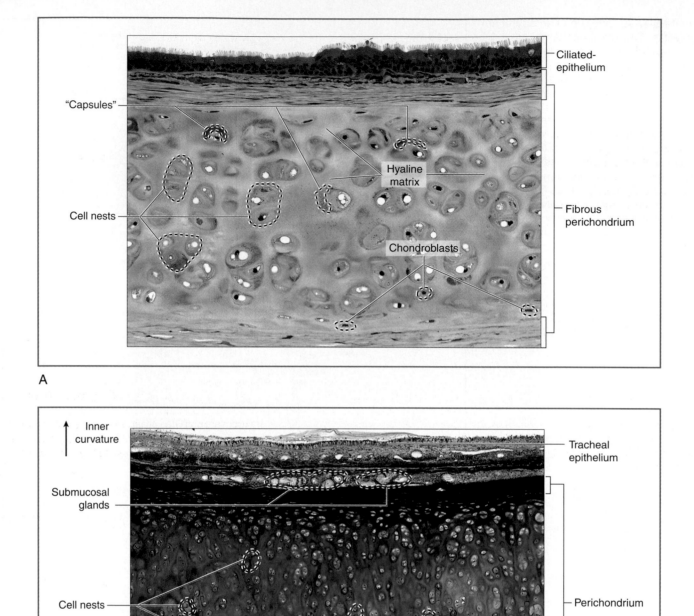

Figure 5-2. Three different examples of hyaline cartilage from the trachea. **A,** H&E stain showing the overall structure of hyaline cartilage clearly. The regions where the matrix is more basophilic (*blue*) than eosinophilic (*pink*) reflects the presence of relatively higher concentrations of the minor collagens, particularly types IX, X, and XI. The pinkest regions of the matrix are where we find the highest relative concentrations of proteoglycan aggregates and type II collagen. This specimen was fixed with modern fixatives and sectioned at 1.5 μm. The chondrocytes are well preserved—they fill their lacunae completely, the empty spaces in some of the cells reflect the former location of nuclei or lipid droplets, several chondroblasts in the field of view have a very distinct partial "capsule" (type VI collagen), and the differences among the three different cells of cartilage (chondrogenic cells, chondroblasts, and chondrocytes) can be seen (180×). **B,** Mallory-azan stain. The structural features are the same as seen in part A, but the matrix stains differently; in particular, the regions that were more blue in part A are brownish-blue in this specimen, whereas the rest of the matrix is deep blue. The inner curvature of the tracheal ring is at the top of the field, and the outer curvature is at the lower part of the field; there is a fairly broad band of chondroblasts near the outer curvature (42×).

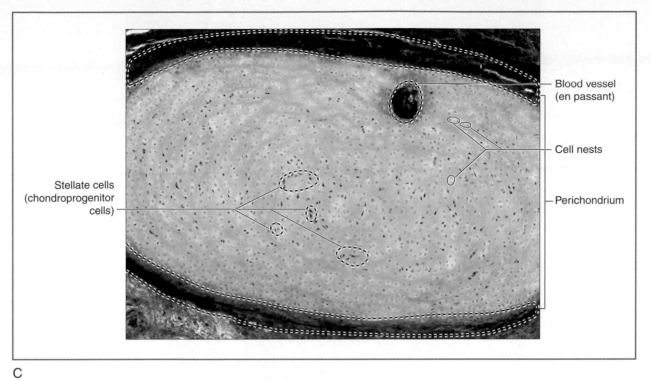

C

Figure 5-2 cont'd. C, Transverse section through one of the tracheal cartilages. The cartilage in this specimen is stained with the Masson trichrome stain, which stains the matrix bluish-green and demonstrates some differential staining of matrix components. Several distinctive features are apparent: (1) there is a complete perichondrium, (2) there is a blood vessel passing through the cartilage near the top of the field, and (3) this section appears to be near the tip of the tracheal C ring (i.e., near the perichondrium) of the cartilage, since some stellate cells and chondroblasts are seen in the midst of the matrix; these would be associated with the inner part of the perichondrium (100×).

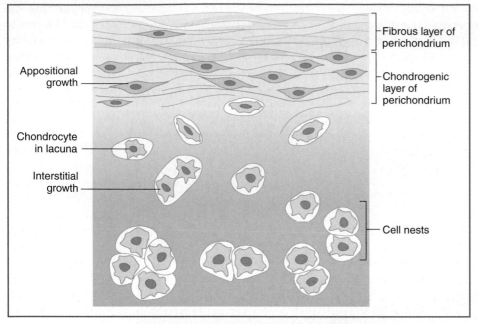

A

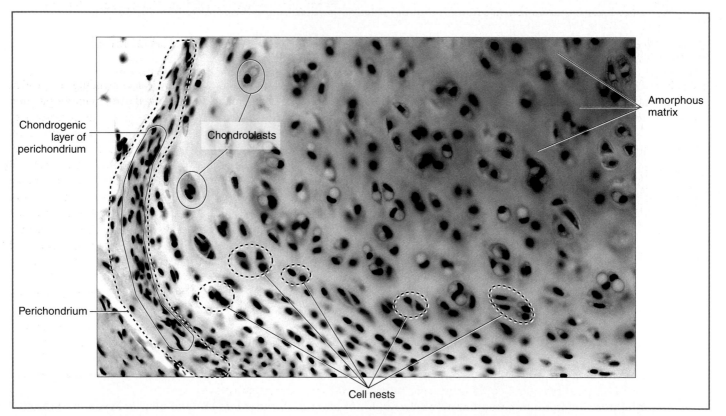

B

Figure 5-3. A, Diagram of a portion of hyaline cartilage representing the inner chondrogenic and outer fibrous layers of the perichondrium, chondroblasts, chondrocytes, and matrix. **B,** Section of tracheal cartilage in which similar features are seen in an actual section—the perichondrium, with its fibrous outer layer and inner chondrogenic layer, chondroblasts, evidence of recent chondroblast mitoses (interstitial growth), cell nests, isogenous groups, and matrix (H&E, 160×).

cells that synthesize and secrete cartilage matrix are called chondroblasts. As the matrix accumulates, the chondroblasts surround themselves by more and more cartilage matrix and become separated from each other. When this happens, the cartilage cells are called chondrocytes. As cartilage grows and develops, the mass of cartilage can grow from within the cartilage matrix (interstitial growth) or by addition of new cartilage at its surface (appositional growth). These two terms refer to cell division and to the addition of new cartilage matrix. Young or fetal cartilage is much more cellular than mature cartilage; compare the adult cartilage images in Figure 5-2 with the fetal cartilage in Figure 5-4.

Chondrocyte Ultrastructure

Mature chondrocytes have a number of defining characteristics. They are rounded polygonal to oval cells with an eccentrically placed spherical nucleus. They have an extensive amount of rough endoplasmic reticulum (rER) that is often dilated if the cell is in an active phase of matrix synthesis and secretion, a prominent Golgi apparatus, and many stubby filopodia. It is not unusual to see numerous large lipid droplets or glycogen granules in the chondrocyte cytoplasm; these two cytoplasmic inclusions reflect storage forms of the precursors of proteoglycan and collagen synthesis. As an avascular tissue, chondrocytes need to store the building blocks of the copious matrix materials they synthesize and secrete (Fig. 5-5). It is important to keep in mind that chondrocytes are living cells; they require energy to maintain themselves and carry out their differentiated functions, and they need to remove the waste products of their metabolism.

Elastic Cartilage

Elastic cartilage (Fig. 5-6) bears many similarities to hyaline cartilage: it is surrounded by a perichondrium, the cells in its matrix are chondrocytes, and much of its matrix is amorphous but it has a considerable content of elastin fibers. The elastin fibers are synthesized and secreted by the chondrocytes.

Fibrocartilage

Fibrocartilage is a mixture or combination of dense regular connective tissue and small numbers of chondrocytes surrounded by scant amounts of hyaline cartilage matrix. Figure 5-7 shows three examples of fibrocartilage stained with two different stains. It can be easy to overlook the small amounts of hyaline cartilage in a specimen of fibrocartilage. The most reliable diagnostic features of fibrocartilage are the presence of polygonal chondrocytes surrounded by scant hyaline matrix intermingled with thick collagen fibers that are characteristically found in tendons or ligaments.

●●● GENERAL PROPERTIES OF BONE

Bone is a mineralized (more specifically, ossified) supporting connective tissue whose major functions are to give the body form and serve as the attachments and support for the skeletal muscles, which in turn allow this system of levers to move about. In addition to these supporting and mobility functions, the structure and composition of bone serves critical and central physiologic roles. Two of most important secondary roles of bone are (1) maintaining serum and tissue fluid concentrations of important ions—calcium (Ca^{++}) and phosphate (PO_4^{2-}), and (2) serving as the primary site of production of the formed elements (red cells, white cells, and platelets) of the circulating blood by virtue of the hemopoietic tissue in the bone marrow–filled cavities of bone.

Mature bone is a remarkably lightweight and strong structure. Its overall strength is determined by its chemical composition and its biochemical and microscopic organization. Bone is a composite material, containing organic and inorganic components organized in a highly structured way. About 90% of its organic components are type I collagen fibers. Nearly all (ca. 95%) of the inorganic components are a specific kind of calcium phosphate crystal—calcium hydroxyapatite ($Ca_{10}[PO_4]_6[OH]_2$). About 5% of bone mineral is in the form of calcium carbonate ($CaCO_3$) and other inorganic materials (magnesium, sodium, potassium, chloride, and fluoride).

●●● BONE STRUCTURE AND COMPOSITION

Bone is described in several ways depending on which structure or function is emphasized. In macroscopic and microscopic terms, bone structure is viewed as consisting of compact or spongy (cancellous) regions; think of this as an architectural description, since it is based solely on what you see when you view a living or dead bone. Bone is prepared for microscopic examination (LM or EM) in two ways: ossified bone is ground to a thickness of about 30–50 μm and viewed unstained, or it is decalcified and prepared for microscopy using conventional techniques. The microscopic appearance of bone reveals several important structural features. Bone is organized into layers or lamellae, there are many lacunae that follow the contours of the lamellae, and the lacunae have many small canals (canaliculi) emanating from their periphery.

Figure 5-8 is a photograph of a hemi-sectioned bone to illustrate compact and cancellous bone, and a diagram labeling the parts of a bone.

Figure 5-9 shows a pair of micrographs of compact bone to illustrate its major features.

The composition of bone is quite different from that of other living tissues. It has a lower water content (10%) than nearly all other tissues (which usually are about 70% to 80% water) and a higher mineral content (65%) than any other tissue except teeth. The organic component of bone is about 25% of its weight, 23% of which is collagen and 2% is other proteins and proteoglycan aggregates. Bone proteoglycan aggregates are much smaller than those of cartilage; the core proteins have only a few glycosaminoglycan chains attached to them, and fewer of them are bound to hyaluronan in the aggregate.

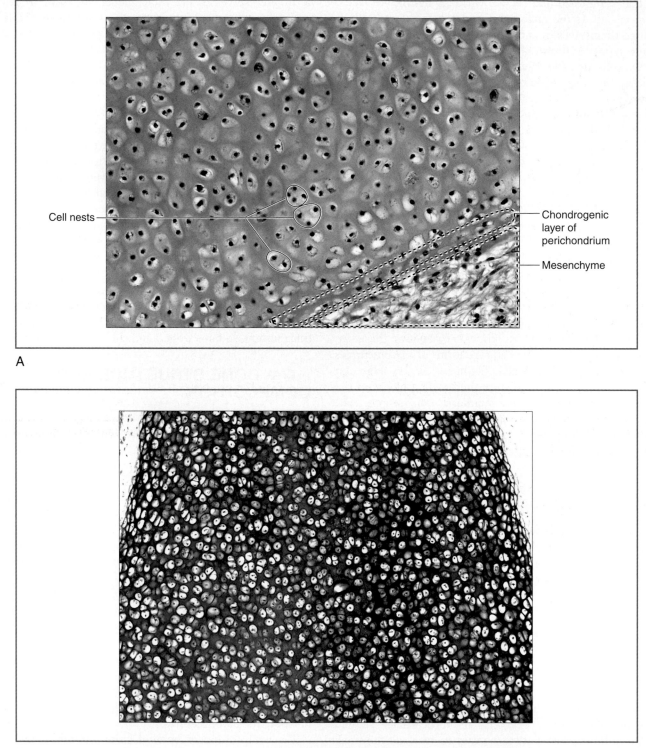

A

B

Figure 5-4. Two different sections of fetal hyaline cartilage stained with H&E. **A,** Mass of cartilage that is much more cellular than mature cartilage is, and a poorly formed perichondrium; the region in which the perichondrium would usually be seen is still mesenchymal connective tissue (200×). **B,** Section through a spinous process of a developing fetal vertebra showing the greater cellularity of fetal cartilage. The matrix is highly basophilic; there are many cell nests and a very thin perichondrium, which is not visible in this image (100×).

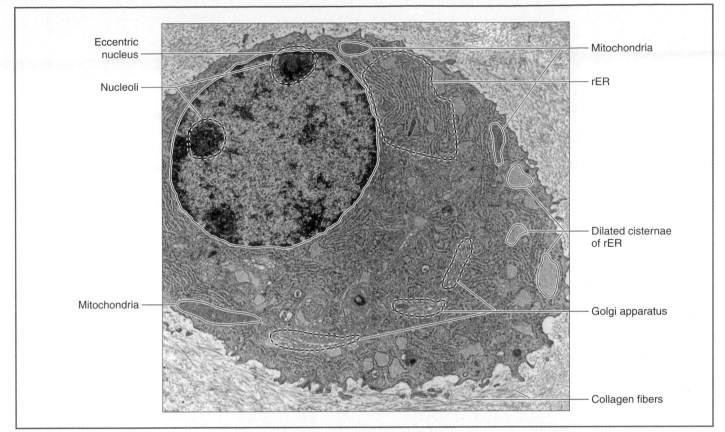

Eccentric nucleus

Nucleoli

Mitochondria

Mitochondria

rER

Dilated cisternae of rER

Golgi apparatus

Collagen fibers

Figure 5-5. Electron micrograph of chondrocytes. Note the eccentric placement of the nucleus, abundant rER with electron-dense cisternal contents, and filopodia on the plasma membrane.

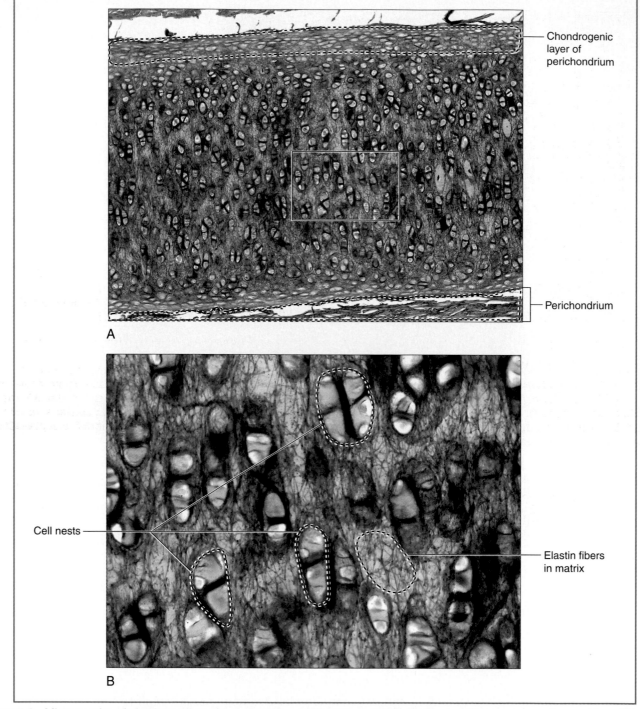

Chondrogenic layer of perichondrium

Perichondrium

A

Cell nests

Elastin fibers in matrix

B

Figure 5-6. Micrographs of elastic cartilage from the pinna of the ear. **A** and **B**, Sections of the same specimen at low (62×) and high (250×) magnification; the stain is orcein—one of the so-called elastic tissue stains.

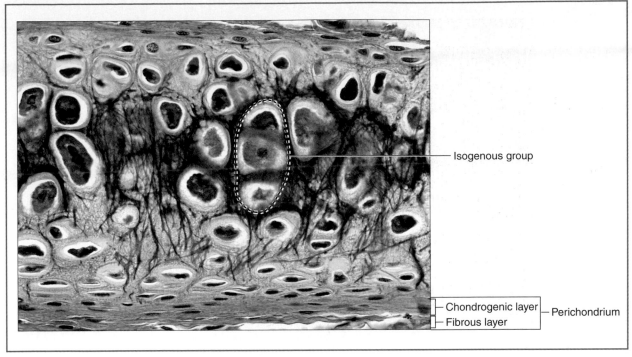

C

Figure 5-6 cont'd. C, Section of monkey ear stained with Milligan's trichrome stain; the cells are well preserved, and the delicate reddish elastic fibers are prominent. The overall character of cartilage is seen in these micrographs—chondrocytes in lacunae, isogenous groups, and a perichondrium. The distinctive difference is the extensive amount of fibrillar material in the matrix. In these specimens, nearly all the elastin fibers are rather delicate, but in some specimens of elastic cartilage, or with different elastin stains, the elastin fibers are more prominent and the fibers give the impression of being more like septae (380×).

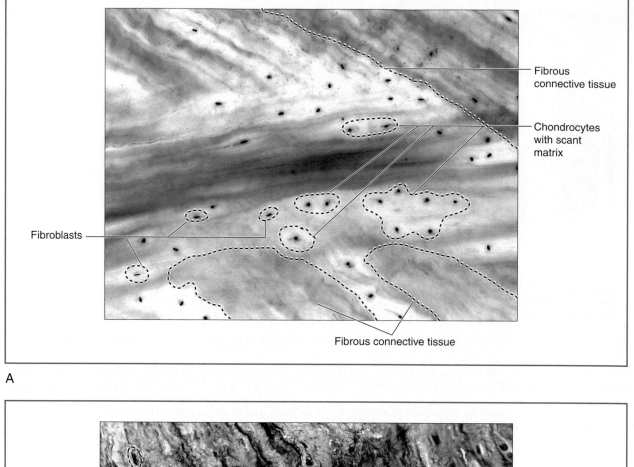

A

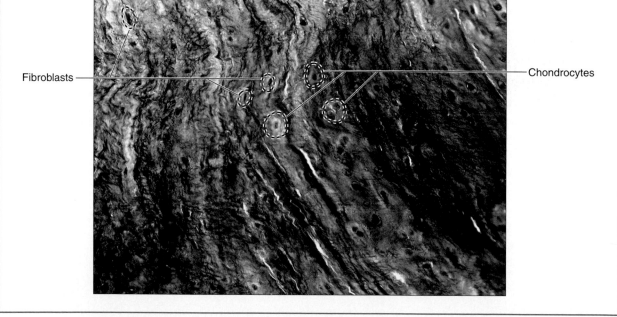

B

Figure 5-7. A, H&E stain of a fibrocartilaginous joint. Most of the cells in this field are chondrocytes with their associated scant matrix. The type I collagenous component is stained more pink and organized at acute angles to one another (180×).
B, Hematoxylin-orange G stain of the fibrocartilaginous joint at the symphysis pubis. The numerous wavy fibrous components predominate in this section, but where chondrocyte nuclei are visible, a light-stained halo indicates the presence of a small amount of hyaline cartilage matrix (70×).

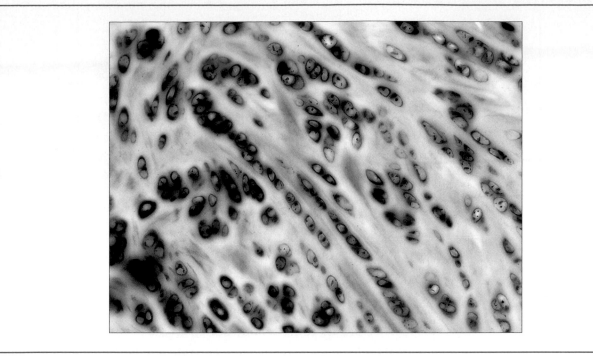

C

Figure 5-7 cont'd. C, Different field of view of the fetal vertebra in Figure 5-4B. Nearly all the cells in this micrograph are chondrocytes; they are lined up in diagonal rows or in small groups. The pale, whitish-pink regions are the fibrous portions of this mass of developing fibrocartilage (180×).

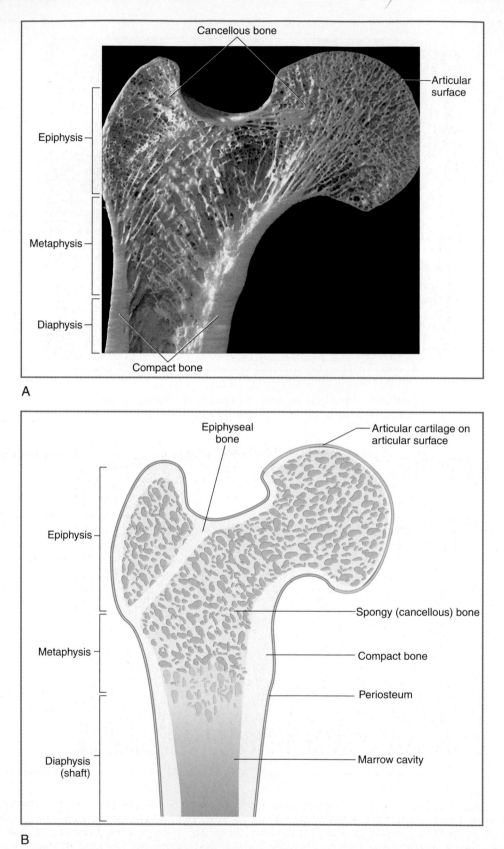

Figure 5-8. A, Section of a dry femur that has been sawed in half lengthwise. The anatomic epiphysis occupies the upper half of the image; the metaphysis and diaphysis (shaft) of the bone are in the lower left quadrant. (From Kerr J. *Atlas of Functional Histology*. St. Louis, Mosby, 1999, p 169.) **B,** Schematic drawing of a similar bone. It includes certain features that are not seen in the photograph in part A, in particular, the periosteum, the cartilage on the articular surface of the epiphysis, and the epiphyseal line. The epiphyseal line is the site of the former epiphyseal growth plate that completely ossifies once the individual completes puberty. After this time an individual no longer grows in height.

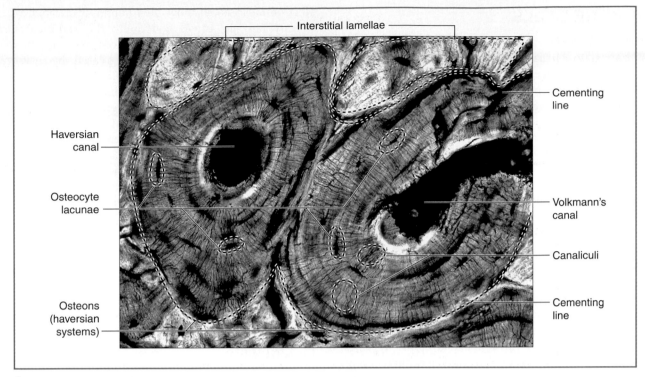

Interstitial lamellae

Cementing line

Haversian canal

Volkmann's canal

Osteocyte lacunae

Canaliculi

Cementing line

Osteons (haversian systems)

A

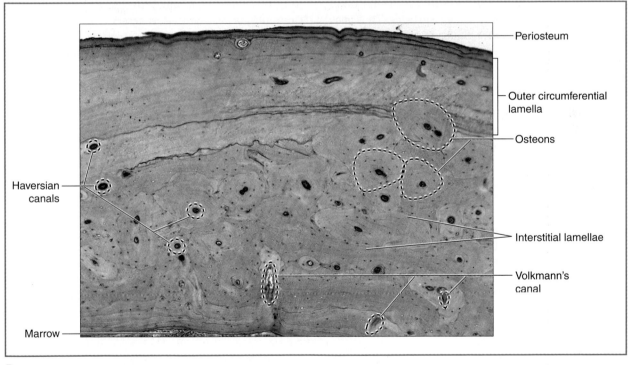

Periosteum

Outer circumferential lamella

Osteons

Haversian canals

Interstitial lamellae

Volkmann's canal

Marrow

B

Figure 5-9. A, Thin ground section of mature, ossified, cortical bone mounted on a slide with no stain added for contrast; the black areas represent air trapped in spaces occupied by osteocytes, haversian or Volkmann's canals, or canaliculi. All cellular materials are lost during specimen preparation owing to the heat generated by the grinding process (210×). **B,** H&E stain of decalcified section of mature cortical bone. The characteristic features of an adult bone are labeled. The lamellar nature of the specimen is seen in the outer circumferential lamella, the osteons, and the interstitial lamellae. Many osteocytes are seen in their lacunae; the cells themselves are not seen because of the low magnification of this photomicrograph (70×).

●●● BONE CELLS

Like cartilage, bone has many cells embedded in its matrix, but in contrast to cartilage, bone is highly vascular and is innervated. Given the fact that the matrix of mature bone is constantly undergoing a process of resorption and redeposition, it is helpful to bear in mind that all bone surfaces are covered or lined with cells. Following the same convention for naming the cells of cartilage (i.e., based on where they are found and what they do), four different types of bone cells are described.

Osteoprogenitor Cells

Osteoprogenitor cells (bone-lining cells, bone-resting cells) are derived from mesenchyme, either mesodermal or ectodermal in origin. In embryonic and fetal life, osteoprogenitor cells are active precursors of osteoblasts. In adult life, they are mostly in a resting state unless they are stimulated to proliferate and differentiate into osteoblasts. In the case of bones that develop from cartilage (see below), the osteoprogenitor cells can be described as osteochondroprogenitor cells, since the cells that comprise the perichondrium become the cells that comprise the periosteum once bone formation has been initiated. They are flattened cells with a small oval nucleus and scant cytoplasm. They are found on the outer (periosteal) and inner (endosteal) bone surfaces. They also line the haversian and Volkmann's canals of mature bone.

Osteoblasts

Osteoblasts are the cells that synthesize and secrete the organic matrix of bone as well as direct ossification of the matrix by secreting small (50–250 nm) matrix vesicles that contain alkaline phosphatase and other calcification-initiating factors. As mentioned above, they differentiate from osteoprogenitor cells; they retain the capacity to divide. They are polygonal to cuboidal cells that directly cover the bone surface they actively deposit. Osteoblasts have a centrally placed, euchromatic, oval nucleus with a prominent nucleolus, abundant rER, Golgi apparatus, and numerous secretory vesicles. The cell surface of the osteoblast has many thin cytoplasmic processes, which fill the canaliculi that permeate bone; many of these processes contact cell processes of nearby osteoblasts and form gap junctions.

Osteocytes

When an osteoblast becomes completely surrounded by woven or lamellar bone, it is called an osteocyte. Osteocytes have a more attenuated cytoplasm than do osteoblasts, which may be a reflection of their lower rate of bone production even though they are metabolically active. The system of canaliculi and lacunae in which osteocytes and their cytoplasmic processes reside are bathed by minute amounts of extracellular tissue fluid. Examination of the fine details of haversian canals and the endosteal surface (by scanning electron microscopy) shows that hundreds of canaliculi open directly into the canals and on to the endosteal surface. Therefore, osteocytes are ideally placed to participate in Ca^{++} homeostasis, which is largely regulated by parathyroid hormone and calcitonin (see discussion later in the chapter).

Normal serum Ca^{++} levels are critical for maintaining the function of all the cells, tissues, and organs of the body. About 99% of all Ca^{++} in the body is in the skeleton, as calcium hydroxyapatite. The concentration of serum (and extracellular tissue fluid) is about 1.0–1.3 mmol/L. Measurements of Ca^{++} exchange between the soluble pool and insoluble pool of Ca^{++} indicate that about 25% of the soluble pool of Ca^{++} is exchanged with the insoluble pool on a daily basis. This exchange is mediated by osteocytes in a process referred to as *osteocytic osteolysis*.

In addition to their important role in Ca^{++} and PO_4^{2-} homeostasis, osteocytes may produce bone matrix, albeit not as much or at the same rate as osteoblasts. Much of the time osteocytes are in a quiescent state with respect to matrix synthesis, but they are metabolically active.

Osteoclasts

Osteoclasts originate from circulating monocyte precursors. Once recruited to a site where bone will be resorbed, 10 to 20 of these monocyte precursors fuse to form a polykaryon. This multinucleate cell forms an attachment to a bone surface mediated by a specific set of integrins, a widely distributed family of cell adhesion molecules. The attachment seals off a small area of bone surface wherein the osteoclasts elaborate an extensive ruffled border and begin to degrade the inorganic matrix by secreting H^+ and the organic matrix by secreting proteases. As a result, they create a small indentation on a bone surface, although osteoclasts are often seen on or near the tips of bone spicules, so the indentation is not obvious. The recess or indentation is called a *Howship's lacuna*. Osteoclasts eventually undergo apoptosis when they have completed their resorption activity. The main function of osteoclasts is to resorb bone, and as such they play a major role in bone development, growth, and remodeling. The small amounts of bone they degrade on a daily basis contribute to the soluble pool of Ca^{++}.

Examples of all three types of bone cells are seen in Figure 5-10. This specimen is a small region from bone developing by the endochondral mechanism (see Endochondral Bone Development).

●●● DETAILS OF BONE STRUCTURE

The outer surface of bone, which typically has smooth contours, is covered by a fibrous sheath—the periosteum—except at the epiphyseal ends if the bone articulates with another bone. In this case the articular surface is covered with hyaline cartilage. The outermost parts of the periosteum have coarse type I collagen fibers containing occasional scattered fibroblasts. The inner portion of the periosteum is somewhat more cellular and is where we find osteoprogenitor cells. The

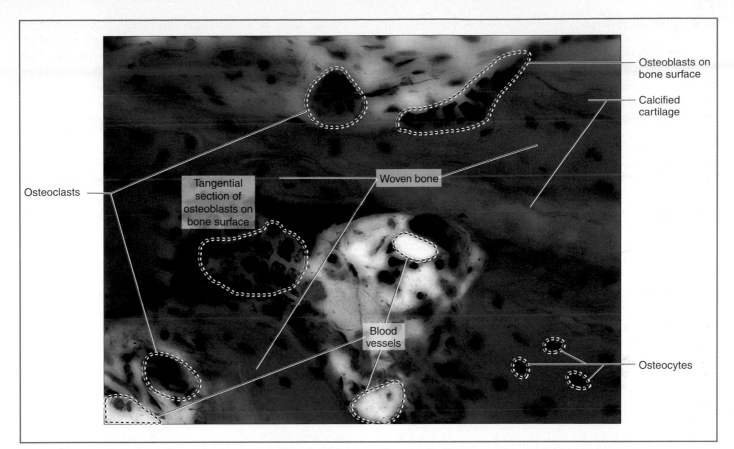

Figure 5-10. H&E stain of decalcified section of developing bone. Three osteoclasts, many osteoblasts, and numerous osteocytes are indicated in this specimen. There are areas of woven (immature) bone in which are embedded remnants of calcified cartilage (H&E, 360×).

PATHOLOGY

Mechanisms of Cancer Metastasis to Bone

Cancer metastasis to bone is a serious complication for about 70% of individuals with advanced cancer of the breast or prostate and about 15% to 30% of those with lung cancer.

The bone metastases are described as osteolytic, owing to activation of excessive osteoclast number and activity, or osteoblastic, as a result of osteoblast activation and excessive bone deposition. Many patients have bone metastasis of both types except for those with multiple myeloma, in which only lytic bone lesions develop. Bone scanning is a useful diagnostic tool in detecting either kind of lesion.

Several factors account for the frequency of bone metastasis:

- Red marrow is a site of high blood flow, so tumor cells arrive in this location at a high rate.
- Tumor cells express adhesion molecules that bind to marrow stroma and to bone matrix.
- The tumor cells stimulate neovascularization and further tumor growth, since bone is a large repository for many growth factors many of which are liberated locally owing to the osteolytic lesions.
- Many of the specific factors that stimulate osteoclast formation are expressed by tumor cells.

Although the specific factors expressed by tumor cells that stimulate osteoblast formation are not identified, it is clear that tumor cells play a role in osteoblastic metastasis as well.

inner (endosteal) surface of bone is lined by osteoprogenitor cells in varying states of activity; the cells may be inactive or may be actively mitotic and produce osteoblasts. The diaphysis of a mature long bone consists of a thick cylinder of compact bone whose inner surface is mostly smooth. The epiphyseal and metaphyseal cavities of the bone are filled with an array of cancellous bone. Bone cavities are filled with red or white marrow; the former is the site of production of the formed elements of blood, and the latter consists of adipose cells (fat tissue). Compact bone and red and white marrow are highly vascular. The blood supply of bone is provided by a nutrient artery near the midpoint of the diaphysis and smaller arteries at the metaphysis. These vessels enter the compact bone via foramina and ultimately make their way to the marrow cavity. The foramina form during bone development and remodeling and are not due to invasion of compact bone by blood vessels.

Mature Bone

All mature compact and cancellous bone is lamellar. The best way to assimilate this fact is to recognize that bone is in a lifelong, constant state of deposition, resorption, and redeposition; this dynamic state begins in utero. Therefore, most, if not all, of the cancellous bone seen at any time in the life of a person was compact bone at an earlier time. The osteocytes in their lacunae are found at fairly regular intervals disposed along the interfaces between adjacent lamellae. Each osteocyte has many cytoplasmic processes that extend into the canaliculi that radiate into the lamellae. In many instances, the cytoplasmic processes from two osteocytes in adjacent lamellae touch each other and have a gap junction (nexus) at the contact site.

The diaphysis of most compact bone consists of circular to oval cylinders, 3–5 cm long, and 100–400 μm in diameter oriented along the long axis of the bone. The cylinders are called osteons or haversian systems. Each osteon has a small canal (the haversian canal), which runs the length of the cylinder and contains a blood vessel or two (a capillary or venule) and often a nerve fiber. The haversian canal has a mean diameter of 50 μm; this arrangement means that osteocytes, on average, are no more than 200 μm from a blood vessel. The haversian canal and all the canaliculi are filled with tissue fluid. It has been estimated that the surface area of the haversian canals and canaliculi is about 300–500 m² throughout the body. The haversian canals of compact bone are interconnected by a smaller number of canals called Volkmann's canals. Most arterial blood reaches the marrow cavity from the circulation and nourishes the

compact bone in a centrifugal direction—from the marrow cavity out. The capillaries in the bone marrow enter Volkmann's and haversian canals as capillaries and small venules and reenter the general circulation. Thus, the blood cells that develop in the red marrow are delivered to the body as well.

The diagram in Figure 5-11 shows a number of structural details that would be seen near the diaphysis-metaphysis region of a long bone. The vascularity of the periosteum is shown on the left side of the figure. Many osteons are depicted in transverse section and a few in longitudinal section. The underlying lamellar organization of compact and cancellous bone is seen by the many alternating lighter and darker yellow layers in each osteon. The orientation of the collagen fibers that comprise each lamella are indicated in the longitudinal sections of three osteons as well as in the outer circumferential lamellae; collagen fibers are oriented more or less orthogonally in adjacent lamellae. This arrangement imparts added strength to the weight-bearing and stress roles that bone plays. The calcium hydroxyapatite crystals, which are small, rod-shaped or plate-like structures (1.5–3 × 30 nm), are arranged along the collagen fibers at regular intervals of about 60 to 70 nm.

Many osteocyte lacunae and canaliculi are seen in the region of a few of the osteons in Figure 5-11. Some of the

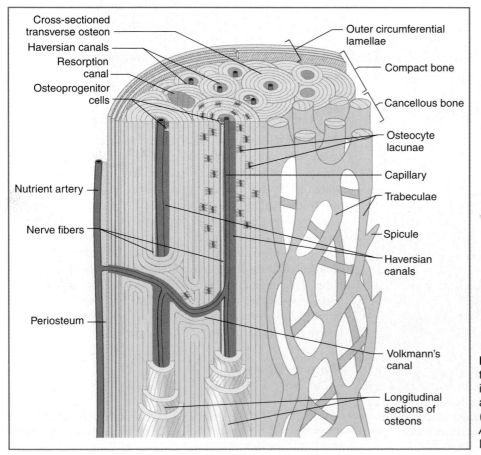

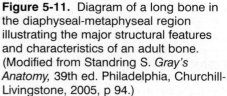

Figure 5-11. Diagram of a long bone in the diaphyseal-metaphyseal region illustrating the major structural features and characteristics of an adult bone. (Modified from Standring S. *Gray's Anatomy,* 39th ed. Philadelphia, Churchill-Livingstone, 2005, p 94.)

osteons are seen with a complete series of concentric lamellae, and others appear to have been partially eaten away (which they were, by osteoclasts) and filled in with a complete (newer) osteon. One place in the diagram shows a resorption canal that has not yet been filled in by a new osteon. Other curved lamellae fill in the spaces between complete and "carved out" lamellae; these are called interstitial lamellae and reflect the presence of earlier (largely resorbed) generations of osteons.

Although most of the cells of bone are omitted from this diagram, many osteoprogenitor cells would line the periosteum; two are seen on the inner surfaces of two haversian canals.

Immature Bone

Newly formed bone in the fetus is called immature or *woven* bone; this type of bone is also found postnatally. It is much more cellular than mature bone, is not organized into osteons, does not consist of recognizable lamellae, and has more randomly oriented osteocytes.

Figure 5-12 shows a transverse section through the diaphysis of a long bone of a growing animal. In this field of view, we see a mixture of lamellar and woven bone. Lamellar bone in osteons and circumferential lamellae are seen in the mature portions of the specimen while the woven, more cellular immature portions are seen in contrast to the mature and more organized regions. There are even places in this specimen where small remnants of calcified cartilage are seen (see Bone Development). Note that most of the osteons and certain groups of lamellae have a slightly more basophilic (darker) outline than the rest of the bone matrix. They are called *cementing lines* and are seen in fully mature bone although they are more prominent in immature bone. They are richer in proteoglycans and noncollagenous proteins than is lamellar bone.

●●● BONE DEVELOPMENT

Bone begins to develop in utero at about the end of the embryonic phase (eighth week) and beginning of the fetal phase of life (ninth week). Among other things, mesenchyme has the capability of differentiating directly into bone or into cartilage. The long bones of the body first appear as cartilage "models" of the mature bones that will replace the cartilage. Thus, bone develops by two mechanisms: mesenchymal bone development and endochondral bone development.

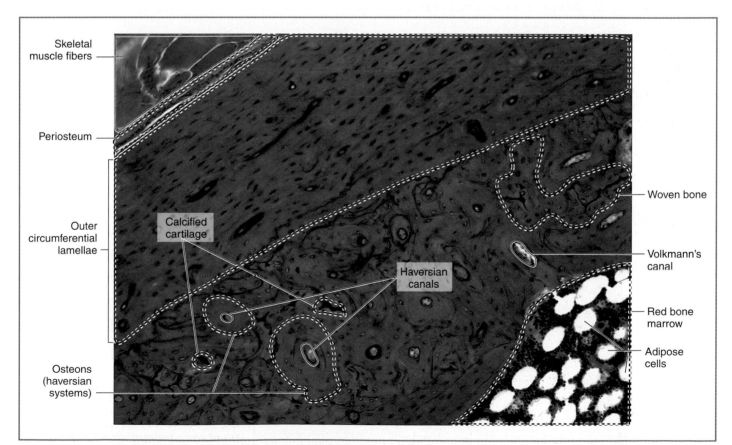

Figure 5-12. H&E stain of a decalcified section of cortical bone from a growing animal. The section shows immature woven bone intermingled with lamellar bone and early osteons. There are a few regions where remnants of calcified cartilage are seen; these are the dark purple–staining regions (H&E, 90×).

Intramembranous Bone Development

In the first case, bone formation begins with a condensation of mesenchyme (i.e., embryonic mesenchymal cells migrate, produce specific cytokines, and aggregate to produce a condensation center where they proliferate into a structure that resembles a "membrane") in a process called intramembranous bone formation, but it might more accurately be called mesenchymal bone formation. The cranial bones and clavicles develop by intramembranous bone formation. The cranial mesenchyme that differentiates into bone is itself derived from neural ectoderm. For this reason, cranial bones are sometimes called ectodermal bone.

The mesenchymal cells initially deposit a cellular sheath of a felt-like mat of collagen fibers called *osteoid*. At this point these cells are called osteoblasts. Osteoid becomes calcified owing to the deposition of amorphous calcium phosphate but only for a brief period, since both the mineral and osteoid are quickly resorbed. Osteoid is rapidly degraded and redeposited into a somewhat more orderly array of collagen fibers. The more orderly array of collagen fibers is called

woven bone. Simultaneously, endothelial cells migrate to the vicinity of the mass of osteoblasts and form capillaries near the woven bone.

The woven collagen fibers become ossified, a subset of calcification that refers to the deposition of calcium hydroxyapatite crystals along collagen fibers. The cycle of osteoid deposition, resorption, woven collagen fiber deposition, and ossification occurs many times over in a short time period until some of the osteoblasts become surrounded by their own woven bone matrix, at which time the cells are called osteocytes. As the osteoblasts become isolated from one another, they leave cytoplasmic processes in the woven bone; bone forms around the cells and their processes, which is how the lacunae and canaliculi that are characteristic of mature bone are formed. The rapid turnover of osteoid is most probably due to the activity of the osteoblasts that first deposited it, but the turnover of woven bone is primarily due to the action of osteoclasts. The bone seen at these early times is described as the primary spongiosa because of its similarity to a sponge. Figure 5-13 shows the process of intramembranous bone formation in a schematic diagram.

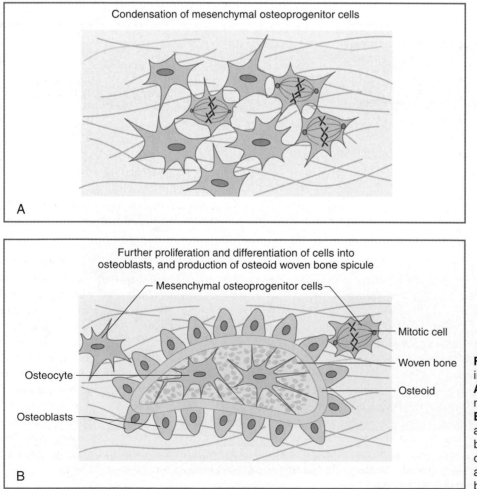

Figure 5-13. Schematic diagram of intramembranous bone formation. **A**, The proliferation and condensation of mesenchymal osteoprogenitor cells. **B**, Osteoblasts have deposited osteoid, and two cells have become surrounded by woven bone and are now called osteocytes. In addition, the immediate area of woven bone formation has become vascularized.

Figure 5-13 cont'd. C, The expanding volume of woven bone spicules just before the spicules and trabeculae grow and join together to form plates of bone. **D**, The new bone has become larger and is being resorbed on one surface by osteoclasts. The surface at left shows some resting bone cells.

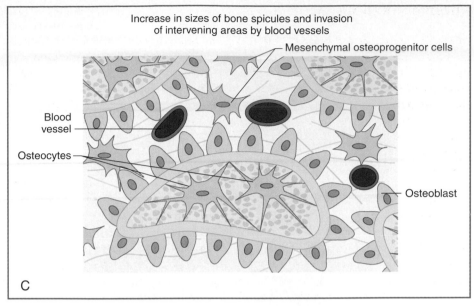

Increase in sizes of bone spicules and invasion of intervening areas by blood vessels

Mesenchymal osteoprogenitor cells

Blood vessel

Osteocytes

Osteoblast

C

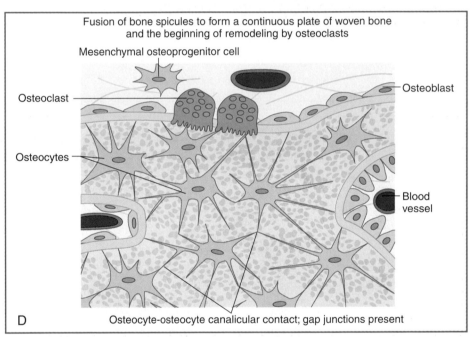

Fusion of bone spicules to form a continuous plate of woven bone and the beginning of remodeling by osteoclasts

Mesenchymal osteoprogenitor cell

Osteoclast

Osteoblast

Osteocytes

Blood vessel

D

Osteocyte-osteocyte canalicular contact; gap junctions present

Figure 5-14 shows two examples of intramembranous bone development in the mandible of a pig embryo; a lighter layer of osteoid is seen between the osteoblasts and the woven bone spicules (spikes). The spicules of bone are covered by osteoblasts and contain a few osteocytes. In Figure 5-14B, six or seven osteoclasts are also seen in the process of resorbing the newly deposited bone. Note that the upper surface of the developing bone is covered by osteoblasts and the lower surface has few (if any) osteoblasts and many osteoclasts; this indicates an upper surface of net bone growth and a lower surface of net resorption.

Bone growth occurs only at a developing or remodeling *surface*, not within the mass of bone itself. That is, bone grows only by appositional (not by interstitial) growth. As the mesenchymal bone primordium grows, the blood vessels in the vicinity of the bone become surrounded by bone, hence the bone becomes vascular. The cranial bones are flat, curved plates with thin shells of compact bone enclosing a small amount of cancellous bone. Through the process of growth and remodeling, these bones become lamellar, and they even develop osteons. Thus, in a small area of bone viewed at medium or high magnification, it is not possible to determine whether the bone developed directly from mesenchyme or by replacement of cartilage. A diagrammatic representation of these events is seen in Figure 5-15. This diagram illustrates the periosteum, a few osteoprogenitor cells, several osteoblasts, a "young" osteocyte, and some osteocyte processes. Note the mat of osteoid fibers and the two layers of lamellar collagen in the upper part of the diagram.

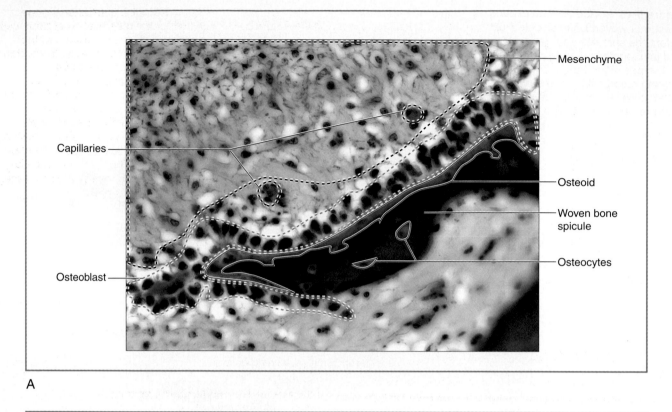

A

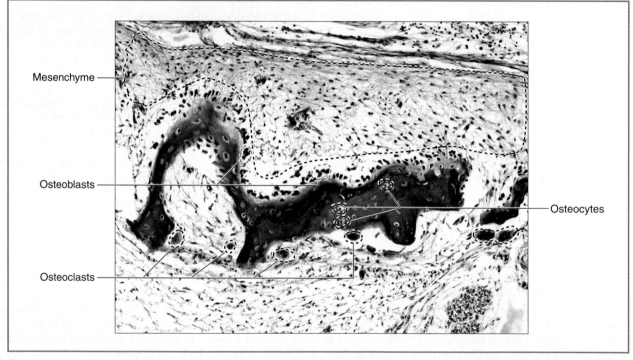

B

Figure 5-14. A and **B**, Two regions of developing intramembranous bone. See text for details (H&E, part A, 260×; part B, 110×).

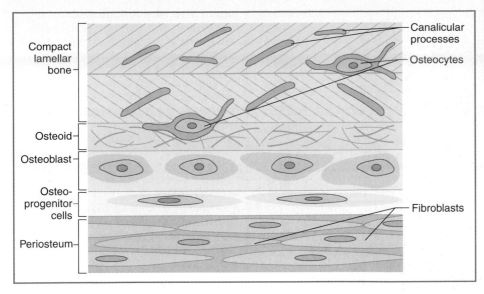

Figure 5-15. Diagram showing the ultrastructural organization of bone cells and matrix as would be seen at the surface of growing bone. At the bottom of the figure, the periosteum and a fibroblast cover the bone surface. Immediately above the periosteum are osteoprogenitor cells, a layer of osteoblasts, and the osteoid they deposit. An osteocyte is shown partially surrounded by osteoid and adjacent to lamellar bone. The two bone lamellae have a number of osteocytic processes and another osteocyte.

Endochondral Bone Development

The long bones of the body develop by replacing a cartilage model—a process called endochondral bone formation. In late embryonic and early fetal life, mesenchyme condenses in a manner similar to that described above for mesenchymal bone formation, but instead of differentiating into osteoblasts, the cells differentiate into chondroblasts under the influence of a number of transcription factors, including *SOX9*, a key gene in early development. The growing mass of cartilage is enclosed by a thin perichondrium. The chondroblasts secrete cartilage matrix and become chondrocytes. The cartilage develops into small "models" of the bones that will ultimately replace them; moreover, they do so in the exact anatomic locations where the bones will develop.

Figure 5-16 is a diagram of the events that occur during endochondral bone formation.

The first appearance of bone in endochondral bone development occurs following changes in chondrocytes in the midst of the diaphysis of the cartilage model. These chondrocytes become hypertrophic, alter their genetic program to secrete large amounts of type X collagen, and attract blood vessels through release of specific growth factors. The hypertrophic chondrocytes also direct adjacent perichondral cells to differentiate into osteoprogenitor cells, which differentiate further into osteoblasts that produce the first bone in the form of a thin collar surrounding the diaphyseal region of the cartilage model. When the collar of woven bone encloses the region of hypertrophic chondrocytes completely (see Figs. 5-16B and 5-16C), the hypertrophic chondrocytes undergo programmed cell death, leaving a small volume to be invaded by osteoblasts, sprouts of capillaries, and hematopoietic tissue. The death of the hypertrophic chondrocytes initiates the mineralization of their own matrix through the release of matrix vesicles containing alkaline phosphatase and other proteins. The

GENETICS

Defects in Tropocollagen Formation— Osteogenesis Imperfecta

Osteogenesis imperfecta (OI) is a group of diseases of mutations of type I collagen genes; over 200 mutations have been described in these genes. OI is inherited as an autosomal dominant disease. There are four types of OI, but they are placed into two classes—tropocollagen underproduction and structurally defective tropocollagen production. The severity of disease depends on the type of OI the individual inherits. The major phenotype associated with OI is moderate to severe bone malformation and fragility (brittleness).

OI type I usually affects the α_1(I) collagen gene as a result of the introduction of stop codons, insertions, or deletions of one or two bases, splicing mutations, or missense codons. Type I mutations lead to an underproduction of tropocollagen molecules because there are not enough α_1(I) chains to allow for the assembly of normal amounts of tropocollagen. Recall that type I collagen tropocollagen has two α_1(I) chains and one α_2(I) chain.

OI types II, III, and IV are mutations in the α_1(I) or α_2(I) chains such that tropocollagen is still formed but the triple helical molecules are structurally defective. All connective tissues are affected, but bone, with its high collagen content, is the most severely affected. The great majority of the mutations in OI types II, III, and IV are a replacement of a glycine in the repeating Gly-X-Y triplet with a bulkier amino acid. These amino acid substitutions disrupt triple helix formation when tropocollagen first forms. Thus, cells still produce tropocollagen molecules, but they are structurally very weak.

The most severe OI phenotype is type II. Individuals with this type of OI usually die in the perinatal period because of extensive bone malformation and fractures. Fractures in the ribs of newborns make breathing virtually impossible, and the infants succumb to respiratory failure.

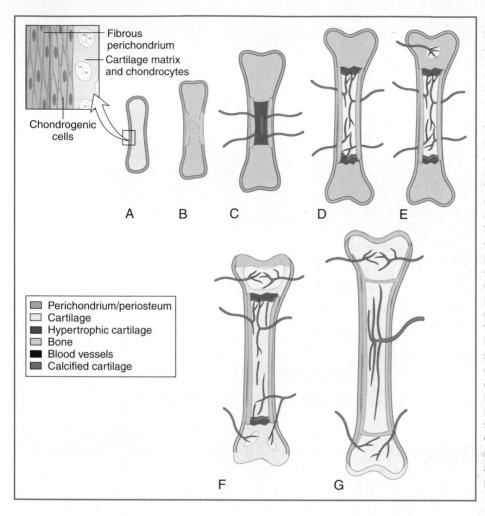

Figure 5-16. **A**, Cartilage model of a future bone. The inset shows the cells and matrix at the mid-shaft region of the perichondrium and their relationship to each other. At this point, the entire cartilage model is covered by a delicate perichondrium. **B**, A thin collar of bone has formed around the diaphysis. **C**, Vascularization of the bone collar and hypertrophy of the diaphyseal chondrocytes. **D**, Blood vessels enter the newly formed medullary cavity and grow toward the epiphyseal ends of the bone, establishing the two growth plates. **E**, A secondary center of ossification has formed, and the whole bone has elongated owing to chondrocyte proliferation and hypertrophy in the growth plate. Up to this time, the entire developing bone is covered by a perichondrium (where cartilage remains) or a periosteum (where bone has formed). **F**, Further lengthening of the bone, appearance of a second center of secondary ossification, and further development of bone vasculature. The cartilage-covered articular surfaces no longer have a perichondrium. **G**, An adult bone. The cortical bone has thickened, the bone has achieved its full length and width, the epiphyseal plates have become ossified ("closed"), and the articular surfaces are free of a perichondrium.

Legend:
- Fibrous perichondrium
- Cartilage matrix and chondrocytes
- Chondrogenic cells
- Perichondrium/periosteum
- Cartilage
- Hypertrophic cartilage
- Bone
- Blood vessels
- Calcified cartilage

monocytic precursors of osteoclasts are attracted to the calcified matrix. The multinucleate osteochondroclasts degrade the calcified cartilage matrix.

At the microscopic level, the cellular changes that take place as the bone collar forms look the same as those seen in the earliest stages of intramembranous bone development; the main difference is that the process occurs on the surface of a cartilage model instead of in a region of condensed mesenchyme.

The capillaries that invade the diaphysis grow, branch, and sprout along the long axis of the cartilage model (see Fig. 5-16D). Osteoblasts deposit osteoid and then woven bone along the remaining spicules of calcified cartilage and the paths created by the combined action of the osteoclasts and capillaries (i.e., the primary spongiosa appears in the developing bone cavity). The chondrocytes toward the epiphyseal ends of the model continue to proliferate and hypertrophy. At about this time, a secondary center of ossification begins within the epiphysis of the cartilage model. Some of the chondrocytes in the metaphysis assume a flattened discoid shape and look much like columns of stacked coins. These

changes result in a cartilaginous disk or plate between the primary spongiosa and the secondary ossification center; this arrangement of cells is called the *epiphyseal*, or *growth*, *plate* (see Fig. 5-16E). The growth plate is the major site of the elongation, growth, and remodeling of the bone until the time of puberty. This is the result of a many year–long cycle of chondrocyte proliferation, hypertrophy, calcification, resorption, and replacement by bone (see Fig. 5-16F) until the epiphyseal plate is completely ossified (or closed), which occurs at the end of puberty. At this time, full adult stature is attained (see Fig. 5-16G).

Epiphyseal Plate

An epiphyseal plate and a diagram based on it are shown in Figure 5-17. The plate is usually divided into four zones (some authors name five) as indicated on the diagram, although the names of the zones may differ in different sources. By convention, the zones are numbered starting farthest away from the diaphysis. In zone 1 are the resting or reserve chondrocytes. Zone 2 is where proliferating chondrocytes are found. Zone 3 is where the chondrocytes mature, deposit

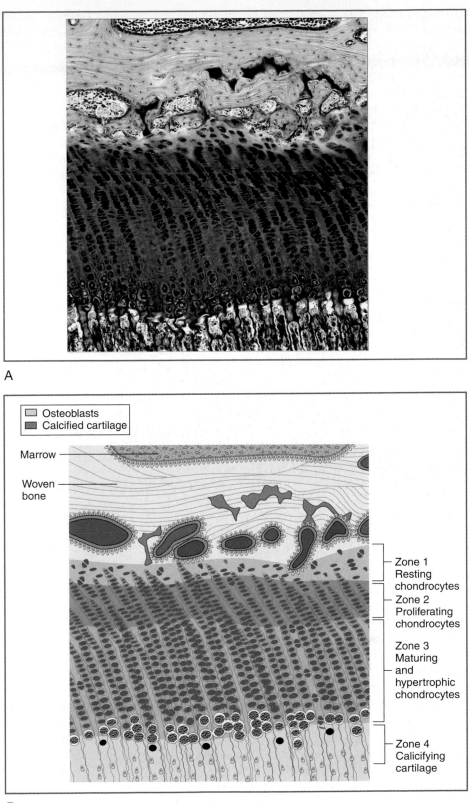

A

B

Figure 5-17. A, Micrograph of an epiphyseal plate (H&E, 50×). **B,** Diagram of the specimen with the four zones and other parts of the epiphysis labeled.

matrix, and begin to hypertrophy. The farther zone 3 chondrocytes are from zone 2, the greater is their rate of matrix deposition; hence, zone 3 is primarily responsible for growth of the epiphyseal plate. The hypertrophic chondrocytes begin to synthesize type X collagen, secrete factors that stimulate microvascularization (ingrowth of capillaries), and undergo programmed cell death. In zone 4, the cartilage calcifies and is invaded by capillaries, osteoblasts, and hematopoietic tissue. The rate of matrix production by hypertrophic chondrocytes (at the zone 3 to zone 4 interface) is what drives bone lengthening—at a considerable rate during fetal life and at a slower rate during postnatal life. Figure 5-18 shows an epiphyseal plate at low magnification and four selected fields at higher magnification to illustrate the different zones.

The molecular characteristics of cartilage and the various genes that are expressed in all cartilage, but especially the epiphyseal plate, are worth noting in the context of an epiphyseal plate. Among the minor protein components of cartilage matrix are proteins called endostatins. These proteins inhibit the growth, motility, and proteases that are characteristic of endothelial cells (the epithelial cells of capillaries that line all blood vessels) when they vascularize any tissue. The cartilage endostatins are thought to be a major factor in maintaining the avascular nature of cartilage. As mentioned above, hypertrophic chondrocytes secrete a specific growth factor (vascular endothelial growth factor, VEGF) that stimulates the local vascularization of cartilage matrix. Therefore, the profound changes that occur in zone 4 of the epiphyseal plate—cartilage matrix deposition, cessation of endostatin synthesis and release, and new secretion of VEGF by hypertrophic chondrocytes—lead to cartilage calcification and vascularization of this zone.

The characteristics of bone growth and development described in the preceding paragraphs and depicted in Figure 5-16 primarily refer to long bones. Many bones that develop by the endochondral mechanism do not become long bones and do not have a "typical" epiphyseal plate even though all the cells and characteristics described above are found in these instances. Many of the specific factors (signaling pathway molecules and the transcription factors they regulate, and various growth factors) that are instrumental for the controlled and coordinated series of events described above have been elucidated. Over 30 such molecules have been identified. Nonetheless, a number remain to be discovered (e.g., what controls the polarity of the columns of chondrocytes and the morphologic and functional changes in the growth plate; what controls the specific morphology of each bone; what controls the coordination of the events associated with the growth plate with the development of joints, ligaments, and tendons).

●●● BONE GROWTH AND REMODELING

Overview of Bone Growth

The elongation of growing bone is due to chondrocyte proliferation and the deposition of new cartilage matrix in zones 3 and 4 of the epiphyseal plate.

Ossified bone matrix grows only by the appositional mechanism irrespective of its initial mechanism of formation (intramembranous or endochondral).

Bone increases in width, diameter, or thickness by cycles of appositional deposition and resorption of compact osteonal and other lamellar bone as well as of cancellous bone. As these cycles of deposition and removal occur, the marrow cavity enlarges by removal of bone at the endosteal surface. Figure 5-19 illustrates these changes.

As compact cortical bone grows in length and diameter in the metaphyseal region, some of the resorbed endosteal compact bone may remain in the form of cancellous bone. This, in part, accounts for the lamellar nature of cancellous bone.

Bone Remodeling

The overall changes in macroscopic bone dimensions summarized above are achieved by a coordinated series of events requiring osteoclastic bone resorption and osteoblastic bone deposition, as shown in Figure 5-20. The leading end of a resorption canal is "younger" than the trailing end. The trailing ("older") end has been filled in with a series of

---

ANATOMY & EMBRYOLOGY

Achondroplasia—Dwarfism

Achondroplasia is a mutation in a gene that affects the fibroblast growth factor-3 receptor (FGFR3), a receptor found on the plasma membrane of chondrocytes. The receptor provides negative growth control, which means that chondrocytes do not respond to FGF properly and do not proliferate normally, thereby inhibiting development of the epiphyseal plate.

Achondroplasia is an autosomal dominant disease. The majority of individuals born with this disease are born to parents of normal stature; this means that a mutation occurs in the germline in one or both parents. These mutations occur with an incidence of about 7 in 250,000 live births. Surprisingly, this new mutation occurs in the same locus in affected individuals with a high incidence, although more detailed molecular genetic analysis indicates that different amino acid substitutions at this codon can cause clinically distinct disorders. A number of other growth plate disorders result from loss-of-function mutations in transcription factors (the homeobox genes), which act very early in development. These are called *SHOX* (for short stature homeobox) gene mutations. Individuals with these disorders demonstrate abnormally short zones of proliferation in the growth plate. Furthermore, within this zone, the chondrocytes are arranged more side-by-side than longitudinally, so they tend to form cell nests rather than columns of chondrocytes. Consequently, the hypertrophic zone is also adversely affected, leading to a phenotypic dwarfism.

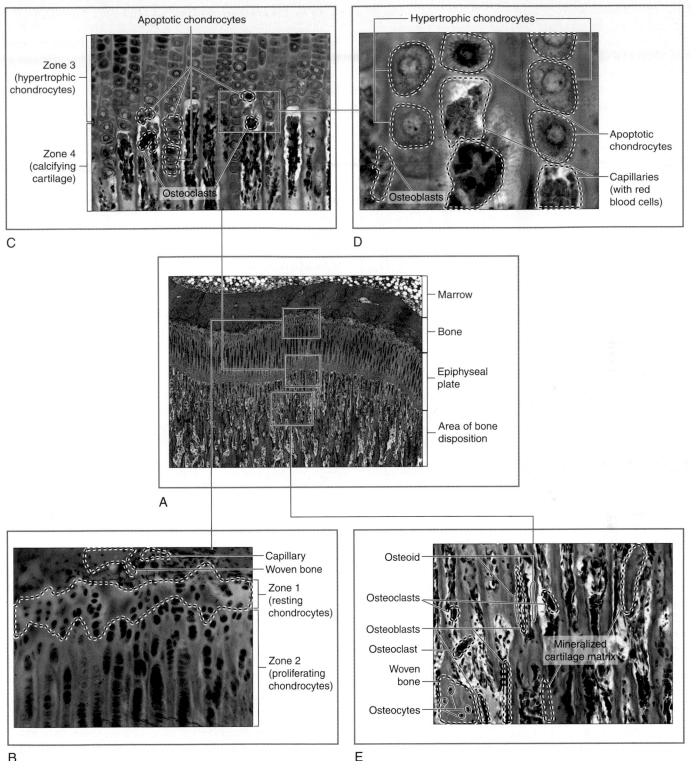

Figure 5-18. Micrographs of an epiphyseal plate. **A,** Low-magnification micrograph of the whole growth zone is at the center. **B,** Higher magnification of zone 1, the resting chondrocytes. The chondrocytes are smaller and distributed more or less randomly in this zone. Just below the resting chondrocytes is the beginning of zone 2 with its many columns of proliferating chondrocytes. **C,** Many hypertrophic chondrocytes (zone 3), some of which are undergoing apoptosis. The bottom part of this panel shows the beginning of zone 4, the zone of calcifying cartilage. The extensive vascular invasion of the columns of apoptotic chondrocytes is seen along with several osteoclasts, osteoblasts (lining the spicules of calcified cartilage), and hemopoietic cells. **D,** A higher magnification of the area indicated in part C. Here are some osteoblasts on the lower left, two hypertrophic chondrocytes undergoing apoptosis, several other hypertrophic chondrocytes, capillaries, and an osteoclast. **E,** View of the spongiosa illustrating many of its important features. There are many osteoclasts, osteoblasts, and osteocytes associated with spicules of calcified cartilage. A thin layer of lighter staining (pink) osteoid is seen in a number of places associated with the layers of osteoblasts.

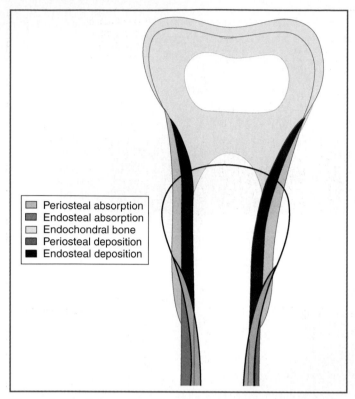

Periosteal absorption
Endosteal absorption
Endochondral bone
Periosteal deposition
Endosteal deposition

Figure 5-19. Schematic of the macroscopic changes that occur during growth and elongation of a long bone. Note the extensive areas of periosteal and endosteal bone resorption and deposition along the bone shaft. The whole epiphysis of the bone undergoes substantial changes in its progress toward becoming ossified (which is not depicted in this diagram).

concentric lamellae, producing a new osteon. As each new lamella of the osteon is deposited, some of the osteoprogenitor cells divide and remain on the endosteal surface to produce the next lamella (i.e., osteons grow in a centripetal direction). This process of compact bone resorption and new osteon formation explains the appearance of adult bone. Three generations of resorption of "old" compact bone and deposition of "new" osteons are depicted in Figure 5-21; as can be seen, each succeeding generation of osteons partially replaces older osteons. The remnants of even older osteons are seen as interstitial lamellae.

Osteons may be found in intramembranous bone, and new osteons may form on periosteal or endosteal surfaces of adult compact bone. Figure 5-22 illustrates how these events occur. The micrograph in Figure 5-22A shows an early stage in intramembranous bone formation. The diagrams in Figures 5-22B, 5-22C, and 5-22D show how the large open space in the early bone plate becomes filled with concentric lamellae to form osteons in a flat bone. Note the capillaries in the middle of the presumptive osteons in Figure 5-22A; these become the vessels of the haversian systems.

●●● BONE PHYSIOLOGY

As mentioned earlier, the inorganic matrix of bone plays a central role in maintaining the serum concentration of Ca^{++} (and PO_4^{3-}) within the normal physiologic range. Many factors act on bone cells to regulate Ca^{++} homeostasis; these include parathyroid hormone, calcitonin, pituitary hormones, thyroid hormone, leptin, vitamin D, estrogen, many cytokines, growth factors, transcription factors, diet, exercise, and doubtless more that remain to be discovered.

From a clinical and physiologic point of view, there is a hierarchy of factors that regulate bone mass. Calcium mobilization overrides other factors regulating skeletal mass and functions. Various "calcium-wasting" diseases (e.g., renal disease, malabsorption, or insufficient dietary Ca^{++} intake) cause a loss in bone mass, highlighting the primacy of maintaining serum Ca^{++} levels over maintaining skeletal mass per se.

As mentioned several times above, there is a balance between bone deposition and resorption, but the two processes do not occur at the same rate. If, for example, it takes 2 to 3 weeks (ca. 15 days) to resorb 20 g of bone, it takes about 3 months (ca. 90 days) to replace that amount of bone (i.e., it takes about six times longer to replace a given mass of bone). In a normal individual where bone mass is at a steady-state level, bone resorption and deposition are in balance, but if resorption increases by a few percent or deposition decreases by a few percent, there will be a measurable amount of osteoporosis in about a year. Each of the hormones discussed in the next section influences bone resorption or deposition, with parathyroid hormone being the most and leptin the least important.

Hormones

Parathyroid hormone (PTH), a polypeptide hormone, is secreted by the parathyroid glands; it acts to increase serum Ca^{++} levels by increasing osteocytic osteolysis and osteoclast activity. Osteocytes and osteoblasts have receptors for PTH on their plasma membranes. The hormone has a short lifetime (ca. 4 minutes) in the circulation, so its effects are rapid. PTH secretion is regulated by a direct feedback of Ca^{++} levels on PTH synthesis and release.

Calcitonin is also a polypeptide hormone and is secreted by cells associated with the follicles of the thyroid gland; they are called parafollicular or C (for "clear") cells. Osteoclasts have receptors for calcitonin; when the hormone is bound to the receptors, bone resorption by these cells is inhibited and osteoclast numbers are diminished.

Estrogen, one of the major hormones of the female reproductive system, has a significant effect on Ca^{++} deposition in bone. Normal levels of estrogen have a slight positive effect on bone deposition, but when estrogen levels decline during menopause, there is a loss in bone mass due to an increased rate of bone resorption. It is this increase in bone resorption that is a factor in the high rate of osteoporosis in postmenopausal women.

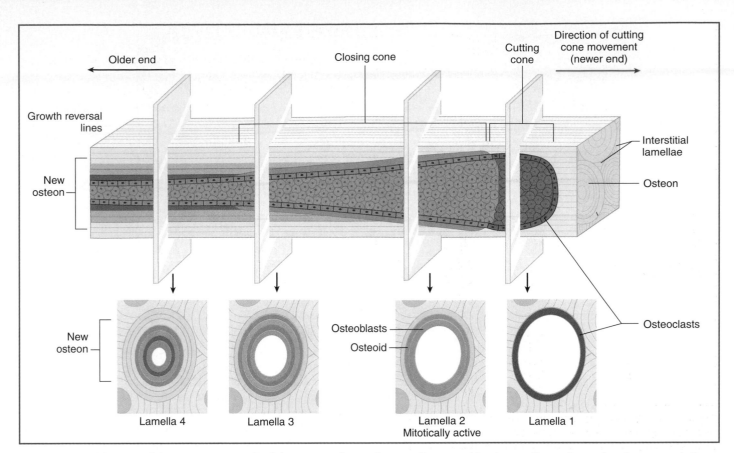

Figure 5-20. Diagram of the appearance of adult compact bone. A resorption canal is given a three-dimensional representation; see text for the process depicted here.

Figure 5-21. Diagrammatic representation of three generations of haversian systems in a small area of compact bone. **A,** First generation of osteons plus some interstitial lamellae (I). The dotted ovals show where the second generation of osteons will be. **B,** The first (*1*) and second (*2*) generations of osteons and where the third generation (*3*) will be. **C,** All three generations and interstitial lamellae. The oldest lamellae (the interstitial lamellae) are the lightest shade of ivory, and each succeeding generation of haversian systems is a darker shade of ivory.

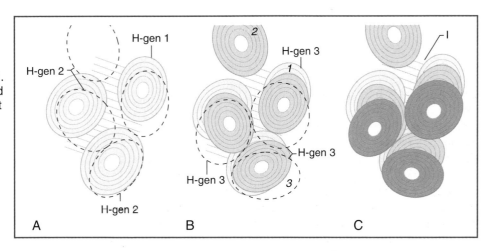

Hormones secreted by the pituitary gland and the releasing factors that regulate the secretion of these hormones regulate bone growth. The pituitary hormone somatotropin (also called pituitary growth hormone) has a direct effect on the growth of the epiphyseal plate. Excessive secretion of somatotropin during childhood years can lead to gigantism, whereas if the excessive secretion occurs during adulthood, a condition known as acromegaly results. This condition is largely due to the continued postpubertal growth of cartilage and other tissues.

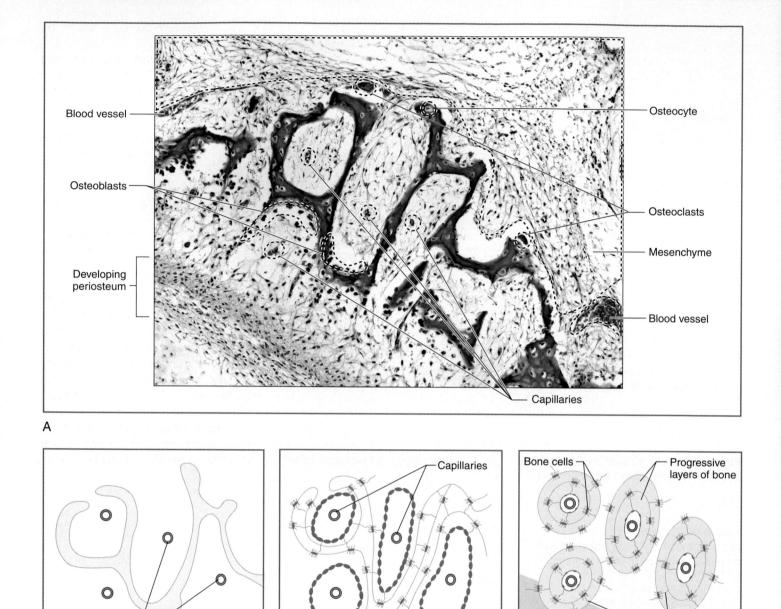

A

B

C

D

Figure 5-22. A, Early stage in a developing intramembranous bone in which some of the developing spicules have fused into a small bit of trabecular bone. The surface at upper right has a few osteoclasts associated with it, and the surface at lower left has many osteoblasts—suggesting a wave of bone formation on one surface and bone resorption on the other. There is a suggestion of the beginning of a periosteum developing in the lower left of the field. Much of the field is filled with mesenchyme; a significant number of small blood vessels and capillaries are also present. **B–D,** Idealized diagrammatic series of events show how this flat bone fills in with osteons and lamellar bone to assume a more mature appearance.

Insufficient thyroid hormone (*hypothyroidism*) during fetal life and childhood years can result in shorter than normal stature (*dwarfism*). Normal levels of the thyroid hormone are required for growth and function of chondrocytes in the epiphyseal plate. Since the levels of thyroid hormone are regulated by tropic hormones secreted by the pituitary gland as well as by synthesis of the hormone itself by the thyroid follicular cells, hypothyroidism can be due to pituitary or thyroid deficiencies.

Leptin is a hormone synthesized and secreted by adipose cells. Its major role is in regulating appetite—high leptin levels suppress appetite and increase energy expenditure. Most current understanding of leptin and its physiologic roles is based on studies with mice; however, several of leptin's actions in mice are not found in humans. Recent studies have shown that leptin-deficient mice have an unexpectedly high bone mass. This effect of leptin seems to be on the sympathetic nervous system via the ventral hypothalamus, which in turn can regulate bone formation. The effects of leptin on humans, and on bone formation in particular, are not fully understood and are the subject of considerable study.

Nonhormonal Factors

The nonhormonal factors discussed below appear in decreasing physiologic and clinical importance.

Vitamin D, in the form of 1,25-dihydroxy-vitamin D_3, is required for efficient uptake of dietary Ca^{++} from the intestines. It also has important roles in mediating the general physiologic effects of Ca^{++} released from bone under the influence of PTH.

In addition to their effects on Ca^{++} homeostasis in bone, PTH, calcitonin and 1,25-dihydroxy-vitamin D_3 influence Ca^{++} uptake and excretion in the gastrointestinal system and the kidneys, respectively.

Adequate dietary intake of Ca^{++} is essential for normal bone homeostasis. Pregnant or lactating women require additional dietary Ca^{++}, since a growing fetus or infant is making bone at a high rate. Children require more dietary Ca^{++} than adults, but the need for dietary Ca^{++} increases with age. Owing to their physiologic osteoporosis, postmenopausal women have an even greater increased requirement for dietary Ca^{++} than men do. In addition to increasing dietary Ca^{++}, many women take estrogen replacement therapy to help prevent osteoporosis, but more recent evidence suggests that other risks are associated with this practice.

A modest but regular exercise program helps maintain bone strength and integrity. Individuals who are confined to bed or are otherwise inactive suffer a loss in bone density. Astronauts, who are subjected to microgravity for extended periods of time, also experience a loss in bone density. Certain athletes during their active periods (e.g., baseball pitchers) have a greater bone mass in their throwing arm than in the other arm. However, women who are competitive distance runners may become amenorrheic and suffer a loss in bone density, since their estrogen levels fall below normal. These examples illustrate some of the hierarchical factors that regulate bone mass.

Nervous System and Special Senses   6

●●● BRAIN

The adult human brain represents an extraordinarily complex conglomeration of cells. It has been estimated that the outermost portion of the brain, the cortex, contains about 21 billion neurons. Since the cortex represents about 40% of the total volume of the brain, the entire brain probably contains approximately 50 billion neurons. Each neuron can receive hundreds of connections from other neurons, and each neuron has its own distinctive anatomy, physiology, and complement of neurotransmitters. This colossal degree of complexity suggests that, in a strict sense, we may never gain a precise and complete understanding of how the brain functions.

Nevertheless, since neurons are organized into specific groups with specific connections and functions, there is some hope that we can eventually gain some approximate knowledge about the brain by understanding how each group contributes to the overall function.

Neuron Grouping

In the cortex, neurons form six layers that all show differences in cell size, shape, and spacing. Moreover, these layers show regional differences that were utilized by the German histologist Korbinian Brodmann to divide the cortex into 52 distinguishable regions, all with different connections and functions.

In subcortical structures such as the thalamus, hypothalamus, midbrain, brainstem, and spinal cord, neurons form irregular clusters of tens of thousands of cells that are called nuclei. Once again, neurons within a nucleus tend to have similar forms and functions. Thus, by analyzing the functions and interrelationships of cortical layers and of brain nuclei, neuroscientists hope to attain a greater knowledge of how the brain functions.

Organization of Brain Neuron Clusters

Originally, the central nervous system (CNS) forms as a simple, hollow tube that invaginates from the dorsal surface of the embryo. By the fourth week of development, this simple tube has developed swellings and constrictions that divide it into forebrain, midbrain, and hindbrain vesicles. Each vesicle, in turn, develops many subdivisions.

Cell Biology of Neurons

Neurons are highly polarized cells in that they have specific regions with different structures and functions (Fig. 6-1). The portion of a neuron immediately surrounding the nucleus is termed the cell body (soma) or perikaryon. The neuronal nucleus within the perikaryon has a number of characteristic features: It is large, typically round, and highly euchromatic and often possesses a large nucleolus. All these features indicate that the nucleus is transcriptionally active and is assembling large numbers of ribosomes. These features are in accord with what we know about gene expression in the brain, which is unusually high. In the cells of most other organs, only about 1000 to 4000 genes out of the total of about 25,000 genes are expressed, but in the brain, as many as 8000 genes may be transcribed. The high levels of protein synthesis within neurons also correlate with extensive

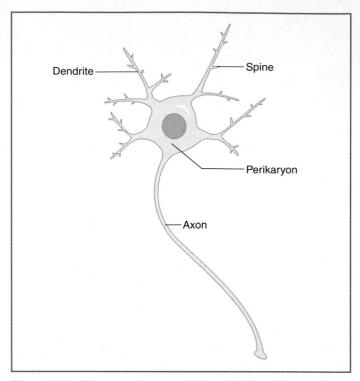

Figure 6-1. Diagram of a neuron showing the perikaryon, tapering dendritic processes, and a single, thin axon.

development of the rough endoplasmic reticulum (rER), which is detectable within perikarya as dense, basophilic masses termed Nissl bodies (Fig. 6-2).

Two different types of cell processes project from the perikaryon. Dendrites are relatively thick, tapering processes that often possess many small, irregular structures called dendritic spines. Dendrites convey electrical impulses toward the cell body (Fig. 6-3). Both dendrites and perikarya receive input from other neurons in the form of synaptic boutons (as noted in Chapter 2; see Figs. 2-7 and 2-8 for electron micrographs of neuronal and synaptic structures).

The other type of cell process is an axon. Neurons typically have only one axonal process, and that process, unlike dendrites, is quite thin, is uniform in diameter (lacking spines), and lacks ribosomes. Axons emanate from a region of the neuronal soma termed an axon hillock and often have synapses at their termini. Both types of processes are supported by elements of the cytoskeleton (microtubules and neurofilaments) that course along them from the perikaryon (see Fig. 1-20).

Neuron Polarization

Specific details are not yet known, but it seems that neurons become polarized in much the same way as epithelial cells. Epithelial cells, for example, may elaborate microvilli and tight junctions at one (apical) surface and a basal lamina at the other (basal) surface. This results from the early accumulation of a protein (PAR3 protein) at the apical end of the cell and a subsequent localized accumulation of the proteins that make up tight junctions and microvilli. Similarly,

PAR3 protein accumulates only in forming axons and seems to induce axon-specific proteins that regulate axonal structure. Henceforth, axons acquire specialized membrane proteins that induce glial cells to myelinate them and that govern the specific electrical properties of axons.

Neurons process information by receiving input from other neurons, by summing and modifying the input, and by generating bursts of electrical impulses that travel along the axon away from the perikaryon. Neurons convey electrical impulses well because they maintain a high membrane potential: the exterior surface of the cell membrane accumulates more positive atoms than does the interior one, leading to a charge separation and an electrical potential (voltage) across the cell membrane. This primarily occurs because neuronal cell membranes constantly leak potassium ions from within the cytoplasm but do not permit the reciprocal import of Na^+ ions. A simplified summary of the structure of a synapse is shown in Figure 6-4.

After a neurotransmitter binds to a postsynaptic receptor, its effects must be terminated to prevent a target neuron from firing indefinitely. One way this is accomplished is via neurotransmitter transporter proteins that take up neurotransmitter molecules from the synaptic cleft and return them to the neuronal cytoplasm for reutilization. Drugs that affect neurotransmitter transporter proteins can have potent effects on brain function. Cocaine, for example, blocks the reuptake of dopamine by dopamine transporters and has a powerful psychostimulant effect. Serotonin reuptake inhibitors are the active agents in antidepression drugs.

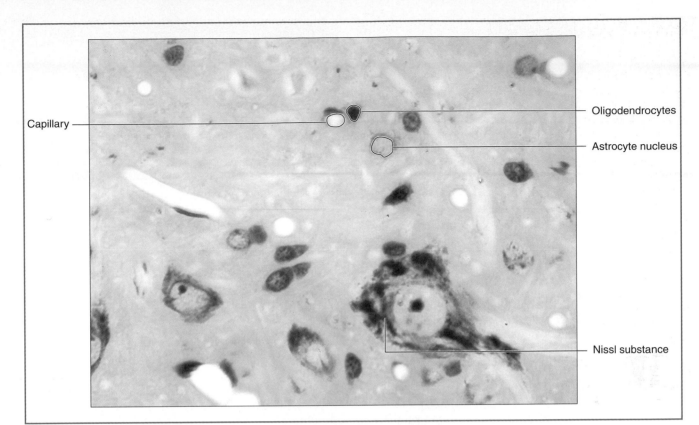

Capillary —

Oligodendrocytes

Astrocyte nucleus

Nissl substance

Figure 6-2. Conventionally stained neural tissue showing basophilic Nissl substance in a neuronal perikaryon. Light-staining nuclei of astrocytes and darker staining nuclei of oligodendrocytes are also visible.

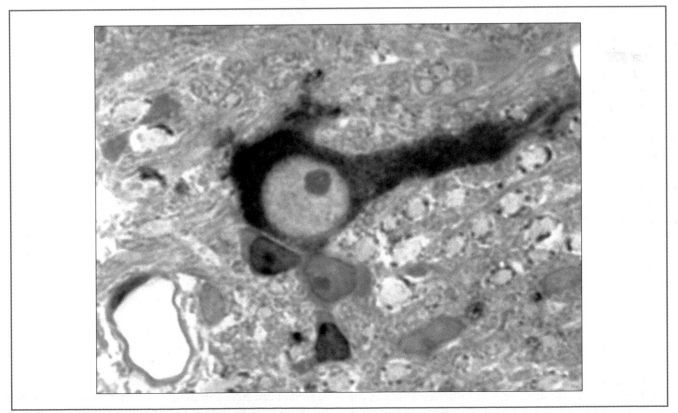

Figure 6-3. Dopaminergic neuron stained for the enzyme tyrosine hydroxylase (TH) (brown) using an immunocytochemical method. The TH enzyme fills the cytoplasm and distinguishes the tapering dendritic process from the surrounding neuropil. Nuclei of glial cells are adjacent to the neuron.

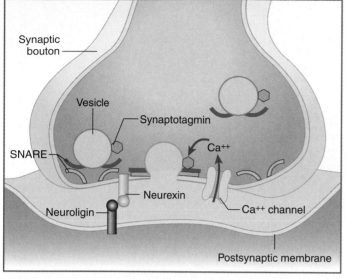

Figure 6-4. Diagram of a synaptic bouton. When Ca^{++} channels in a bouton are activated by an action potential, Ca^{++} enters the cell and binds to synaptotagmin. Synaptotagmin, in turn, alters the function of vSNARE proteins so that they bind to tSNARE proteins and cause fusion of a synaptic vesicle with the presynaptic membrane. Neurotransmitter molecules released from vesicles diffuse into the synaptic cleft to bind to postsynaptic receptor proteins. Other postsynaptic proteins such as neuroligin bind to presynaptic neurexins to keep the synaptic membranes in close apposition.

The mechanism by which a neuron generates action potentials and activates other neurons is subject to a wide variety of influences. One important influence appears to be the overall anatomy of the cell itself. Each neuron in each portion of the CNS has a distinctive arrangement of the dendritic processes that grow out of it. (Figs. 6-5 to 6-7). Pyramidal neurons of the cerebral cortex derive their name from a distribution of dendritic processes that form a rough triangle around the perikaryon; neurons of the cerebellum have their own distinctive dendritic "tree;" and so on. How this comes to be is uncertain, but studies indicate that homeotic proteins influence the precise geometry of the dendrites that a developing neuron will grow in each portion of the CNS.

The shape and branching pattern of this dendritic tree has a profound influence on the distribution of electrical charge on the neuron and can determine whether a neuron is a rapidly firing neuron with sudden bursts of action potentials, or a slowly firing neuron. So, in part, structure determines function in the CNS, and the overall anatomy of a neuron is not merely of incidental interest.

The chemical synapses described above are not the only means by which neurons communicate with each other. In addition, many neurons synthesize gap junctions between themselves composed of a protein called connexin-36. These gap junctions permit the flow of ions between neurons and allow large groups of neurons to fire in a synchronous manner. About 10% of most cortical neurons possess such electrical synapses, whereas in other brain regions, such as

PHYSIOLOGY

Synaptic Transmission

Activated synapses release chemical neurotransmitters into the synaptic cleft separating two nerve cells, and the neurotransmitters diffuse across the cleft to bind to postsynaptic receptors. A common excitatory neurotransmitter is glutamate; a common inhibitory transmitter is γ-amino butyric acid (GABA). A number of transmitters are catecholamines (e.g., norepinephrine or dopamine). Others are peptides (neuropeptide Y, substance P, orexin). At least 40 other neurotransmitters have been identified. When a neurotransmitter binds to a receptor two things can result:

- The cell is hyperpolarized by chloride entry. This increases the voltage difference between the exterior and interior of the cell, resulting in an inhibitory postsynaptic potential (IPSP). It also effectively lowers membrane resistance, making it harder to excite.
- The cell is depolarized by sodium entry. This decreases the voltage difference between the exterior and interior of the cell, resulting in an excitatory postsynaptic potential (EPSP).

If the dozens of synapses on the cell contribute more EPSPs than IPSPs to the membrane voltage, the overall membrane voltage of the entire cell will decrease. If this decrease is sufficient, it will activate voltage-gated sodium channels present in the axon and axon hillock. The result is a runaway influx of sodium into the axon and the propagation of a wave of depolarization (action potential) down the axon.

When the action potential reaches synaptic terminals at the end of the axon, it activates voltage-gated calcium channels in the membrane. As a result, calcium enters the synaptic bouton. Calcium modifies the function of so-called SNARE proteins on synaptic vesicles (vSNARES); the presynaptic membrane (tSNARES), and synaptic vesicles then fuse with the presynaptic membrane to release their contents.

Chemicals that degrade SNARE proteins block synaptic transmission. One such chemical is the toxin produced by bacterium *Clostridium botulinum*, which is now widely used in treatments of facial nerves. By blocking nerve transmission to facial muscles, skin wrinkling can be diminished.

Postsynaptic membranes also have an array of specialized proteins. Neuroligin proteins help keep the pre- and postsynaptic membranes attached to each other while other proteins anchor neurotransmitter receptors in place and help maintain the integrity of the synapse.

the hippocampus or inferior olive, as many as 90% of the neurons are capable of this alternative means of communication (see Fig. 2-5 for an overview of the hippocampus). Electrical synapses are more abundant in the brains of newborns and may play a role in brain development.

In addition to axons and dendrites, most CNS neurons elaborate another type of process that is rarely mentioned in most texts of histology or neuroscience. The process is a single nonmotile cilium that is thought to have some sort of additional sensory function. It is called a primary cilium.

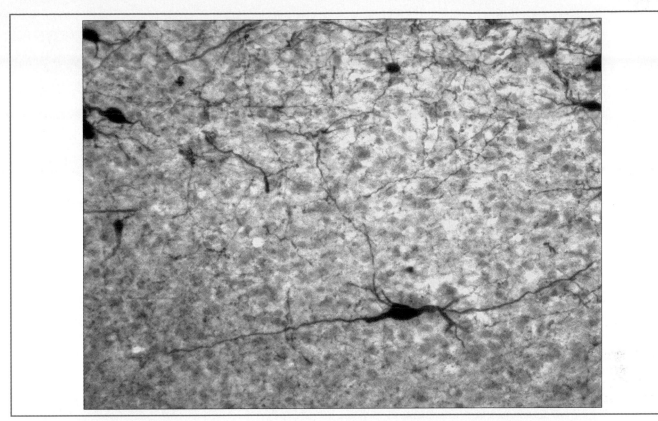

Figure 6-5. Dopaminergic neuron of the zona incerta of the hypothalamus, stained for tyrosine hydroxylase using an immunocytochemical method. Long, dendritic processes of this neuron extend in two directions only. No axons are visible in this micrograph.

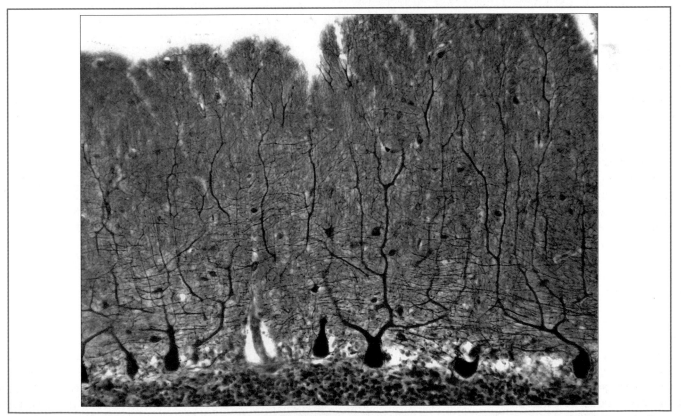

Figure 6-6. Purkinje cell neurons of the cerebellar cortex, stained with a Golgi silver stain. The dendritic arbor of these cells forms a flattened, fan-like pattern of processes.

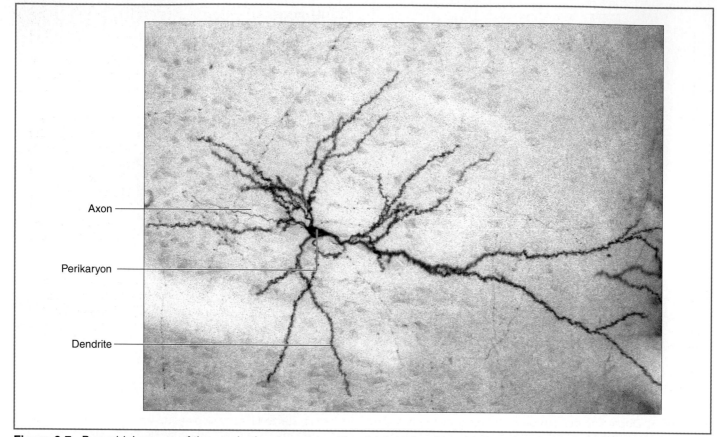

Figure 6-7. Pyramidal neuron of the cerebral cortex, stained for atrial natriuretic peptide using an immunocytochemical method. Tapering, apical, and lateral dendritic processes of this neuron occupy a pyramid-shaped space around the perikaryon. A single thin axonal process is also visible. (Courtesy of Dr. James McKenzie.)

Neuronal cilia have been ignored for many years, but it is now clear that they are abundant and functional in the CNS. Neuronal sensory cilia are particularly important for the function of the retina (see Retina). Their importance is also illustrated by a genetic disorder, Bardet-Biedl syndrome. In this rare syndrome (incidence of 1 in 150,000), abnormal ciliary function in neurons can lead not only to visual impairment but also to obesity and an impaired general functioning of the brain.

Another feature of nerve cells, plasticity of function, sets them apart from other tissue types such as muscle or epithelia. When stimulated, contractile cells of muscle or secretory cells of glandular epithelia typically react again and again in a predictable, stereotyped way: they always do the same thing. Nerve cells, however, can be trained to alter their responsiveness to a stimulus. This is the basis for learning and memory.

A classical example of the capacity of the brain for learning was first investigated by the Russian physiologist, Ivan Pavlov. Pavlov was studying the secretion of saliva in dogs, which commonly produced saliva in response to the taste of meat powder. During his experiments, Pavlov's apparatus made a ringing sound each time the dog was presented with meat powder. Subsequently, Pavlov was surprised to find that dogs had learned to salivate in response to the ringing sound alone even in the absence of the taste of meat. He termed this response a conditioned reflex, and the ringing sound was a conditioning stimulus.

Neuron Behavior

The activity of a single neuron can be visualized deep within the brainstem (salivatory nucleus) that controls the salivary glands (Fig. 6-8). This neuron may receive dozens of synapses from all over the CNS, but one synapse (*A* in Fig. 6-8), conveying a response to the taste of meat from gustatory brain centers, will have a particularly strong influence on the neuron's activity and will provoke a signal initiating salivation. If another synapse (*B*) from auditory regions conveying a response to a ringing noise is activated at the same time, that synapse will gradually acquire the strong potency of synapse A, so that a ringing sound will become associated with the taste of meat. Thus, simply put, a dog has learned to salivate in response to a bell, and a neuron has learned to fire in response to a ringing sound as well as in response to the taste of meat. The long-lasting change in synaptic function is a type of so-called long-term potentiation.

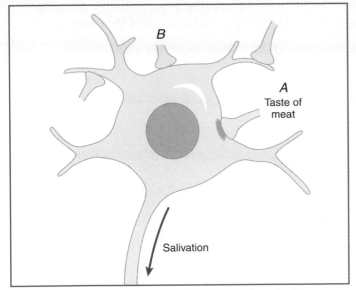

Figure 6-8. Diagram of a neuron that controls salivation. Synapse *A* conveys taste information and is a powerful stimulus to the neuron. Synapse *B* conveys sound information and can acquire the strength of synapse *A* if it is activated simultaneously with the activation of synapse *A*. This diagram depicts a paradigm of the learning process termed a conditioned reflex.

NEUROSCIENCE

Learning and Memory

The cell biology of learning is incompletely understood, but a number of principles are becoming clear. First, when a pair of synapses are activated for a long time, these synapses are labeled by a number of proteins.

The mRNA for a protein called activity-related cytoskeletal associated protein (ARC) specifically accumulates in activated synapses, and the ARC protein becomes incorporated into the synapse and may play a role in strengthening it.

Fragile X mental retardation protein (FMRP) also accumulates in activated synapses and regulates mRNA translation there. Genetic defects in a region of the X-chromosome containing the gene for the FMRP protein cause learning disabilities and can affect as many as 1 in 4000 male children.

Finally, when glutamate receptors are activated in a synapse, they cause the release from the synapse of a protein called CREB (cyclic AMP response element binding protein). CREB travels to the neuronal nucleus and stimulates the transcription of learning-related genes.

Neuron Learned Response

It is known that neurons that have undergone some types of "learning" actually display anatomic changes (e.g., numbers and sizes of dendritic spines increase). In many cortical neurons, about 10% of synapses are remodeled or removed each week! For this to have a meaningful, functional consequence, only specific synaptic areas of a neuron must be modified. For one thing, the neuron must "recognize" that two synapses are activated at precisely the same time. Secondly, only the activated synapses out of hundreds of inactive ones must somehow be labeled. Third, the labeled synapses must somehow be made permanently more effective so that the learned reflex is preserved. Some of the molecules involved in solving some of these challenges have been identified only recently.

Cell Biology of Neuroglia

In addition to neurons, about 60% of the cells in the brain are supporting cells called neuroglia. Three varieties of CNS glial cells are known.

Astrocytes

Astrocytes are cells with small, ovoid, euchromatic nuclei and numerous branching processes that extend away from the cell nucleus. Each process is supported by cytoskeletal intermediate filaments composed of glial fibrillary acidic protein (GFAP) (Fig. 6-9). Once regarded as merely occupying the space between neurons, astrocytes are known to have a number of important functions:

- Astrocytes induce endothelial cells of capillaries to construct extremely tight junctions that prevent the free passage of material from the blood into the brain (the blood-brain barrier). One secreted astrocytic protein that seems to participate in this induction is called *src*-suppressed *c*-kinase substrate.
- Astrocytes take up excess glutamate from neurons, transform it to glutamine, and export glutamine back to neurons for reconversion to glutamate. Astrocytes also scavenge excess potassium and other ions that are released from neurons.
- Astrocytes are a major site of glucose utilization in the brain and metabolize glucose into lactate, which is exported to neurons as a major nutrient.
- Astrocytes secrete a number of molecules into their environment, including cholesterol, that appear to regulate the ability of neighboring neurons to create synapses.
- Astrocytes respond to neurotransmitters released from activated neurons by secreting lipid molecules (epoxyeicosatrienoic acids) that dilate blood vessels. Dilated blood vessels provide more nutrients and oxygenated hemoglobin for rapidly firing neurons.
- Astrocytes possess a metal-binding protein, metallothionein I, and appear to protect the brain from toxic effects of metals such as mercury or cadmium.

After a brain injury that kills cells, astrocytes, but not neurons, have the capacity to undergo cell division and

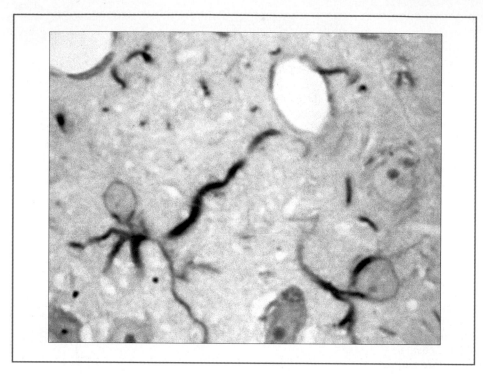

Figure 6-9. An astrocyte, stained by an immunocytochemical method, to illustrate cytoskeletal intermediate filaments of glial fibrillary acidic protein (GFAP).

migrate to the injury to replace the missing cells and form a glial scar. This structure may actually prove to be as much a hindrance as a help, since it seems to prevent the regrowth of new axonal sprouts through a damaged area. Glial scarring is one reason that spinal cord injuries may cause permanent paralysis: motor neurons of brain regions above the injury cannot establish renewed communications with spinal neurons that innervate the limbs. There is some hope, however, that this barrier to recovery can be overcome. Specialized glial cells found in the olfactory bulbs of the brain called olfactory ensheathing cells seem to create tunnels for regenerating axons and may allow them to pass through damaged regions, at least in experimental animals. If cells like these ensheathing cells could be transplanted into an injured CNS region, there might be an enhanced possibility of some recovery of function. Studies performed by a number of researchers have shown that implantation of ensheathing cells into the injured spinal cord of a rat can enhance the recovery of normal spinal anatomy and function.

Axonal Growth

Glial cells from one brain region (olfactory bulb) and astrocytes from other regions promote axonal growth. Neurons of the olfactory epithelium are virtually unique: unlike most other neurons, they have the capacity to undergo cell division. This means that newly formed neurons constantly have to insert axons from the olfactory epithelium, through the cribriform plate of the nasal cavity, and into the olfactory bulb of the brain. This constant remodeling of axons and connections, absent from most of the brain, demands that accessory cells permit the ability of axons to grow and make new connections.

Oligodendroglia

The main function of oligodendrocytes is to create the layer of insulating lipid and protein (myelin) that they wrap around axons. Iron atoms seem to be important for this process, and Perls' test for iron demonstrates the stubby, short, iron-rich cytoplasmic processes of oligodendroglia (Fig. 6-10). Oligodendrocytes have small, round, heterochromatic nuclei and make a number of specialized proteins, such as myelin basic protein and proteolipid protein, that stabilize the myelin sheath. In peripheral nerves, similar cells called Schwann cells myelinate axons in a similar fashion, but unlike oligodendroglia, Schwann cells can myelinate only one axon at a time rather than multiple axons from multiple neurons.

Microglia

Microglia have an anatomic appearance that makes them difficult to distinguish from oligodendrocytes in routine preparations. These cells, however, are functionally quite different. Unlike the other glial cells, which are derived from the neural tube, microglia develop in the bone marrow and are members of the mononuclear phagocytic cell population. Microglia have many proteins and properties in common with monocytes of the blood, and like monocytes, function as phagocytic cells that ingest and clean up debris within the brain. Perhaps the most important role of microglia takes place early in development. The new developing brain with an excess number of neurons. Many of these neurons fail to make proper connections with their targets in the brain or body and consequently undergo apoptotic cell death. Microglia phagocytose all of this cellular debris and prepare the brain for further maturation.

Figure 6-10. An oligodendrocyte, stained with Perls' test for iron, to show branching processes that myelinate axons.

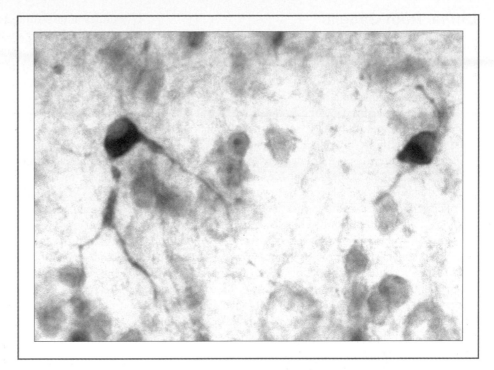

One unfortunate consequence of the monocyte-like phenotype of microglia is that these cells are prey to the same vulnerabilities as their counterparts in the immune system. Thus, they are easily infected with the AIDS virus (HIV) and may release cytokines such as interleukin-1 and tumor necrosis factor, which can damage adjacent neurons. This process may partly explain the abnormal brain function and dementia that may afflict patients in the later stages of HIV infection.

●●● SPINAL CORD AND PERIPHERAL NERVES

The spinal cord contains the same components as the brain: neurons organized into clusters called nuclei, and associated glial cells. In the adult, the spinal cord is 44 cm in length and has a diameter of about 12 mm. On this basis, the cord can be expected to contain hundreds of millions of neurons and therefore contains an appreciable fraction of all the neurons of the CNS.

The spinal cord is organized into an interior gray matter, containing neuronal perikarya, and an overlying white matter, containing mainly axonal processes. This ordering of layers in the spinal cord is the reverse order from that in the brain. The gray matter is subdivided into a dorsal horn that receives sensory input and a ventral horn where motor neurons are located. A major function of the spinal cord is to interact with associated structures that do not play nearly so important a role in the function of most of the rest of the brain. These structures are dorsal root ganglia and peripheral nerves.

PATHOLOGY

Alzheimer's Disease

Alzheimer's disease is an age-related degenerative brain disorder that currently affects 4 million North Americans. Symptoms include dementia and memory loss and are associated with neuronal cell death in specific CNS regions such as the hippocampus and nearby cortical regions. These brain regions contain extracellular structures called amyloid plaques that are mainly composed of a protein, amyloid-β protein. These aggregations of amyloid have a toxic effect on neurons.

A membrane protein called amyloid precursor protein (APP), along with proteins that stimulate its cleavage into plaque-forming fragments (β- and γ-secretases, presenilins), seem to have a central role in the disorder. Mutations in the APP and presenilin genes have been found among a relatively rare subset of individuals with Alzheimer's disease who show early onset of symptoms (often before age 55). The disease seems to segregate in an autosomal dominant manner in early-onset families as well.

A lipid-binding protein called apolipoprotein E (ApoE) somehow influences the course of the disease. If a specific isoform is inherited (ApoE4), the risk of developing the disease late in life increases from 20% to 90%. ApoE is produced mainly by astrocytes but is also present in selected neurons in the cortex and hippocampus. This distribution of ApoE may be one reason why only selected brain regions degenerate in this disease.

An aging-associated accumulation of oxidative stress in mitochondria, inflammatory brain processes, or age-related increases in obesity and diabetes may be related to the progression of the disease.

Dorsal Root Ganglia

Dorsal root ganglia originate as masses of neural crest cells that form alongside the developing neural tube (Fig. 6-11). These aggregations of specialized sensory neurons develop in response to a protein called brain-derived neurotrophic factor (BDNF) that is secreted by the neural tube. If this effect of BDNF is experimentally blocked in developing mice, the mice mature without any dorsal root ganglia.

While most neurons are noteworthy for the elaborate and complicated shapes of their dendritic trees, sensory neurons of the dorsal root ganglia are noteworthy for the relative simplicity of their anatomy: they are shaped like smooth, spherical balls and emit only a single, slender axonal process into the surrounding mass of axons (called the *neuropil*) (Fig. 6-12). Each axonal process bifurcates into two branches that grow in different directions. The first branch grows toward the neural tube and eventually will carry sensory information to the CNS. The second branch grows toward peripheral organs such as the skin and will carry sensory information toward the dorsal root ganglion. These unusual axons break the rule that axons only carry an action potential *away* from the perikaryon, since the second branch does send an impulse from the skin toward the dorsal root ganglion. In fact, however, this impulse bypasses the perikaryon and con-tinues uninterrupted into the spinal cord. Sensory neurons of the dorsal root ganglia were formerly called pseudounipolar neurons. In fact, these cells are unipolar, since they possess only one process at one pole of the cell, but since during development they often possess another process that subsequently degenerates, the term pseudounipolar was first applied to these cells (Fig. 6-13).

Once inside the spinal cord, sensory axons typically synapse on interneurons located in the dorsal region of the cord. These interneurons, in turn, can send processes that ascend or descend within the cord to innervate other neurons. Occasionally, these processes directly innervate motor neurons located in the ventral portion of the cord. These motor neurons then send their axons out of the CNS again. These three elements—a sensory neuron, an interneuron, and a motor neuron—constitute the simplest nervous circuit and are responsible for very simple, fast reflexes such as the knee jerk reflex. Efferent motor axons that leave the cord are gathered together with afferent sensory axons into bundles that form peripheral nerves.

Peripheral Nerves

Peripheral nerves contain a mix of various types of axons (large diameter, small diameter, myelinated, unmyelinated,

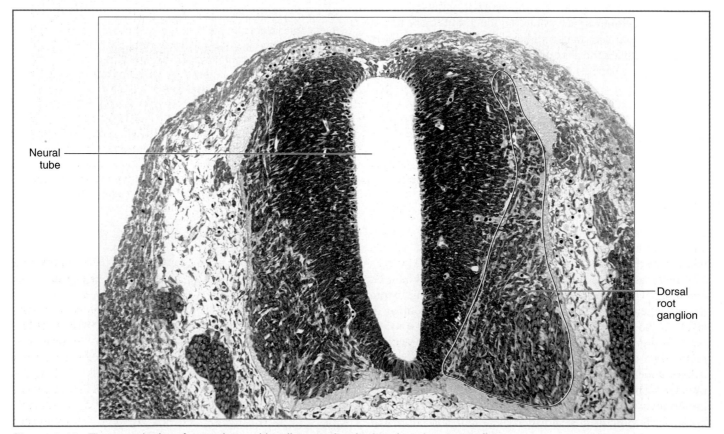

Neural tube

Dorsal root ganglion

Figure 6-11. The neural tube of an embryo with adjacent, developing dorsal root ganglia.

Figure 6-12. Diagram of spinal cord showing the ventral horn of gray matter, a dorsal root ganglion containing sensory pseudounipolar neurons, and a mixed peripheral nerve containing both sensory and motor axons.

Ventral horn

Dorsal root ganglion

Mixed peripheral nerve

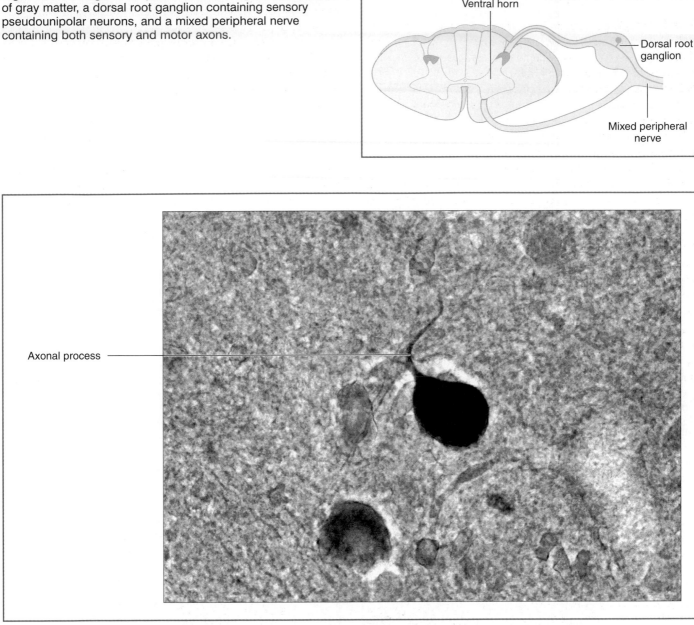

Axonal process

Figure 6-13. View of a sensory pseudounipolar neuron giving off its bifurcating axonal process. These neurons have both an unusual anatomy and an unusual metabolism, in that, unlike CNS neurons, they are able to accumulate glycogen. This glycogen, which fills the cell, was stained by the periodic acid–Schiff procedure that stains carbohydrates.

sensory, and motor) but no dendrites (Fig. 6-14). All peripheral nerve axons are enclosed by the cytoplasm of glial cells called Schwann cells. In some cases, Schwann cells wrap repeating layers of membrane around an axon to form a myelin sheath; in other cases (unmyelinated fibers), the axons merely pass along simple invaginations of Schwann cell cytoplasm (Fig. 6-15). Schwann cells are stimulated to differentiate and add myelin to axons by a protein, neuregulin, which is secreted by neurons.

One fortunate feature of Schwann cells is that these glia, unlike CNS glia, do not form obstacles to axonal regrowth after damage to a peripheral nerve. This means that a sub-stantial recovery of function can take place after injury to a peripheral nerve, unlike the events that take place after damage to a central nerve tract.

Glial cells myelinate axons. The advantage of a myelin sheath is that myelinated axons can conduct an electrical impulse more quickly and efficiently than unmyelinated axons. In an unmyelinated axon, a wave of depolarization slowly activates voltage-gated sodium channels all along the length of the axonal plasma membrane. In myelinated axons, such channels are 40-fold more concentrated at intervals along the axon, at sites between adjacent Schwann cells called nodes of Ranvier, than in the rest of the axonal mem-

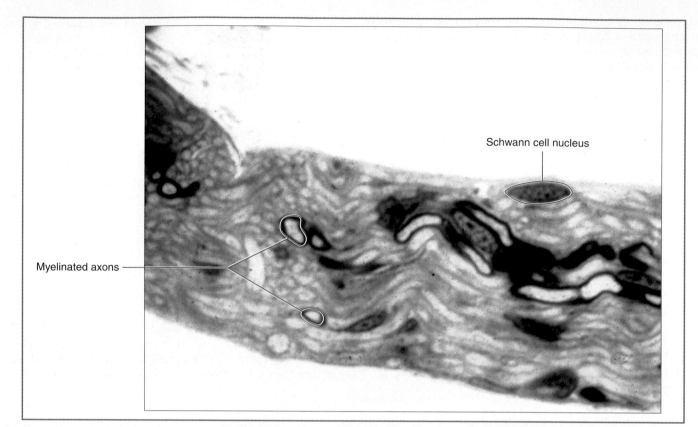

Figure 6-14. Longitudinal section through a peripheral nerve showing Schwann cell nuclei. The myelin sheaths of myelinated axons are dark-staining here owing to prior exposure to osmium tetroxide, which has an affinity for lipids in myelin. (Courtesy of Kate Baldwin.)

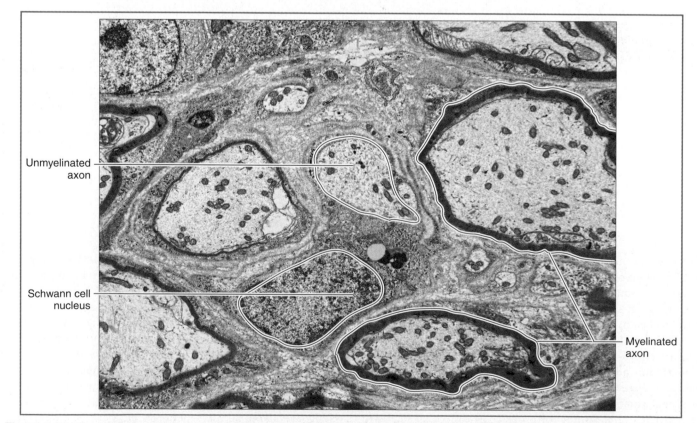

Figure 6-15. Transmission electron micrograph of a peripheral nerve showing myelinated axons and an unmyelinated axon encircled by the cytoplasm of a Schwann cell. (Courtesy of Enrico Mugnani.)

brane. When the sodium channels at one node of Ranvier open, a major change in extracellular ion concentrates at the node and quickly propagates through the low-resistance environment of the extracellular fluid until it activates the next node of Ranvier. This means of transmission, called saltatory transmission after the Latin word for jumping, is much more rapid and efficient than in unmyelinated axons. The insulating properties of myelin, formed of membrane lipids and at least nine myelin-specific proteins, make this form of conduction possible.

Additional components of a peripheral nerve are formed by three different layers of connective tissue: endoneurium, perineurium, and epineurium (Fig. 6-16; see also Fig. 3-6). The endoneurium is composed of sparse wisps of collagen plus fibroblasts and mast cells that directly touch the Schwann cells. The perineurium is a capsule-like structure formed by flattened fibroblasts and myofibroblasts that completely encloses a bundle of axons (typically 30 to 60 in number) and associated endoneurium. This perineurium layer is not easily penetrated by circulating molecules and constitutes the blood-nerve barrier that prevents harmful substances from penetrating nerves, just as the blood-brain barrier, composed of tightly sealed capillaries, prevents harmful material from entering the brain. Finally, located exter-nally to the perineurium, the epineurium is a sheath of dense, irregular connective tissue that binds together many bundles of axons to form a peripheral nerve. The large amounts of collagen in the epineurium and the special structure of the epineurium give a nerve the structural strength that prevents it from snapping when it is pulled or stretched.

Sensory Axons

The sensory axons present in a peripheral nerve terminate in skin, muscle, or connective tissue. These termini can function in the absence of any specialized sensory structures (nonencapsulated endings) or as axons enclosed in elaborate sensory structures such as pacinian corpuscles, muscle spindles, or Meissner's corpuscles (encapsulated endings). The functions of encapsulated endings are described in the preceding chapters on muscle and skin, but it is appropriate to briefly discuss the nonencapsulated endings here. These bare nerve endings respond primarily to pain, temperature, and pressure.

One striking feature of peripheral nerves is that they are typically accompanied by arteries, veins, and lymphatics, which constitute a neurovascular bundle. This is a direct consequence of the developmental and angiogenic properties of nerves.

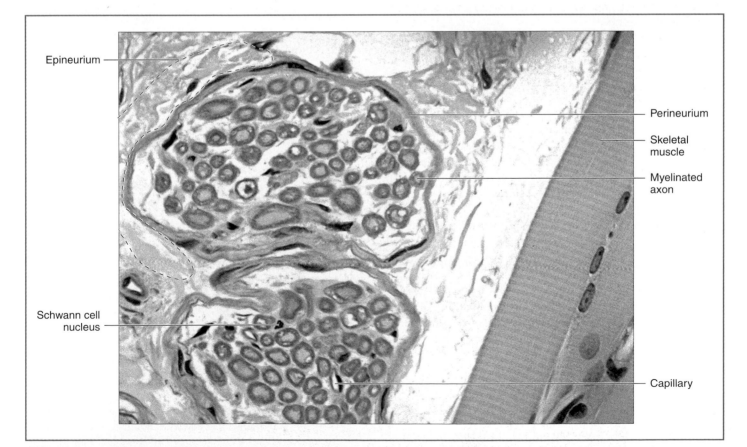

Figure 6-16. Light micrograph of a cross-section through a peripheral nerve showing the dense connective tissue of the epineurium, the perineurium, and the endoneurium. One probable Schwann cell is visible at the periphery of a myelinated axon. Skeletal muscle is visible at right.

NEUROSCIENCE

Sensory Nerve Endings

Pain-sensing nerve endings within the skin are presented with a serious challenge: how to discriminate between normal, nondamaging stimuli and destructive stimuli. Destructive stimuli injure cells and signal a sensation of pain that triggers a protective reflex withdrawal from the stimulus. Nerve endings respond to destructive stimuli by releasing ATP, and this reaction occurs when a living, active cell is damaged and bursts.

A subset of dorsal root ganglion cells synthesize so-called purinergic receptor proteins and transport them down to pain-sensitive nerve endings. These receptors, after binding ATP released from injured cells, signal a sensation of pain to the CNS. Other receptors on these endings bind histamine that is released from mast cells during inflammation.

Temperature-sensitive nerve endings have only recently been understood, thanks, curiously enough, to studies utilizing food flavorings. One flavoring that strongly mimics the sensation of heat is called capsaicin, the active ingredient found in chili peppers. It is now known that capsaicin evokes a feeling of heat by binding to temperature-sensitive membrane proteins that react to heat by allowing the entry of calcium and depolarizing a nerve ending.

Similarly, cold-sensitive neuronal proteins bind another flavoring, menthol, which mimics the sensation of cold. These food flavorings are all variants of vanillin, a molecule found in vanilla beans. Accordingly, the temperature-sensitive receptors of nerve endings have been named transient receptor potential vanilloid receptors.

During embryogenesis, axons grow out from the CNS in search of targets to innervate. The pioneering tip of an axon is called a growth cone, an active zone of the axonal cell membrane that constantly extends filopodia in all directions. As axons migrate, they secrete angiogenic factors such as vascular endothelial growth factor (VEGF), which stimulate the differentiation of nearby mesenchymal cells into arteries.

Axons are guided to their targets by a variety of extracellular molecules such as laminin and semaphorin. Once an axon has contacted a target, it responds to localized growth factors such as nerve growth factor, which stimulate the activity and survival of the far-away perikaryon. Neurons that fail to make such an axonal contact with their target undergo apoptosis and die. This process sculpts the anatomy of dorsal root ganglia: those ganglia innervating target-rich body areas such as the limbs remain fairly large, whereas the ganglia innervating target-sparse areas such as the thorax diminish in size.

Autonomic and Cranial Nerve Ganglia

Dorsal root ganglia are not the only accumulations of neurons that can be found associated with the peripheral nervous system. The autonomic nervous system also possesses two types of ganglia: parasympathetic ganglia (clusters of neurons buried deep within organs such as the salivary glands and the heart) and sympathetic ganglia, positioned as an interconnected chain along both sides of the vertebral column (Fig. 6-17). In all these ganglia, a specialized subtype of Schwann cell, the satellite cell, forms a layer that invests the surface of neuronal perikarya. Also, some of the cranial nerves that originate in the midbrain and brainstem and innervate the face have sensory ganglia with neurons that in many ways resemble those of the dorsal root ganglia. These sensory cranial nerve ganglia are the trigeminal (semilunar) ganglion of cranial nerve V, the geniculate ganglion of nerve VII, the glossopharyngeal ganglion of nerve IX, and the inferior (nodose) ganglion of nerve X.

●●● EYE

While the eye can be regarded as a sensory structure of the face, in many ways the eye is also an extension of the brain surrounded by a compartment of highly specialized connective and epithelial tissues. This viewpoint is borne out by examining the developmental process that creates the eye.

The eye develops from a spherical outgrowth from the forebrain called the optic vesicle. As this vesicle approaches the overlying ectoderm, it folds in about itself to form a cup-shaped structure (Fig. 6-18). This optic cup then induces another vesicle—the lens vesicle—to pinch off from the ectoderm and become attached to the margins of the cup. The anterior cells of the lens vesicle are simple cuboidal epithelial cells. However, the posterior cells of the vesicle are exposed to molecules such as fibroblast growth factor that are secreted by the optic cup. These cells respond by becoming transformed into extremely long and specialized lens fiber cells (see Lens). The optic cup itself differentiates into the retina, iris, and other structures.

ANATOMY & EMBRYOLOGY

The Eye

If all the steps in eye embryogenesis fail to go smoothly, a number of developmental anomalies can arise:

- Optic vesicle formation is under the control of a number of homeotic proteins called RX, PAX6, and PTX2. If these proteins are experimentally disrupted in mice, eye formation fails. These proteins may also underlie some human malformations of the eye.
- For two eyes to form from two optic vesicles, neural tissue must be subdivided along the midline via the action of a signaling molecule called sonic hedgehog (Shh). If Shh is inactivated or is not properly bound to cholesterol, the embryo develops a single, midline eye (cyclopia). This can commonly occur in sheep embryos after maternal ingestion of a plant with a toxin that affects Shh function. Very likely, cyclopia in sheep may have been a factual basis for the Greek myth of the sheep-herding Cyclops that threatened Odysseus.

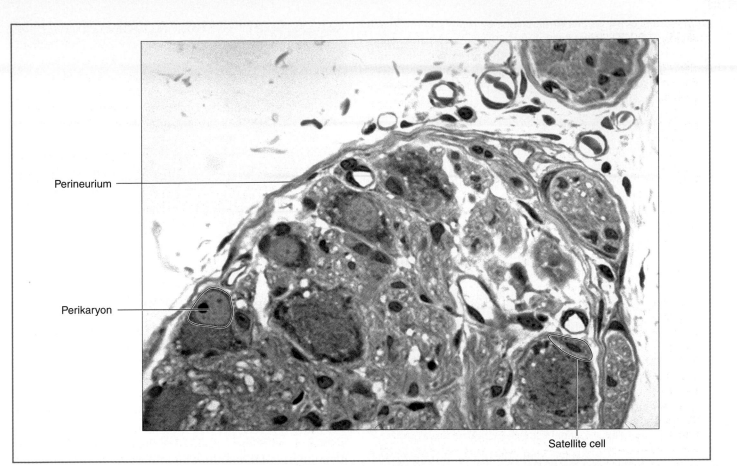

Figure 6-17. Sympathetic ganglion showing the perineurium, a neuronal perikaryon, and an adjacent satellite cell.

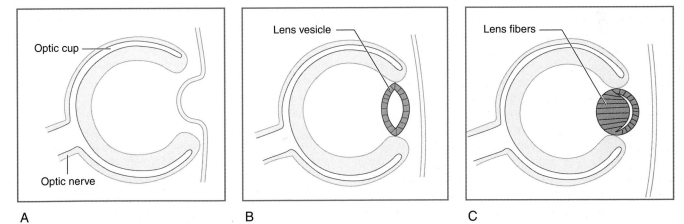

A   B   C

Figure 6-18. Diagram of eye development from the optic vesicle. **A,** The developing optic cup induces an infolding from the overlying ectoderm that becomes the lens vesicle at **B. C,** The posterior epithelial cells of the lens vesicle elongate to form lens fibers.

The adult eye contains three layers, or tunics, with distinct functions for each (Figs. 6-19 and 6-20). The outermost tunic of connective tissue is divided into the posterior sclera and the anterior, transparent cornea. Deep to this outermost layer is a vascular layer, or uvea. The uvea is also divided into a posterior choroid and into more anterior structures that form the ciliary body and iris. Finally, the innermost tunic of the eye is formed by the retina and a melanin-containing pigment epithelium that underlies the retina. This pigment epithelium is continued anteriorly to cover the ciliary body and a portion of the iris. All these structures have unique morphologies and functions that are discussed in the next section.

Cornea

Histologically, the cornea is a relatively simple structure: it is mainly composed of a dense regular connective tissue (stroma) covered on the exterior surface by a stratified squamous corneal epithelium and on the interior surface by a simple squamous epithelium (corneal endothelium) (Fig. 6-21). The rather thick basement membranes of these epithelia have been awarded distinctive names by early histologists (Bowman's membrane for the corneal epithelium basement membrane and Descemet's membrane for that of the endothelium). The anterior corneal epithelium, on encountering the margins or the cornea at a junctional landmark called the limbus, continues onto the surface of the sclera and also is reflected onto the inner surface of the eyelids as the conjunctiva. The connective tissue cells of the stroma also bear a special name—keratocytes.

The ordinary appearance of these structures under the microscope gives no clue about their transparency to light. One feature that helps make the cornea transparent is that it is totally avascular: no blood vessels or blood cells are present to scatter or absorb light. This avascularity is an unusual feature of corneal connective tissue (and cartilage). Both these tissues contain molecules that suppress the growth of capillaries. One such molecule, a transmembrane protein called tenomodulin, has been shown to suppress angiogenesis in the cornea and also in the lens of the eye.

Another basis for the transparency of the cornea is that stromal keratocyte cells deposit collagen fibers in their environment that all have the same diameter and are all spaced 20 nm apart. When photons enter this crystal-like, extremely regular arrangement of collagen, two things can happen: the photons can pass between the collagen fibers or bounce off the fibers at a 45-degree angle. When a photon bounces off at one angle, it invariably interacts with another photon bouncing off at an opposite angle, owing to the precision of collagen spacing. This phenomenon, called destructive interference, cancels out both photons. This mechanism is thought to be the basis for transmission of light through the cornea that is uncomplicated by diffuse rays that would make images hazy.

The regular spacing and orientation of collagen fibers in the cornea is critical for maintaining the transparency of the cornea. Two factors play an important role in this spacing:

PATHOLOGY

The Cornea

Corneal scarring or an imperfect corneal shape can lead to visual impairment, since the cornea is responsible for at least 70% of the refraction of light entering the eye. The avascularity of the cornea makes corrective corneal surgeries more feasible.

Corneal transplants from cadavers are widely used to replace damaged corneas. Such transplants are possible because the lack of blood vessels in the donor cornea protects it from attack by the immune system of the host.

LASIK (laser-assisted in situ keratomileusis) surgery utilizes lasers to reshape the contours of the cornea and enhance the visual acuity of a patient. An early variant of this procedure, radial keratotomy, was discovered by an ophthalmologist, Svyatoslav Fyodorov. Fyodorov found that the vision of a patient after corneal injury due to an automobile accident had mysteriously improved. He was prompted to repeat this accidental corneal reshaping with surgical cuts into the cornea that also reshaped it. Fortunately, the corneal epithelium and stroma react to injuries like these with a vigorous healing response.

spacing is adjusted by a glycosaminoglycan called lumican that binds to collagen fibers (mice lacking this glycosaminoglycan display cloudy corneas), and spacing is dependent upon the proper degree of hydration of the cornea. Since the cornea is rich in protein and since it is in constant contact with the fluid (aqueous humor) in the anterior portion of the eye, the cornea naturally tends to absorb water and expand like a sponge. To prevent this and to avoid disturbances in collagen spacing, the corneal endothelium constantly transports sodium, bicarbonate, and water out of the stroma and back into the aqueous humor.

One final special feature of the cornea is that all of its cells must be nourished by simple diffusion of molecules present in the tears or in the aqueous humor. As a consequence, any interference with tear production, such as damage to nerves innervating the lacrimal glands, can cause serious corneal damage. Such patients must continually apply solutions of artificial tears to their eyes to help lubricate and nourish the cornea.

Ciliary Body and Iris

Located just posterior to the limbus, the ciliary body is a wedge-shaped mass of smooth muscle and loose connective tissue (uveal layer) covered by a stratified cuboidal epithelium (retinal layer) that is thrown into a number of finger-like processes (ciliary processes) (see Fig. 6-20). This epithelium is unusual in that the innermost layer of nonpigmented cells (touching the aqueous humor) is upside down relative to the outermost layer of pigmented cells, so that the two cell layers touch each other at their apical surfaces. This is a

Figure 6-19. Diagram of the major structures of the adult eye. Three layers of the eye are shown. The outermost layer is composed of the anterior transparent cornea and the opaque sclera. The cornea joins the sclera at a landmark called the limbus. The second layer is composed of the posterior choroid and the anterior ciliary body, which holds the lens in place, and the iris. The third layer is the retina and pigment epithelium.

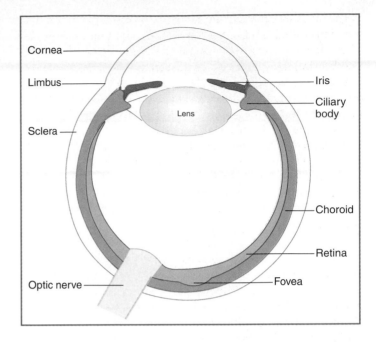

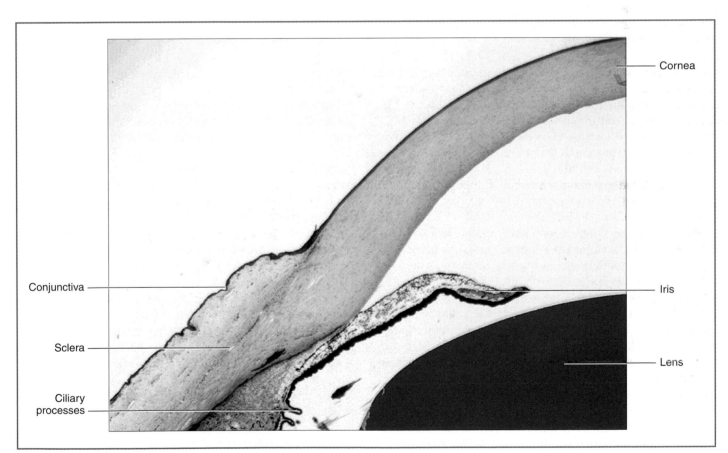

Figure 6-20. Low-magnification view of the anterior portion of the eye showing the cornea, iris, lens, and ciliary processes that extend into the aqueous humor from the ciliary body. The sclera is covered by an epithelial layer termed the conjunctiva, which is continuous with the epithelium covering the cornea.

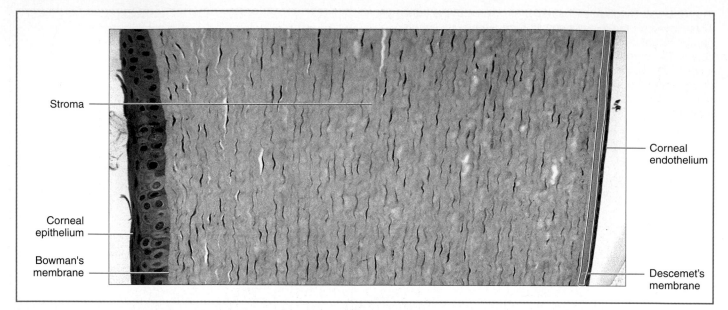

Stroma

Corneal epithelium

Bowman's membrane

Corneal endothelium

Descemet's membrane

Figure 6-21. View of the cornea showing the corneal endothelium, Descemet's membrane, stroma, Bowman's membrane, and the outermost corneal epithelium.

consequence of the invagination of the optic vesicle to form the optic cup during development, which brings together the two cell layers that will form the ciliary epithelium. The arrangement of cells in the ciliary epithelium represents a simple version of that found in the retina, where the apical surface of pigmented cells faces the apical surface of the photoreceptor cells (Fig. 6-22).

The ciliary epithelium has a number of important secretory functions. One of these—the production of aqueous humor—is achieved by transporting sodium, chloride, and water through basal infoldings of both cell types, across the cells, and into the aqueous humor. Aqueous humor in many ways represents an ultrafiltrate of plasma escaping from the fenestrated capillaries present within the ciliary body, with one prominent exception: the concentration of proteins in aqueous humor is almost a thousand-fold less than in plasma. This low level of proteins is important, since some protein molecules are large enough to scatter light and interfere with vision. To prevent serum proteins from entering the aqueous humor, ciliary epithelial cells are sealed together by tight junctions that form a functional blood-eye barrier.

The nonpigmented layer of the ciliary epithelium has another function—the secretion of molecules comprising the zonular fibers that make up the suspensory ligament of the lens. This ligament anchors the lens to the ciliary body. A major component of zonular fibers is a protein called fibrillin, which is also abundant in elastic fibers of connective tissue (see Fig. 4-8A). These fibers insert into the basal lamina of the ciliary epithelium and also into the basement membrane that surrounds the epithelial cells of the lens (also called the lens capsule). In Marfan syndrome, a genetic disorder, fibrillin production is abnormal. This leads both to inelasticity of

connective tissues and to displacement of the lens from its proper position.

Beneath the ciliary epithelium and associated loose connective tissue is a mass of smooth muscle, the ciliary muscle. This muscle has several subdivisions organized in complicated ways; the major subdivision is composed of bands of smooth muscle that run in a circular direction, parallel to the margins of the cornea and organized in the same way as a purse-string that opens and closes an old-fashioned money bag or purse. When these smooth muscles contract in response to parasympathetic innervation, the overall diameter of this muscular circle decreases and the tension on the lens lessens. This allows the lens to assume a more rounded shape, shortening its focal length, so that light from nearby objects can be focused on the retina (a process called accommodation). This arrangement makes sense: the eye at rest naturally focuses on distant objects, and muscular effort need be applied only when close-by objects are examined.

An anterior projection of the ciliary body is a flat plate of connective tissue called the iris (Fig. 6-23). The iris is pierced at the center by an opening, the pupil, which admits light into the eye. The posterior surface of the iris is covered by a stratified cuboidal epithelium that, unlike the ciliary epithelium, produces pigment granules of melanin in both layers. This posterior epithelium stops at the pupillary margin, so that the anterior surface of the iris is bare of epithelium and the connective tissue (stroma of the iris) is in direct contact with the aqueous humor.

The iris is not a static plate of tissue but can change its shape to allow more light or less to enter the eye. Two muscles accomplish this. The constrictor pupillae muscle is a circular band of smooth muscle located in the iridial stroma at the

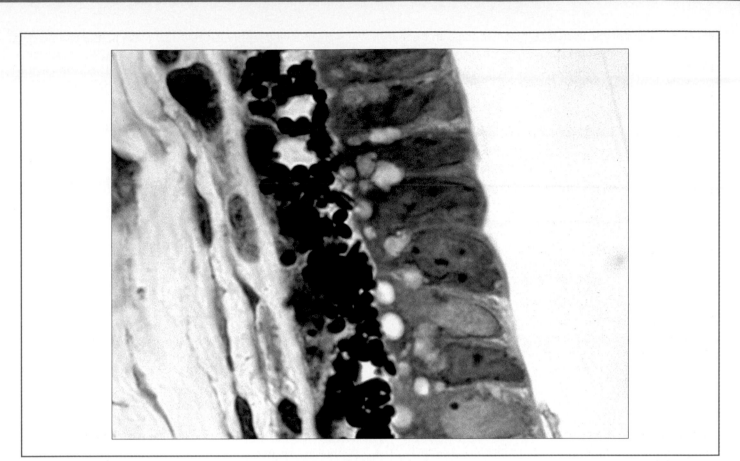

Figure 6-22. High-magnification view of the epithelium covering the ciliary processes showing the innermost nonpigmented cells and the outermost cells containing pigment granules filled with melanin.

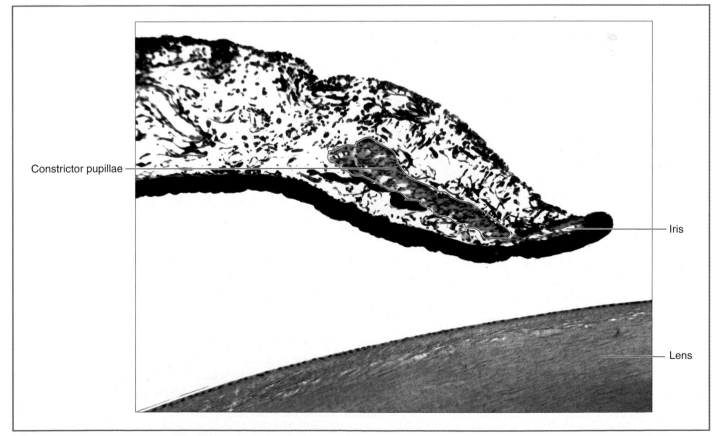

Constrictor pupillae

Iris

Lens

Figure 6-23. View of the iris showing the constrictor pupillae muscle embedded within the stroma. (Courtesy of Kate Baldwin.)

pupillary margin of the iris. This muscle contracts in response to parasympathetic stimulation. Fibers of the other muscle, the dilator pupillae muscle, have an unusual origin and morphology: they are formed within the basal compartment

of pigmented myoepithelial cells that make up the basal layer of the posterior epithelium of the iris (Fig. 6-24). These cells extrude thin, irregular cell processes rich in myosin and actin into the iridial stroma, and they contract upon stimulation by sympathetic nerves. The balance of activity of these two muscles determines the diameter of the pupil and the amount of light entering the eye.

Trabecular Meshwork

Just anterior to the iris is a specialized patch of tissue called the trabecular meshwork. This is composed of thin strands of connective tissue (collagen and fibroblasts) that are covered by a thin, simple squamous epithelium that is continuous with the endothelium of the cornea. The trabecular meshwork functions as a filter and outflow channel for aqueous humor, which originates in the posterior chamber of the eye at the ciliary body and percolates forward around the lens to enter the anterior chamber of the eye via the pupil. Aqueous humor enters the trabecular meshwork and then leaves it to enter a hollow tube embedded in the connective tissue of the sclera called the canal of Schlemm (Fig. 6-25).

The task of removing aqueous humor from the eye without breaching the blood-eye barrier is accomplished by the simple squamous epithelial cells of the canal of Schlemm via macropinocytosis, in which huge pinocytic vesicles form on the meshwork side of the epithelium, pinch off to enclose a

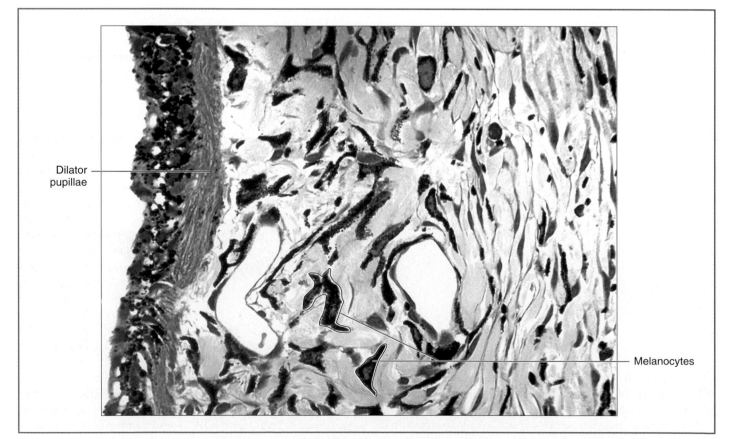

Figure 6-24. High-magnification view of the iris showing melanocytes within the stroma. Processes from the posterior epithelial cells of the iris form the dilator pupillae muscle.

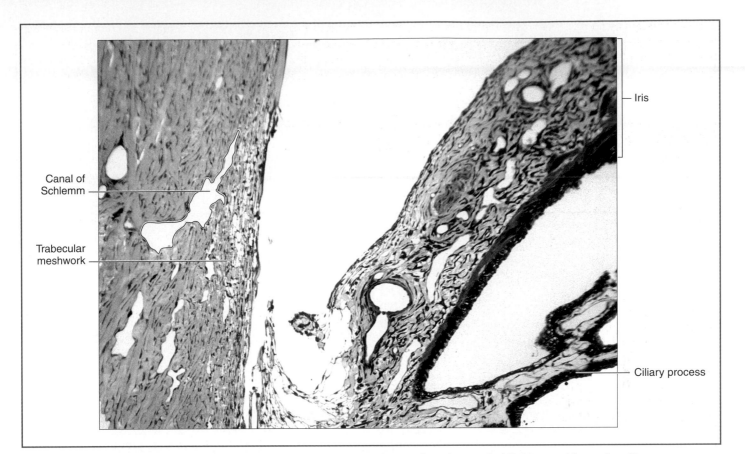

Figure 6-25. View of the iridocorneal junction showing the trabecular meshwork, canal of Schlemm, iris, and a ciliary process.

PATHOLOGY

Glaucoma

Glaucoma is an extremely common condition, affecting an estimated 75 million people worldwide (1.9% of North Americans over the age of 40 may have this condition). There appear to be multiple causes.

One cause is an abnormality in a gene for a protein called myocilin, which is abundant in cells of the trabecular meshwork. Mutated forms of myocilin appear to be folded improperly and accumulate within cells of the trabecular meshwork.

Another stimulus for glaucoma occurs when pigmented epithelial cells of the iris degenerate and release melanin granules into the aqueous humor. These granules appear to clog up the passageways within the trabecular meshwork and impede the drainage of aqueous humor.

drop of fluid, and move to the luminal side of the canal to release the fluid into the interior. This fluid, in turn, is drained off via venules that directly connect to the canal of Schlemm.

If an imbalance between the formation and the removal of aqueous humor develops, intraocular pressure will gradually increase and can have damaging effects on the retina and the optic nerve. This condition is called glaucoma.

Lens

As noted previously, the lens is composed of extremely long cells that form from the epithelial cells on the anterior surface of the lens. They multiply and differentiate at the margins of the lens (bow of the lens) (Fig. 6-26). These cells, like many other cells of the eye, are unusual. When fully differentiated, these cells destroy all of their membranous organelles, including even the nucleus. Only a very few other cells in the body (e.g., erythrocytes and keratinocytes) undergo such a drastic transformation. The process of destruction of a lens cell nucleus shows similarities to events that take place during programmed cell death (apoptosis) and, indeed, a number of apoptotic enzymes that destroy DNA (caspases, DNAase) are active in lens cells. Somehow, however, this destructive process is limited so that the entire cell does not die.

Even if lens cells are not dead, they cannot be viewed as vigorously alive either. Lacking rER or mitochondria, they cannot synthesize new proteins or carry out oxidative metabolism. They survive by anaerobic glycolysis of glucose and other molecules, utilizing sparse amounts of cytosolic

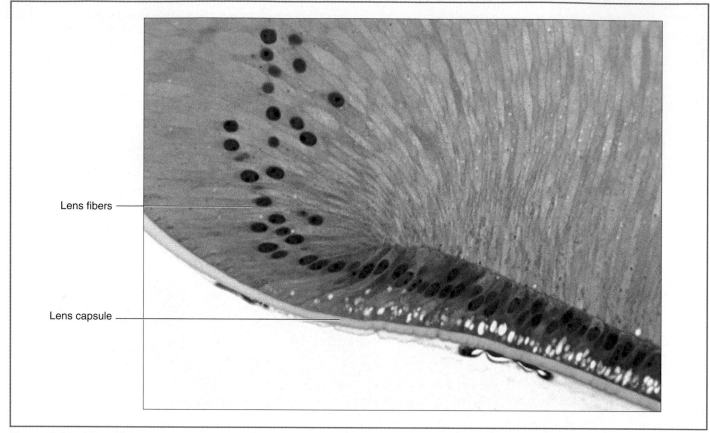

Lens fibers

Lens capsule

Figure 6-26. View of the margin of the lens showing the transition from short, anterior epithelial cells to the elongated, posterior epithelial cells known as lens fibers. All these epithelial cells are surrounded by a thick basement membrane called the lens capsule.

glycolytic enzymes. Since cells deep within the lens are far from the aqueous humor, they depend on the transfer of nutrient molecules from other lens cells via gap junctions between cells. Most of the protein within lens cells is in the form of crystallin proteins. Once again, an orderly arrangement of crystallin proteins appears to be critical for the maintenance of lens transparency.

Retina

The retina is composed of three layers of nerve cells—two layers of nerve processes that interconnect them and an underlying pigment epithelium (Figs. 6-27 and 6-28). Each layer of neurons is complex enough to justify an in-depth look.

Photoreceptor Layer

Human eyes possess two types of neurons in the photoreceptive layer that directly respond to light: rods (responsive to dim light) and cones (responsive to colors in bright light). Each eye has about 7 million cones and 100 million rods. Photoreceptor neurons are unusual in that they possess a single, highly modified cilium instead of dendrites that receive signals from other cells.

PATHOLOGY

The Lens

When the lens of the eye becomes cloudy or opaque, this condition is called cataract. Cataract surgery to remove cloudy lenses and replace them with artificial plastic lenses is the most common operation for adults aged 65 and older and, in 2002, accounted for 12% of the U.S. Medicare budget. Although this condition can be corrected, efforts to avoid cataract formation are desirable. There are two important risk factors for cataract:

- Exposure to ultraviolet (UV) light. A study of Maryland fishermen some years ago showed that those who did not wear a brimmed hat or sunglasses during exposure to summer sunlight had a three-fold increase in the risk for developing cataracts. UV light can cross-link crystallin proteins and impair their function. Thus, simple attention to eye protection can have beneficial results.
- High levels of blood glucose. Diabetics have an elevated risk for developing cataracts. This seems due to a process called nonenzymatic glycosylation, in which glucose molecules become added to crystallin proteins. Improved control of blood glucose diminishes this risk.

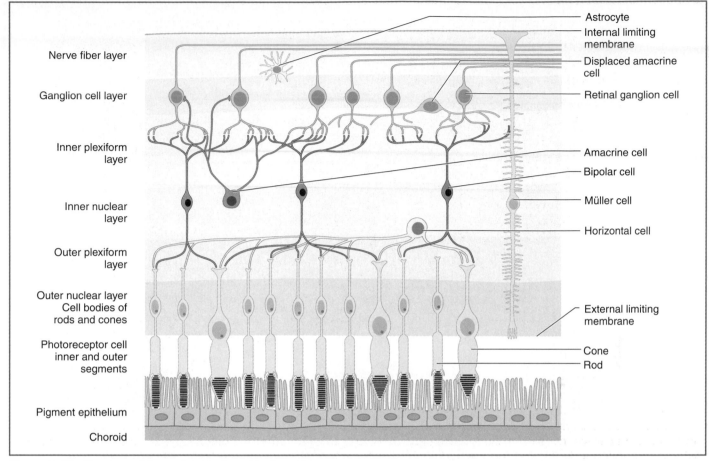

Nerve fiber layer

Ganglion cell layer

Inner plexiform layer

Inner nuclear layer

Outer plexiform layer

Outer nuclear layer
Cell bodies of rods and cones

Photoreceptor cell inner and outer segments

Pigment epithelium

Choroid

Astrocyte

Internal limiting membrane

Displaced amacrine cell

Retinal ganglion cell

Amacrine cell

Bipolar cell

Müller cell

Horizontal cell

External limiting membrane

Cone

Rod

Figure 6-27. Diagram of the cell types found in the retina.

BIOCHEMISTRY

Vision

In rods, the targets are monomers of a specialized membrane protein called opsin. Opsin spans the plasma membrane of each disc seven times; it is associated with retinol (a form of vitamin A). When retinol is combined with opsin, the overall rod molecule is called rhodopsin. Each rod contains some 10 million rhodopsin molecules, which account for 90% of the protein present within rod disc membranes.

Retinol has many carbon-carbon double bonds and, like many similar compounds such as dye molecules, readily absorbs light. Unlike other compounds, however, retinol changes its shape (straightens out) when it absorbs light (i.e., cis-retinol changes to trans-retinol). This causes a change in configuration and function of the opsin protein.

Activated rhodopsin, in turn, activates a series of other proteins called transducin and phosphodiesterase. The main consequence is a fall in cytoplasmic concentrations of the signaling molecule, cyclic GMP (cGMP).

A reduction in cGMP causes cation channels in the plasma membrane to close, thereby hyperpolarizing the cell and reducing the amount of glutamate liberated at the axonal end of the rod. Thus, photoreceptor cells react to light by inhibiting their activity.

The system is reset to respond to another photon in two ways: trans-retinol pops off the opsin protein and is replaced by a fresh molecule of cis-retinol, and the activated opsin protein is reconfigured to its inactive form by a number of other proteins.

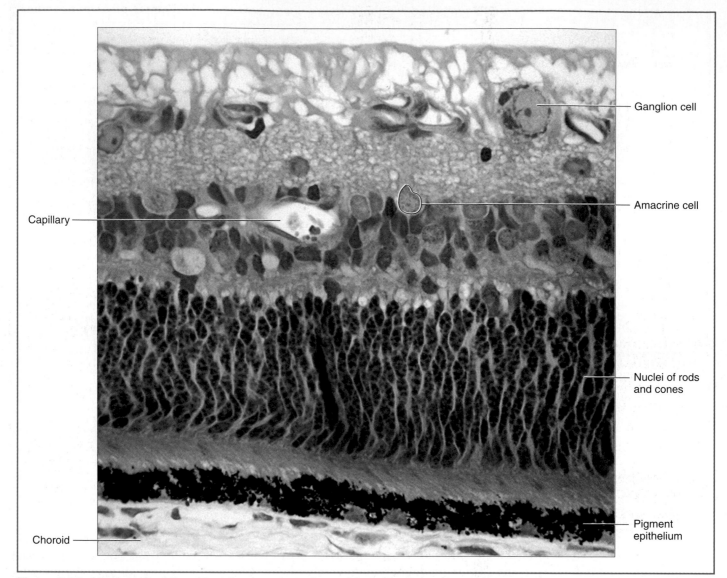

Figure 6-28. Micrograph of the retina showing a ganglion cell, an amacrine cell, a retinal capillary, nuclei of rods and cones, and the pigment epithelium.

The wide cytoplasmic space within this cilium is filled by over a hundred flattened, membranous discs derived from infoldings of the plasma membrane. The modified cilium of rods is cylindrical, whereas in cones, it is conical. This portion of a photoreceptor neuron is called the outer segment. It is connected to a more conventional portion of cytoplasm (the inner segment) by a modified basal body–like structure (containing nine microtubule doublets but no central microtubules). Finally, the inner segment of each cell is connected via a constriction in the cell to a region containing the cell nucleus (forming the outer nuclear layer of the retina) and the axonal terminal of the cell (called a spherule for rods and a pedicle for cones) (Figs. 6-29 and 6-30).

The membranous discs within the outer segment of the photoreceptors are positioned perpendicular to the pathway of light through the cell, maximizing the possibility that a photon will strike a target in the discs before it passes through the cell.

Light Targets

The basis for rod reactivity to light (rhodopsin) has been reasonably well understood for a number of years. Cone function, in contrast, was more mysterious until the genes coding for the visual pigment of cones were analyzed. These genes, coding for three types of cone opsin (iodopsin), have slight differences in amino acid sequence. In the portion of the opsin protein that binds retinal, the total electrical charge on the nearby amino acids varies among the three iodopsin isoforms because of the differing amino acid sequences. This varying charge near the retinal molecule influences its double bonds and "tunes" retinal to absorb mainly blue, red, or green light. This is the basis for color vision.

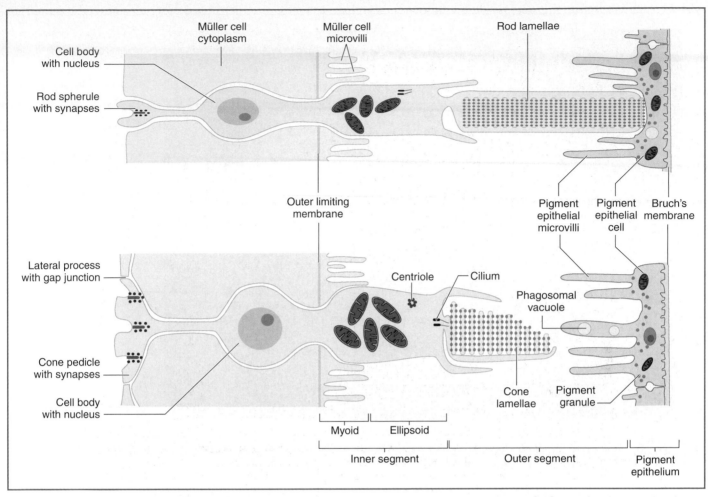

Figure 6-29. Diagram of the structures of rods and cones in the retina. (Modified from Standring S. *Gray's Anatomy,* 39th ed. Philadelphia, Churchill-Livingstone, 2005, p 714.)

Cones are not randomly distributed over the retina but are concentrated in a small portion called the fovea. The high numbers of cones in the fovea, plus an attenuation of the other layers of the retina, allows the fovea to be the region of the retina with the highest visual acuity.

Inner Nuclear Layer

Retinal photoreceptor cells synapse onto a variety of other neurons; the nuclei of these neurons inhabit a layer called the inner nuclear layer. There are three neuronal subtypes within this layer. The first type, the bipolar cell, receives synaptic input from rods or cones. Where this synaptic information goes depends on where it comes from: bipolar cells connected to cones pass information directly to ganglion cells; bipolar cells connected to rods pass information either directly to ganglion cells or to a second type of neuron in the inner nuclear layer termed an amacrine cell. In actuality, there are many types of amacrine cells with many shapes and neurotransmitters. These cells form part of the circuitry that immediately processes visual information even before it reaches the brain.

The third type of cell within the inner nuclear layer, the horizontal cell, extends long processes on each side of the perikaryon that contact both photoreceptor neurons and bipolar cells (Fig. 6-31). These cell types are responsible for the phenomenon of lateral inhibition, in which illuminated rods suppress the activity of neighboring unilluminated rods. Lateral inhibition increases the perceived contrast between light and dark areas of the visual field and makes perception more acute.

Ganglion Cell Layer

All the information gathered by the outer neurons of the retina converges on large ganglion cells in the innermost layer of the retina (see Fig. 6-28). One type of ganglion cell may receive information from as many as 100 rods. This means that this ganglion cell can be activated by as little as several photons of light, but the exact location of the photons among 100 rods is indeterminate. Such ganglion cells provide for sensitive vision in dim light that is not especially accurate concerning the location of a visual stimulus. Another type of ganglion cell may receive information from only a single cone. This cell requires that many photons excite the single cone before an event is perceived, but that event will be located precisely. These ganglion cells provide for accurate color vision in bright light.

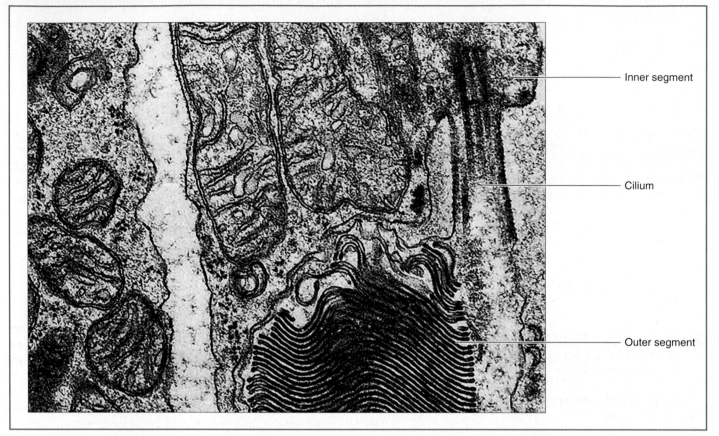

Figure 6-30. Transmission electron micrograph of the membranous discs of a rod cell. (From Standring S. *Gray's Anatomy,* 39th ed. Philadelphia, Churchill-Livingstone, 2005, p 715.)

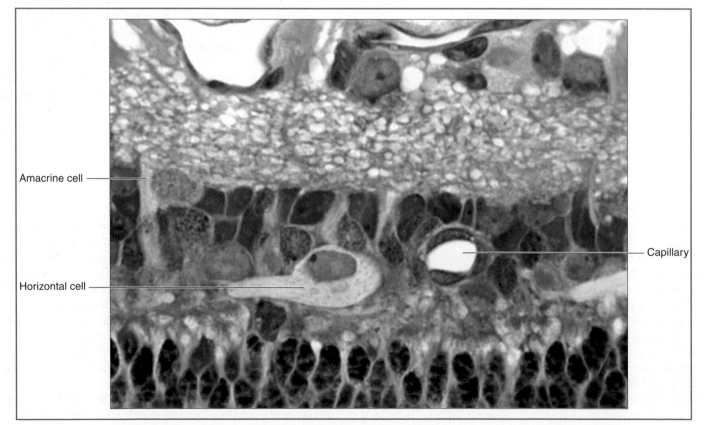

Figure 6-31. Horizontal cell in the retina.

PATHOLOGY

Retinal Capillaries

Although capillaries do not normally interfere with visual processes, they can pose a problem in certain circumstances. One example is a disorder that was inadvertently caused by physicians, and another arises from the metabolic disturbances seen in diabetes mellitus.

During the 1950s, when incubators were introduced to aid the breathing of premature babies, reports of retrolental fibroplasia became more numerous. In this condition, an overgrowth of retinal capillaries appears and causes permanent blindness. Suddenly, 400 to 500 newborns became afflicted with this condition each year. It was found that exposure of the developing retina to high levels of oxygen suppressed the growth of capillaries. When newborns were returned to a normal atmosphere, the retinal capillaries compensated by growing excessively. Curtailment of the practice solved the problem. Ironically, improved methods of preserving the life of extremely premature babies, involving respirators, are now provoking a resurgence of this problem.

In diabetes mellitus, bleeding and aneurysms of retinal capillaries occur and can impair vision. These abnormalities are provoked by high levels of glucose, which cause a decrease in the tight junction protein, occludin, in endothelial cells. The precise mechanisms whereby glucose causes capillaries to make abnormal tight junctions and to become leaky are uncertain. They may involve alterations in vascular endothelial growth factor (VEGF) or a transformation of glucose into intracellular deposits of sorbitol, catalyzed by an enzyme called *aldose reductase*.

It was recently discovered that a subpopulation of ganglion cells possess a unique form of visual pigment, melanopsin, which allows these cells to respond to light independently of any input from rods and cones. About 1% of the ganglion cells in the rodent retina possesses this primitive type of visual pigment; these cells project to a portion of the hypothalamus, the suprachiasmatic nucleus, that governs 24-hour rhythms in the brain and body. Apparently, these special ganglion cells are not devoted to processing optical details of the visual field but simply record whether ambient light is bright or dim (i.e., daytime or nighttime light).

Other cell types within the retina provide often overlooked, but still important, functions. Müller cells, long cells that span the entire width of the retina, function like astrocytes and help nourish neuronal cells. They possess high-capacity GLUT2-type glucose transporters, like cells in the liver. These transporters enable an elevated import of glucose into Müller cells. The glucose is converted to lactate and exported to neurons as a fuel molecule.

An important pathologic state of the retina is found in a retinal cancer called retinoblastoma. This cancerous overgrowth of photoreceptor cells or Müller cells appears in newborns (about 1 in 20,000 births). It is caused by a mutation in the retinoblastoma protein, an inhibitor of mitosis that is present in all cells of the body. It is normally inactivated (phosphorylated) by a cyclin-dependent kinase (cdk4 + cyclin D) to promote cell division. Tumors resulting from a mutated retinoblastoma protein can be aggressive and may require removal of the eye.

Endothelial cells of capillaries are also common in the retina and of course provide a blood supply.

The eyes constantly shift position slightly, so that images of the outside world never stay on the same place in the retina for very long. If the eye is experimentally immobilized and an image is shown on the retina for minutes at a time, the retina "learns" to ignore it and it will disappear from view! This seems to explain why images of the retinal capillary bed, which never shift position, are not apparent in our visual field. This rule can be broken, however, in a simple ophthalmologic procedure: if a dim penlight is brought close to the cornea and is used to shine light on the retina briefly, flashes of the tree-like branching pattern of retinal capillaries can briefly appear in the visual field as the shadows they cast change their positions.

Retinal Pigment Epithelium

Underlying the retina is a layer of melanin-containing, simple cuboidal epithelial cells called the pigment epithelium (see Fig. 6-28). The melanin in this layer absorbs light that would otherwise be reflected to reenter the retina and interfere with vision. Pigment epithelial cells also phagocytose the rhodopsin-containing membranous discs that are continually shed from the apical portions of rods and cones.

The pigment epithelium is not attached to photoreceptor cells by junctional complexes, so that the two cell types are rather easily torn away from each other. This condition, called retinal detachment, can be corrected by lasers that "tack down" the retina by creating small, focal burns and scar tissue. One ocular structure that helps to prevent retinal detachment is the vitreous humor, a mass of viscous fluid, rich in hyaluronic acid, which occupies most of the space behind the lens. This fluid helps to keep the retina in place and helps maintain normal ocular pressure and shape. If, during development of mouse eyes, small tubes are placed into the eyeballs to drain off this fluid, the eyes never attain their normal size, and the retina detaches to form a folded, useless layer.

Additional ocular structures include the highly vascular connective tissue just beneath the retina, a layer termed the uvea. This layer contains many highly pigmented melanocytes that also help absorb stray beams of light. Enclosing most of the eye is the dense connective tissue of the sclera. It is pierced posteriorly by axons of the optic nerve, which is formed when all the fibers from the ganglion cells are collected at the back of the eye at the optic disc (Fig. 6-32). This area represents the "blind spot" in the visual field. Since no photoreceptors are present in the optic papilla, it cannot detect any objects in this portion of the visual field. In addition, the sclera is the point of attachment of six extraocular muscles that rotate the eye.

Finally, the eye itself is protected by the eyelid, a flap of skin containing skeletal muscle fibers of the orbicularis oculi; a dense, semirigid mass of connective tissue called the tarsal plate that gives the upper eyelid stiffness; rows of sebaceous

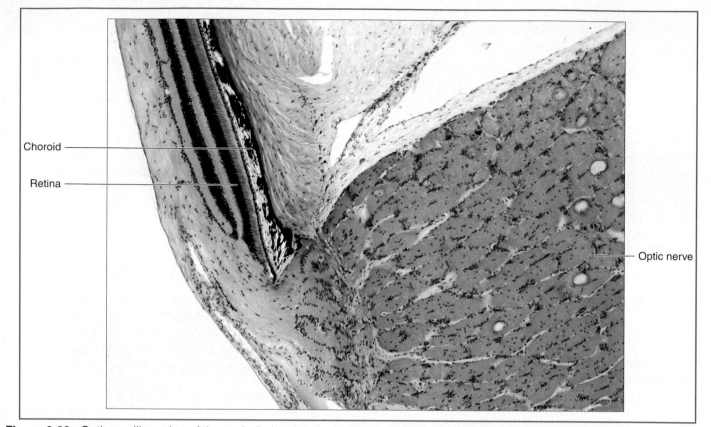

Figure 6-32. Optic papilla region of the eyeball showing the optic nerve, the retina, and the highly pigmented choroid.

Choroid

Retina

Optic nerve

glands called meibomian glands, which are unusual in that they are not associated with hairs. They contribute an oily secretion to the tears that helps lubricate the surface of the eye. The margins of the eyelids bear large hairs, eyelashes, which are associated with sweat glands (glands of Moll) (Fig. 6-33). The interior of the eyelid is lined by a stratified squamous epithelium that possesses goblet cells (conjunctiva). The conjunctiva reflects off of the interior of the eyelid onto the surface of the sclera and eventually becomes continuous with the epithelium of the cornea.

A final consideration is a fundamental question of how the eye came to exist. It is so complicated a structure that it is difficult to imagine how it could evolve from a simpler precursor. Darwin himself expressed concern that the eye posed a serious challenge for his theory of evolution. Even worse, eyes of other animals such as flies or octopuses have radically different structures from the mammalian eye, suggesting that they all might have evolved independently.

A more recent examination of the homeotic genes governing eye development puts these considerations into a more balanced perspective. Even if eye structures vary among species, the homeotic genes that govern eye development are surprisingly similar among flies, humans, mollusks, and even jellyfish. This genetic similarity suggests that primitive eyes may have evolved only once in a distant ancestor common to all sighted species. The anatomy of simple eyes of jellyfish or ciliated invertebrate larvae suggest that eyes might have originated from a simple epithelium possessing pigmented

cells and interspersed photosensitive cells. Some of the photosensitive cells may have possessed visual pigment at the apical cytoplasms and detected only the presence or absence of light. These probably evolved into ganglion cells, amacrine cells, bipolar cells, and horizontal cells. The remaining photosensitive cells possessed visual pigment within cilia, evolved into rods and cones, and detected more subtle variations in light directionality and frequency.

●●● EAR

Inner Ear

Although at first glance it would not seem likely, the inner ear shows many anatomic and functional similarities to the eye. The inner ear, like the eye, is derived in the embryo from a hollow, fluid-filled epithelial sac (otic vesicle). The eye conducts two functions: a simpler, probably ancestral, function of determining the presence or absence of light, and a more complex function of determining the frequency (color) and directionality of light. Similarly, the ear is devoted to a simple, primitive function of detecting vibrations in fluid that are caused by shifting the position of the head, and a more complex function of detecting fluid vibrations caused by sound and determining the frequency and directionality of that sound. Unlike in the eye, the primitive and sophisticated functions of the ear are carried out by two anatomically

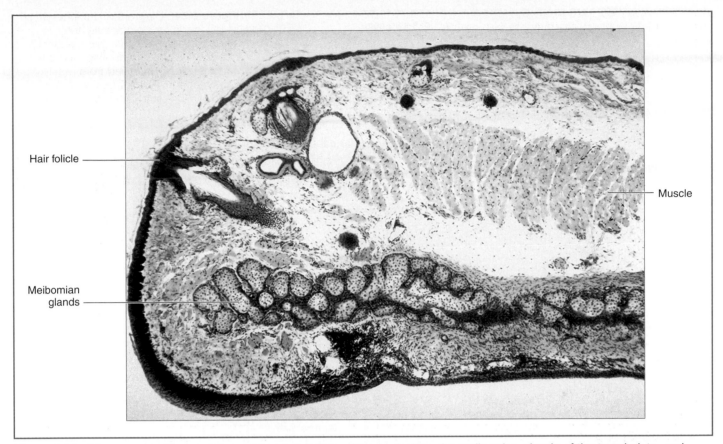

Hair follicle

Muscle

Meibomian glands

Figure 6-33. Micrograph of the eyelid showing a hair follicle of the eyelashes, the meibomian glands of the tarsal plate, and skeletal muscle of the orbicularis oculi muscle.

distinct divisions of the inner ear, the vestibular apparatus and the cochlea, respectively.

During development, the vestibular apparatus first becomes distinguishable as the dorsal division of the otic vesicle and forms under the influence of a homeotic protein called Hmx2. Shortly after, thin epithelial tubes, the semicircular canals, grow out of the vestibular sac under the influence of another protein, Prx1. The ventral division of the otic vesicle, meanwhile, is stimulated by another homeotic protein called Pax2 to form a long, coiled tube, the cochlear duct. All of these complicated, hollow epithelial tubes constitute the membranous labyrinth.

As portions of the membranous labyrinth develop, they become surrounded by hyaline cartilage. This cartilage is gradually replaced by bone in a peculiar and poorly understood process: unlike in cartilage replacement in long bones, epiphyseal plates never form around the inner ear. These may not be required in the ear, which, unlike long bones, does not need to grow substantially after birth. Apparently, an erosion of cartilage by macrophages takes place even in the absence of an epiphyseal plate, and then osteoblasts arrive via the vasculature to lay down bone in place of cartilage. The bone that finally encloses the adult structures of the ear is termed the bony labyrinth. Fluid found within the membranous labyrinth is called endolymph, and it

contains high concentrations of potassium, much like intracellular fluid. Fluid found within the bony labyrinth (surrounding the membranous labyrinth) is called perilymph. It contains high concentrations of sodium, like most extracellular fluid.

During the maturation of the inner ear, the vestibular portion subdivides into two small sacs: the small, spherical saccule and the larger, ovoid utricle. Three semicircular canals sprout from the utricle and rejoin it; each canal has, at one basal connection with the utricle, a swelling called an ampulla (Fig. 6-34). Within each ampulla is a sensory device called the crista ampullaris. This is not the only sensory structure within the utricle, which also possesses a patch of sensory epithelial cells called the macula. The adjacent sac, the saccule, also possesses a macula. These two vestibular sacs communicate with the cochlear duct via a small tube called the ductus reuniens. Finally, another small tube, the endolymphatic duct, projects away from the saccule and utricle to terminate blindly in the subdural space of the brain.

As the vestibular structures and the cochlear duct mature, they attract sensory axons from two ganglia. Vestibular structures promote the survival of vestibular ganglion neurons that innervate them by secreting BDNF, in rather the same way as the developing spinal cord promotes the

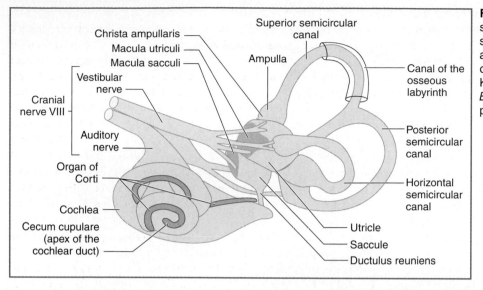

Figure 6-34. Diagram of the inner ear showing the utricle, saccule, the semicircular canals that join the utricle at swellings called ampullae, and the cochlear duct. (Modified from Kierszenbaum A. *Histology and Cell Biology*. Philadelphia, Mosby, 2002, p 253.)

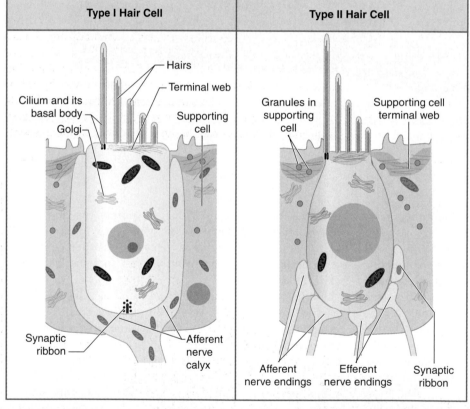

Figure 6-35. Diagram of the two types of hair cells found in maculae.

development of dorsal root ganglia. The cochlear duct utilizes another protein, neurotrophin-3, to support the growth of the spiral ganglion that innervates it. The spiral and vestibular ganglia send axons into the brain as the vestibulocochlear nerve (VIIIth cranial nerve).

One overriding principle can be used to understand the ear: all the sensory portions of the inner ear rely on sensory hair cells that have stereocilia (elongated microvilli) embedded in an overlying gelatinous matrix. When vibrations shake this matrix, the sensory cells in contact with it depolarize to

send a signal to the brain. This basic function is simply more sophisticated in the cochlea than in the vestibule.

Macula

Sensory hair cells in the maculae of the saccule and utricle are designed to respond to gravity or to steady movement (linear acceleration). These sensory cells are present in a patch of stratified columnar epithelium (macula) along with adjacent support cells. Sensory cells come in two types (Fig. 6-35). Type I cells are almost enclosed by an enveloping calyx formed by afferent nerve axons, and they seem to fire steadily and continuously in response to a steady movement. Type II cells receive numerous, and smaller, synaptic boutons on their basal surfaces from both afferent and efferent axons. These cells seem to fire only intermittently and only when there is a drastic change in movement or perceived gravity (as in falling). The apical surfaces of the sensory cells are decorated by 50 to 60 stereocilia and a single, nonmotile cilium termed a kinocilium.

Lying beneath both of these sensory cell types are cytoplasmic processes of supporting cells. Supporting cells contain abundant amounts of intermediate filaments, which give them substantial structural strength. Sensory cells, in contrast, are peculiar in that they are almost totally depleted of intermediate filaments. They thus represent fragile cells enclosed by strong cells, much like soft-boiled eggs nestled in an egg carton.

In the maculae of the utricle and saccule, both the sensory and support cells are covered by a gelatinous mass of extracellular molecules (protein fibers and glycosamino-glycans) of uncertain composition called the otolithic membrane (Fig. 6-36). Embedded in this gelatinous mass of protein are numerous crystals of calcium carbonate called otoliths or otoconia. These apparently form around a protein core that is secreted by support cells. When the otolithic membrane shifts in response to gravity or to acceleration, the stereocilia embedded into it bend, triggering depolarization of the sensory cells.

Crista Ampullaris

Within the ampullae at the base of each semicircular canal is a raised mass of epithelial tissue (crista) that is similar in appearance to a macula and contains sensory and support cells resembling those in the macula (Figs. 6-37 and 6-38). One difference is that the gelatinous mass of extracellular material covering a crista, called a cupula, is taller and lacks otoconia. The cupula is wafted to and fro within the ampulla when fluid moves within a semicircular canal, much like a swinging door. Since semicircular canals are oriented at roughly 90-degree angles to each other, fluid flow in each one is maximal only at a specific angle of rotation of the head for each canal. An analysis of the neural output of all three semicircular canals by the brain allows an instantaneous calculation of exactly how the head is rotating at any one time.

This information is particularly important for the control of eye movement. When the head is turned from side to side but the eyes are kept fixed on a distant object, the eyes must rotate in the opposite direction and then snap back to remain on the object (this sudden movement is called nystagmus). This automatic correction of eye movement to adjust for head movement is carried out by neurons of the brainstem nuclei of cranial nerves III, IV, VI, and VIII, all of which are interconnected and influence the activity of one another. The function of all these nuclei can be simply tested by intro-ducing ice water into one ear: the resultant cooling and shift-ing of the endolymph within the semicircular canals results in nystagmus of the eye even in the absence of head movement.

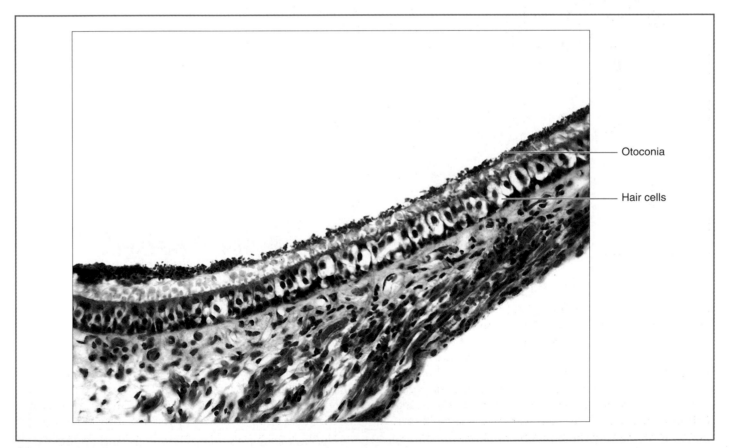

Figure 6-36. Macula, showing sensory hair cells and otoconia embedded in the otolithic membrane.

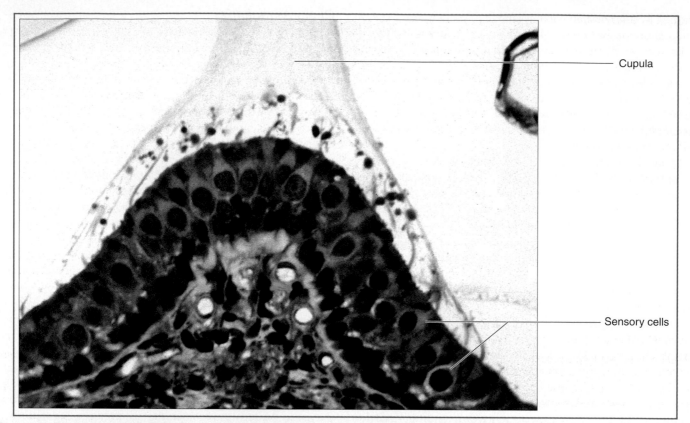

Cupula

Sensory cells

Figure 6-37. Crista ampullaris at the base of a semicircular canal. Sensory hair cells, intermingled with support cells, send stereocilia up into a gelatinous mass called a cupula.

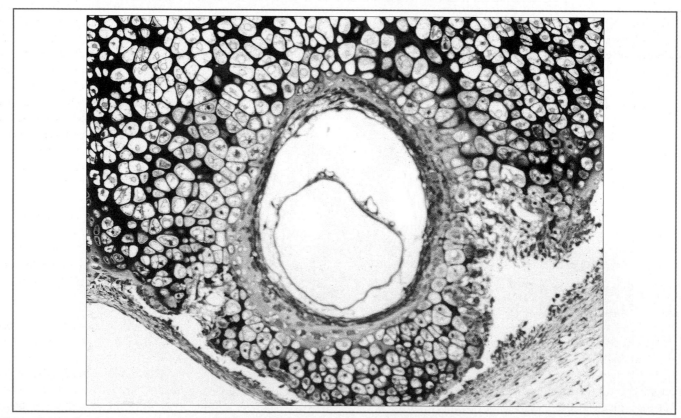

Figure 6-38. Semicircular canal in a newborn rat. A thin rim of bone has grown around it, forming the bony labyrinth, but the bulk of the tissue surrounding the canal is still hyaline cartilage that will be replaced by bone in the adult.

Figure 6-39. Diagram of the cochlea.

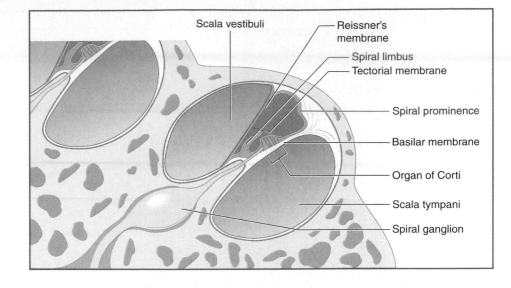

Scala vestibuli

Reissner's membrane

Spiral limbus

Tectorial membrane

Spiral prominence

Basilar membrane

Organ of Corti

Scala tympani

Spiral ganglion

Cochlea

The cochlear duct (also called the scala media) begins its existence as a straight, blind-ending epithelial tube, but by 25 weeks of embryonic life, it has completed a spiral containing two and one-half turns. The cochlea gradually acquires many complex anatomic features, described by a specialized nomenclature that can be a bit confusing (Fig. 6-39).

Within the center of the spiral, a tapering bony process called the modiolus, shaped rather like a wood screw, forms to support the medial curve of the cochlear duct and to enclose the masses of nerve cells that form the spiral ganglion. The roof of the cochlear duct is formed by a layer of simple squamous epithelium called Reissner's membrane, which separates it from a perilymph-filled space above called the scala vestibuli. The floor of the cochlear duct is formed by a more complex layer of epithelial cells (the organ of Corti, first described in detail by the Italian anatomist Alfonso Corti) (Fig. 6-40).

The organ of Corti lies atop a thin layer of connective tissue called the basilar membrane, which stretches from the lateral wall of the cochlear duct (spiral ligament) to the medial wall of the cochlear duct (spiral limbus, overlying the bony spiral lamina of the modiolus). Finally, below the organ of Corti is another perilymph-filled space called the scala tympani. The two perilymph-filled spaces communicate with each other at a junction called the helicotrema, which is located at the apex of the cochlea. The overall volume of these spaces (76 μL) is substantially larger than the overall volume of the cochlear duct (7 μL).

Organ of Corti

In the embryo, the organ of Corti initially appears rather similar to a macula and contains a patch of sensory hair cells surrounded by numerous, ordinary-appearing support cells. As in the macula, the support cells secrete a mass of gelatinous material that covers over the surface of the sensory cells. Subsequently, however, the support cells drastically change their shapes, shorten, and retract from the gelatinous mass of protein, which now is termed the tectorial membrane. This membrane, containing type II collagen, proteoglycans, and a protein called tectorin, becomes attached to the medial wall of the cochlear duct and projects laterally to lie upon the apical surfaces of the sensory hair cells (Figs. 6-41 and 6-42).

The sensory hair cells of the cochlea are similar to those elsewhere in the ear except that they lack a kinocilium. In any given cross-section, three lateral sensory cells (outer hair cells) and one more medial sensory cell (inner hair cell) can be seen, supported by an enclosing cytoplasm of support cells called phalangeal cells. These two groups of hair cells are separated by peculiar cells called pillar cells, which are densely filled with keratin filaments and which are very strong. Tips of the stereocilia of the outer hair cells are actually embedded into the tectorial membrane, whereas the stereocilia of the inner hair cells merely brush up against the tectorial membrane at a site called Hensen's stripe (Figs. 6-42 and 6-43). The tips of the stereocilia are connected to each other by thin filamentous structures called tip links (Fig. 6-44).

Even though the outer hair cells are much more numerous than the inner hair cells in the organ of Corti, they receive innervation from only 5% of the nerves projecting to the organ. Most of the afferent axons of the cochlea, which arise from about 30,000 neurons, innervate the inner hair cells.

Structure and Function

The first mysterious feature of the cochlea is that it is more sensitive to quiet sounds and responds more accurately to specific frequencies than would be predicted by a simple mathematical analysis of the movements of the basilar membrane. A feature of the cochlea is that 5–20 ms after a series of sharp clicking sounds were directed into the ear, small noises called otoacoustic emissions could be detected emanating from the ear via the eardrum. In other words, the

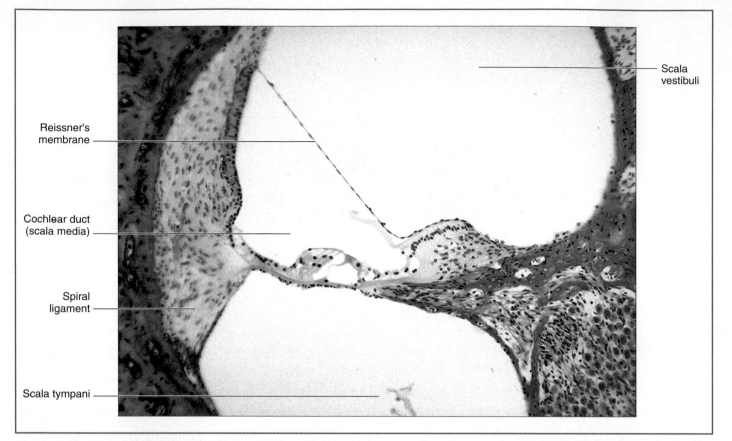

Reissner's membrane

Cochlear duct (scala media)

Spiral ligament

Scala tympani

Scala vestibuli

Figure 6-40. Low-magnification view of the cochlea showing the scala vestibuli, Reissner's membrane, cochlear duct (scala media), scala tympani, spiral ganglion, and spiral ligament.

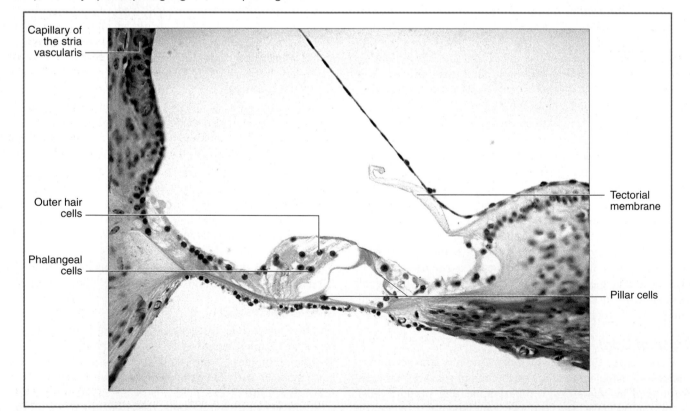

Capillary of the stria vascularis

Outer hair cells

Phalangeal cells

Tectorial membrane

Pillar cells

Figure 6-41. Higher magnification view of the cochlea showing the components of the organ of Corti. The tectorial membrane has been pulled away from the hair cells as a result of artifactual shrinkage during tissue preparation. The basilar membrane supports a variety of cells visible here, including outer hair cells, phalangeal cells, and pillar cells. A capillary is visible within the epithelium of the stria vascularis.

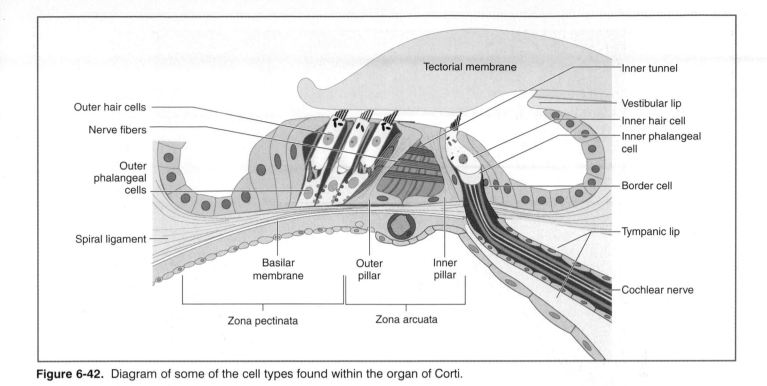

Figure 6-42. Diagram of some of the cell types found within the organ of Corti.

PATHOLOGY

Sound Perception

Sound vibrations enter the outer ear, pass through the middle ear, and enter the inner ear via a membrane-covered opening called the oval window. Vibrations of the oval window create waves within the perilymph of the scala vestibuli, which in turn cause the cochlear duct and organ of Corti to vibrate.

Collagen fibers within the basilar membrane are much shorter at the base of the cochlea (150 μm long) than at the apex of the cochlea (450 μm long). These regional differences in the width of the basilar membrane affect its responses to vibration, so that low tones primarily affect the basilar membrane at the apex of the cochlea, and high frequency tones affect the cochlea at its base. This effect of basilar membrane width can be visualized by imagining that you have clamped one end of a yardstick and one end of a pencil to a table and then have hit them both on their free ends. The tip of the yardstick will vibrate much more slowly than the tip of the pencil. This means that a pure tone entering the organ of Corti will have a maximal effect in a specific row of 40 contiguous

inner hair cells out of a total of about 3500 inner hair cells stretched out along the entire 32 mm length of the basilar membrane.

When the tectorial membrane bounces along the apical surface of an inner hair cell, it pulls on the stereocilia. All of these stereocilia are interconnected by thin strands called tip links, containing cadherin-23. When the stereocilia bend in one direction, they exert tension on the tip links, which seem to be connected to K^+ channels embedded in the plasma membrane. The K^+ channels respond to this tension by opening and depolarizing the cell. On the other hand, when the stereocilia bend in the opposite direction, the tip link strands slacken and reduce tension on the K^+ channels. These recently identified channels are called transient receptor potential A1 receptors.

Mutations in tip link proteins or in at least 30 other proteins found in stereocilia (e.g., myosin isoforms 6, 7, or 15) can provoke hereditary deafness syndromes such as Usher's syndrome.

PATHOLOGY

Hearing Loss

Hearing loss affects hundreds of millions of people worldwide and is one of the most common disabilities. It is often, though not always, due to an age-related accumulation of damage to hair cells by loud sounds, which can injure hair cells and cause their death. These damaged cells are not replaced by new hair cells; by age 60, about 50% of the original 13,000 outer hair cells are gone. If this injury could somehow be repaired, hearing could potentially be restored.

Some animals, such as chickens and fish, can regenerate new hair cells after damage. A potential therapeutic goal would

be to replicate this ability in mammalian hair cells.

The genes that regulate mammalian hair cell differentiation and cell division are gradually being identified. A transcription factor called Math-1 stimulates the differentiation of hair cells from supporting cells.

In addition, the retinoblastoma protein regulates the ability of cells to undergo mitosis. If it is experimentally deleted in mice, these mice recover the ability to make new hair cells. However, since a generalized reduction in the retinoblastoma protein can lead to cancer, any therapeutic approach would have to restrict changes in this protein to the inner ear.

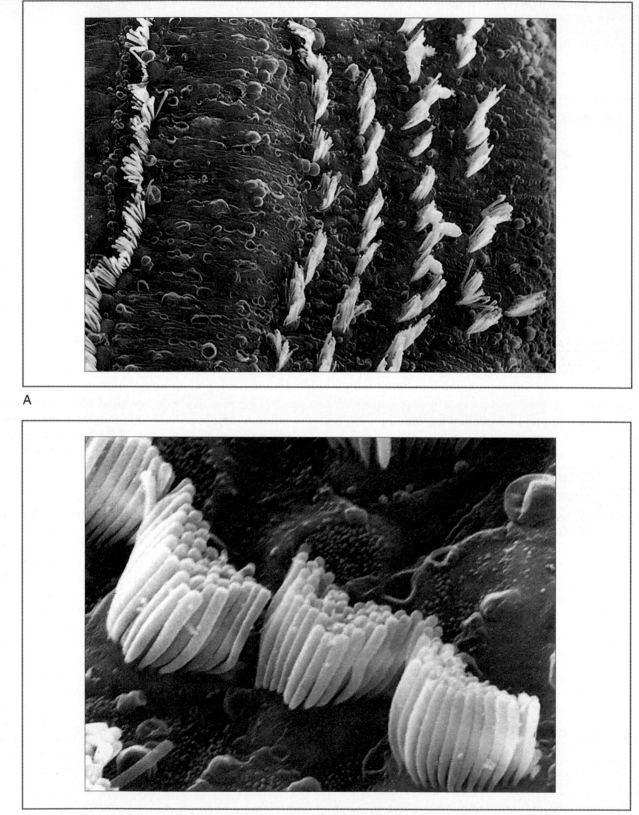

A

B

Figure 6-43. Scanning electron micrographs showing the stereocilia visible at the surfaces of the inner (**A**) and outer (**B**) hair cells of the cochlea. (From Standring S. *Gray's Anatomy,* 39th ed. Philadelphia, Churchill-Livingstone, 2005, p 643.)

Figure 6-44. Diagram of the apical portions of sensory hair cells. **A,** The stereocilia are not bent by sound vibrations, and the tip links connecting them to each other are relaxed. **B,** The stereocilia are bent by sound vibrations and exert tension on the tip links. The taut tip links activate K$^+$ channels that depolarize the cell.

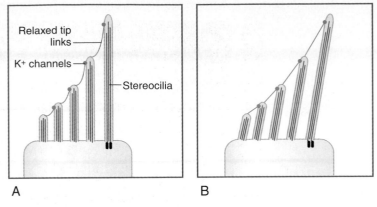

ear can function both as a microphone and as a speaker, so that ear structures can produce sounds and respond to them.

Both mysteries are related to an unusual property of outer hair cells. When these cells are depolarized, they can rapidly change their height by as much as 5% to vibrate up and down on the inferior surface of the tectorial membrane. These movements are what cause the otoacoustic emissions of sound from the cochlea. These movements, by vibrating the tectorial membrane, also appear responsible for the previously unexplained high sensitivity and selectivity of nearby inner hair cells. The piston-like movements of the outer hair cells in response to sound enhance the function of the inner hair cells. Efferent axons that terminate on the outer hair cells adjust their activity to improve hearing.

This remarkable functional motility of the outer hair cells also has a unusual anatomic component. These cells, unlike most other cells of the body, do not adjust their length by utilizing the sliding of myosin and actin filaments. In fact, the entire cell membrane of these cells actively contracts. This appears due to contraction of an abundant integral membrane protein called prestin, which also functions as a channel for anions to cross the membrane. When these proteins contract, they exert tension upon interconnecting filaments of spectrin just beneath the cell membrane and cause the shape of the cells to change. Thus, these cells of the cochlea violate many of the rules for the behavior of most cells.

The high concentrations of K$^+$ in the endolymph appear crucial for the proper function of the organ of Corti. The composition of the endolymph is regulated by a patch of epithelial cells on the lateral wall of the cochlear duct called the stria vascularis (see Fig. 6-41). This epithelial structure is composed of three cell layers: a superficial layer of so-called marginal cells, an intermediate layer composed mainly of melanocytes, and a third layer of basal cells. The most eccentric aspect of the stria vascularis is that, in addition to these three cell types, it possesses *intraepithelial capillaries*. The stria vascularis is thus the only vascularized epithelium in the body. This comes about because, during development, the basal lamina separating the epithelial cells from the underlying connective tissue is somehow dismantled, allowing capillaries to enter the epithelium. The melanocytes in direct contact with these capillaries possess membrane K$^+$ channels

that allow them to extract K$^+$ ions from the bloodstream and export them into the endolymph. Various types of experimental damage to these melanocytes lead to an abnormal endolymph and to deafness.

All the sensory information leaving the ear passes through either the spiral ganglion that innervates the cochlea (see Fig. 6-39) or the vestibular ganglion that innervates the maculae and cristae (Fig. 6-45).

The overall anatomy of the cochlea is rather similar in all mammals and birds. In fish and reptiles, however, the cochlear duct may be a short, uncoiled, blind ending tube that extends straight out from the saccule and which apparently has a diminished ability to discriminate between sound frequencies relative to the more elaborate cochlea of mammals.

Middle Ear

The middle ear is mainly occupied by three small bones, or ossicles: the malleus, attached to the eardrum (tympanic membrane), the intermediate incus, and the stapes, attached via its footplate onto the surface of a membrane covering the oval window that leads into the inner ear (Figs. 6-46 and 6-47). These bones convey sound vibrations from the eardrum to the inner ear. Not all animals possess all three ossicles: fish, for example, have only a single stapes that connects the eardrum to the oval window. The two additional bones—malleus and incus—appear to have been derived, during evolution, from small bones of the jaw that were displaced into the ear. Movements between these two additional bones exert further leverage on the eardrum and increase the sound-induced force on it. The hole above the footplate of the stapes (obturator foramen) is formed by the passage of a small artery (stapedial artery) through the bone. In humans, but not in all mammals, this artery disappears during embryogenesis.

The reason that bones transmit sound relates to the higher viscosity of fluid relative to air. Sound travels through air easily, alternatively compressing and rarifying it to create vibrations. In fluid, however, the transmission of vibrations is more attenuated and requires more energy. The resistance of fluid to sound transmission is called *impedance*. The inner ear ossicles have the function of impedance matching between air and inner ear fluid. Sound striking the tympanum exerts a

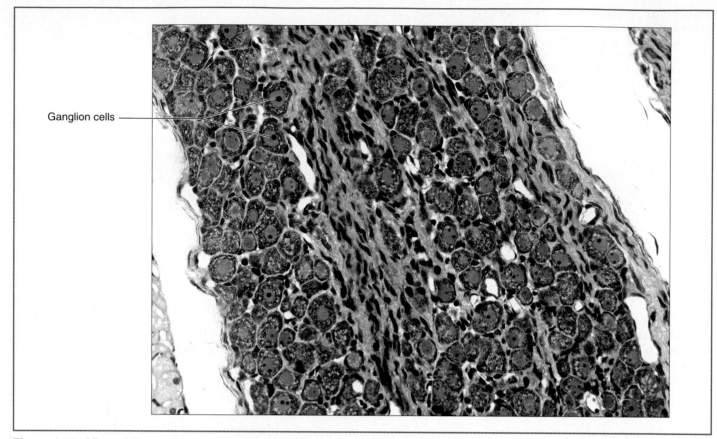

Figure 6-45. View of the vestibular ganglion. Hundreds of sensory ganglion cells contribute axons to the vestibular nerve.

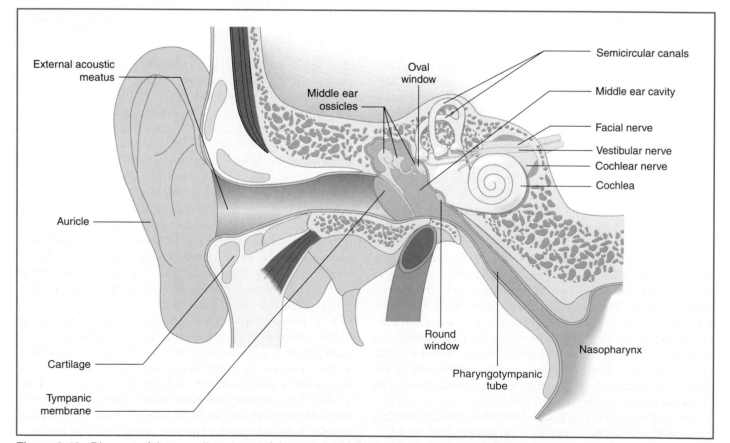

Figure 6-46. Diagram of the overall anatomy of the outer, middle, and inner portions of the ear.

Figure 6-47. Diagram of the middle ear showing the tympanic membrane (TM), the malleus (M), incus (I), and stapes (S), the round window (RW), and the location of the stapedius muscle (SM). A semicircular canal (SC) and portion of the utricle (U) are also shown.

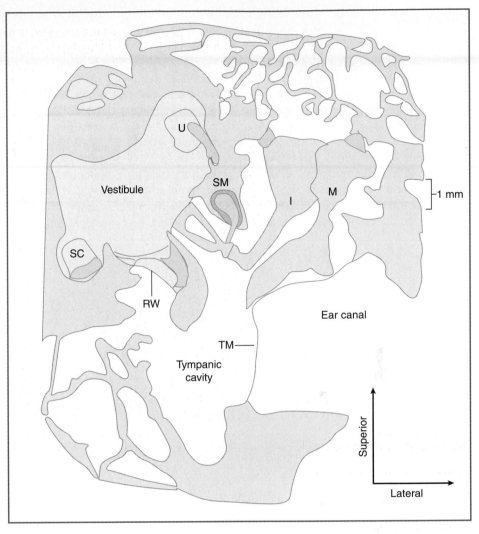

force across some 60 mm². This energy is transmitted by the ossicles onto the membrane covering the oval window, which is much smaller (3.2 mm²). Thus, a sound exerts a much greater force per square millimeter on the oval window than on the eardrum and so can overcome the greater impedence of fluid for the transmission of vibrations. After vibrations depress the oval window and course through the endolymph of the inner ear, they emerge again at another opening, the round window, which conveys them back into the middle ear. In this way, displacement of the incompressible fluid of the inner ear is moved from the oval window to the round window.

The stapes is also important for the acoustic reflex that protects the ear from damage due to sudden, loud noises. A loud sound causes a reflex contraction of the stapedius muscle that inserts on the stapes and tightens the ligament that holds the stapes in place. This dampens the vibrations of the stapes and protects the inner ear. Another muscle, the tensor tympani, inserts into the neck of the malleus, but its function is uncertain. It does not seem to play a major role in protecting the ear from loud sounds.

A long tube, the auditory or eustachian tube, connects the middle ear with the nasopharynx. Its terminal opening can be enlarged via contractions of the tensor veli palatini muscle of the nasopharynx, which serves to equalize the air pressures in the pharynx and middle ear. This can sometimes be accomplished by voluntary yawning when needed (e.g., during an airplane ride). The auditory tube is lined by a pseudostratified columnar epithelium and strengthened by a layer of hyaline cartilage.

Outer Ear

The outer ear is composed of the pinna (or auricle—skin supported by elastic cartilage) and the external auditory meatus. The latter is basically an irregular tube lined with skin and possessing a normal complement of hairs and sebaceous glands. In addition, specialized apocrine sweat glands called ceruminous glands are present that secrete a mixture of proteins and lipids termed cerumen. This material, mixed with sebaceous secretions, constitutes earwax.

The stratified squamous epithelium of the auditory meatus continues onto the surface of the eardrum. It resembles thin skin in all ways except one: epithelial cells on the center of the eardrum can be observed to gradually migrate toward the periphery of the eardrum. This is a useful activity, since it tends to remove debris from the eardrum, but the mechanism whereby these skin cells are directed to move in this way is unknown.

An examination of the ears of fish and other organisms shows clearly how the cochlea arose as an extension of the saccule. Recent data once again suggest that the fundamental structures making up the ear may have been present in ancestors common to both vertebrates and invertebrates. The auditory organs of flies, present in Johnston's organ of fly antennae, require a number of proteins for development and function that are also found in vertebrate ears (e.g., myosin 7, prestin). Thus, tissues making up the ear may have had a very ancient origin.

Cardiovascular System, Blood, and Blood Cell Formation

7

●●● OVERVIEW OF THE CARDIOVASCULAR SYSTEM

The cardiovascular system includes the blood and lymphatic vascular systems. Blood consists of cells, proteins, dissolved gasses, nutrients, hormones, metabolic waste products, and fluids. Lymph consists of the cells of the lymphoid system and fluids.

The primary function of the cardiovascular system is to distribute blood to the entire body and to collect lymph from peripheral organs and tissues. The blood vascular component consists of a pump, the heart, and an extensive system of tubes, the blood vessels, that make up a closed, circular system. The vessels that leave the heart are called arteries, and those that return blood to the heart are called veins. Pumping of the heart generates an arterial blood pressure of about 100 mm Hg while venous blood returns to the heart at a pressure of about 5 to 10 mm Hg.

As the arteries reach their target organs (brain, kidneys, intestines, etc) or other end points (areas of loose connective tissue, mesenteries, pia mater, etc) their diameter becomes smaller and smaller and their wall thickness thinner and thinner until the tube is composed of single cells that form a cylinder, the capillaries. A schematic diagram of the cardiovascular system is seen in Figure 7-1. This diagram illustrates the closed circular nature of the blood vascular system and its tributaries and the unidirectional flow of lymph in the lymphatic vascular system.

The heart and blood vessels have three layers. In the heart the layers are called *endocardium*, *myocardium*, and *epicardium*. The analogous layers in blood vessels are *tunica intima*, *tunica media*, and *tunica adventitia*.

In a normal, healthy individual, many components of the blood, e.g., nutrients (glucose, amino acids, O_2), vitamins, hormones, and proteins, exchange with tissue fluids and gases (with the exception of the red blood cell [RBC]). There is one significant exception regarding RBCs in the spleen (see Chapter 8). A certain amount of tissue fluid and white cells are taken up by blind-end capillaries of the lymphatic circulation, carried through an extensive branching system of thin-walled vessels, the lymphatic vessels, and returned to the blood vascular circulation via the larger veins near the heart.

The exchange of fluid-containing nutrients and oxygen with tissue fluids containing metabolic waste products and CO_2 occurs in capillary beds, which are often referred to as microvascular beds or as the microcirculation. Normally, many white cells leave the bloodstream in the microcirculation. Most of the fluid is taken up in the distal or venous end of a microvascular bed by a subset of vessels called postcapillary venules. Remaining fluid and those white cells of the immune system that have been immunologically stimulated or are engaged in *immune surveillance* are taken up by lymphatic capillaries and thereby travel to the lymphoid organs.

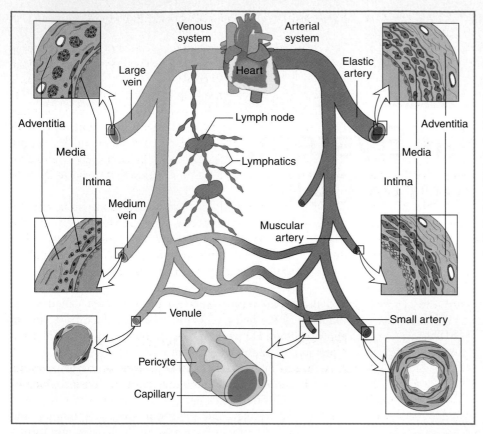

Figure 7-1. Diagram of the cardiovascular and lymphatic circulatory systems. The arterial side is shown in red-colored vessels, the venous side in blue-colored vessels, and some lymph nodes and the lymphatic circulation in purple-colored vessels. Note that the lymphatic circulation drains into the inferior vena cava through the thoracic duct, the largest diameter lymphatic vessel; this is the major site for lymph to re-enter the blood circulation although there are others. A schematic representation of the wall structure of typical arteries and veins are shown near their location in the diagram. The three layers of the vessel walls are colored to correspond to their basic tissue type.

●●● GENERAL STRUCTURE OF THE HEART

The heart has four chambers: the right atrium and right ventricle and the left atrium and left ventricle. The chambers are arranged to support a two pump–two circuit circulatory system—the pulmonary circulation and the systemic circulation. The right atrium receives blood from the peripheral systemic circulation and delivers it to the right ventricle, which pumps it to the lungs for reoxygenation. Blood is returned to the left atrium from the lungs and then to the left ventricle. The reoxygenated blood is distributed to the body by contraction of the muscular left ventricle. The atria are relatively thin-walled chambers of about equal size and wall thickness. The left ventricle is a thick walled conical chamber; the right ventricle has a thinner wall and can be thought of as a large cone-shaped covering of the outer surface of the left ventricle. The right ventricle has a larger capacity than the left ventricle, but the wall of the left ventricle is two to three times thicker than the right ventricle (Fig. 7-2). Heart muscle itself is nourished by an extensive network of coronary arteries.

The majority of the mass of the heart is cardiac muscle (see Chapter 4). Compared with skeletal muscle, cardiac myocytes are surrounded by more endomysium-like connective tissue. In further contrast to skeletal muscle, cardiac muscle fibers are not organized into parallel fascicles or long bundles of muscle fibers. The long-range organization of cardiac muscle fibers reflects two underlying characteristics: bundles of

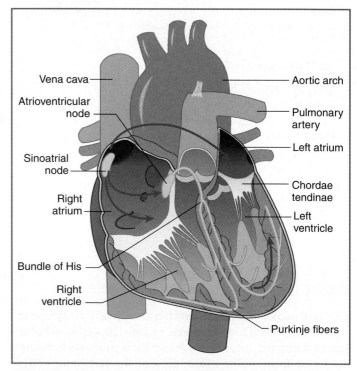

Figure 7-2. Diagram of the heart shows both atria and ventricles, the ascending and descending vena cava, the aortic arch and its three branches that carry blood to the head, and the conducting system of the heart (shown in yellow)—the sinoatrial node, atrioventricular node, the bundle of His, and the Purkinje fibers. The direction of conduction is shown by the dark blue arrows. The supporting structures of the valves, the chordae tendinae, are also shown.

different sizes are organized into many oblique groups that appear as long, intertwined spiral bundles, and when the ventricles contract, they do so with a wringing-like motion which forcefully ejects blood into the pulmonary artery and the aorta.

Heart Valves

The openings of the atria into the ventricles are guarded by valves that prevent backflow. The valve between the right atrium and ventricle is called the tricuspid valve and the one between the left atrium and ventricle is called the bicuspid (or mitral) valve. A large artery leaves each of the ventricles—the pulmonary artery from the right ventricle and the aorta from the left ventricle, each having a set of valves called the semilunar valves. These four-valved openings of the heart are in about the same anatomic plane and are supported by dense fibrous connective tissue rings. The valves are made of thin, tough connective tissue and are covered with endocardium. The innermost part of the valves is continuous with the fibrous rings. The atrioventricular valves have connective tissue extensions, the chordae tendinae, which connect to muscular extensions of the inner heart wall called papillary muscles. The fibrous rings are called the cardiac skeleton and in some species have a cartilage-like appearance (Fig. 7-3A). Figure 7-3B is a diagram of the atrioventricular valves and cardiac skeleton.

●●● HEART AS A PUMP

Contractile Properties of Cardiac Myocytes

Individual cardiac myocytes can be isolated from a heart and grown in tissue culture. They retain the cylindrical shape they have in situ, including the step-like ends where they had intercalated disks. If the culture medium has the correct Ca^{++} concentration and nutrient supply, the individual cells beat in a synchronized rhythmic manner. Thus, the cells are shown to have intrinsic contractile properties.

Contraction of the Heart

Because of its intrinsic contractility, the heart beats in the absence of external stimuli. Furthermore, specialized structures (nodes and fibers) within the walls of the heart regulate the contraction rate. The specialized structures are modifications of cardiac muscle. The nodes are called the sinoatrial (S-A) node and the atrioventricular (A-V) node. The S-A node is also called the *pacemaker node*. The A-V node continues into the A-V bundle (of His), which bifurcates into right and left bundle branches, which are further subdivided into specialized conducting cells called Purkinje fibers. A wave of contraction is initiated by the S-A node, which forces blood from the atria into the ventricles. A subsequent wave of contraction begins at the apex of the heart causing the ventricles to forcibly expel blood into the pulmonary artery and the aorta.

Systemic Regulation of Heart Rate

The heart is subject to exquisite regulation of its pumping (beating) rate by the autonomic nervous system (ANS). Both divisions of the ANS innervate the heart. Parasympathetic fibers delivered by the vagus nerve (cranial nerve X) terminate mainly in the S-A and A-V nodes but also innervate the myocardium. Sympathetic fibers also innervate both nodes, the myocardium, and the coronary arteries that supply the heart with blood. The sympathetic component causes an increase in heart rate, and the parasymphatics cause the rate to diminish.

Specialized receptors are found in the carotid sinus and the aortic arch. One set of receptors are *baroreceptors* and the other are *chemoreceptors*. The former sense and respond to fluctuations in blood pressure, and the latter respond to oxygen, carbon dioxide, and pH changes.

●●● BLOOD VESSELS

General Structure of Blood Vessels

All blood vessels larger than capillaries have three layers: *tunica intima, tunica media,* and *tunica adventitia.* Each of

---

PATHOLOGY

Hypertrophic Cardiomyopathy

The most common cause of sudden cardiac death in children and adolescents is hypertrophic cardiomyopathy. It is also the most common cause of sudden cardiac death in younger athletes, accounting for about one-third of sudden deaths in these individuals. About 10% of these cardiomyopathies are congenital.

The congenital forms are the most common monogenic cardiac disorders and are transmitted as autosomal dominant disorders. Hundreds of point mutations have been described in more than 10 structural proteins of the sarcomere. Two of the more common mutations that lead to hypertrophic cardiomyopathy are in the β-myosin heavy chain and in the troponin I subunit of troponin. Other mutations have been described in the cardiac muscle isoforms of actin, α-tropomyosin and titin. The mechanism of the hypertrophy is thought to be an increase in the contractile force of the sarcomere, which leads to hypertrophy of the myocytes. At the microscopic level, the normal organization of cardiac myocyte bundles is highly disrupted owing to enlarged, disorganized myocytes and infiltrations of leukocytes. These hypertrophic changes probably lead to sudden death as a result of electrically unstable myocardial function and ventricular tachyarrhythmias. The pathologic presentation is marked left ventricular hypertrophy often with a massively thickened ventricular septum, atrial enlargement, and a small left ventricular cavity. Interestingly, there is another group of mutations in structural proteins of the sarcomere that leads to a different form of cardiomyopathy—dilated cardiomyopathy.

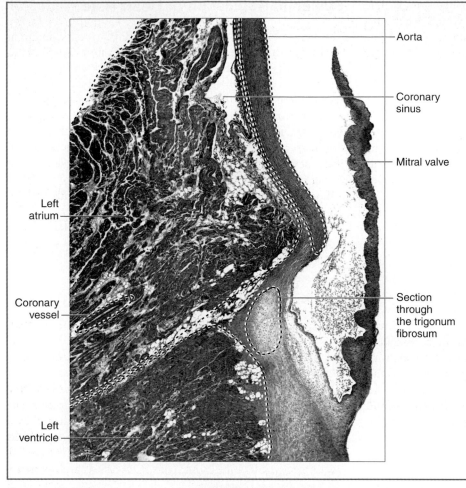

Aorta

Coronary sinus

Mitral valve

Left atrium

Coronary vessel

Section through the trigonum fibrosum

Left ventricle

A

Figure 7-3. A, Section of the left ventricle and left atrium of a monkey heart near the mitral valve (Milligan's trichrome stain, 17.5×). One flap of the mitral valve and the beginning part of the aortic arch are seen. A section through the left ring of the trigona fibrosa is seen in the lower central part of the field. The characteristics of the connective tissue in this specimen are suggestive of cartilage. **B,** Diagram shows the trigona fibrosa, both atrioventricular valves, the aorta and pulmonary trunk. The approximate section plane of this diagram is indicated in the heart diagram on the left.

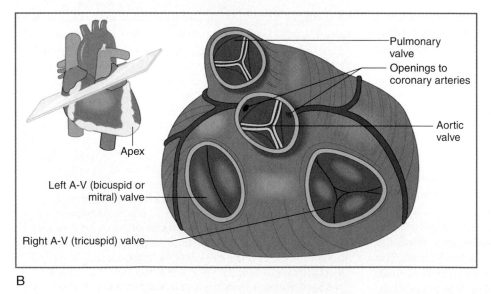

Pulmonary valve

Openings to coronary arteries

Aortic valve

Apex

Left A-V (bicuspid or mitral) valve

Right A-V (tricuspid) valve

B

the layers is characterized or dominated by a single cell type, and each layer has a characteristic matrix (Table 7-1). It is important to remember that the entire cardiovascular system is lined by a single cell type, the endothelial cell. This specialized simple squamous epithelial cell lines the endocardium of the heart, lines all the arteries and veins, and makes up all the capillaries. Like the heart, larger blood vessels receive a blood supply from outside their structure through a system of small vessels called the *vasa vasorum*.

Several features of blood vessels are helpful when one is identifying them in sectioned material. It is common to see *paired* (or *companion*) *vessels* in sections of organs or in

TABLE 7-1. Cellular and Matrix Composition of Blood Vessels

Tunica	Predominant Cell Type	Matrix Characteristics	Other Features
Intima	Endothelial cells and associated basal lamina. The endothelial cells have occluding junctions between them	—	Small amounts of subendothelial loose connective tissue containing fibroblasts and a few smooth muscle cells are found in largest vessels
Media	Smooth muscle cells and associated lamina externa	Collagen types I and III, many elastin fibers, proteoglycans NB: the matrix components are synthesized by smooth muscle cells	Larger vessels contain smallest termini of vasa vasorum. In larger vessels, occasional gap junctions may be seen between smooth muscle cells of the tunica media and endothelial cells of the tunica intima
Adventitia	Fibroblasts	Loose connective tissue	Vasa vasorum, occasional nerves

neurovascular bundles that are readily dissected in a cadaver. The paired vessels are an artery and vein that are approximately equidistant from the heart and the capillary bed each vessel serves. The artery in such sections is usually more circular than the vein and has a thicker wall and smaller caliber than its companion vein. In other words, the ratio of the caliber of an artery to its wall thickness is always smaller than the same ratio for its companion vein.

Blood Vessel Classification

The structure of the walls of blood vessels and their inner diameters (caliber) varies in a more or less continuous manner from the largest artery (the aorta), which has a diameter of about 25 mm, down to capillaries, which have diameters of about 5 μm, and back to the vena cava, whose diameter is about 30 mm. Blood vessels are classified by reference to their wall structure and thickness and to a lesser extent, their caliber. Furthermore, the classification is based on the arterial side of the circulatory system; for each arterial category, there is a comparable venous category whose structural characteristics and appearance are more variable than its arterial "partner." The following are the major categories of blood vessels.

Elastic Arteries

The tunica intima of these vessels usually has a thin, subendothelial layer of loose connective tissue with a few fibroblasts and a rare smooth muscle cell. They have a relatively thick tunica media with spirally arranged smooth muscle cells, thick collagen fibers, and many elastin fibers. The elastin fibers are arranged into concentric fenestrated lamellae. It is hard to be precise about the thickness of the tunica adventitia, since it blends into the surrounding connective tissue; it has numerous blood vessels that supply the tunica media (the vasa vasorum) and some nerves. The caliber of elastic arteries ranges from about 10 mm to 25 mm. Figure 7-4 shows four sections of elastic arteries stained with three different stains

to highlight the cellular composition and the matrix content of the tunica media of elastic arteries.

Large Muscular Arteries

The tunica intima is a single layer of endothelial cells with a scant or absent subendothelial layer of connective tissue. The boundary of the tunica intima and media is demarcated by a prominent layer of elastic fibers called the inner elastic lamina (IEL). The tunica media has circularly oriented smooth muscle cells and collagen and elastin fibers. At the boundary of the tunica media and adventitia, another prominent layer of elastin fibers is seen—the external elastic lamella (EEL). A thin tunica adventitia is present. The caliber of the large muscular arteries ranges from about 2 mm to 10 mm. Sections of muscular arteries and companion veins are seen in Figure 7-5.

PATHOLOGY

Aneurysms and Elastic Arteries

A rather common abnormality of elastic arteries is an aneurysm, a weakening of the tunica media leading to dilatation of the vessel wall. Aneurysms are found in about 10% of autopsies. Most aneurysms are fusiform, and some are saccular (balloon-like). Many are dissecting aneurysms in which there is a longitudinal splitting of the tunica media by a hematoma, or hemorrhage, into the muscular layer of the vessel wall. The underlying cause is a weakening of the tunica media. The weakening may be due to a focal bacterial infection or a congenital factor. Laboratory studies have shown that the amount of elastin in the dilated part of the vessel is significantly less than in the uninvolved part and that the amount of elastin mRNA is also reduced. The incidence of aneurysms increases with age, hypertension, and the presence of an atherosclerotic plaque.

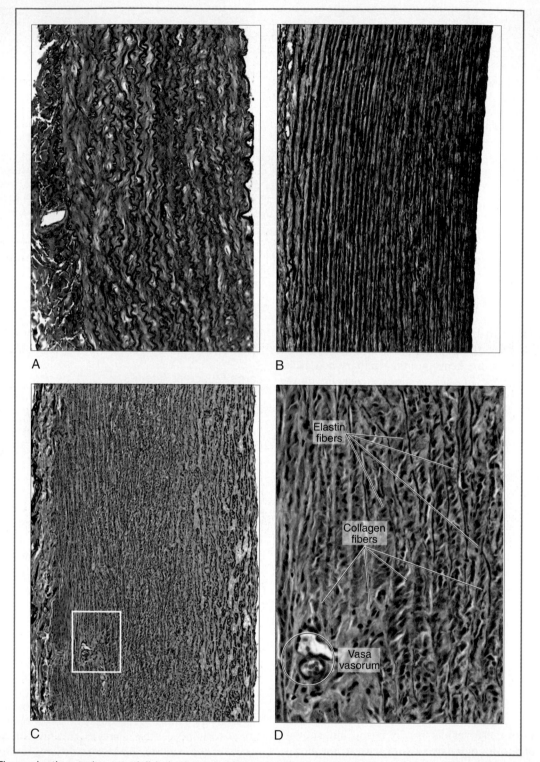

Figure 7-4. Three elastic arteries are visible in these sections; in all cases, the tunica intima is to the right and the tunica adventitia is to the left. None of the endothelial cells of the tunica intima are visible. **A,** H&E stain of the carotid artery (140×). The smooth muscle cells, and their nuclei, of the tunica media are readily identifiable. The fenestrated elastic lamellae of the tunica media are the dark red–stained, wavy fibers throughout the tunica media. This vessel has a more prominent inner elastic lamella than the aorta, which is indicative of its transition to the morphology typical of a large muscular artery. Some coarse collagen fibers of the tunica adventitia, including a cross-section of a vasa vasorum, are visible on the left margin of the specimen. **B,** Orcein stain of the aorta (160×). The extensive elastic lamellae of the tunica media are well demonstrated. Essentially no cellular features are discernable with this stain, although some of the tunica adventitia, with several vasa vasorum, is recognizable. The collagen fibers are stained a much lighter brown than the elastin fibers. **C** and **D,** Sections of monkey aorta stained with Milligan's trichrome stain (**C,** 80×; **D,** 280×). The cellular and matrix components are well differentiated with this stain. The tunica adventitia, with many vasa vasorum, at left in part C is stained light aqua blue. Part D shows the area in the box in part C at higher magnification; the elastin fibers are stained bright red-orange, the collagen is aqua blue, and the smooth muscle cells are reddish magenta. A small arteriole and venule are seen at lower left, illustrating the intimate intermingling of the cells and matrix components of the tunica media.

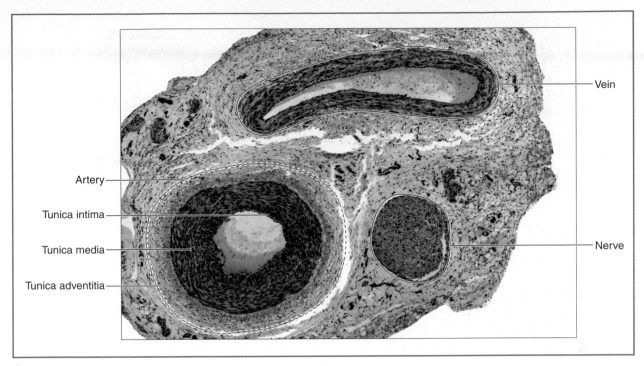

Vein

Artery

Tunica intima

Tunica media

Tunica adventitia

Nerve

A

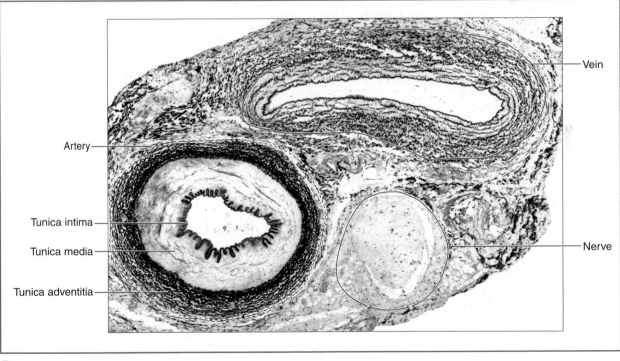

Vein

Artery

Tunica intima

Tunica media

Tunica adventitia

Nerve

B

Figure 7-5. A and **B,** The same neurovascular bundle (part A, H&E, 31×; part B, orcein, 31×). **C,** Resorcin-fuchsin elastic stain of the femoral artery and vein of a small mammal (80×). In part A, the thick muscular walls of the artery and the vein are evident; the arterial wall is thicker, rounder, and of smaller caliber than the vein. The nerve fiber is also well stained. In part B, the amount and distribution of elastin fibers in the artery are well demonstrated; a prominent IEL and EEL are seen. In contrast, the companion vein has a significant elastin content, but the elastin fibers are seen throughout the tunica media and the tunica adventitia with no particular distribution. The nerve is noticeable because of its round, unstained shape. The paired vessels in both sections illustrate the relationship of wall thickness, caliber, shape, and elastin content and the distribution of companion arteries and veins. The three layers of the arteries in both sections are readily identifiable. The companion muscular artery and vein in part C are larger than those in parts A and B, so the elastin fiber content is more pronounced. The structural characteristics of paired vessels are well demonstrated in this specimen. Several nerve bundles are seen above the vessels. A bundle of skeletal muscle fibers is also seen at bottom right.

Continued

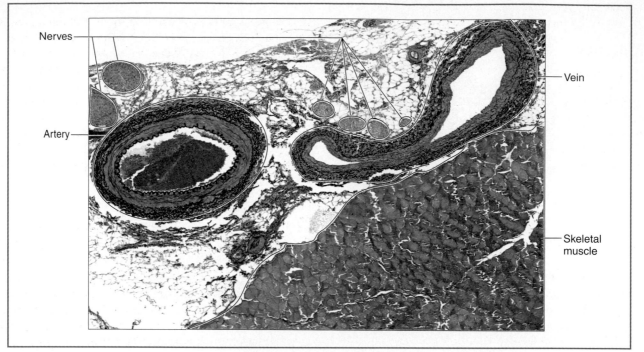

Nerves

Artery

Vein

Skeletal muscle

C

Figure 7-5 cont'd.

BIOCHEMISTRY

Atherosclerosis and Muscular Arteries

Many elastic, large- and medium-sized muscular arteries may become occluded by intimal deposits of lipids, accumulations of smooth muscle cells and macrophages, matrix proteins, and calcifications. The disease that results from this process is called atherosclerosis. The major complications of atherosclerosis are ischemic heart disease, myocardial infarction, stroke, and peripheral vascular disease, which can lead to gangrene of the extremities.

The pathogenesis of atherosclerosis is complex, and many factors contribute to its progression. A major factor is a high blood serum level of cholesterol, a lipid component of the diet as well as a molecule synthesized by all cells of the body, in particular by the hepatocytes, the parenchymal cells of the liver. Dietary cholesterol is metabolized by the *exogenous pathway*, and cholesterol synthesized by the liver and other cells is metabolized by the *endogenous pathway*. In both cases, cholesterol travels in the blood in lipoprotein particles—lipid droplets surrounded by several protein (apolipoprotein) molecules.

Four major classes of lipoprotein particles are described:
- Chylomicrons are particles containing cholesterol and triglycerides, which are assembled in the intestinal epithelial cells and delivered to lymphatic capillaries in the lamina propria of intestinal villi.
- Very low density lipoproteins (VLDLs), particles that are produced in hepatocytes and secreted directly into the bloodstream.
- Low-density lipoproteins (LDLs), the major form of atherogenic lipoproteins, which are taken up predominantly by the liver
- High-density lipoproteins (HDL).

The triglycerides in chylomicrons are removed in capillaries and by the cells in adipose and muscle tissue. This leaves a smaller version of lipoprotein particle rich in cholesterol and protein called intermediate-density lipoprotein (IDL) and LDL.

IDL and LDL particles are taken up by hepatocytes and other cells wherein the cholesterol is metabolized for excretion or for other cellular use (e.g., cellular membranes, hormones).

Impaired ability to remove the lipoprotein particles from the circulation leads to increased serum cholesterol levels and a higher incidence of atherosclerosis.

Of at least four monogenic diseases that affect cholesterol uptake, the best characterized is familial hypercholesterolemia, which causes a deficit in the number of LDL receptors (LDLRs) per cell. It is an autosomal dominant disease, the gene for which is located on the short arm of chromosome 19. More than 600 mutations have been identified in the LDLR gene. One in 500 people is heterozygous for one such mutation, but only one in one million is homozygous for a mutation at a single locus. Individuals who are heterozygous produce half the normal number of LDLR proteins and have serum cholesterol levels two to three times normal. Homozygous individuals have extremely low levels of LDLR proteins and serum cholesterol levels six to ten times normal. The disease affects children in the first decade of life.

Essentially all named arteries (and veins) are in the elastic and muscular categories.

Small Muscular Arteries

The tunica intima is a single layer of endothelial cells. The tunica media has a prominent IEL but no EEL, circularly arranged smooth muscle cells, and more collagen fibers than elastin fibers. A thin tunica adventitia is present. The caliber of the small muscular arteries ranges from about 0.1 mm to 2 mm. Two specimens of small muscular arteries and companion veins are seen in Figure 7-6.

Arterioles and Metarterioles

The tunica intima is a single layer of endothelial cells. The tunica media has a few layers of circularly arranged smooth muscle cells and some collagen fibers. A thin tunica adventitia is present. These vessels are found at the beginning of microvascular beds. The smooth muscle cells have receptors for epinephrine and norepinepherine (potent vasoconstrictors), which contract, thereby occluding the vessel and closing down the microvascular bed. Thus, they are important regulators of the microcirculation. Their caliber ranges from about 10 μm to 100 μm. A whole mount preparation of small vessels from the pia mater is seen in Figure 7-7.

Capillaries

The wall of a capillary consists of a single cell endothelial layer and its basal lamina. Occasionally a special cell called the pericyte is seen (see Pericytes). Important variations of capillary structure are also discussed below. Their caliber ranges from about 5 μm to 10 μm. Two small capillary beds are seen in Figure 7-8.

Postcapillary Venules

These vessels have a simple wall made of a single endothelial cell layer, its basal lamina, an occasional smooth muscle cell, and pericytes. They are the primary site for the transmural migration of lymphocytes from the circulation to the interstitial space and back. Their caliber ranges from about 10 μm to 50 μm.

Venules

The tunica intima is a single layer of endothelial cells. The tunica media has one to two layers of circularly arranged smooth muscle cells. The tunica adventitia is thicker than the tunica media. Their caliber ranges from about 50 μm to 100 μm. Several venules and postcapillary venules are seen in Figure 7-8.

Small Veins

The tunica intima is a single layer of endothelial cells with one to two layers of smooth muscle cells. The tunica media has two to four layers of circularly arranged smooth muscle cells (continuous with the smooth muscle cells of the tunica intima) and collagen fibers. The tunica adventitia is thicker than the tunica media. Their caliber ranges from about 0.1 mm to 2 mm. A good example of a small vein is seen in Figure 7-9.

Medium Veins

The tunica intima is a single layer of endothelial cells and some smooth muscle cells. These veins have valves made of a thin elastic connective tissue flap covered on both surfaces by endothelial cells. The tunica media has four to ten layers of circularly arranged smooth muscle cells, collagen fibers, and elastin fibers. The larger veins in this category may have an incomplete IEL. The tunica adventitia is thicker than the tunica media. The larger veins in this category have isolated bundles of longitudinally oriented smooth muscle cells. Their caliber ranges from about 2 mm to 10 mm. Veins of this type are seen in Figure 7-5.

Large (Elastic) Veins

The tunica intima is a single layer of endothelial cells and subendothelial connective tissue. Large veins may also have valves. The tunica media has ten or more layers of circularly arranged smooth muscle cells, many collagen fibers, and elastin fibers. The elastin fibers are not organized into distinct lamellae. The tunica adventitia is much thicker than the tunica media and has numerous isolated bundles of longitudinally oriented smooth muscle cells. Their caliber ranges from about 10 mm to 30 mm. Some examples of the vena cava are seen in Figure 7-10.

Capillary Structure

Capillaries are the smallest and most numerous of the blood vessels; estimates tell us there are thousands of miles of them in our bodies. Their average diameter is about that of an RBC, 7 to 8 μm, but some are only about 5 μm in diameter, so in the smallest of capillaries RBCs become distorted, squeezing their way through the lumen. Yet their total cross-sectional area is about 600 times that of the aorta. The implications of this geometry impart significant advantages to capillary function because

- The flow rate of blood through a capillary is very slow.
- Capillary hydrostatic pressure is nearly zero.
- The diffusion path for the exchange of gases, nutrients, fluids, and waste products is minimized.
- The ratios of capillary volume to endothelial surface area and to thickness favor efficient bidirectional exchange of materials between the capillary and the extracellular space.

From a structural point of view, there are three types of capillaries:

- *Continuous capillaries* are found in all types of muscle, the central nervous system, the lung, exocrine glands, connective tissue layers of the skin, etc.
- *Fenestrated capillaries* are found in the intestines, gallbladder, endocrine glands, and kidney. There are two kinds of fenestrated capillaries—those with closed fenestrations (the most common) and those with open fenestrations, which are found only in the glomerular capillaries of the renal corpuscle.
- *Discontinuous capillaries* are found only in the liver.

Capillaries are difficult to see in sections in the light micro-

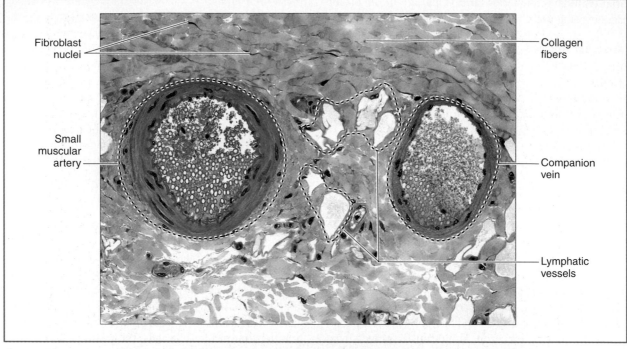

A

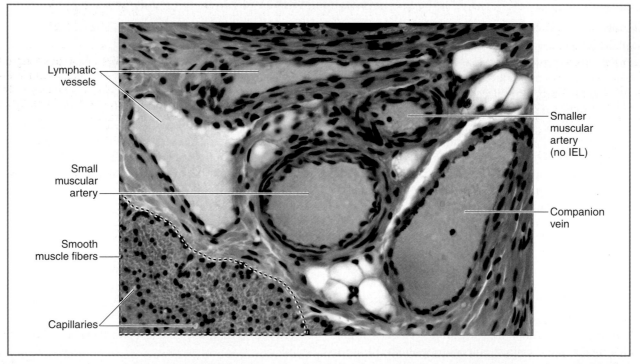

B

Figure 7-6. Companion arteries and veins of the small category are seen in these H&E-stained sections. Part A is from the submucosa of the colon (200×), and part B from the submucosa of the jejunum (240×). **A,** The vessels are of comparable caliber although the artery has a thicker wall and is somewhat rounder than its companion vein—a reminder that rules in biology are replete with exceptions. The IEL of the artery is visible as a wavy red line with a few endothelial cell nuclei visible on the luminal surface. The nuclei of smooth muscle cells of the tunica media are seen in both vessels. A number of lymphatic vessels are seen near the blood vessels; in a few of these, the endothelial cell nuclei can be identified. **B,** The paired vessels in this section are about 20% smaller than those in part A (note the difference in magnification). In this case, the IEL of the artery is barely visible, but its presence is evident by the slight clear line under the endothelial cells and the wavy luminal border of the vessel. The much thinner wall and larger caliber lumen of the vein (allowing for the fact that the vein is probably obliquely sectioned), are also evident. There are many lymphatic vessels in this section, some filled with slightly different amounts or concentrations of lymph fluid.

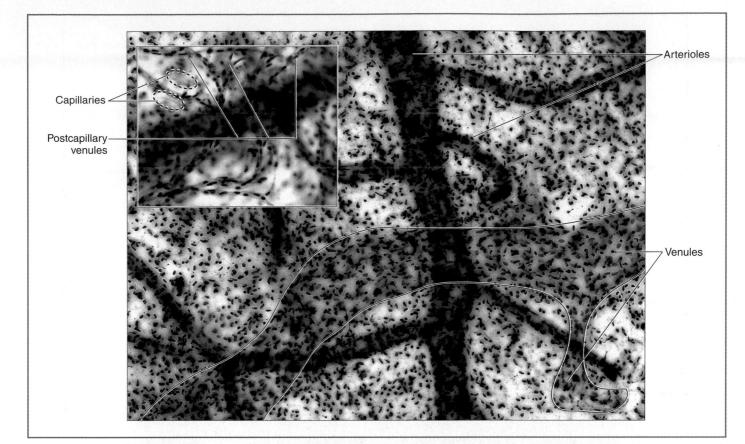

Figure 7-7. Whole-mount preparation of the pia mater (110×), a thin, tough, vascular sheet of connective tissue covering the brain. Small arterioles, metarterioles, and postcapillary venules can be seen. Since both walls of the vessels are visible in this preparation, it is possible to identify them on the basis of their diameter and their relative staining "density." Essentially only the nuclei are stained, so endothelial and smooth muscle nuclei can be identified on the basis of their shape and position. Short segments of several capillaries and postcapillary venules are seen at higher magnification in the inset (200×).

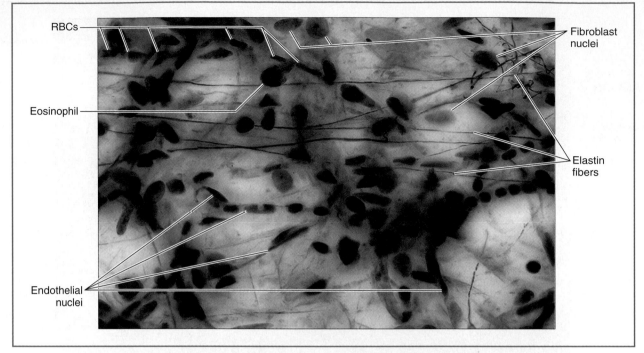

RBCs

Fibroblast nuclei

Eosinophil

Elastin fibers

Endothelial nuclei

A

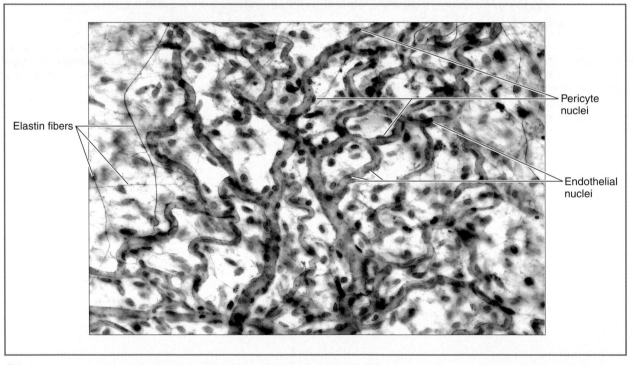

Elastin fibers

Pericyte nuclei

Endothelial nuclei

B

Figure 7-8. Two small capillary networks in spread preparations are seen in this figure. **A,** A high magnification of several small arterioles and capillaries stained with H&E (360×). The vessel walls are barely stained, but the erythrocytes and endothelial cell nuclei are seen. Several fibroblast nuclei and elastin fibers are seen in the connective tissue. A tissue eosinophil is seen in the central upper left part of the field. **B,** A network of small arterioles, capillaries, and venules (iron hematoxylin stain, 190×). A few elastin fibers are in the field of view. Many endothelial cell and pericyte nuclei are seen in or on most of the vessels; the two cell types can be distinguished based on whether their nuclei follow the contour of and are bounded by the endothelial cell wall or whether they appear as bulges on the outer wall of the vessel wall.

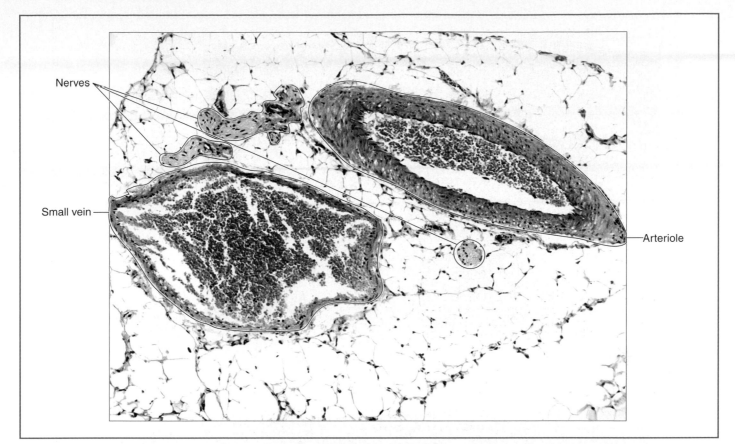

Figure 7-9. A pair of small companion vessels embedded in adipose tissue are seen in this H&E-stained section. Both vessels are sectioned obliquely. Note the appearance of the smooth muscle cells in the tunica media at the upper left end of the vessel compared with the central part. The vein is thin walled and filled with blood.

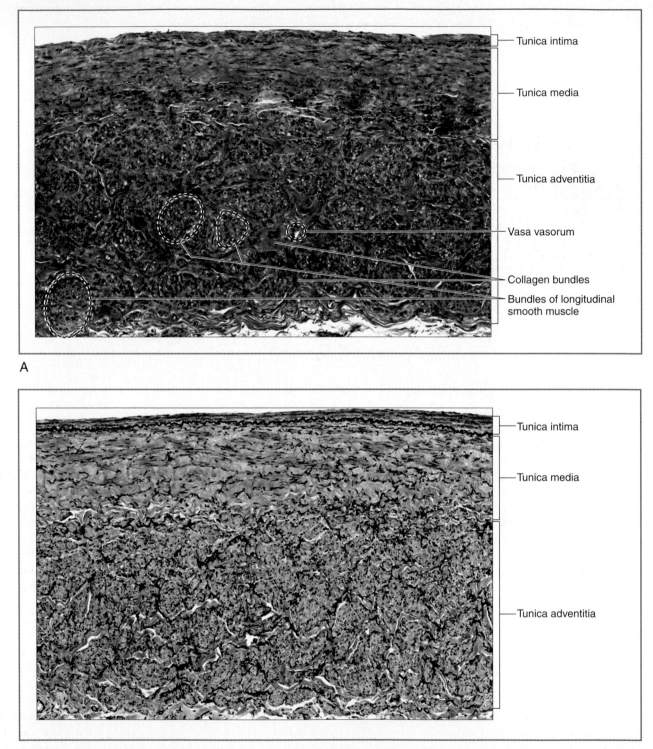

A

B

Figure 7-10. Three full-thickness sections of human vena cava. **A,** H&E stain, 50×; **B,** resorcin-H&E stain, 62.5×; **C,** Milligan's trichrome stain, 25×. The relative thickness of the three tunics is seen in parts A and B—the tunica adventitia is much thicker than the tunica media and has many longitudinally oriented bundles of smooth muscle in it. The tunica media contains relatively more collagen than the tunica media of the aorta, but the entire wall thickness of the vena cava has substantially less elastin than the aorta. The tunica intima is about the same thickness as that of the aorta. The vena cava has a prominent, thin, inner elastic lamina (part B); there are also a number of elastin fibers throughout the wall. The section in part C shows a distinctive feature of large elastic veins—an intimal thickening. These are large expansions of connective tissue under the endothelium and are the sites of the valves in these vessels; since the thickenings are so long and large, it is common to not see the valve cusps in a section, as is the case here.

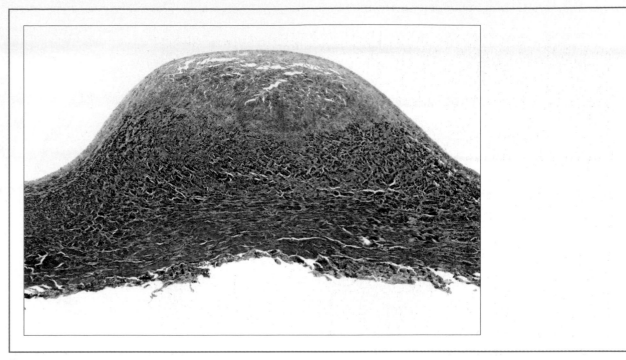

C

Figure 7-10 cont'd.

scope but can be seen in spread preparations more readily, as in Figure 7-8. Capillary structure is best understood at the electron microscopic level as discussed and shown below.

The endothelial cell, and its basal lamina, of continuous capillaries consists of a thin sheet of cytoplasm that either wraps around to contact itself to form a tube or forms one by contacting adjacent endothelial cells. Electron micrographs reveal many important features of these tiny vessels. Figure 7-11 shows that adjacent contact surfaces of the plasma membranes form occluding (tight) junctions; cytoplasmic (marginal) folds are often seen projecting into the lumen near the junctions. Many plasmalemmal (pinocytotic) vesicles are seen in the thin cytoplasmic rim; these represent the major site of bidirectional transport of fluids and solutes between the blood and the interstitial space. A nucleus may or may not be seen, depending on the plane of section. When the nucleus can be seen, it bulges into the lumen of the capillary.

Fenestrated capillaries have the same characteristics as continuous capillaries (including plasmalemmal vesicles), except the endothelial cell walls have hundreds of small fenestrations (little windows) 80 to 100 nm in diameter (Fig. 7-12). Nearly all fenestrated capillaries have a thin, non-membranous (i.e., nonlipid) diaphragm across each individual fenestration (i.e., they are "closed" fenestrations). The fenes-trations are thought to increase the rate of bidirectional movement of materials across the capillary wall. This inter-pretation is supported by two facts: fenestrated capillaries are found in locations where material moves across the capillary wall at a high rate or where a large amount of material moves across the wall; and studies have shown that capillaries in the intestines and gallbladder have a thicker wall and fewer plasmalemmal vesicles and fenestrations when they are not actively absorbing material from their lumens.

The capillaries in the kidney are mostly of the closed fenestrated type, but those in the renal corpuscle have open fenestrations. The open fenestrations of these capillaries are part of the glomerular filter and help explain how the large volume of provisional urine (ca. 120 L/day) is formed in the kidneys.

Discontinuous capillaries are found lining the sinusoids of the liver. They have large openings in their endothelial cell walls that permit the blood flowing through them (a large proportion of which comes from the intestines and is rich in nutrients) to directly come into contact with the many short filopodia of the underlying hepatocytes without having to traverse the cytoplasmic wall of the endothelial cell or to rely on the plasmalemmal transport process (Fig. 7-13). Only a sparse basal lamina is associated with the cytoplasm of discontinuous capillaries, and none with the discontinuities.

A diagrammatic representation of all three capillary types is seen in Figure 7-14.

Sinusoidal Capillaries

There are several locations where capillary caliber is much larger than is typical. Some have diameters in the range of 20 to 80 μm and are usually described as being *sinusoids* or

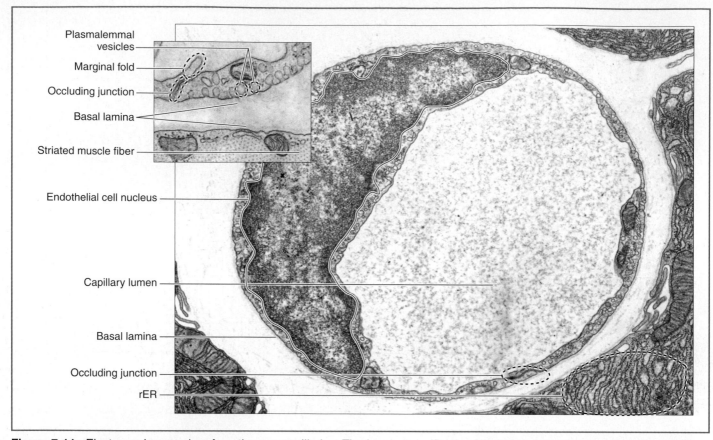

Plasmalemmal vesicles

Marginal fold

Occluding junction

Basal lamina

Striated muscle fiber

Endothelial cell nucleus

Capillary lumen

Basal lamina

Occluding junction

rER

Figure 7-11. Electron micrographs of continuous capillaries. The lower magnification image is a transverse section of an entire continuous capillary from a serous exocrine gland. The thin cytoplasmic rim of the endothelial cell has many plasmalemmal vesicles, a few mitochondria, a cell junction, and a large nucleus. The inset is a higher magnification of a portion of a capillary wall from striated muscle showing the occluding junction and a marginal fold. The basal laminae are faint but visible in both micrographs—surrounding the entire vessel and adjacent to the exocrine cell fragments in the lower magnification image, as well as being associated with the endothelial cell and muscle fiber fragments in the inset. (Courtesy of Don W. Fawcett.)

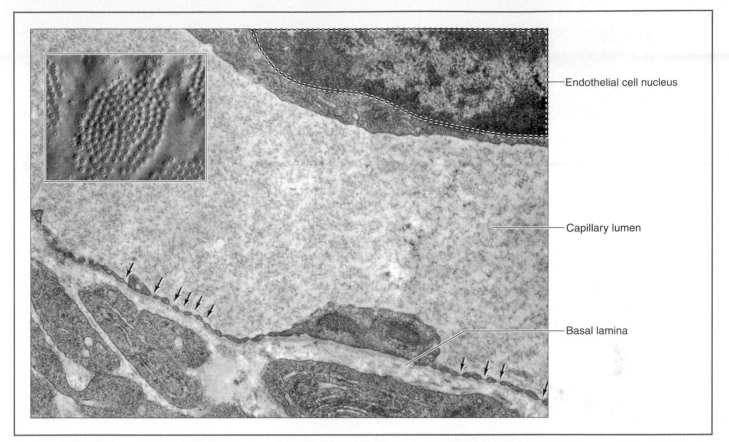

Endothelial cell nucleus

Capillary lumen

Basal lamina

Figure 7-12. Electron micrographs of fenestrated capillaries. A portion of a closed fenestrated capillary is seen in the TEM; the fenestrations are indicated by arrows. The delicate basal lamina is also seen on the abluminal surface of the capillary. The inset shows a freeze-fracture etching electron micrograph; this is an *en face* view of the luminal surface of the capillary. The fenestrations are seen to occur in oval groups with a regular spacing among them. (Courtesy of Don W. Fawcett.)

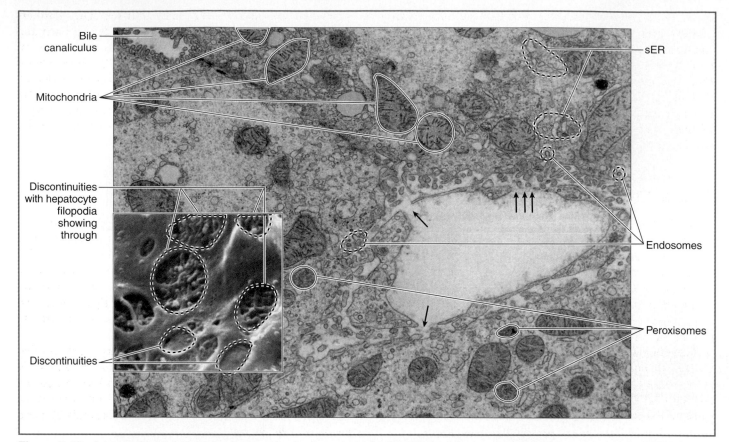

Figure 7-13. A transmission electron micrograph of a liver sinusoid (10,000×) and a scanning electron micrograph (SEM) (inset, 12,725×). In the TEM, discontinuities in the sinusoid are indicated by arrows. Numerous mitochondria, peroxisomes, endosomes, profiles of smooth endoplasmic reticulum (sER), and a bile canaliculus are labeled. (Courtesy of Patricia C. Cross, Stanford University Medical School.) The discontinuities in the wall of the endothelial cell can be seen more clearly in the SEM inset; this is a view from the lumen of the sinusoidal capillary looking toward the hepatocyte. The filopodia of the hepatocyte are visible through several of the discontinuities. (Courtesy of Richard G. Kessel and Randy H. Kardon, Iowa University Hospital and Clinic.)

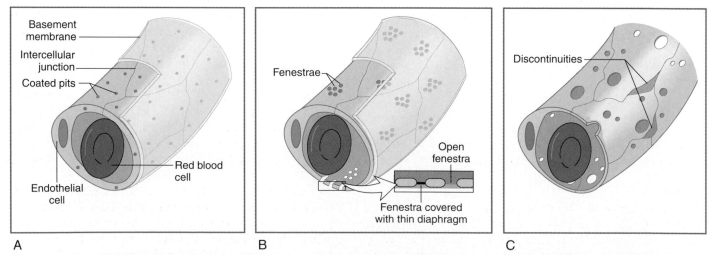

Figure 7-14. Diagrams of the three types of capillaries. **A,** Continuous capillary. Note the elongated shape of the endothelial cells and the diameter that is approximately the same as that of the erythrocyte in the lumen. **B,** Fenestrated capillary showing both closed fenestrations (the most abundant kind of fenestration) and open fenestrations. **C,** Discontinuous capillary showing the many shapes and arrangements of the discontinuities. (Modified from Boron W, Boulpaep E. *Medical Physiology*. Philadelphia, WB Saunders, 2003, p 465.)

sinusoidal capillaries; they are found in the bone marrow, adrenal cortex, liver, and a few other places. Nonetheless, the sinusoidal capillaries of bone marrow are of the continuous type, those of the adrenal cortex are of the closed fenestrated type, and as mentioned above, liver sinusoids have discontinuous capillaries. Thus, it is most appropriate to describe capillary types on the basis of the structure and appearance of their walls, not their caliber. Use of the term sinusoid should refer *only* to the caliber or luminal diameter of a capillary.

Special Characteristics of Blood Vessels

Endothelial Cells

Although the endothelial cell is morphologically a simple squamous epithelial cell, it has many specialized functions in the circulatory system. Among the more important are

- The tight junctions that help hold the endothelial cells together and thereby regulate transmural exchange of materials.
- The marginal folds often seen near the junctions, which play a role in the transmural migration of white blood cells (WBCs).
- Expression of adhesion molecule receptors (addressins) that bind to adhesion molecules (selectins) on circulating WBCs and cause them to slow down, roll, and bind to the adluminal surface of postcapillary venules to facilitate the transmural migration of white cells.
- Plasmalemmal vesicles, which are found in the endothelia of all vessels and are largely responsible for fluid and solute exchange. The number of vesicles per square micrometer of endothelial cell surface area varies with the type of vessel (capillaries may have about $1000/\mu m^2$, larger arteries down to arterioles about $200/\mu m^2$, and venules about $600/\mu m^2$).
- Special cytoplasmic granules called Weibel-Palade bodies that store a glycoprotein (von Willebrand factor) that is important in the early steps of blood clotting. This factor is released at the site of injury to blood vessels in response to the presence of a number of cytokines; it promotes the adherence of platelets to collagen underlying the endothelial cells. Weibel-Palade granules also store platelet-synthesized cytokines.
- Synthesis of a potent smooth muscle relaxing factor, nitric oxide (NO), from L-arginine.
- Synthesis and release of endothelium-derived relaxing factor (EDRF), another smooth muscle relaxing factor.

Pericytes

Many capillaries and most postcapillary venules have an occasional cell intimately associated with their tissue (abluminal) surface. This cell is a pericyte; it is surrounded by a basal lamina, and its nucleus bulges out from the vessel wall (see Fig. 7-8B). It has a dendritic structure and is thought to have contractile properties. In fact, the pericyte may be a mesenchymal vascular stem cell, since it is known to give rise to smooth muscle cells in normal vascular growth or during

regeneration of blood vessels following tissue injury. Furthermore, in experiments done on mice during fetal growth and development, the existence of pericytes is dependent on platelet-derived growth factor-β (PDGF-β). Mice whose PDGF-β gene has been deleted do not develop pericytes, exhibit extensive microaneurysms of capillary beds, and die in late fetal life. Therefore, it is safe to say that the pericyte is a cell whose full function and significance in vascular homeostasis is yet to be understood.

Special Vascular Arrangements

Portal Systems

The most common arrangement of blood vessels is artery–capillary bed–vein. In three major anatomic locations, there are variants of this arrangement: the gastrointestinal (GI) system, the cortex of the kidney, and the pituitary gland. In all three cases, there are two capillary beds with an intervening vein (in the GI system) or artery (in the other two cases) between the two capillary beds. These are referred to as *portal systems*.

Blood is delivered to the GI system by many arteries that ramify into many capillary beds. The blood is ultimately collected in a large vein, the portal vein, which brings the blood to the liver, where it once again flows into the system of discontinuous capillaries of the hepatic sinusoids. This is a *venous portal system*.

The portal systems in the kidney and pituitary gland are *arterial portal systems*.

Arteriovenous Shunts

In a number of locations, blood passes directly from the arterial circulation to the venous circulation, bypassing a capillary bed. This vascular arrangement is called an arteriovenous (AV) shunt or anastomosis. The shunts have three segments: an initial arterial segment typical of small arterioles, an intermediate segment of similar or smaller caliber to the arteriole but with a much thicker muscular wall than is typical of its caliber, and a terminal segment typical of a small vein. The intermediate segment may be coiled and is richly innervated.

When smooth muscle in the wall of the intermediate segment is relaxed, blood flow bypasses the capillary bed; when it is contracted, the blood flows through the capillary bed. This is in contrast to the usual function of a precapillary sphincter, which delivers blood to a capillary bed when it is open.

AV shunts are found in the skin, lips, penis, and clitoris. They are common and extensive in the skin of marine and arctic mammals, where they have important roles in thermoregulation. When an AV shunt is open, heat is conserved because the warm blood is not dispersed to capillary beds, and when it is closed, a much larger volume of blood flows through capillary beds allowing heat to be lost throughout the body surface. AV shunts in humans are not so extensive as those in other mammals. The role of AV shunts in erectile tissue is somewhat different, since contraction of the intermediate segment traps blood in cavernous venous sinuses causing the tissue to become engorged with blood, hence more rigid (i.e., erect).

Atypical Vessels

Variations in the typical organization of blood vessels are found in many locations in the body. Several examples are described in Table 7-2; two examples of atypical vessels are shown in Figure 7-15.

●●● LYMPHATIC VESSELS

Lymphatic Capillaries

Lymphatic capillaries are closed tubes that begin as blind-end cylinders of endothelial cells. They collect excess tissue fluid and lymphocytes from interstitial tissue spaces. They drain the periphery in a one-way flow, not a circulation, ultimately into the great veins (e.g., inferior vena cava) close to the heart. They tend to run in parallel with blood capillaries in most locations. They are present in all but a few organs (e.g., the brain, bone marrow, eyeball).

The caliber of lymphatic capillaries may range from 1.5 to 10 times that of capillaries. At the ultrastructural level they have many plasmalemmal vesicles and may have openings near cell junctions. They have a very thin to absent basal lamina and are anchored to the surrounding connective tissue by integrin-containing focal contacts. Figure 7-16 shows lymphatic capillaries in intestinal villi and a larger lymphatic vessel in a lymph node. Several small lymphatic capillaries can be seen in Figure 7-6B.

Collecting and Main Lymphatic Vessels

As the lymphatic capillaries coalesce into larger vessels, they acquire thin tunics of smooth muscle and connective tissue (i.e., a tunica media and a tunica adventitia). However these

TABLE 7-2. Atypical Blood Vessels

Location or Type of Vessel	Tunica Intima	Tunica Media	Tunica Adventitia	Comment
"Typical" artery	Endothelium and its basal lamina Little or no connective tissue	Several layers of circumferential smooth muscle cells	Loose and dense irregular connective tissue, vasa vasorum, fibroblasts, and macrophages	All three tunics are present
Umbilical arteries (two) and vein	Typical	Of the muscular type but lack inner and external elastic laminae Thick muscular walls have circular, spiral, and some longitudinal smooth muscle	Essentially absent Tunica media is surrounded by mucous connective tissue of cord	The vein is most centrally located and has a large caliber lumen
Splenic artery	Typical	May contain two layers of smooth muscle: inner longitudinal and outer circular	Typical	This modification is common in arteries that may bend significantly
Small penile arteries	Longitudinal thickenings made of smooth muscle bundles	Typical	Typical	Intimal thickenings help control local blood flow and occlude the lumen
Venous sinuses of the spleen	Rod-shaped endothelial cells oriented in the direction of blood flow, incomplete basal lamina arranged in bands around outer circumference of endothelial cells	None	None	These vessels lack pericytes, and their structure can be likened to a barrel, where the endothelial cells are staves and the basal lamina is a hoop
Postcapillary venules of lymph nodes	Cuboidal to low columnar endothelium cells with very thin basal lamina	None	None	Also called high endothelial venules (HEVs) Major site of lymphocyte diapedesis that occurs between endothelial cells

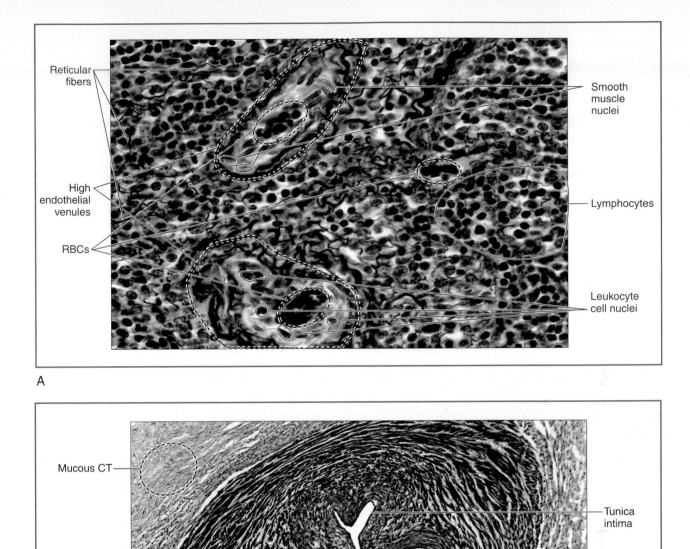

A

B

Figure 7-15. A, Section of the deep cortex of a lymph node stained with a silver-eosin stain (360×) shows two examples of specialized venules found in lymph nodes—high endothelial venules (HEVs). Erythrocytes and leukocytes that have passed through the cortical part of a lymph node are collected in these specialized vessels. They have a high, almost cuboidal, endothelium and one or two layers of smooth muscle in their walls. The endothelial cell nuclei are parallel to the axis of the venule and are not flattened as they are in most other blood vessels. The smooth muscle cells are wrapped around the venule in a circular fashion. In this specimen, little or none of the cytoplasm of any of the cells can be seen, but the nuclear shape and orientation can be used to identify most of the cells in the field of view. Since this specimen has been stained with silver-eosin, the reticular fibers are evident; in fact, the tunica adventitia of both HEVs is seen to be invested with a prominent array of reticular fibers. **B,** Transverse section of one of the umbilical cord arteries (Milligan's stain, 35×). There are several distinctive features of this highly coiled, thick-walled muscular artery: there is no internal or external elastic lamina, the lumen of the vessel is highly folded, and the tunica media is very thick and has several atypical layers of smooth muscle fibers—an inner longitudinal layer and several spiral layers with different pitches. The tunica media has a higher than typical content of unstained proteoglycans in this specimen although their distribution can be inferred by the unstained spaces in the tunica media. There is no tunica adventitia proper, only the mucous connective tissue of the umbilical cord itself.

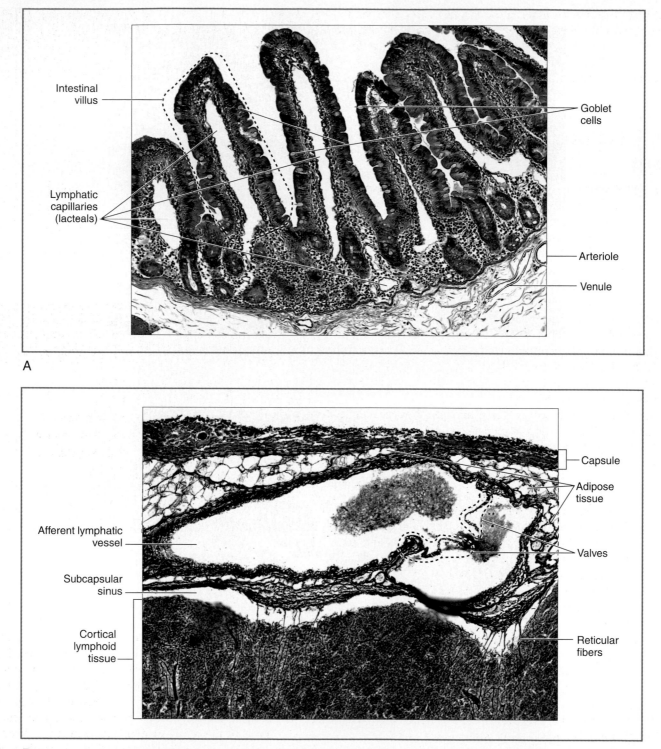

A

B

Figure 7-16. A, Section of intestinal villi of the jejunum (Milligan's stain, 70×). Several of the villi have elongated openings, which are the blind-end origins of lymphatic capillaries (called lacteals) found in the small intestines. **B,** Section of the capsule and outer cortex of a lymph node (silver stain, 90×). The large oval structure is a large lymphatic vessel just under the capsule of a lymph node. Both flaps of a lymphatic valve can be seen toward the right side of the vessel. The slightly less stained amorphous material in the lumen of the vessel is lymph. The endothelial cells of the lymphatic vessels cannot be distinguished in either of these micrographs partly because of the low magnification and the silver stain, which reveals little cellular detail. The endothelial cells lining the lymphatic capillaries in Figure 7-6B (H&E stain in a higher magnification micrograph) are readily identifiable.

additional layers are thinner, more irregular, and less clearly demarcated than blood vessels of similar caliber. The tunica intima of these lymphatic vessels has many long, thin valves—more than are found in veins. Even these larger lymphatics are quite small; the largest lymphatic vessel is the *thoracic duct* and is about 4 to 6 mm in diameter.

●●● BLOOD AND BLOOD FORMATION

Blood

Blood is a highly specialized and atypical fluid connective tissue; it is pumped around the body by the heart via the system of blood vessels. It consists of *formed elements*, erythrocytes (RBCs) and leukocytes (WBCs), suspended in a protein-rich fluid called plasma. In the adult, all erythrocytes and nearly all leukocytes develop in the bone marrow (see later in the chapter). The formed elements of blood make up about 45% of its volume; about 1% of the formed elements is WBCs. The remaining 55% consists of plasma.

The numbers of RBCs and WBCs in a cubic millimeter (μL) of blood from a normal, healthy individual are given in Table 7-3. Leukocytes are classified into three main groups based largely on their morphology and less on their composition and biochemistry.

Since mature erythrocytes lack a nucleus (they extrude it late in their differentiation) and platelets are cell fragments (which are shed from their precursor cell in the bone marrow directly into the blood), some authors decline to regard these two components of blood as "cells." This is an overly narrow distinction, and they are referred to as cells in this text.

The blood cells seen in sectioned specimens are in the lumina of arteries and veins (more commonly in arteries) and are usually packed or clustered closely together, making it difficult to discern the different types of cells as well as any of their specific characteristics. Furthermore, the most widely used stain, hematoxylin and eosin, reveals few differences among the different WBCs. Consequently, the most useful way to study blood cells is to place a drop of fresh blood on a slide and use the edge of a second slide to spread (smear) the drop across nearly the entire surface of the slide. Furthermore, two special stains are used to stain the cells—Wright's stain or Giemsa's stain—which are mixtures of several acidic and basic dyes. Each of these stain WBCs in a predictable and characteristic manner, permitting their differentiation and identification with considerable accuracy.

Plasma

The fluid compartment of blood is a protein-rich solution of many proteins and other solutes. The majority of the proteins are synthesized and released by hepatocytes and antibody-producing lymphocytes. Table 7-4 is a list of the major solutes in the plasma.

TABLE 7-3. Formed Elements of Blood

Formed Element	Cells/μL	Percent (of All) Leukocytes
Erythrocyte	$4.3-5.7 \times 10^6$ (males)	—
	$3.9-5.0 \times 10^6$ (females)	
Leukocyte	$3.5-10.5 \times 10^3$	100
Agranulocyte		30–35
Lymphocyte	$0.9-2.9 \times 10^3$	25–28
Monocyte	$0.3-0.9 \times 10^3$	5–8
Granulocyte		65–70
Neutrophil	$1.7-7.0 \times 10^3$	50–67
Eosinophil	$0.05-0.5 \times 10^3$	1.5–5
Basophil	$0-0.03 \times 10^3$	0–0.3
Platelets	$150-450 \times 10^3$	—

TABLE 7-4. Blood Plasma Composition

Component	Percentage (%)
Water	91–92
Proteins	6.5–8.0
Albumin	60 (of protein)
Globulins	35–38 (of protein)
Others—e.g., clotting factors	2–3 (of protein)
Hormones and other ligands	0.1–0.2
Nutrients and waste materials (glucose, urea, amino acids, catabolic products, vitamins)	1–2

Blood Cells

Erythrocytes

The living, undehydrated erythrocyte is 8.6 μm in diameter, 7.6 μm in blood smears, and about 5.0 to 6.0 μm in sectioned tissue. The protein content of the RBC is nearly all hemoglobin (ca. 95% of the dry weight), the pigmented protein that binds oxygen upon its passage through lung capillaries, delivers it to the body, and then carries carbon dioxide back to the lungs for elimination in the expired air. The RBC is a biconcave disk, a shape that is a nearly perfect geometric compromise between a sphere (the ideal shape for minimizing surface area of a given volume) and a disk (the ideal shape for maximizing surface area of a given volume). Thus, the RBC is highly adapted to transport gases (O_2 and CO_2) to and from the tissues and organs of the body. The shape of the RBC is maintained by a group of specialized integral and internal peripheral proteins of its plasma membrane. The cell is highly elastic, permitting it to squeeze through capillaries whose caliber is smaller than that of the RBC itself.

Leukocytes

There are three groups of WBCs, two of which are nucleated: *agranulocytes* (or *nongranulocytes*) and *granulocytes*. The third group is the platelet, a cell fragment of a large precursor cell in the bone marrow, the megakaryocyte (see Platelet Development [Thrombopoiesis]). WBCs are named on the basis of their appearance in blood smears stained with Wright's (or Giemsa's) stain. The criteria used to classify them arc size of the cell, shape of the nucleus, presence or absence of cytoplasmic granules, and color of stained granules in those cells that have them.

Agranulocytes

There are two types of agranulocytes in the circulation: lymphocytes and monocytes.

Lymphocytes are the most abundant of the agranulocytes, about 26% to 28% of all leukocytes. Although their size range is about 8 to 12 μm, most are a bit larger than an RBC, namely, 8 to 9 μm. They are spherical (round) cells with a large heterochromatic nucleus; the nucleus usually appears to be spherical although it has a small indentation that may not be noticed in a blood smear. The nucleus is surrounded by a thin rim of homogenous cytoplasm that contains no granules although at high magnification (using an oil immersion objective), occasional small, azurophilic granules may be seen. (Azure is one of the several dyes used in Wright's stain.) These are lysosomes and are called nonspecific granules in blood cells. When lymphocytes are examined in the transmission electron microscope (TEM), few organelles are seen—a few free ribosomes, an occasional mitochondrion, and more infrequently, a small Golgi apparatus or a centrosome. Lymphocytes and their precursors proliferate in the bone marrow, lymph nodes, and thymus gland.

There are three functional kinds of lymphocytes in the circulation—B lymphocytes (B cells), T lymphocytes (T cells), and natural killer (or cytotoxic) lymphocytes (NK cells), but they cannot be distinguished from one another on the basis of their morphology. They each have a distinctive set of cell surface molecules (CD markers) that can be labeled with fluorescent agents, permitting their ready identification. The main functions of lymphocytes occur in the lymphoid organs and other tissues and organs where they are key components of the immune system. B cells are responsible for the humoral immune response (i.e., they synthesize and secrete several types of immunoglobulins following activation, proliferation, and distribution around the body). T cells are responsible for the cell-mediated immune response. NK cells are programmed during their development to destroy certain virus-infected cells and some tumor cells. However, few if any of these functions take place in the blood. The blood vascular and lymphatic circulations distribute and collect lymphocytes to and from the entire body.

Monocytes make up about 5% to 8% of all leukocytes. Their size ranges from about 9 to 18 μm in diameter. Their nuclei can be ovoid to U-shaped and usually have an obvious indentation; the nucleus contains more euchromatin than a lymphocyte nucleus and therefore is lighter staining. The indented region near the nucleus is unstained in the light micrograph (LM), but upon examination in the TEM, this region is seen to contain the centrosome and Golgi apparatus. Mitochondria, rough and smooth endoplasmic reticulum, and other organelles are also commonly seen. The monocyte has many electron-dense lysosomes, which can also be recognized at high magnification in the LM as azurophilic (nonspecific) granules. Monocytes proliferate in the bone marrow.

Monocytes have long been known to be the precursors of connective tissue macrophages as well as other phagocytic cells in other organs. In this regard, they are described as members of the *mononuclear phagocytic system*. Other members of this system include lung alveolar macrophages,

IMMUNOLOGY

Leukocyte Diapedesis

Most leukocytes in the circulation may enter tissue spaces following specific signaling events, which usually are triggered by injury or inflammation. The process of the selective entry of activated leukocytes into tissue space is called leukocyte homing and is mediated by a number of adhesion molecules and their ligands. The adhesion molecules are expressed by leukocytes, endothelial cells, and some of the tissues underlying the endothelium.

The three main families of adhesion molecules expressed by the leukocytes are called homing receptors: selectins, integrins, and molecules in the superfamily of immunoglobulins. These molecules are distinct from antigen receptors. The ligands for these molecules, expressed on the surface of endothelial cells, are called addressins.

Chemokines are the signals that stimulate the adhesion events. The chemokines are synthesized by the endothelial cells or the underlying tissue cells. Those produced by the endothelial cells are stored in distinctive granules, the Weibel-Palade granules. Those from underlying cells cross the endothelial cell and bind to its luminal surface.

The majority of leukocytes that exhibit leukocyte homing, primarily polymorphonuclear leukocytes and T lymphocytes, and that leave the circulation do so in postcapillary venules. Once the process is initiated, it may be described as occurring in four steps:

- The leukocytes become loosely tethered to the endothelium and roll on the endothelial cell surface, events mediated by E-selectins.
- The chemokines then trigger the leukocytes to engage in the next step.
- The leukocytes then latch onto the luminal surface of the endothelial cells, a process that involves specific integrins.
- Lastly, the leukocytes migrate across the endothelial cell wall (diapedesis), not through the tight junctions it forms with adjacent endothelial cells but through large pores that open in the endothelial cell wall.

perisinusoidal macrophages of the liver (Küpffer cells), and macrophages of lymph nodes, the spleen, and bone marrow. Monocytes are also precursors of osteoclasts, the multinucleated cells responsible for bone resorption and degradation. The osteoclast arises near bone surfaces by the fusion of 5 to as many as 20 monocytes. On the basis of cell kinetic studies, monocytes remain in the blood only for about 3 days.

Recent evidence suggests that a small population of monocytes remains in the blood for very long periods of time and furthermore that these cells are stem cells. It is widely accepted that there are hemopoietic stem cells in the circulation. It is likely there are also stem cells for other tissues and organs in the circulation, but it has been difficult to demonstrate what they may be precursors to and whether they are truly capable of restoring damaged tissues or repopulating functional cells in an organ.

Granulocytes

There are three types of granulocytes in the circulation: polymorphonuclear neutrophils (neutrophils, PMNs), eosinophils, and basophils. Each of the three types has distinctive staining characteristics in the LM in terms of nuclear shape and the number, color, and nature of their cytoplasmic granules. When the granulocytes are studied in the TEM certain common features as well as several distinctive features are noted. Although nuclear shape differs among the three types of granulocytes, the nuclear envelope of each type has a "generous lining" of heterochromatin and central areas of euchromatin. Their ultrastructure, often combined with histochemical techniques, shows that each granulocyte type has a *type-specific granule* and *lysosomes*, which correspond to the azurophilic granules in the LM.

Neutrophils

As shown in Table 7-3, neutrophils are not only the most abundant of the granulocytes, they are also the most abundant leukocyte. They are larger than an RBC with a diameter of 12 to 15 µm. They have many small, pale granules in their cytoplasm and a distinctive, multilobed nucleus. The nucleus may have three to five lobes, which are interconnected by thin strands of chromatin; based on observations of living neutrophils, the number of lobes and their orientation in the cell are dynamic. They leave the circulation in great numbers daily, most commonly inhabiting loose connective tissue. Living cells are motile, actively moving about like amebae. Their life in the circulation is short—8 to 12 hours; once in connective tissue, they live for a week or less. Because of their relatively large numbers (among the leukocytes) and their short life span, they are replaced daily by the bone marrow. Indeed, a significant fraction (ca. 33%) of the bone marrow is devoted to the production of neutrophils.

Neutrophils are important members of the innate immune system, and as such, they play a central role in the inflammatory response. Their primary function is phagocytosis and degradation of bacteria and other foreign materials. The degradation products often are further processed by lymphoid organs and the lymphocytes that inhabit them; these steps may lead to the synthesis and secretion of antibodies by B cells and initiation of the cellular immune response by programmed T cells.

In the TEM, the cytoplasm of neutrophils is filled with many small granules (all of which are variants of lysosomes), a small Golgi apparatus, and relatively few other organelles. The granules are classified into three types: specific (secondary) granules, azurophilic (primary) granules, and tertiary (tertiary) granules. All three types contain granule-specific groups of enzymes. The specific granules are the most abundant, outnumbering azurophilic granules by about two to one. As is the case for other leukocytes, azurophilic granules are typical of lysosomes in other cells.

Eosinophils

It is relatively easy to find and identify eosinophils in blood smears because of their abundance, but especially because of their distinctive staining characteristics and morphology. Eosinophils are about 10 to 15 µm in diameter and have a bilobed nucleus and a cytoplasm filled with bright red, refractile eosinophilic granules. Examination of eosinophils in the TEM reveals an explanation of the refractile nature of the granules—they are ovoid and have a prominent rectangular crystalloid inclusion.

Eosinophils play a prominent role in the body's reaction to parasitic infections. Their numbers in the circulation and in loose connective tissues increase significantly in individuals infected with protozoans and helminthic parasites. The contents of the eosinophil-specific granules (Table 7-5) have strong cytotoxic effects on parasites. They also have a general role in the innate immune response and the allergic response. They populate the loose connective tissues that lie under the epithelial cells of the gut and upper respiratory tree.

Basophils

Basophils are the least numerous of the leukocytes and can be difficult to find in a blood smear. They are about 8 to 14 µm in diameter. Their cytoplasm is filled with intensely blue-staining granules; the granules are so numerous as to nearly obscure the nucleus. Basophils arise from the same hemopoietic cell lineage as mast cells (see Chapter 4), but they are distinct cells. Basophils leave the circulation and enter connective tissue following appropriate stimuli.

Like eosinophils they have an important role in the allergic response. Both of these granulocytes have cell surface receptors (F$_c$ receptors) for one of the immunoglobulins, IgE. When the IgE molecules bind to the granulocyte plasma membrane, they cause it to degranulate, releasing enzymes and other bioactive molecules that help modulate the vasodilation characteristic of an allergic response or anaphylactic shock.

Figure 7-17 shows a set of LMs of all the leukocytes. Figure 7-18 shows TEMs and a drawing of each of the leukocytes.

Platelets

Platelets (*thrombocytes*) are small (ca. 2 to 3 µm), ovoid disks that play a key role in blood clotting and hemostasis. Platelets

Table 7-5. Contents of Granulocyte Granules

Type of Granulocyte Granule	Content
Neutrophil	
Specific granules	Phospholipase A$_2$ Myeloperoxidase Cationic proteins Acid hydrolases Elastase Cathepsins
Azurophilic granules	Phospholipase A$_2$ Lysozyme Alkaline phosphatase Type IV collagenase Lactoferrin Vitamin B$_{12}$–binding proteins
Tertiary granules	Metalloproteinases (e.g., gelatinase and cathepsins)
Eosinophil	
Specific granules	Crystalloid contents: major basic protein, eosinophil cationic protein, eosinophil peroxidase, and eosinophil-derived neurotoxin Histaminase Arylsulfatase Collagenase Cathepsins
Azurophilic granules	Acid hydrolases Collagenase Other eosinophil-specific hydrolases
Basophil	
Specific granules	Preformed mediators of the inflammatory response including histamine, heparan sulfate, and chondroitin sulfate Synthesis of leukotriene and other mediators upon stimulation
Azurophilic granules	Acid hydrolases

The *structural* or *cytoskeletal region*. The discoid shape of the circulating platelet is maintained by a circumferential ring of microtubule bundles (the bundles contain from 10 to 25 microtubules). Also found in this region are many actin filaments and myosin II filaments. These proteins play a critical role in the shape changes that occur when platelets are activated to form a clot.

The *organelle* region. The bulk of the central region of the platelet is filled with many organelles and granules, some of which are common to most cells and a few of which are platelet specific. The common organelles are mitochondria, peroxisomes, and glycogen granules. There are three types of granules that are specific to platelets. The most numerous and largest are α-granules, which contain many proteins including coagulation factors, fibrinogen, PDGF, and others. Next are the less numerous and smaller δ-granules, which contain agents that facilitate cell adhesion and vasoconstriction. The third type are the λ-granules, which are platelet lysosomes.

The *canalicular* and *tubular membrane* region. The open canalicular membrane system is a remnant of the plasma membrane invaginations in the megakaryocyte that facilitated platelet shedding. Parts of this membrane system connect with the platelet plasma membrane. The tubular membrane system does not connect with the platelet plasma membrane but occasionally may fuse with the open canalicular membrane system. The tubular membrane system is derived from the endoplasmic reticulum of the megakaryocyte, and its major function in the platelet is to store calcium ions.

When platelets are activated to initiate a clot (the primary hemostatic platelet plug), they undergo a dramatic change in shape to become flattened structures with numerous pseudopodia. The activated platelets adhere to the injured endothelial plasma membrane and to each other. They release the contents of α- and δ-granules, leading to vasoconstriction and formation of a secondary platelet plug (or definitive clot). The actomyosin system in platelets is responsible for clot retraction. Other bioactive compounds released by activated platelets facilitate further steps that result in healing of the injured vessel and surrounding tissue. One important factor in tissue healing is PDGF, mentioned earlier in regard to pericyte differentiation.

Blood Cell Formation

are highly structured cytoplasmic fragments of a large polyploid cell in the bone marrow, the megakaryocyte (see Platelet Development [Thrombopoiesis]). They are shed into the sinusoidal capillaries of bone marrow in long, "beaded strands"; the "beads" separate into individual platelets while still in the sinusoidal capillaries. The platelet has four characteristic structural regions:

The *plasma membrane* or *peripheral region*. This region consists of the plasma membrane, which has many external associated glycoproteins and glycosaminoglycans, giving the platelet a thick glycocalyx. These carbohydrate-rich macromolecules are critical to the initial phases of platelet adhesion to endothelial cells at the site of vascular damage.

In the adult, RBCs and WBCs are formed in the red bone marrow. During embryonic life, they form in the yolk sac, and during fetal life the major site is in the liver (with a lesser contribution from the spleen). The process is called hemopoiesis or hematopoiesis; these terms collectively refer to the proliferation and differentiation of all the formed elements of blood—erythrocytes and leukocytes. Much of the bone marrow in the adult does not contain hematopoietic tissue; instead the marrow cavity is filled with adipose tissue and is called white bone marrow. It is common to refer to red cell development as erythropoiesis, white cell development as leukopoiesis, and platelet development as thrombopoiesis. Two other terms are also used to refer to red cell and white

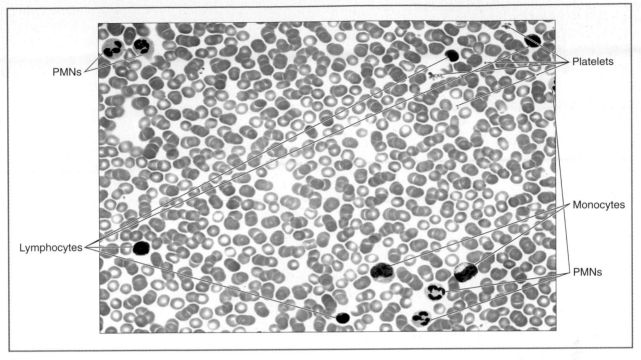

A

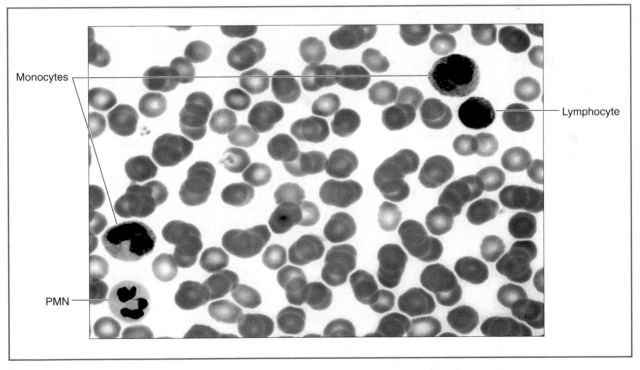

B

Figure 7-17. Light micrographs of blood smears stained with Wright's or Giemsa's stain. **A,** Medium-power field (320×) of a blood smear showing many erythrocytes and four types of leukocytes: polymorphonuclear (PMN) leukocytes, monocytes, lymphocytes, and platelets. **B,** Higher magnification field (640×) containing two monocytes, a PMN, and a lymphocyte. Somewhat more detail can be seen in these four leukocytes than in the lower magnification field.

Continued

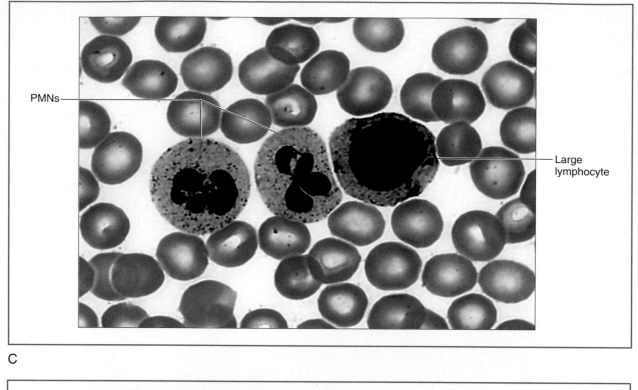

PMNs

Large lymphocyte

C

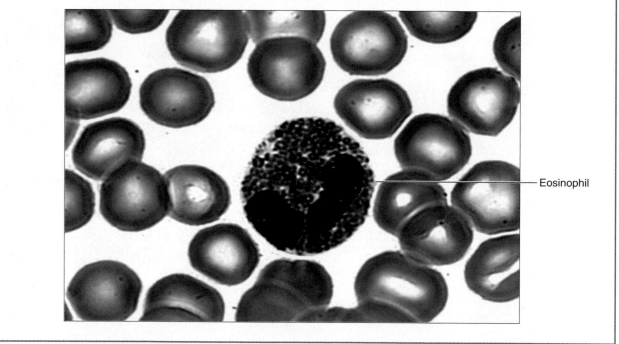

Eosinophil

D

Figure 7-17 cont'd. C, Two PMNs and a large lymphocyte (1250×). Azurophilic granules can be seen in both cell types. There are a large number of unstained (neutrophilic) granules in the cytoplasm of the PMNs. **D,** An eosinophil showing its characteristic bilobed nucleus and the bright red granules that fill the cytoplasm of this cell type (1600×).

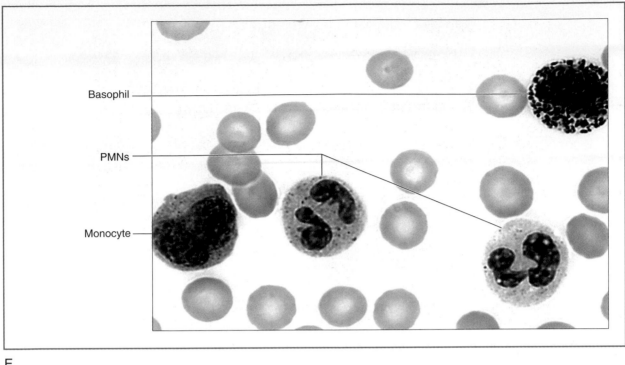

Basophil

PMNs

Monocyte

E

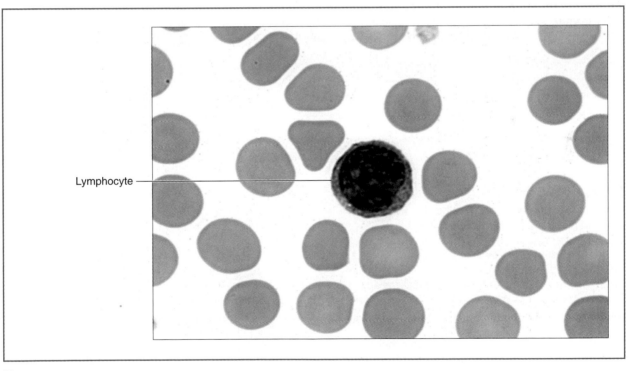

Lymphocyte

F

Figure 7-17 cont'd. E, Four leukocytes: a basophil, two PMNs, and a monocyte (1700×). All four cells show the characteristic nuclear and cytoplasmic features of each type. The basophil is slightly less filled with granules than is typical, allowing the nucleus to be seen even though little sense of nuclear shape can be ascertained. **F,** Small lymphocyte. The typical large, nearly spherical nucleus with a thin cytoplasmic rim is readily seen (1400×). Compare the appearance of this lymphocyte with those in part A to appreciate the higher resolution of an oil immersion micrograph. *Continued*

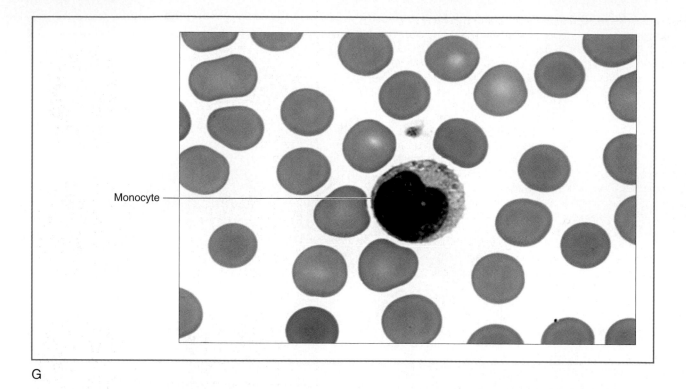

G

Figure 7-17 cont'd. G, Monocyte in its most "typical" appearance—a large indented nucleus with a lighter staining region (the Golgi apparatus) near the indentation and only the faintest suggestion of cytoplasmic granules (1400×).

BIOCHEMISTRY

Hemostasis

Hemostasis refers to the normal mechanisms that maintain blood in one of two states: a freely flowing (clot-free) fluid state, or rapid production of a localized clot at the site of vascular injury or activation. Each of these states reflects sets of two highly regulated processes. In pathologic terms, the opposite of hemostasis is thrombus formation—formation of clots that do not function to control bleeding (e.g., at an atherosclerotic site) or to excess such that tissue or organ function is compromised.

Normal hemostatic clotting has four stages:

- Vasoconstriction, a transient neurogenic event that also involves release of endothelin by nearby endothelial cells.
- Platelet adhesion to exposed collagen, activation, and granule release. A strong mediator of this process is von Willebrand factor, a constitutive glycoprotein product of normal endothelial cells stored in Weibel-Palade granules. ADP and thromboxane A₂ are also released; these molecules actively contribute to the next step. The immediate consequence of these events is formation of the primary hemostatic plug.
- Local activation of the blood clotting cascade, which results in fibrin polymerization and expansion of the clot to form the secondary (or definitive) hemostatic plug. More platelets

become activated (they secrete their granular contents and change shape) and adhere to the growing clot and contract. The clotting cascade is a highly regulated, multistep process involving many proteins (about 13), cofactors (e.g., Ca^{++}, phospholipids), and proteolytic events (about nine). A major step toward the end of the cascade is thrombin activation, which catalyzes the conversion of fibrinogen to fibrin, which in turn polymerizes and stabilizes the clot.

- Clot limitation and ultimate dissolution. These events occur after neutrophils and red cells become entrapped near the surface of the definitive plug. The endothelial cell secretes *tissue-type plasminogen activator* (t-PA) which begins to dissolve the fibrin polymers. Heparin-like proteoglycans on the endothelial cell surface help limit further expansion of the clot. Endothelial cells release thrombomodulin, which binds to thrombin, converting it from a procoagulant to an anticoagulant form. The entrapped neutrophils contribute to clot dissolution by further degrading fibrin polymer fragments.

Thus, the endothelial cell is seen to have both *anticoagulant* and *procoagulant* properties and functions.

Figure 7-18. Electron micrographs and diagrammatic drawings of the leukocytes. **A,** PMN in which the polymorphic nuclear shape and many cytoplasmic granules are seen. **B,** Eosinophil showing its characteristic bilobed nucleus and large, crystalloid-containing cytoplasmic granules. **C,** Basophil. The granules and bilobed nucleus are seen to greater advantage in the EM compared with the LM. **D,** Monocyte showing its many cytoplasmic details (e.g., the indented nucleus and associated Golgi apparatus, the centrosome and one of the centrioles, numerous profiles of rER and sER, lysosomes, and peroxisomes). (Courtesy of Patricia Cross, Stanford University School of Medicine.) **E,** Small lymphocyte. Note the round nucleus and relatively uncomplicated cytoplasm of this cell compared with the other leukocytes. **F,** Composite micrograph of two platelets in two planes of section. A peripheral bundle of microtubules can be seen in both section planes. Many dense granules, some profiles of the platelet canalicular system, and a cluster of glycogen granules are also visible. (EMs for parts A, B, C, and E from Kierszenbaum A. *Histology and Cell Biology.* Philadelphia, Mosby, 2002, pp 150–153. EM for part F from Pollard TD, Earnshaw WC. *Cell Biology.* Philadelphia, WB Saunders, 2002, p 483.)

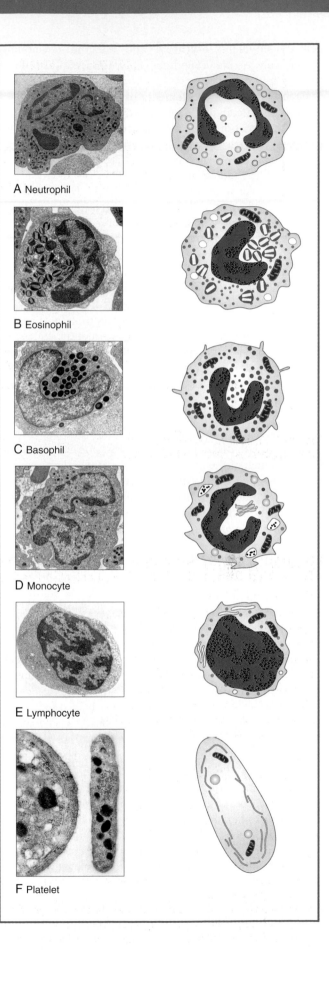

A Neutrophil

B Eosinophil

C Basophil

D Monocyte

E Lymphocyte

F Platelet

cell development, erythroid and myeloid development, respectively. As mentioned above, lymphocytes also develop in lymphoid organs.

Each of the formed elements of blood has a specific life span in the circulation, a cell-specific lineage of proliferation and differentiation, and a characteristic length of time to progress from each stem cell precursor to the mature form of the cell that enters the circulation. Table 7-6 lists the blood cells and the lifetime of mature cells in the blood and how long they take to mature in the marrow. Different sources may give different cell lifetimes and different maturation times in the marrow, so the student should recognize that the absolute number of days given in Table 7-6 is less important than the relative lifetimes of each cell type.

Each blood cell type is replenished in large numbers daily to maintain a steady state level of each cell in the circulation within the "normal" range. The general scheme of hemopoiesis is mediated by a group of glycoprotein factors that bind to cell lineage–specific surface receptors, followed by several rounds of proliferation and a distinctive series of cytodifferentiation events that results in the mature (or nearly mature) cell leaving the marrow compartment and entering the circulation.

The formed elements pass through the walls of the continuous sinusoidal capillaries of the bone marrow by a process called diapedesis. There was considerable debate through much of the 20th century about whether each blood cell developed from its own stem cell precursor (the *polyphyletic* theory of hemopoiesis) or whether there was a single stem cell that could give rise to all the formed elements of blood (the *uniphyletic* theory of hemopoiesis). Many lines of experimental evidence have demonstrated that the uniphyletic theory is correct. A single cell gives rise to all the blood cells; it is called the pluripotent stem cell (PPSC). It is useful to bear in mind that stem cells are a self-renewing population of cells that divide rarely throughout life. When they do divide, one of the two sibling cells retains its properties as a stem cell and the other continues to divide, differentiate, and ultimately gives rise to one of the mature cells in the circulation. These cells can be isolated from bone marrow or even from circulating blood.

The experimental approach that has been used to study and identify hemopoietic stem cells is based on the ability of donor (potential) stem cells to proliferate in the spleens of specially treated (irradiated) mice or a special strain of recipient mice (an immunotolerant strain called the nude mouse). In more recent years it has been possible to grow most hemopoietic stem cells in tissue culture. In either case, as a cell proliferates it gives rise to colonies of individual mature blood cells or groups of blood cells (e.g., erythrocytes and neutrophils, or neutrophils and monocytes, or granulocytes and megakaryocytes). These studies have led to such cells being named colony-forming units (CFUs). After further cloning of such splenic or tissue culture colonies, a lineage of hemopoietic stem cells has been defined.

The techniques used to grow mouse (or chicken) hemopoietic CFUs in tissue culture have been adapted to the study

TABLE 7-6. Blood Cells and Developmental Kinetics

Cell	Time to Maturation in Bone Marrow	Lifetime in Circulation	Lifetime in Tissue
Erythrocyte	7–8 days	120 days	—
Lymphocyte (B cell)		Days	Variable, days to years (as plasma cells)
Lymphocyte (T cell)		Days to decades	Weeks to decades
Monocyte	2–3 days	Most—16 hours, some —years	Variable duration; present as members of the mononuclear phagocytic system
Neutrophil	Ca. 2 weeks	6–8 hours	1 to 2 days
Eosinophil	Ca. 2 weeks	8–12 hours	A few days?
Basophil	Ca. 2 weeks	9–18 months (in mice)	?
Platelet	Ca. 5 days	10 days	—

of human hemopoietic CFUs as well. These studies may result in significant therapeutic benefits by providing a source of lineage-specific hemopoietic stem cells. A current understanding of hemopoiesis lineage is presented in Figure 7-19.

Each cell lineage is under the control its own set of glycoprotein growth factors (cytokines). About a dozen of the cytokines belong to a group called interleukins; many of the interleukins are produced by lymphocytes, but some are made by endothelial cells, stromal cells in the bone marrow, fibroblasts, or end-product cells in the myeloid lineage. Except in a few cases, the growth factors act on more than a single cell and often on more than one cell line.

Erythropoiesis is regulated by erythropoietin, a glycoprotein synthesized and secreted by interstitial cells (fibroblasts) in the cortex of the kidney. Erythropoietin acts on the erythroid stem cell, CFU-E and its precursor, the granulocyte-erythroid-monocyte-megakaryocyte (CFU-GEMM) multipotential stem cell, as well as the subsequent dividing cells in the erythroid line.

Myeloid cell development is regulated by several growth factors: granulocyte-macrophage colony-stimulating factor (GM-CSF), granulocyte colony-stimulating factor (G-CSF), and several of the interleukins. GM-CSF acts on CFU-GEMM and cells downstream of it in the granulocyte and monocyte lines. G-CSF acts on CFU-E, CFU-GM, eosinophil (CFU-Eo), basophil (CFU-Ba), and megakaryocyte (CFU-Meg).

Thrombopoiesis is regulated by *thrombopoietin*, a glycoprotein synthesized in the bone marrow. It stimulates the CFU-Meg stem cell to undergo endomitosis (karyokinesis

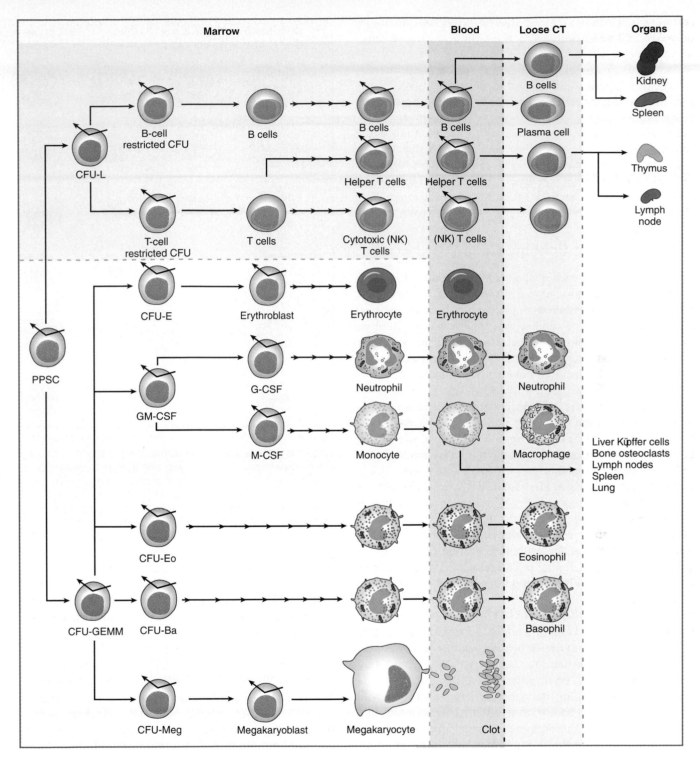

Figure 7-19. This chart presents a schematic view of the development of all the formed elements of blood. The vertical columns are grouped into four compartments: the bone marrow, the circulation, a loose connective tissue compartment, and the final tissue or organ destination of the fully differentiated cells, if that is their ultimate disposition. The upper one third of the marrow compartment shows lymphopoiesis (B- and T-cell development); the lower two thirds of the marrow compartment shows erythroid and the rest of myeloid development. From the perspective the cells depicted, all four compartments are separated from one another by capillary endothelial cells. Stem cells are represented on the left part of the diagram; their capacity to divide and reproduce the stem cells are indicated by bent arrows pointing to the left.

without cytokinesis), a process that results in a 30- to 50-μm polyploid cell and continues to affect the mature megakaryocyte.

The development of B cells occurs in the bone marrow, spleen, lymph nodes, and mucosa-associated lymphoid tissue (see Chapter 8). B-cell development is largely influenced by specific interleukins.

T cells develop in the bone marrow and populate the thymus gland early in life. They proliferate in the thymus, enter the circulation, and remain there for decades; they also populate the T cell–rich regions of lymph nodes. Like B cells, their proliferation and development are regulated by interleukins.

Development of Specific Cells

The development of each of the formed elements of blood is described by a number of cell divisions and a continuous series of cell differentiation steps. The first one or two cell divisions in each of the cell lineages are "stem cell" divisions (i.e., one of the two siblings remains a stem cell and the other initiates and continues its progress toward becoming one of the mature blood cells). Red bone marrow may be studied in sectioned material or by removing a small specimen of marrow (via a needle biopsy) and preparing a smear; in either case, the same two stains are used for marrow as for blood smears—Wright's or Giemsa's. The task of identifying individual cell lines and the sequential cells developing in each line can be difficult, even for experts.

When the number and life-time of RBCs and WBCs in the circulation are factored together with the amount of time it takes for each lineage to develop in the bone marrow, the observed distribution of developing red and white cells in red bone marrow is better understood. Erythroid cells are about one-third of the developing cells, neutrophils another third, and the remaining WBCs the remaining third.

Erythrocyte Development (Erythropoiesis)

Once a CFU-E has been stimulated by erythropoietin and other growth factors to divide further, a series of cells can be found in the marrow that are characteristic of the erythroid line. The developing erythrocyte is a cellular factory that synthesizes hemoglobin; its cytoplasm becomes filled with free polyribosomes, hemoglobin mRNA, hemoglobin, and relatively little else. The erythroid cell undergoes a series of changes that are summarized schematically in Figure 7-20. This figure shows six characteristic cells in the erythroid line: *erythroblast, basophilic erythroblast, polychromatophilic erythroblast, orthochromatophilic erythroblast, orthochromatophilic erythrocyte* (reticulocyte), and the *erythrocyte*. The primary size, cytoplasmic, and nuclear changes are shown. The cell becomes progressively smaller. Initially the cytoplasm has a pronounced azure color (due to high ribosomal RNA and mRNA content), which gradually changes to the typical orange-red color of the erythrocyte (due to the increasing hemoglobin content). The chromatin becomes more and more condensed, and the nucleus gets smaller and

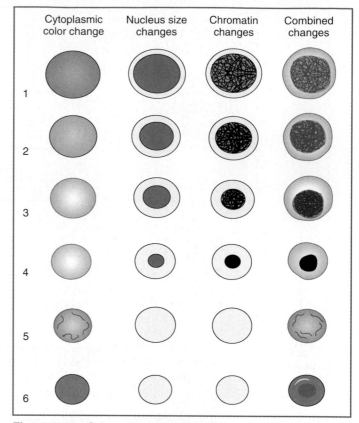

Figure 7-20. Schematic of steps in the erythroid line. Three sets of erythroid-specific parameters highlighted in this figure are cytoplasmic color changes, changes in nuclear size and staining intensity, and changes in chromatin pattern. An accurate composite set of drawings of the actual erythroid cells is shown at right. Mitotic divisions may take place at any of the stages with a nucleated cell (1–4).

smaller until it becomes pyknotic and is extruded from the cell between stages 4 and 5. Many of these changes are also seen and named in the series of electron micrographs in Figure 7-21.

Granulocyte Development (Granulopoiesis)

The three types of granulocytes share a few common stem cell CFUs during development but soon branch into the individual granulocyte (CFU-G, CFU-Eo, and CFU-Ba) lineages. The terminology for the cells in all three lineages is similar. Since the neutrophils are the most numerous of the granulocytes in the marrow and the circulation, their development is best understood. Cells in this line are the *myeloblast, promyelocyte, neutrophilic myelocyte, neutrophilic metamyelocyte, band* (or "*stab*") *neutrophil,* and *neutrophil.* The developing eosinophils and basophils are named similarly but prefaced by eosinophilic or basophilic. There are substantial changes in the appearance of the cytoplasm owing to the acquisition of the lineage-specific granules as well as to the shape and size of the nucleus that is characteristic of each mature granulocyte.

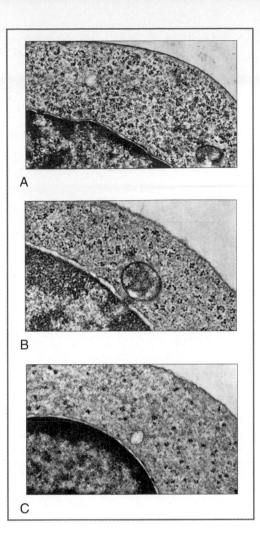

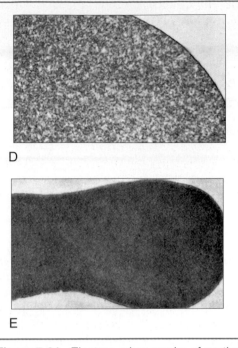

Figure 7-21. Electron micrographs of portions of cells in the erythroid line. The most striking changes are the decreasing numbers of ribosomes from the top to the bottom and the increasing hemoglobin content. **A,** Basophilic erythroblast. **B,** Polychromatophilic erythroblast. **C,** Orthochromatophilic erythroblast. **D,** Reticulocyte. **E,** Erythrocyte. (From Fawcett DW. *Bloom and Fawcett: A Textbook of Histology*, 11th ed. Philadelphia, WB Saunders, 1986.)

Monocyte Development (Monocytopoiesis)

Monocytes develop from a CFU-GM progenitor under the influence of a monocyte-colony stimulating factor (M-CSF) and of several of the interleukins. Individual intermediate-stage cells are not recognizable; the mature monocyte in the bone marrow is about 20 μm in diameter. They enter the bloodstream and end up in their target locations, where they develop into one of the many further differentiated cells they are capable of becoming, a major one of which is the macrophage.

Platelet Development (Thrombopoiesis)

The cellular progenitor of platelets is the megakaryocyte, the largest cell in the bone marrow, ca. 60 μm or greater in diameter. The megakaryocyte is derived from the CFU-GEMM, which gives rise to a CFU-Meg under the influence of thrombopoietin and other cytokines. The DNA in the nucleus of the CFU-Meg undergoes two to six rounds of replication, but the cell does not undergo cytokinesis, a process called *endomitosis*. As a result the megakaryocyte has a multilobulated nucleus with a DNA content of 4–32 N. In specimens of bone marrow, the megakaryocyte and the osteoclast may be confused, but the megakaryocyte has a *multilobulated* nucleus and the osteoclast is *multinucleated*.

Lymphocyte Development (Lymphopoiesis)

Lymphocytes develop from a CFU-L multipotent stem cell; this cell is derived from the PPSC. The CFU-L is the progenitor for B lymphocytes, T lymphocytes, and NK lymphocytes. Consequently, all the lymphocytes that develop in the bone marrow develop from a CFU that is different from the CFU-GEMM, the progenitor of erythroid and other (nonlymphocyte) myeloid cells. As is the case for developing monocytes, intermediate stages in the differentiation of lymphocytes are difficult to identify in the marrow. The most characteristic features of differentiating and mature lymphocytes are the large nucleus to cytoplasm ratio and the relatively unstained thin rim of cytoplasm. The expansion of functional populations of B, T, and NK lymphocytes occurs in the lymphoid organs—lymph nodes, spleen, and thymus.

Lymphoid System 8

The central function of the lymphoid system is to protect the body from pathogens. This function is accomplished by a disseminated array of molecules, cells, and organs.

Components of the lymphoid system are distributed throughout the body. They include peptides, proteins, lymphocytes, and other cells in the blood and lymph vascular system and connective tissue compartments. They may be part of the stroma and parenchyma of most organs of the body. They also include relatively unorganized or highly organized accumulations of lymphoid cells, as well as the solid lymphoid organs.

●●● IMMUNE SYSTEM FUNCTION

From a functional perspective, the lymphoid system is called the *immune system*. The immune system has two responses to infection: the *innate* (nonspecific) response and the *adaptive* (specific) response. Components of the innate immune response are in place prior to exposure to microbial pathogens, other antigens, or similar challenges. The cells, or their precursors, responsible for the adaptive response are also present, but they are in a preimmune functional state until challenged. Functional aspects of the immune system are beyond the scope of this book, but a familiarity with certain basic terms and their meaning is useful in understanding the structure of the lymphoid system.

Innate Response

The innate response involves physical barriers (epidermal, other epithelial surfaces, and materials secreted onto the surfaces) to the entry of pathogens and the phagocytic cells of connective tissue—macrophages, polymorphic neutrophils, as well as organ-dwelling phagocytes, those of the *phagocytic mononuclear system* (e.g., Küpffer cells of the liver, alveolar macrophages of the lung, microglia of the central nervous system). It also involves inflammatory cells of connective tissue—mast cells and eosinophils. A distinct type of lymphocyte, the natural killer (NK) cell, is also part of the innate response; it has the capacity to kill cells that have been infected with various microbes, especially viruses. The NK cell differentiates from bone marrow–derived large lymphocytes in peripheral blood.

The liver synthesizes many proteins that are part of the innate immune response. The majority of these are *complement proteins*. One of the others is C-reactive protein (CRP). CRP is an early marker of infection; its serum level may increase several thousand–fold following an infection.

The innate response is an early reaction to tissue infection; it occurs within a few hours of exposure to microbes. A defining characteristic of the innate immune response is that the cells and their responses do not change (adapt) even when presented with repeated challenges by the same stimulants or pathogens.

Adaptive Response

The adaptive response of the immune system is tailored or directed toward specific pathogens or antigens. The adaptive response is characterized by a high degree of specificity toward specific microbes and antigens, high diversity of the response, "memory" of the initial immune challenge, and the ability to distinguish "self" from "non-self" (a characteristic called *tolerance*). It takes days to weeks to be expressed, and its effects may persist for years.

Lymphocytes are the key players in the adaptive response; there are two main arms of the adaptive response—the humoral and the cell-based response. Both types involve cell division and the synthesis and expression of differentiated characteristics in the expanded cell populations. The humoral response refers to the production of many specific antibodies to antigens by B lymphocytes, which become programmed to produce the antibodies. There are five major types of immunoglobulins, several of which have a number of subtypes. Immunoglobulins are found in the serum, interstitial tissue fluid, and on epithelial surfaces.

The cell-based adaptive response involves T lymphocytes, which also become programmed to respond to specific immune challenges. There are two major functional subsets of T lymphocytes. One is the helper T lymphocyte (T_H); the other is the cytolytic or cytotoxic T lymphocyte (CTL). Furthermore, there are two types of T-helper lymphocytes: T_H1 and T_H2 cells, both of which secrete cytokines. T_H1 cells are largely involved with the humoral immune response and T_H2 cells with the cell-mediated immune response. There are many functional varieties of T cells, which can be distinguished from each other by monoclonal antibodies made to the external domains of integral membrane proteins (surface markers). The markers are called CD4+, CD8+, CD11+, etc. The CD abbreviation stands for cluster of differentiation, a terminology introduced when monoclonal antibodies were made to surface markers of human leukocytes. Each of the surface markers was recognized by a group (cluster) of monoclonal antibodies. Initially, the markers were used to study the lineage and differentiation of leukocytes, but as more monoclonal antibodies were developed to these markers, it became possible to identify the many kinds of leukocytes from each other. Currently, CD markers are used for qualitative and quantitative identification of leukocytes in research and clinical settings.

The cells and organs of the immune system communicate with each other via an elaborate system of peptide ligands and receptors. Examples of the peptide components include many cytokines, interferons, interleukins, and other cell recognition or cell-signaling molecules. The signaling molecules are typically found in connective tissue compartments or in lymphoid organs where they carry out their myriad functions. The receptors are the CD molecules, the major histocompatibility complexes (MHC I and II), and numerous others.

●●● LYMPHOID (IMMUNE) SYSTEM STRUCTURE

The structure of the lymphoid system ranges from a population of highly disseminated individual cells (e.g., lymphocytes, macrophages, antigen-presenting cells) to morphologically recognizable aggregates of cells to discrete solid organs.

Distribution of Individual and Aggregate Lymphoid Cells

Diffuse Lymphoid Tissue

The cells of the lymphoid system (lymphocytes) are derived from stem cells in the bone marrow. The lymphocytes enter the bloodstream until they leave the circulation to carry out their many functions. They are frequently seen in compartments of loose connective tissue and are particularly abundant in mucosal lamina propria. As discussed in Chapter 3, the basal lamina serves as a barrier to movement of nearly all cell types into an epithelium—except for lymphocytes.

Lymphocytes readily cross the basal lamina and are often found among epithelial cells in an epithelial sheet. Figure 8-1 shows examples of individual lymphocytes in epithelia, moderate numbers of lymphocytes in lamina propria, and accumulations of lymphocytes obliterating the lamina propria and completely surrounding adjacent epithelial tissue. Lymphocytes and macrophages in these locations are exposed to many antigens; typically they travel to lymph nodes to initiate the next steps in the immune response. This type of lymphoid tissue is called diffuse lymphoid tissue.

Lymphoid Nodules

Lymphocytes in or near mucosal surfaces may form aggregates, which show a greater degree of organization and differentiation than diffuse lymphoid tissue does. The aggregates are called lymphoid nodules and may be single nodules or accumulations of nodules; some authors refer to them as *follicles*. The nodules have a lighter staining, eccentrically placed region called a *germinal center*; the germinal center is surrounded by a denser accumulation of lymphocytes called the *mantle zone*. A germinal center contains lymphoblasts, lymphocytes, plasma cells, macrophages, and antigen-presenting cells (APCs). Lymphoid nodules are both a storage site and source of B lymphocytes. Figure 8-2 shows four examples of lymphoid nodules, three from the digestive system and one from the lung.

Tonsils

The tonsils form a ring of lymphoid tissue at the entrance to the oropharynx. There are three sets of tonsils: *pharyngeal tonsils* (known as the *adenoids* when they are diseased), *palatine tonsils*, and the *lingual tonsil*. Tonsils have two major histologic features: they are in close proximity to an external epithelium and they usually display deep epithelial invaginations called *tonsillar crypts* (and *tonsilar pleats* in the pharyngeal tonsil). Although it can be difficult to distinguish the tonsils from each other at the microscopic level, a useful identifying feature is the type of epithelium associated with the tonsillar lymphoid nodules. Pharyngeal tonsils have the pseudostratified ciliated columnar epithelium with many goblet cells characteristic of the upper respiratory tract; palatine tonsils have a thin, partially keratinized stratified squamous epithelium; and the lingual tonsil has a rather thick nonkeratinized stratified squamous epithelium and often has skeletal muscle bundles deep to the epithelium, a characteristic of the tongue. Examples of pharyngeal and lingual tonsils are seen in Figure 8-3.

None of the three types of lymphoid tissues described above have afferent lymphatic vessels, but all are either drained by efferent lymphatics or are in close proximity to lymphatic capillaries (e.g., the lacteals of intestinal villi) (Fig. 8-4).

Lymphoid Organs

Lymph Nodes

Lymph nodes are bean-shaped, solid organs of the lymphoid system. They are found as solitary nodes or in clusters

Text continued on page 242

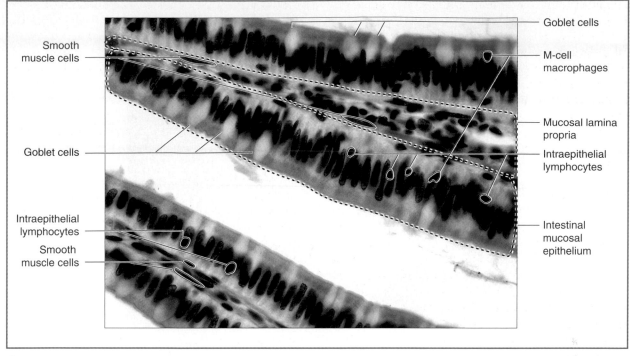

A

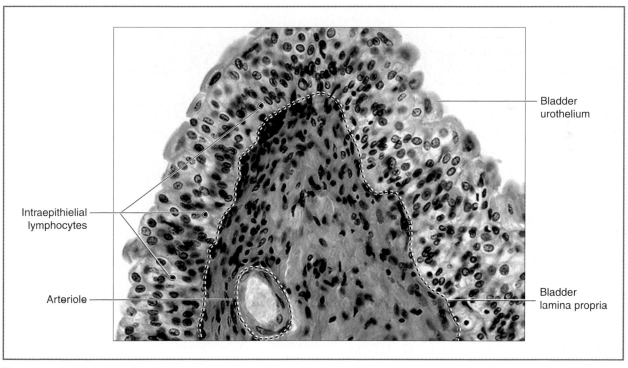

B

Figure 8-1. Micrographs illustrating the extensive presence of diffuse lymphoid tissue in mucosa. **A,** H&E-stained section of jejunal intestinal villi (400×). The simple columnar epithelium of the villi, which contain intestinal absorptive and goblet cells, demonstrate a number of individual isolated lymphocytes. One or two of the nuclei in the epithelium *may* be a specialized intraepithelial macrophage of the immune system, the M cell. It is the appearance and location of the nuclei in the epithelium that are the primary bases for identifying the specific cell types. **B,** H&E-stained section of bladder epithelium (180×) showing a number of individual lymphocytes; not all the lymphocytes are labeled.

Continued

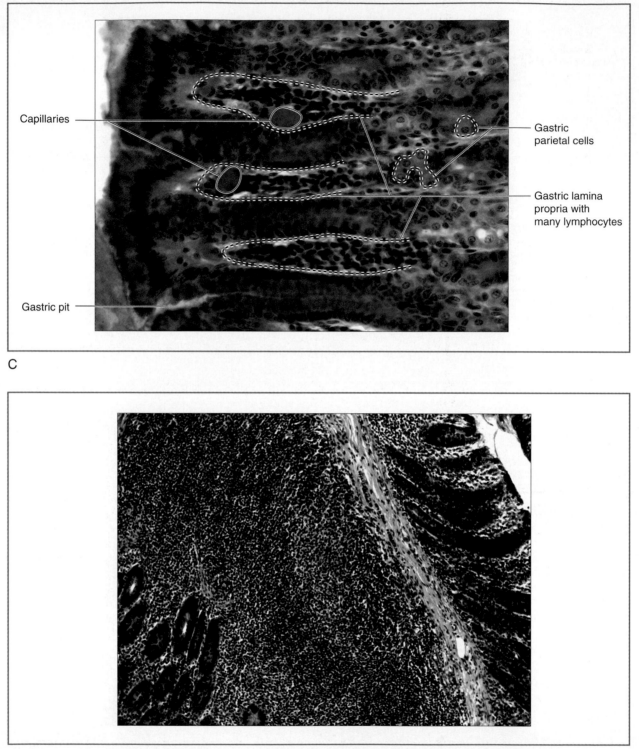

Capillaries

Gastric parietal cells

Gastric lamina propria with many lymphocytes

Gastric pit

C

D

Figure 8-1 cont'd. C, H&E-stained section of fundic stomach (250×) showing many lymphocytes in the connective tissue of the lamina propria. Most of the nuclei in the lamina propria are lymphocytes, and some are macrophages. **D,** H&E-stained section of colon (80×) showing thousands of lymphocytes in this location; the huge mass of lymphocytes in the central part of the field may be a tangential section of a lymphoid nodule (see Fig. 8-2). The lymphocytes nearly completely obscure the boundaries and cellular characteristics of the mucosa and submucosa.

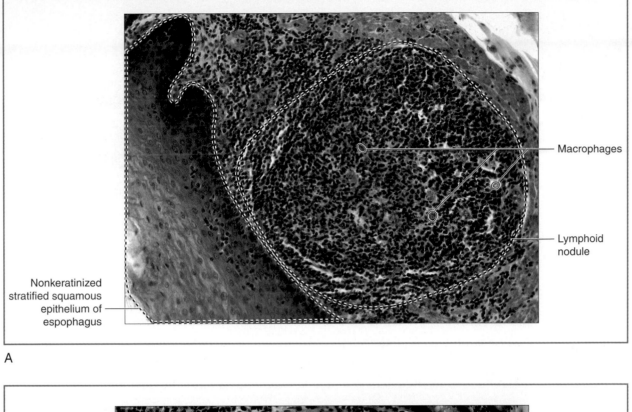

Macrophages

Lymphoid
nodule

Nonkeratinized
stratified squamous
epithelium of
espophagus

A

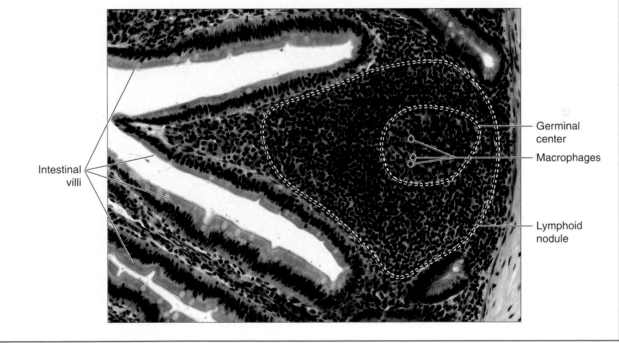

Germinal
center

Macrophages

Lymphoid
nodule

Intestinal
villi

B

Figure 8-2. Micrographs illustrating the appearance of lymphoid nodules in mucosa. **A,** H&E-stained section of esophagus (150×). The solitary lymphoid nodule in this micrograph fills the entire lamina propria. The central part of the nodule shows a germinal center, lymphoblasts, plasma cells, and several macrophages. The macrophages are relatively easy to identify, but the other cell types are identifiable primarily on the basis of their location and lighter staining. **B,** H&E-stained section of cat jejunum (160×) showing another solitary lymphoid nodule. One of the intestinal villi is distended by the nodule, which has a small germinal center with the same cell types as seen in part A. *Continued*

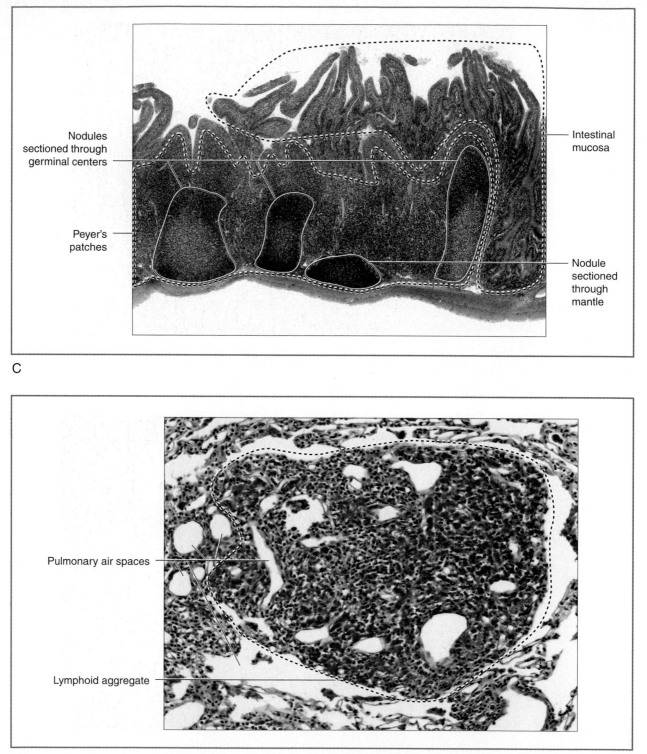

Nodules sectioned through germinal centers

Intestinal mucosa

Peyer's patches

Nodule sectioned through mantle

C

Pulmonary air spaces

Lymphoid aggregate

D

Figure 8-2 cont'd. C, H&E-stained section of ileum (20×). The ileum has a particularly massive aggregation of lymphoid nodules called Peyer's patches. They are located in a region of the ileum that is opposite the attachment of the digestive tube to the mesentery. Some of the nodules are sectioned through the mantle cells and others through germinal centers. **D,** H&E-stained section of a lung nodule with a large lymphoid aggregate (125×). The aggregate does not have the characteristics of the lymphoid nodules seen in the three preceding micrographs, but it is an aggregate of lymphoid cells interspersed among lung tissue. It has many macrophages filled with brown material seen in individuals who live in large cities or are smokers.

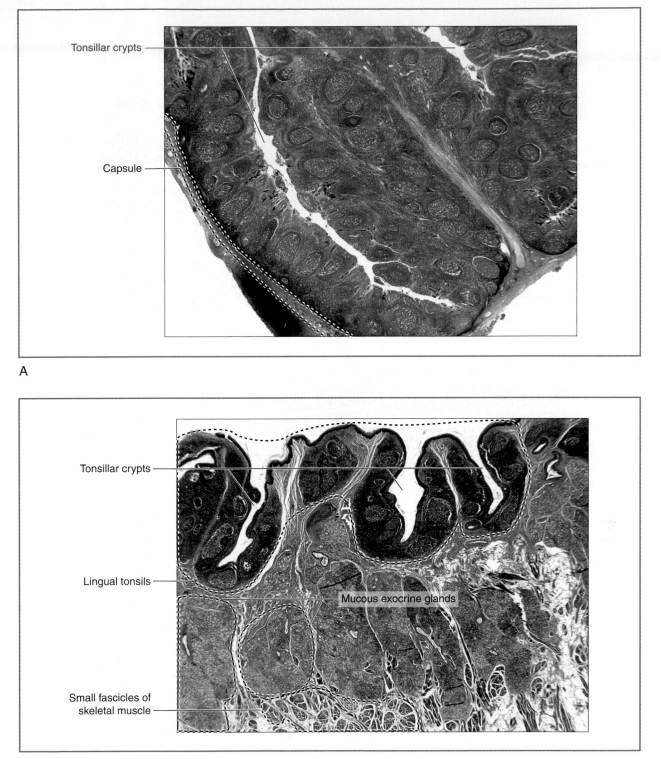

Tonsillar crypts

Capsule

A

Tonsillar crypts

Lingual tonsils

Mucous exocrine glands

Small fascicles of skeletal muscle

B

Figure 8-3. Low-magnification views of pharyngeal and lingual tonsils. Both specimens have deep tonsillar crypts and many lymphoid nodules. **A,** H&E-stained section of pharyngeal tonsils (8×); the tonsillar epithelium is not seen in this micrograph. Note the crypts and the large number of lymphoid nodules, most of which have a germinal center. **B,** H&E-stained section of lingual tonsils (8×); the tonsillar epithelium is seen in this micrograph. The region of the tongue just below the tonsils is replete with mucous exocrine glands; bundles of skeletal muscle fibers are seen below the glands.

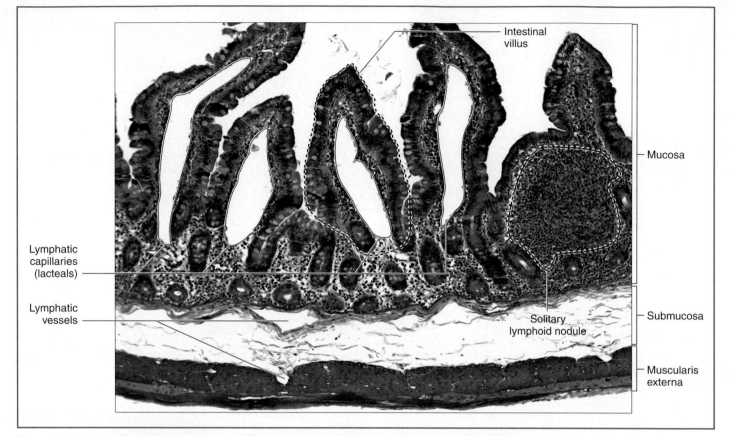

Figure 8-4. Micrograph of jejunum from a small mammal (Milligan's trichrome stain, 80×). There are several intestinal villi with dilated lacteals, a lamina propria with many lymphocytes, one villus with a solitary nodule, and a large lymphatic vessel at the boundary between the mucosa and the submucosa. It appears that this same vessel penetrates the muscularis externa. Note the goblet cells, stained pale green in this specimen; several can be seen emptying their mucous secretions into the intestinal lumen.

throughout the body and range in size from about 1 to 2 mm to 20 mm in their long dimension. As a solid organ they have a capsule with trabeculae penetrating the cortex, a cortex and medulla, parenchymal and stromal cells, and a hilum. Lymph nodes are interconnected by the extensive lymphatic vascular system of the body. Recall that lymphatic vessels are supplied with many valves to prevent backflow. In regions where many lymph nodes are found, many of the nodes are interconnected, in series, by lymphatic vessels. A diagram of a lymph node is seen in Figure 8-5; the upper half of the diagram illustrates the lymphatic circulation through the node while the lower half illustrates the blood vascular circulation of the node. The small indentation on the side of the lymph node, the hilum, is the locus of the blood supply to and from the node, the efferent lymphatics, as well as a small nerve.

Lymph is a clear or yellowish fluid that originates from the interstitial fluid of the body. It contains lymphocytes and other cells of the lymphoid system (e.g., APCs and macrophages). Lymph is delivered to the lymph nodes at the outer curvature of the cortex via many *afferent lymphatic vessels*. The lymph and its cellular contents percolate through the node via the subcapsular (cortical) sinus, along the trabecular

sinuses, around the cortical nodules, and through the deep cortex and medullary sinuses, and they exit the node at the hilum via one or two *efferent lymphatic vessels*. This flow of lymph—entering the node via cortical afferent vessels and exiting the node via efferent vessels at the hilum—is unique to lymph nodes and is an important feature of their function (Fig. 8-6). As the lymph flows through the lymph node, the lymphocytes exchange with those of the node. APCs and macrophages may take up residence in a node, thereby delivering their antigens to a major site of the adaptive immune response. The many interactions among soluble and cellular components of the lymph and the parenchyma of the lymph node are described as a kind of biochemical and cell recognition/signaling filtration of the lymph, or more concisely as immune surveillance. In addition to the filtered lymph and its cells, the lymph leaving via an efferent lymphatic has a higher antibody concentration than it did upon entering the node owing to the synthesis and secretion of antibodies by plasma cells in germinal centers.

The stroma of lymph nodes consists of *reticular fibers*, a delicate network of fine type III collagen fibers, and associated glycoproteins. The fibers stain a dark brown-black color with stains that contain Ag$^+$ (reticular stains) such as are

Figure 8-5. Diagram of a lymph node, with major structural features indicated. (Modified from Gartner LP, Hiatt JL. *Color Textbook of Histology*, 2nd ed. Philadelphia, WB Saunders, 2001, p 288.)

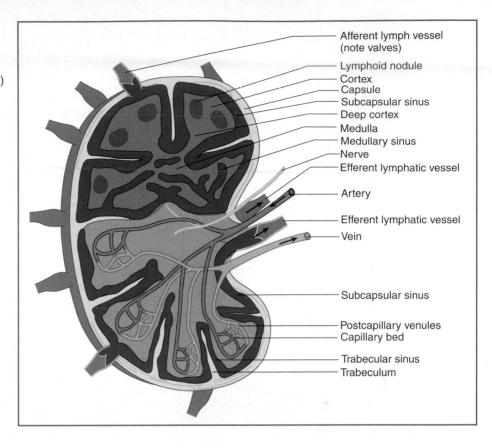

Afferent lymph vessel (note valves)
Lymphoid nodule
Cortex
Capsule
Subcapsular sinus
Deep cortex
Medulla
Medullary sinus
Nerve
Efferent lymphatic vessel
Artery
Efferent lymphatic vessel
Vein
Subcapsular sinus
Postcapillary venules
Capillary bed
Trabecular sinus
Trabeculum

PATHOLOGY

Chronic Lymphocytic Leukemia of B Lymphocytes (B-CLL)

There are many different kinds of leukemia, a lymphoproliferative disease. One of the most common is chronic lymphocytic leukemia. It is the most common leukemia in the Western world, comprising about 30% of all cases.

While the exact cell of origin of CLL is not known, current thinking indicates that it originates from a mantle zone–based B lymphocyte. It is diagnosed on the basis of a lymphocyte count > 5000/μL. A subset of individuals with B-CLL become anemic and thrombocytopenic as a result of the production of autoantibodies to red blood cells and to platelets. The abnormal B lymphocytes have receptors for glucocorticoids. When glucocorticoids bind to the lymphocytes, the abnormal lymphocytes lyse, providing a rather simple and effective way to manage the disease.

seen in Figures 8-7A and 8-7B. The fibers are synthesized by reticular cells, which are actually fibroblasts on the basis of morphologic and biochemical criteria. The reticular fibers are largely encased by thin cytoplasmic sheaths of the fibroblasts.

The parenchyma of lymph nodes is largely made of all types of lymphocytes and associated lymphoid cells in their numerous functional forms (e.g., B and T lymphocytes, lymphoblasts, plasma cells, macrophages, and APCs; see Fig. 8-7C). The parenchyma of the lymph node has a characteristic

organization. The region of the cortex closest to the capsule contains many lymphoid nodules (the *nodular cortex*), which are rich in B lymphocytes. Just under the nodular cortex is a region of closely packed lymphoid tissue called the deep cortex (paracortex); this is a T lymphocyte–rich region. The nodular and deep cortex both contain dendritic APCs, but the deep cortex has many-fold more, since these cells are largely involved in T lymphocyte interactions. The medulla of the lymph node has many large sinuses and loosely packed lymphocytes. The organization of the medullary lymphocytes is described as a network of *medullary cords*. The sinuses interspersed among the medullary cords are the beginnings of the efferent lymphatic vessels of the node. Many activated or partially activated lymphocytes that encountered macrophages and APCs in the cortex enter the medullary sinuses and leave the node via an efferent lymphatic vessel.

The blood vessels and the blood vascular circulation through a lymph node have special characteristics. Arterial blood, which enters the node at the hilum, travels first to the nodular cortex, where the vessels ramify into a network of capillaries around the nodules. The capillaries coalesce into a number of postcapillary venules, which have an unusual endothelium. The endothelial cells are not squamous as in most other locations but rather are cuboidal to low columnar; consequently, these vessels are called high endothelial venules (HEVs) (Figs. 8-8 and 8-9). Lymphocytes in the blood enter the deep cortex via the HEVs, interact with the lymph and its cells, and leave the node via the medullary sinuses and efferent lymphatic vessels. Some of the lymphocytes in

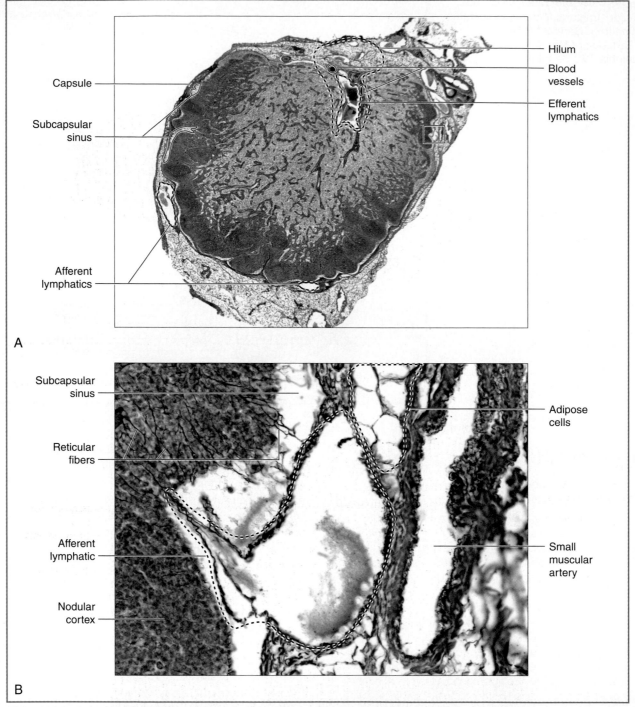

Figure 8-6. **A,** Micrograph of a lymph node sectioned in the transverse plane, stained with a reticulin stain (11×). In addition to the labeled features, the nodular and deep cortex and the medulla are clearly seen. **B,** Higher magnification of the region of the box in part A (240×). It is an afferent lymphatic; a valve flap and its communication with the subcapsular sinus can be seen.

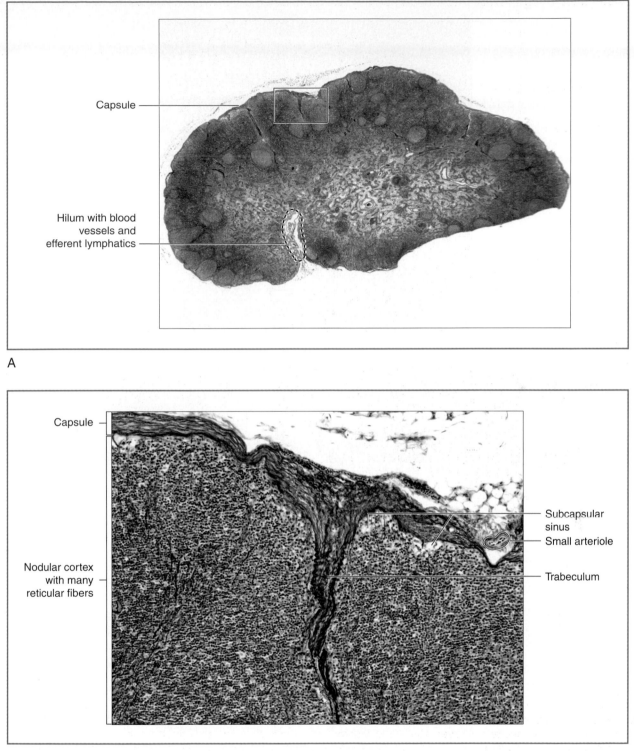

A

B

Figure 8-7. A, Micrograph of a lymph node, sectioned in the longitudinal plane, stained with a silver stain (10×). The hilum with its blood and lymphatic vessels can be discerned even at this low magnification. **B,** Higher magnification of the region in the box in part A (200×) showing the dense nodular cortex, many fine reticular fibers, a trabeculum, and a small region of the subcapsular cortex.

Continued

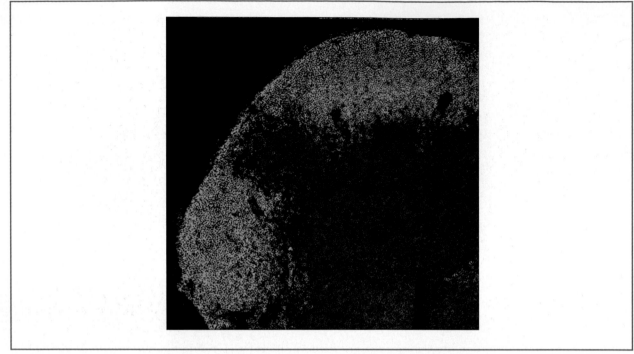

C

Figure 8-7 cont'd. C, Immunochemical stain of a lymph node illustrating the distribution of B lymphocytes (*green*) in the nodular cortex and T lymphocytes (*red*) in the deep cortex. (From Abbas AK, Lichtman A. *Cellular and Molecular Immunology*, 5th ed. Philadelphia, WB Saunders, 2005, p 29.)

PATHOLOGY

Lymphatic Filariasis

Helminths—worms—are among the most common human pathogens. From 25% to 50% of the world's population is infected with one or more species of worm. About 100 to 200 million people are infected with one of two species of filarial (thread-like) roundworms. The infection is spread by bites from several different species of mosquito that carry infectious worm larvae. Hundreds of bites, presumably to build up the parasitic load, are usually required for infection. The larvae migrate to the lymphatic vessels and lymph nodes, where they mature into adult worms. They accumulate in regions with large numbers of lymph nodes. After male and female worms mate, the female releases microfilariae into the lymphatics and bloodstream. The pathologic and physiologic consequences are the result of the immune response to degenerating adult worms. These responses include activation of T_H2 lymphocytes and accumulation of lymphocytes, eosinophils, macrophages, and plasma cells. The infections persist for years, and many asymptomatic individuals have antibodies to the worms. About 5% of infected individuals have near-total blockage of the lymphatics of the arms, legs, or testes. Such individuals have massive lymphedema, called elephantiasis, of the limbs or scrotum. Engorgement of the scrotum (male hydrocele) is about 10 times as common as that of the limbs. Male hydrocele can be alleviated by a simple surgical procedure, but this is generally unavailable in affected parts of the world. Infection with filarial worms can be prevented by the addition of one of several drugs to table salt.

the deep cortex enter the HEVs and leave the node in the venous circulation.

Spleen
Structure

The spleen is the largest organ of the lymphoid system; it weighs about 150 g and is located in the upper left quadrant of the abdominal cavity. The spleen is a solid organ with a connective tissue capsule and trabeculae; the capsule contains fibroblasts and myofibroblasts and in some species, but not in humans, smooth muscle cells. The splenic stroma consists of fine reticular fibers and the cells that make them, reticular cells. It has a hilum, which is the site for the passage of the splenic artery and vein, nerves, and one or more efferent lymphatic vessels. In contrast to lymph nodes, the spleen has no afferent lymphatics; the efferent lymphatic vessels originate in the vicinity of trabeculae.

The parenchyma contains lymphocytes, plasma cells, macrophages, and APCs. The splenic parenchyma does not have a cortex and a medulla; instead it is organized into *white pulp* and *red pulp*, designations based on the appearance of the fresh-cut surface of the organ. The white pulp appears as circular to elongated oval grayish areas owing to the presence of dense accumulations of white blood cells. The red pulp that occupies the rest of the parenchyma has a sponge-like appearance and is red because of the presence of many red blood cells. There is a transitional region of about 80 to 100 μm at the interface between the white and red pulp called the marginal zone.

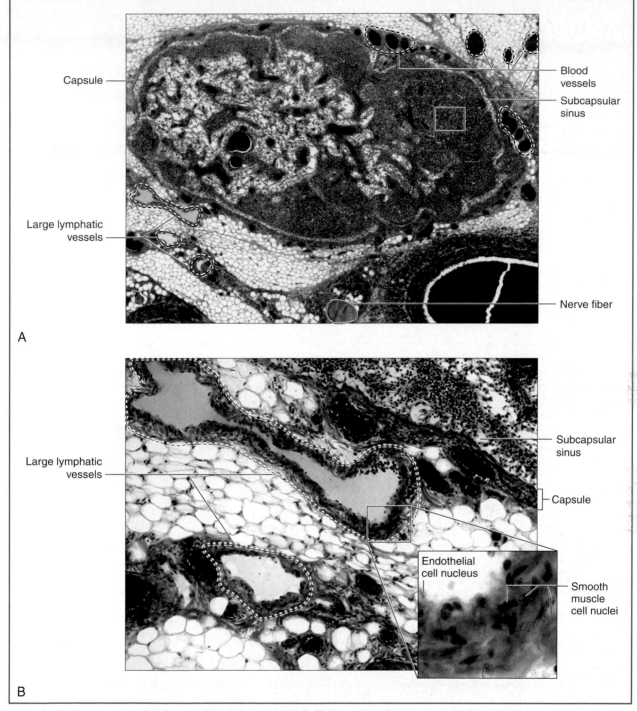

Capsule

Blood vessels

Subcapsular sinus

Large lymphatic vessels

Nerve fiber

A

Large lymphatic vessels

Subcapsular sinus

Capsule

Endothelial cell nucleus

Smooth muscle cell nuclei

B

Figure 8-8. **A,** Mallory-azan stain of a small lymph node (23×). This section does not pass through the hilum or any afferent or efferent lymphatics, but the substantial blood supply to a node, HEVs, and large lymphatic vessels is well illustrated in this specimen. **B,** Higher magnification of the two large lymphatic vessels (90×). Both vessels are filled with lymph; a small number of lymphocytes can be seen near the endothelial surface of each vessel. Both vessels have a thick wall characteristic of larger lymphatics; hence, it is possible to see some smooth muscle cells in their walls (inset, 1000×).

The key to understanding the structure and function of the spleen is to appreciate its vascularization. Blood enters the spleen via the splenic artery that branches extensively to the trabeculae, from which it is distributed to the parenchyma of the spleen via many small arteries. The small arteries are sheathed with a relatively thick layer of T lymphocytes called the periarterial lymphatic sheath (PALS). There are several small lymphoid nodules distributed along each PALS; the nodules are aggregates of B lymphocytes, some of which have a germinal center. In a transverse section of a PALS in a region with no nodule, the artery is in the center of the lymphocyte sheath; hence, it is called the central artery. The

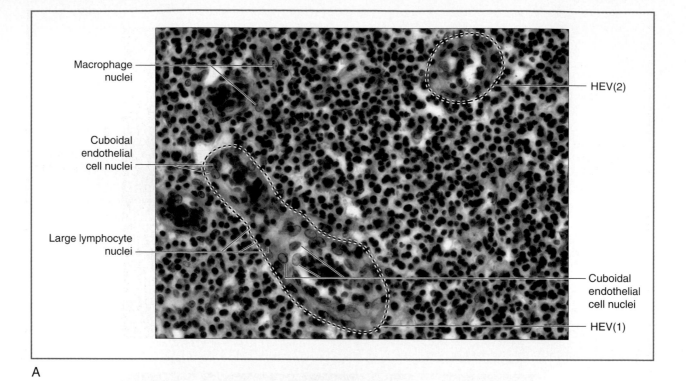

A

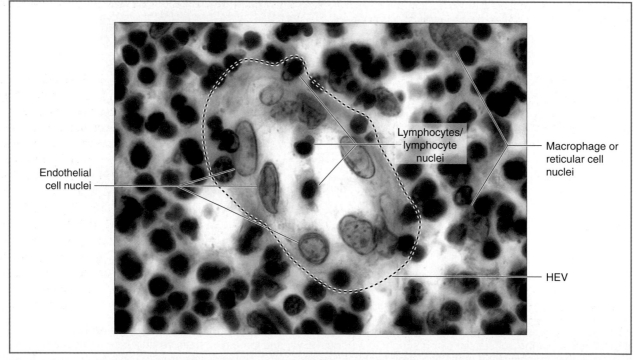

B

Figure 8-9. A, Two HEVs are seen, at a higher magnification (370×) of the area indicated in Figure 8-8A. One of the venules is sectioned transversely, and the other is a tangential section of a curving HEV. The thick endothelium of the venules with lymphocytes passing across the vessel wall can be seen. **B,** Oil immersion micrograph (1000×) of another HEV. The venule is surrounded by many lymphocytes. Several endothelial nuclei of the high endothelial cells are evident as well as several lymphocytes in the vessel wall and lumen.

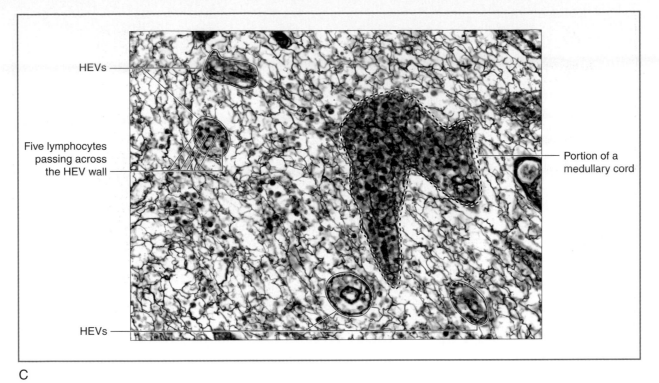

C

Figure 8-9 cont'd. C, Higher magnification (240×) of the reticulin-stained node in shown in Figure 8-6. Most of the field is occupied by medullary sinuses; a small portion of a medullary cord is indicated. There are four HEVs in the field, one of which has five lymphocytes that appear to be in transit across the vessel wall.

lymphatic sheath and nodules are supplied with many capillaries that originate from the central artery. If the PALS is sectioned through one of its associated nodules, the central artery is eccentrically placed. Figure 8-10 shows three sections of the spleen, in low, medium, and higher magnification views.

Immunochemical staining of lymphoid tissue is a particularly useful way of visualizing the underlying distribution of different populations of lymphoid cells. The distribution of B lymphocytes and APCs in the spleen is seen in Figure 8-11. The majority of the APCs are in T lymphocyte–rich PALS, but the nodular areas, which are B lymphocyte–rich areas, also show a small number of APCs.

The caliber of the central artery becomes smaller and smaller and its lymphatic sheath becomes thinner, finally leaving the white pulp where, now in the red pulp, it branches into a parallel series of very small arterioles (40–50 µm in diameter), the *penicillar arterioles*. The penicillar arterioles have three regions: the pulp arteriole; the sheathed arteriole, which has a sheath of macrophages; and the terminal arteriolar capillaries. Blood from the terminal arterial capillaries either drains directly into *venous sinuses* (the "closed circulation") or terminates in the red pulp (the "open circulation"). Both modes of circulation, open and closed, coexist in the red pulp, although the majority is thought to be of the closed type.

The venous sinuses (also called venous sinusoids or splenic sinusoids) have a highly specialized structure. They consist of elongated endothelial cells, positioned lengthwise along the vessel, which resemble the staves of a wooden barrel;

there are large gaps (and regions of close cell-cell contact) between the staggered parallel endothelial cells. They have a discontinuous basal lamina organized into thin, interconnected strands oriented at right angles to the endothelial cells; hence the sinuses have a discontinuous basal lamina. The endothelial cells may also be wrapped by thin strands of reticular fibers in a similar orientation to the basal lamina. Therefore, the venous sinuses have a structure similar to a (leaky) barrel with staves and hoops (Figs. 8-12 to 8-15). Macrophages are always associated with the venous sinuses but not in the numbers seen with the sheathed capillaries.

The spaces between all the vessels of the red pulp are filled with splenic parenchyma; in sections, the parenchyma of the red pulp appears as cords (splenic cords, cords of Billroth), but in three dimensions they are curved, anastomosing plates of cells.

Function

The spleen has many important functions, yet it is not essential to life. Individuals may have their spleen removed surgically and survive for years, albeit with somewhat impaired immune function. There is a great deal of immune activity in the spleen owing to interactions between dendritic cells and T lymphocytes and between macrophages carrying ligands bound to MHC complexes and B lymphocytes. Resting B lymphocytes can be activated to become lymphoblasts, which differentiate into plasma cells. The plasma cells may synthesize and secrete immunoglobulins in the spleen, or

Text continued on page 255

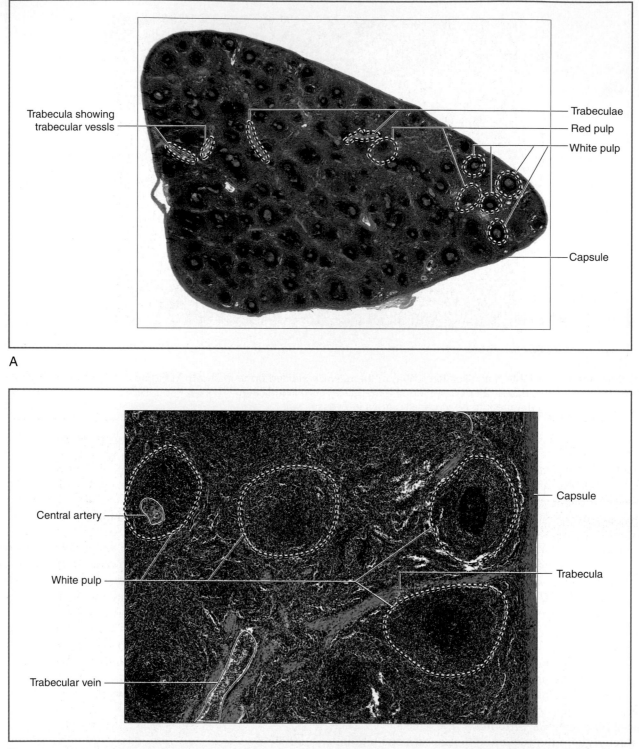

A

B

Figure 8-10. A, Transverse section of a spleen at low magnification (H&E, 7.5×). The organ is surrounded by a thick connective tissue capsule from which emanate numerous trabeculae. The capsule of the human spleen has some myofibroblasts and possibly some smooth muscle cells; their functional significance is not clear, since unlike several other mammals, the human spleen does not contract. The dense blue-stained areas are the white pulp (PALS) and the less dense red-stained areas are the red pulp of the spleen. At low magnification some of the unstained regions adjacent to the white pulp (i.e., the marginal zone) can be discerned. Some areas of the white pulp are sectioned through nodules in the PALS. **B,** A higher magnification (50×) section of the same specimen. In addition to the features labeled in part A, a central artery and trabecular vein are labeled.

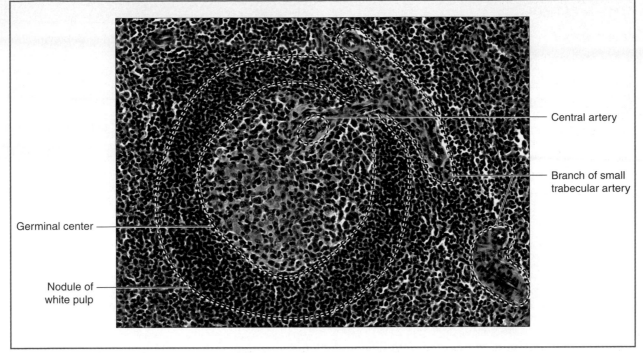

— Central artery

— Branch of small
trabecular artery

Germinal center —

Nodule of —
white pulp

C

Figure 8-10 cont'd. C, Section of a nodular part of the PALS in which a small trabecular artery, germinal center, and central artery are seen.

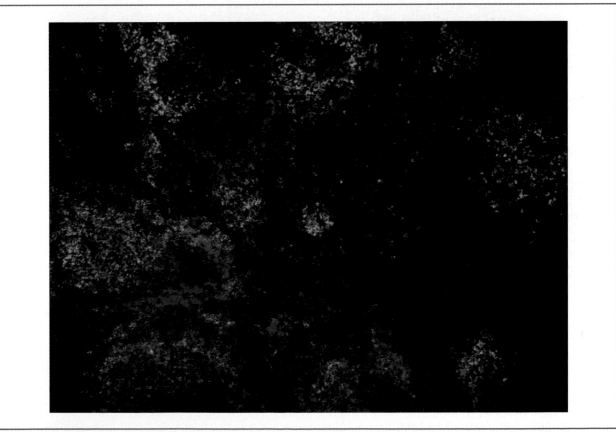

Figure 8-11. Immunofluorescence stain of a frozen section of mouse spleen. The green color shows the localization of a highly specific monoclonal antibody to B lymphocytes—CD45r, a pan–B cell marker. The red color shows the distribution of dendritic cells (APCs plus other dendritic cells) labeled with the CD11c+ monoclonal antibody, a pan–dendritic cell marker. The dark regions represent blood vessels and the distribution of T lymphocytes. (Courtesy of Samantha Bailey and Stephen Miller.)

GENETICS & PATHOLOGY

Sickle Cell Disease

Sickle cell disease is an autosomal recessive disease that results from a single nucleotide mutation in the gene for the β-chain of hemoglobin (Hb). The mutant form of hemoglobin is called HbS. It leads to severe anemia and splenomegaly. The mutation causes valine to be substituted for glutamic acid in the sixth amino acid position of the β-chain of hemoglobin. At physiologically normal low O_2 tension, particularly in venous blood, homozygous individuals experience dramatic and painful microvascular occlusion owing to the polymerization of HbS-containing hemoglobin tetramers. The red cells containing the hemoglobin polymers (fibers) become sickle shaped. Some of these cells become trapped in capillary beds while others persist in the circulation. Because of the major role in filtering blood of splenic venous sinuses, the spleen becomes pathologically enlarged (splenomegaly). The splenomegaly may be so severe that even at the age of 10 to 12 months, the affected individual becomes functionally asplenic. This further exacerbates the anemia and associated clinical problems.

IMMUNOLOGY

Autoimmune Diseases and Molecular Mimicry

Molecular mimicry is one of several explanations for the range of autoimmune diseases seen in humans. Molecular mimicry seems to be a mechanism whereby helper T lymphocytes and the specific antibodies synthesized by programmed B lymphocytes are normal. However, the antibodies produced react against host proteins, thus overcoming normal immune tolerance mechanisms. The disease in which this mechanism is most often cited is rheumatic heart disease; others, such as the myocarditis that follows infection with *Chlamydia* or *Trypanosoma cruzi* and type I diabetes in viremic individuals, have been suggested.

The production of specific antibodies typically involves recognition of 10 to 18 amino acids as the "antigen" in the partially degraded foreign pathogen. The antibodies generated may recognize primary, secondary, or tertiary structural features of the antigen. However, the smaller the antigenic epitope may be, the greater the likelihood that a specific antibody may recognize a host protein. An extreme example would be the case of a single amino acid or a dipeptide epitope. Antibodies to such small epitopes could cross-react with many host proteins. In the case of molecular mimicry, the antigenic epitopes are thought to be four to six amino acids or small, common secondary or tertiary structural motifs in proteins.

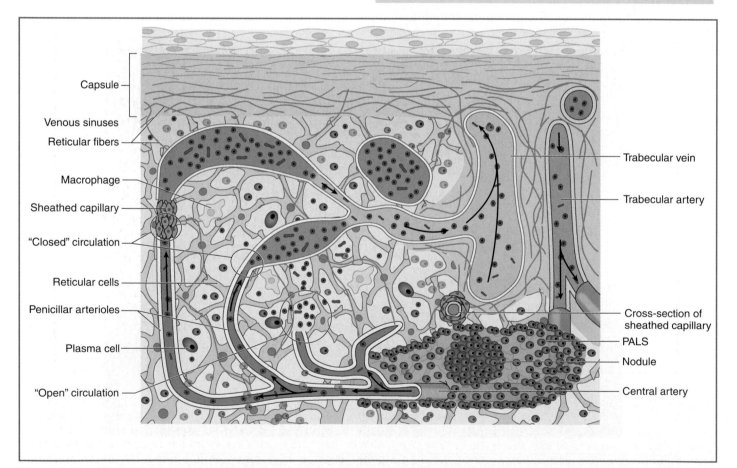

Figure 8-12. Diagram of the spleen. The capsule, a trabecula, reticular fibers, and reticular cells occupy much of the field. Lymphocytes are the small nucleated circular cells, and erythrocytes are the small bright red cells. Note the large number of macrophages and plasma cells in the red pulp. Blood flow is represented by the black arrows and can be traced through the following seven locations: (1) a trabecular artery, (2) a central artery, (3) penicillar arterioles, (4) sheathed capillaries, (5a) the *closed circulation* into a venous sinus, (5b) the *open circulation* into a venous sinus, (6) a collecting vein, and (7) a trabecular vein. (Modified from Standring S. *Gray's Anatomy*, 39th ed. Philadelphia, Churchill-Livingstone, 2005, p 1242.)

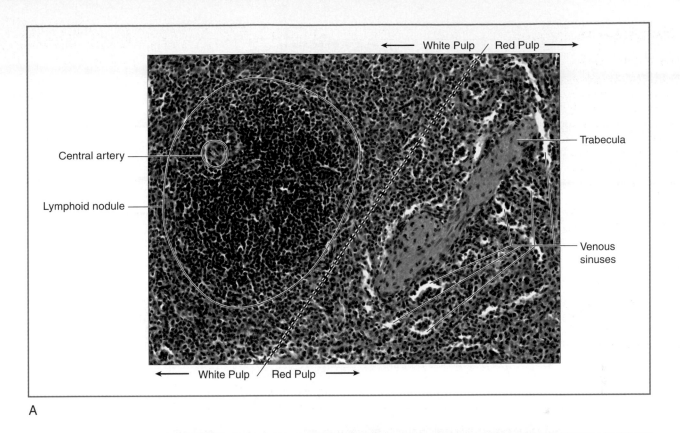

A

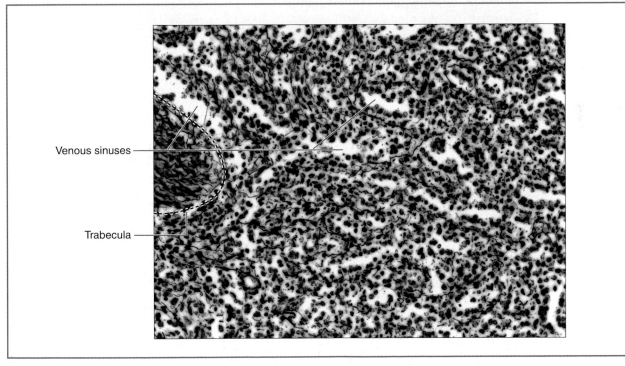

B

Figure 8-13. A, H&E stain of spleen (160×). White pulp occupies approximately the upper left half of the field, and red pulp occupies the lower right half. A lymphoid nodule, lacking a germinal center, with its eccentrically placed central vein is seen in the white pulp. There are many venous sinuses near the trabecula in the red pulp. **B,** Reticulin (silver) stained section of spleen (180×). Many venous sinuses are seen in this section. Many reticular fibers are seen in this specimen including in the trabecula. Most of the sinuses have reticular fibers running parallel along their length; in a few instances, it is possible to see a suggestion of fibers at right angles to the axis of the sinus.

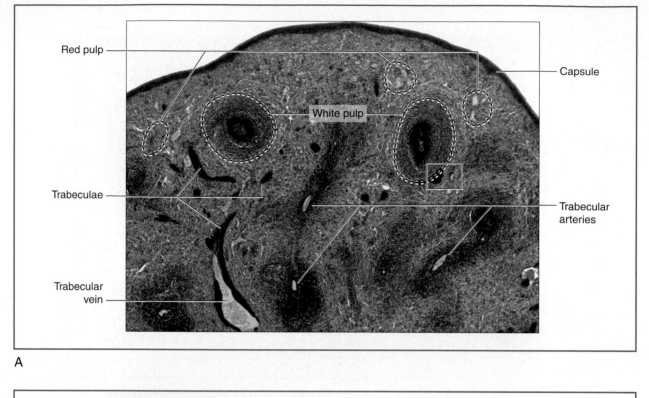

Red pulp

Capsule

White pulp

Trabeculae

Trabecular arteries

Trabecular vein

A

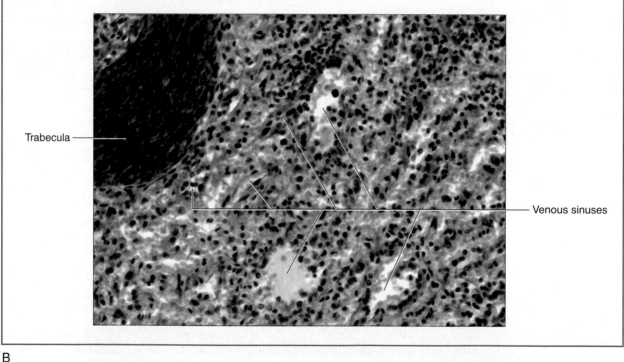

Trabecula

Venous sinuses

B

Figure 8-14. A, Mallory-azan stain of spleen (17×). The capsule, trabeculae, trabecular arteries and veins, and white and red pulp are seen in this section (note that nuclei stain red with Mallory-azan so the white pulp is dark red). **B,** Higher magnification (220×) of the area in the box in part A. This stain permits a distinction between fibroblasts and myofibroblasts in the trabecula. Nuclei of fibroblasts are elongated with little or no visible cytoplasm while myofibroblasts are the larger fusiform cells. Several good examples of venous sinuses are labeled in the middle part of the field.

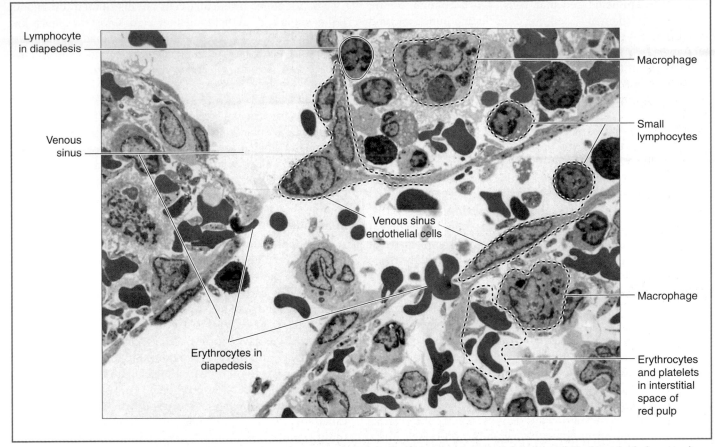

Figure 8-15. Electron micrograph of a splenic venous sinus (1600×). Red blood cell and white blood cell diapedesis is seen in several locations near the sinus endothelial cells. It is possible to identify many of the specific cells in the red pulp at this relatively low magnification. (Courtesy of Judith Taggert Rhodin.)

they can leave the spleen and travel to remote sites to carry out this function.

A major function associated with the red pulp is the removal and destruction of aged or abnormal platelets and erythrocytes. Platelets and erythrocytes are found in extravascular spaces in the red pulp because of its open circulation. Normal platelets and erythrocytes reenter the blood vascular circulation by squeezing through the gaps between the elongated endothelial cells of the venous sinuses while the defective ones are unable to pass through the gaps and are phagocytosed by macrophages. Defective or aged platelets and erythrocytes in the lumen of the venous sinuses that attempt to move into extravascular spaces are also phagocytosed by nearby macrophages. The spleen also serves as a site for the clearance of bacteria and immune complexes that may be in the circulation. This filtration function of the spleen serves many important physiologic roles.

Thymus
Structure

The thymus is a bilobed lymphoid organ located in the superior mediastinum anterior to the heart and the great vessels. At about 6 to 7 weeks of development, the endodermal epithelium begins to develop. Marrow-derived multipotential lymphocyte

stem cells (CFU-Ls), the future T lymphocytes, populate the tubular outgrowth of the developing organ at about 9 to 10 weeks of fetal development. The thymus is fully developed at birth and persists as an active lymphoid organ for about the first two decades of life. Its lymphoid tissue begins to become replaced with adipose tissue in the late teen years, a process largely complete by the time a person reaches the mid-30s.

The thymus has a connective tissue capsule, which divides the organ into lobules. Connective tissue trabeculae, which originate from the capsule, penetrate the lobules, carrying blood vessels with them. The thymus has no distinct hilum, but blood vessels and nerves enter the lobules from the many invaginations between the lobules. There are no afferent lymphatics, but numerous efferent lymphatics, which originate in the thymic parenchyma, leave the organ at a number of sites. In addition to fibroblasts, the capsule has variable numbers of macrophages, plasma cells, and lymphocytes and small numbers of other connective tissue cells.

The stroma of the thymus is unlike the other lymphoid organs (and nearly all other organs as well) in that it is an *epithelial reticular system* rather than a set of organized connective tissue cells and fibers. As the organ develops, the CFU-L cells occupy spaces between the developing tubular epithelial rudiment, resulting in the mature lymphoepithelial organ. The epithelial reticular cells, which contain keratin intermediate filaments and form occluding junctions and desmosomes—general characteristics of epithelial cells—play an important role in isolating the CFU-L cells from the blood and the rest of the body. This arrangement, which is discussed in more detail below, is referred to as the *blood-thymus barrier*. Since the thymus is the organ in which the majority of T lymphocytes initially develop, the isolation of T-lymphocyte precursors and their immunocompetent progeny from the rest of the body is of considerable significance. T lymphocytes are the long-term memory cells of the lymphoid system and play a major part in the body's self-recognition mechanisms.

Six types of epithelioreticular cells have been described on the basis of electron microscope and immunochemical studies. EM studies show differences in the overall shape of the epithelial reticular cells, their nuclei, and cytoplasmic appearance. Immunochemical studies have used antibodies to a number of specific keratin intermediate filaments and other cell markers to determine their distribution and immunochemical differences. The details of the morphology of the six cell types is beyond the scope of this book, but it is worth noting the differences in their distribution and function. The first three types are found in the cortex, and the last three are located in the medulla.

Type I epithelial reticular cells are found just under the connective tissue capsule of the thymus, among the cortical parenchyma and surrounding the cortical blood vessels. Their major function is thought to be to provide a barrier between the connective tissue of the capsule and the blood vessels. They are confined to the outer parts of the cortex.

Type II epithelial reticular cells are found throughout the cortex. They are stellate cells and elaborate numerous desmosomes with neighboring epithelioreticular cells. They express class I and class II MHC glycoproteins on their surface, a characteristic not shared by the other epithelial reticular cell types. They are involved with instructing the developing T lymphocytes.

Type III epithelial reticular cells are found at or near the corticomedullary boundary. They have a sheet-like cytoplasm and have occluding junctions and desmosomes between them.

Type IV epithelial reticular cells are also found at the corticomedullary boundary but are predominantly in the medulla. Type III and type IV cells have a similar appearance and perform similar barrier functions.

Type V epithelial reticular cells are distributed throughout the medulla and are held together by desmosomes much like type II cells, but they are fewer in number than type II cells.

Type VI epithelial reticular cells are found in distinctive ball-shaped structures called Hassall's corpuscles. They consist of tightly wrapped, flattened epithelioreticular cells that may have a keratinized core.

Except for Hassall's corpuscles, the different types of epithelial reticular cells are difficult to recognize in conventionally stained sections in the light microscope. Figures 8-16 to 8-18 show examples of thymus glands from infants and from a 35-year old man. Figure 8-19 is a diagram of part of a thymus gland.

Function

As mentioned above, the organization of the blood-thymus barrier, particularly for smaller vessels and capillaries, plays a central role in the development and production of T lymphocytes. The capillaries that supply the thymic cortex are of the continuous type with a complete basal lamina. The capillaries have a sheath of connective tissue about 20 to 30 μm thick; there are often macrophages in the sheath. The sheath itself is surrounded by another basal lamina and the cells that secrete it, the type I epithelioreticular cells. Figure 8-19 is a drawing of this special vascular arrangement.

The cortex of the thymus is packed with CFU-L cells, often called thymocytes, which become "instructed" or "educated" to differentiate into immunocompetent T lymphocytes. There is a substantial expansion of the number of T lymphocytes during this "education" process. The immunocompetent T lymphocytes enter the circulation and are distributed to lymph nodes, solitary nodules, and sites of diffuse lymphoid tissue.

About 98% of the maturing T lymphocytes undergo programmed cell death on the way to becoming immunocompetent T lymphocytes. The apoptotic cells are phagocytosed by the abundant population of macrophages in the thymic cortex. During the process of T lymphocyte education, the cells express a large number of cell specific CD markers. Many regulatory factors play a role in T-lymphocyte education—cytokines, interferons, and cell-cell interactions. In addition to expected interactions between lymphocytes and macrophages, there are specific interactions between lymphocytes and epithelioreticular cells. Many of the "educated" lymphocytes persist in the body for decades as T lymphocyte memory cells.

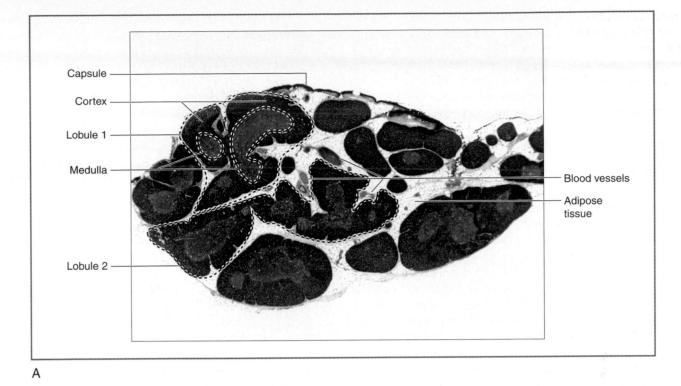

Capsule
Cortex
Lobule 1
Medulla
Blood vessels
Adipose tissue
Lobule 2

A

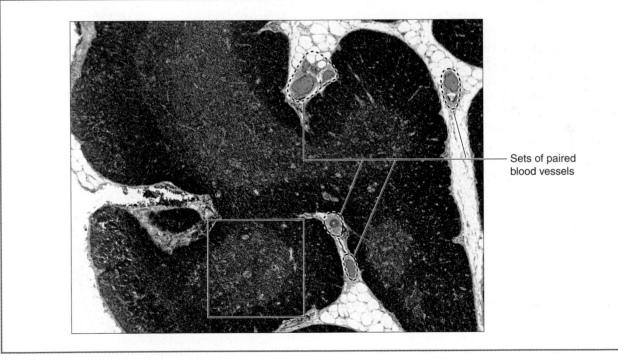

Sets of paired blood vessels

B

Figure 8-16. **A,** Mallory-azan stain of thymus gland (8×). The thymic lobules and part of the capsule are evident. There are many blood vessels in the connective tissue near the lobules, most of which are paired vessels. The darker cortical and lighter medullary areas can be seen in most lobules. Two of the lobules are circled because they show the confluence of the medulla from one part of a lobule to another particularly well. In fact, this arrangement illustrates the fact that the lobules are not lobules in the strict sense. **B,** Lobule 1 (from part A) rotated 90 degrees counterclockwise (40×). The delicate connective tissue capsule can be seen surrounding the lobule. Several blood vessels, surrounded by a rather thick connective tissue sheath (tunica adventitia), can be seen in the thymic parenchyma.

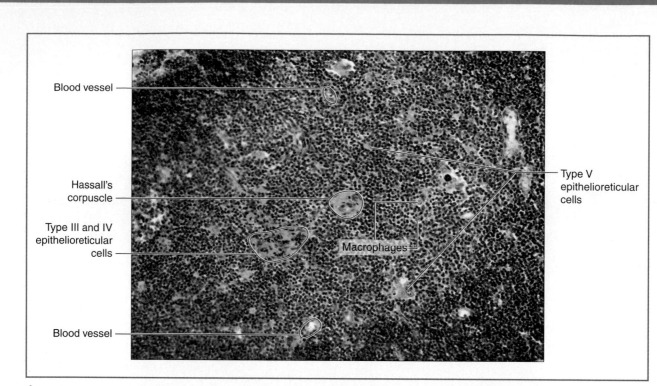

A

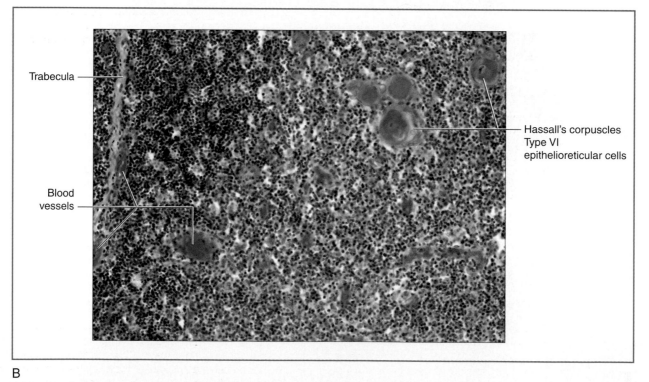

B

Figure 8-17. A, Higher magnification (150×) of the boxed area in Figure 8-16B. Most of the field shows the medulla surrounded by the more lymphocyte-dense cortex. Two good examples of Hassall's corpuscles (consisting of type VI epithelioreticular cells) are seen; several other types of epithelioreticular cells are labeled, although precise identification of these cells depends on immunochemical staining and electron microscopy. **B,** H&E stain of thymus gland from an infant (180×). Several Hassall's corpuscles are seen in the upper right corner of the field. A connective tissue trabeculum and nearby blood vessels are seen at the left. There are several locations where epithelioreticular cells can be seen, but their identification as specific types is even more difficult to make in an H&E section.

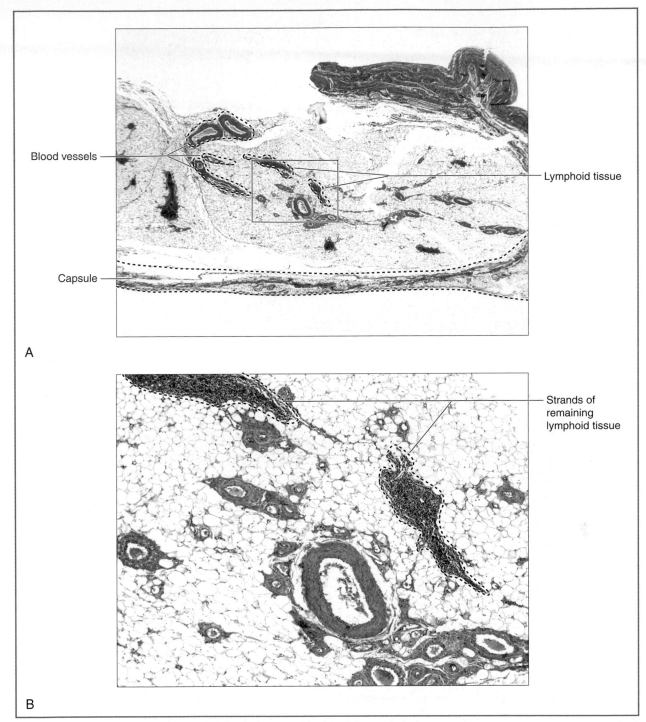

Figure 8-18. A, Low magnification (9×) of the thymus of a 35-year-old human (H&E stain). The capsule is seen along the bottom edge of the specimen. The extensive replacement of lymphoid tissue by adipose tissue is evident. Blood vessels are circled, and the remaining lymphoid tissue is labeled. **B,** Higher magnification (45×) of the boxed area in part A showing some of the blood vessels, remaining lymphoid tissue, and adipose tissue in greater detail. The blood vessels range in size from a large muscular artery (in the lower central part of the field) down in size to a few capillaries (near the upper right corner).

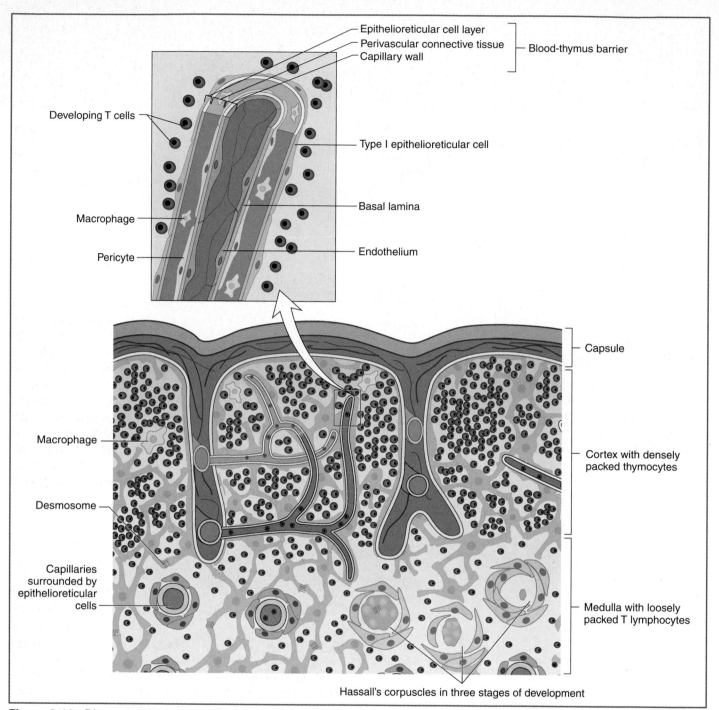

Figure 8-19. Diagrammatic representation of the cortex and part of the medulla of a thymus gland. The capsule and two trabeculae with reticular fibers and blood vessels are represented. The densely packed thymocytes, macrophages, and specially isolated blood vessels are shown in the cortex of a lobule in the upper center of the field. The more loosely packed medulla, with fewer T lymphocytes and macrophages, is represented in the lower part of the field. The epithelioreticular cells (in various shades of orange-brown) are seen throughout. Note the pattern of the epithelioreticular cells and the fact that they touch one another; in several instances, the contact points are shown to have desmosomes, but most cells have occluding junctions (not shown). This drawing does not represent the six types of epithelioreticular cells, although three stages in the formation of a Hassall's corpuscle are shown in the lower right quarter of the field. The earliest stage is at right and the latest at left. (Modified from Standring S. *Gray's Anatomy*, 39th ed. Philadelphia, Churchill-Livingstone, 2005, p 982.)

Integumentary System

9

●●● FUNCTIONS OF THE INTEGUMENT

The skin has many important functions:
- It serves as a major water barrier to the environment—tissue fluids do not leave the body through the skin, and fluids in the environment are prevented from entering the body by the skin. The barrier function is entirely attributable to the epidermis.
- It is a major thermoregulator by virtue of its large surface area and large number of sweat glands, which serve this function by the evaporative cooling of the secreted sweat. When the body surface becomes too hot from a high ambient temperature, by exercising, or from a fever, over a liter of sweat can be produced per day.
- It serves as a protection from many environmental insults—chemical and physical, particularly the harmful ultraviolet wavelengths in sunlight.
- It is the first line of defense of the immune system.
- It has many sensory functions, mediated by several kinds of specialized nerves and nerve endings.
- It performs a variety of endocrine functions by secreting hormones and cytokines and by producing the active form of vitamin D.

●●● GENERAL PROPERTIES OF THE INTEGUMENT

The integument (skin, cutis), as an organ, consists of two principal layers: an outer epithelial layer called the epidermis and a deeper connective tissue layer called the dermis. The epidermis is a keratinized, stratified squamous epithelium consisting of four structural and functional layers (five in some locations). The thicker and deeper dermis consists of two layers: the papillary dermis and the reticular dermis. There is a subcutaneous fascia under the integument called the hypodermis that connects the skin to underlying organs; it is a layer of loose, fatty connective tissue. Certain skin structures, such as the hair follicle bulbs and the secretory parts of sweat glands, originate in the hypodermis (Fig. 9-1).

Thickness

Although the skin is thought of as a fairly uniform body envelope, its structure is quite variable. Its thickness ranges from about 1 mm to 5 mm in different body regions, it has hair on most but not all of its surface, there are different amounts of pigment in different regions, and sweat glands are not uniformly distributed. Histologically, skin is described as being *thick* or *thin*, a distinction usually, but not always, based on the thickness of the epidermis. The thickest skin on the body is on the upper back, but the thickest layer in this region is the dermis, not the epidermis. Skin with the thickest epidermis is found on the palms of the hands and soles of the feet—the palmar and plantar surfaces.

Hair

Skin can be described as *hairy* or *hairless*. However, there is a great variety in the amount, characteristics, thickness, and length of hair, depending on the body region. Several locations are hairless: the palmar and plantar surfaces, the lips, and regions around the urogenital openings. Certain hairs have a distinct length and shape (e.g., the eyelashes), others are highly variable in length and shape (e.g., scalp hair and a man's beard). Still other hairs are very fine (e.g., on the inner surface of the arm and the eyelids). There are also significant differences in the amount and characteristics of

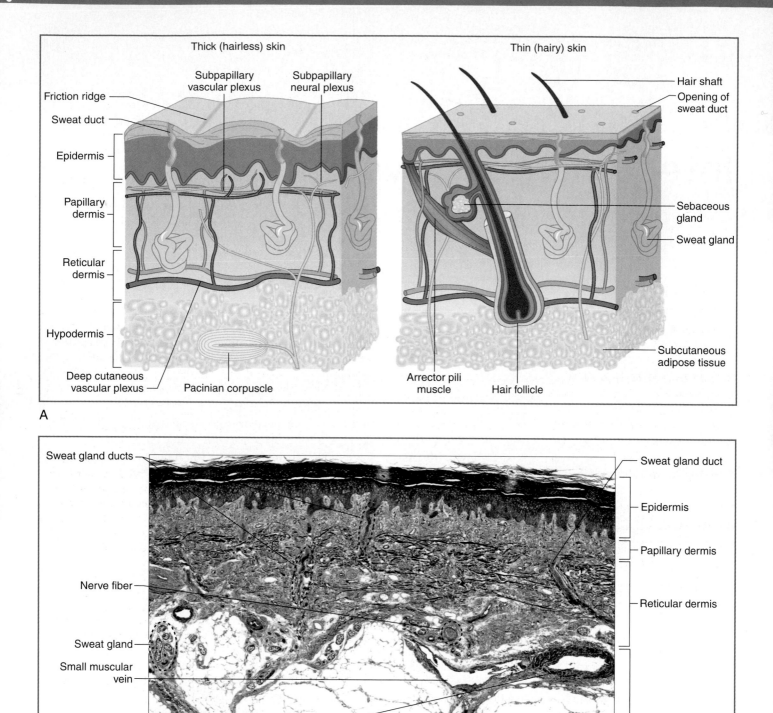

A

B

Figure 9-1. **A,** Structures of the skin. (Redrawn from Standring S. *Gray's Anatomy*, 39th ed, Philadelphia, Churchill-Livingstone, 2005, p 158.) **B,** Full-thickness section of thin skin (trichrome stain, 20×). Many features of skin are labeled in this micrograph.

hair in the same body regions between the two sexes. Hair (and nails) are made up almost entirely of the fibrous protein keratin.

●●● LAYERS OF THE SKIN

Epidermis

General Characteristics

The epidermis of thin skin has four layers (strata); thick skin has five layers. The layers are named from the deepest to the surface, as follows:

- Stratum basale
- Stratum spinosum
- Stratum granulosum
- Stratum lucidum (thick skin only)
- Stratum corneum

Figure 9-2 illustrates all five layers of the epidermis. Even though the cells in each layer have a characteristic appearance, all of them are called *keratinocytes.*

The postmitotic cells in the three (or four) upper layers of the skin undergo a programmed series of cellular differentiation as they move slowly from the stratum basale to the stratum corneum. These events take about 2 to 3 weeks. In each layer, different keratin genes are expressed as the cells progress toward the free surface of the skin while those expressed in lower layers are shut down. Keratin filaments (a major type of intermediate filament) comprise about 85% of the protein of keratinocytes. More than 20 keratin genes are expressed in the epidermis as the keratinocytes differentiate and move from the basal to the superficial layer. The epidermal keratins are usually described as *soft keratin.*

The stratum basale is the single layer of cells at the base of the epidermis; it produces hemidesmosomes and a basal lamina, both of which anchor the epidermis securely to the underlying dermis (Fig. 9-3). As indicated in the diagram, the hemidesmosome has proteins that link the keratin filament component of the cytoskeleton, via proteins of the plakin family, to integral membrane proteins, one of which is a specific form of the cellular adhesion protein integrin ($\alpha6\beta4$); the other is BP180. One of the plakins (BP230) and BP180 have been identified as two of the immunogens in the autoimmune disease bullous pemphigoid. Three plasma membrane proteins (integrin; BP180; and CD151, a member of the tetraspanin family of membrane receptors) bind to laminin, a component of the basal lamina. In turn, laminin and other proteins bind to type VII collagen in the basal lamina. This illustrates how the hemidesmosome serves as an adhesion complex and as a signal transduction mediator between the extracellular matrix and the cytoskeleton.

The stratum basale is the layer from which the cells that make up the more superficial layers of the epidermis originate. Certain cells in the stratum basale (epidermal stem cells) divide in a controlled temporal and spatial manner to ensure an adequate supply of new cells for the entire epidermis as cells are shed from the surface of the skin. About

PATHOLOGY

Blistering Diseases of the Skin

There are a number of blistering (bullous) diseases of the skin. Most of these diseases are difficult to treat. Their degree of severity ranges from relatively mild blistering to severe cases; if the latter are untreated, they may be fatal. At least two blistering diseases are autoimmune diseases and have been well studied.

One of the most common is pemphigus vulgaris. Affected individuals have antibodies to desmoglein III. Desmogleins are membrane proteins of the E-cadherin family. They have a short cytoplasmic domain, a membrane-spanning domain, and a large extracellular domain. The extracellular domain of desmogleins of adjacent desmosomes have a high affinity for one another and serve a major role in the cell-to-cell adhesion of desmosomes. Higher concentrations of desmoglein III are found in the lower part of the epidermis. The pemphigus vulgaris antibodies bind to desmoglein III, largely in the stratum spinosum, causing blisters (bullae) in this epidermal layer. The antigen-antibody complexes may also cause the release of plasminogen activator and production of the protease called plasmin. These factors lead to lysis of cells of the stratum spinosum. Accordingly, pemphigus vulgaris causes blisters in suprabasal layers of the epidermis.

A less common but well characterized blistering disease is called bullous pemphigoid. Affected individuals have antibodies to at least two proteins associated with hemidesmosomes. The immunogens in bullous pemphigoid are called BP180 and BP230 (a member of the plakin family of proteins). These proteins form strong associations with keratin intermediate filaments and integral membrane proteins of the hemidesmosome. In fact, plakins serve as linkers between all three components of the cytoskeleton and between the cytoskeletal filaments and the plasma membrane. BP180 is one of the integral membrane proteins of the hemidesmosome. When bullous pemphigoid antibodies are in the tissue fluid near the epidermis, the basal cells of the epidermis are disrupted, both in the membrane region of the hemidesmosome and intracellularly. It is postulated that these events involve complement activation and degranulation of mast cells followed by eosinophil degranulation, but the postulate has not been proved. Accordingly, blisters form at the level of the basal lamina. This effectively leads to a splitting of the epidermis from the papillary dermis.

10% of the stratum basale cells are the stem cells of the epidermis.

In addition to the stratum basale keratinocytes, there are two other cell types in the stratum basale: *melanocytes,* which are dendritic (highly branched) cells and produce the dark brown-black pigment of the skin, and *Merkel cells,* which are sensory cells.

The stratum spinosum may be a few to many cell layers thick depending on the overall thickness of the epidermis. The cells of the stratum spinosum synthesize large amounts of keratin filaments, many of which are associated with the

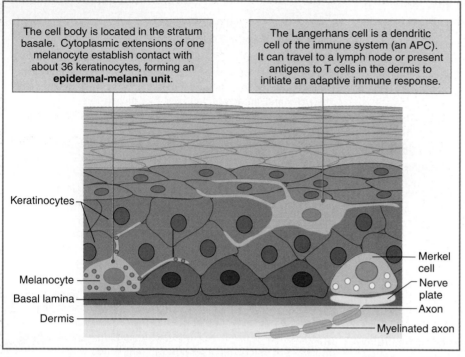

The cell body is located in the stratum basale. Cytoplasmic extensions of one melanocyte establish contact with about 36 keratinocytes, forming an **epidermal-melanin unit**.

The Langerhans cell is a dendritic cell of the immune system (an APC). It can travel to a lymph node or present antigens to T cells in the dermis to initiate an adaptive immune response.

Keratinocytes

Melanocyte

Basal lamina

Dermis

Merkel cell

Nerve plate

Axon

Myelinated axon

A

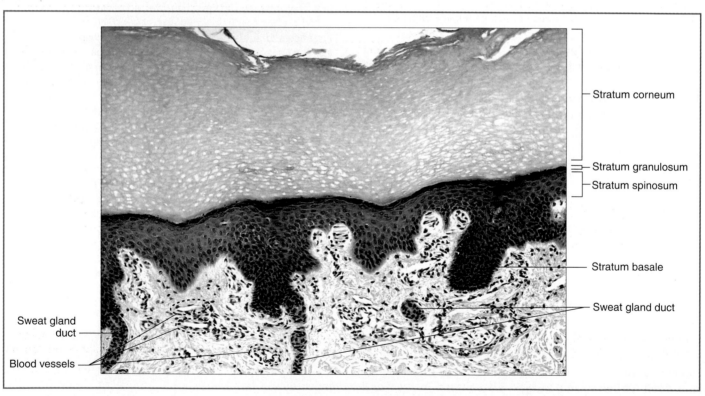

Stratum corneum

Stratum granulosum

Stratum spinosum

Stratum basale

Sweat gland duct

Sweat gland duct

Blood vessels

B

Figure 9-2. A, Melanocytes originate from the neural crest in the embryo and are visible by the eighth week of development. Merkel cells are tactile mechanoreceptors that also derive from the neural crest and appear in the palmar and plantar epidermis at about 8 to 12 weeks. Langerhans cells are mostly found in the stratum spinosum; they originate from bone marrow cell precursors and are present in the skin of the embryo 4 to 5 weeks following the arrival of melanocytes. **B,** Section of the epidermis of a fingertip (H&E, 100×). The four layers of the epidermis are labeled. Even though this specimen has a rather thick epidermis, it lacks a stratum lucidum and is therefore classified as thin skin.

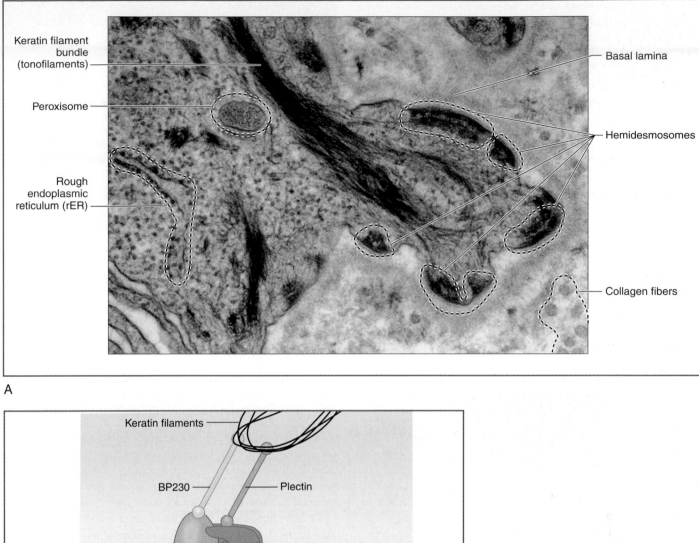

A

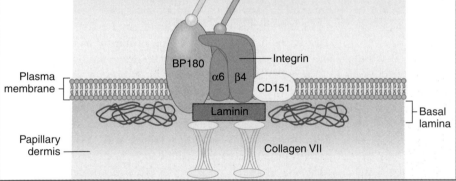

B

Figure 9-3. A, Electron micrograph of several hemidesmosomes in an epidermal basal cell. **B,** Diagram of a hemidesmosome showing how cytoplasmic keratin filaments are anchored to the underlying connective tissue. (Both courtesy of Jonathan Jones.)

numerous desmosomes these cells elaborate. Each keratinocyte of the stratum spinosum may have several hundred desmosomes; it is common for cells to shrink slightly during specimen preparation while the desmosomes hold fast to neighboring cells. This leads to the cells having a "spiny" or "prickly" appearance (Fig. 9-4). The cytoplasm of the keratinocytes becomes filled with bundles of tonofilaments (keratin filaments) as the cells move slowly toward the epidermal surface. They also possess membrane-coating granules (lamellar granules), although these granules appear in greater numbers in the stratum granulosum. There is a specialized cell of the immune system found mostly in the stratum spinosum—the *Langerhans cell* (see Specialized Cells).

The stratum granulosum is only about 2 to 5 cell layers thick in all thicknesses of skin. The keratinocytes in this layer have two types of specialized granules: *keratohyalin granules* and *membrane-coating granules* (also called *lamellar bodies*). As these cells continue to differentiate, they degrade most of their major cell organelles: nucleus, mitochondria, endoplasmic reticulum, lysosomes, and peroxisomes. However, they retain most components of their cytoskeleton. The degradation of organelles is a specialized variant of programmed cell death, since the entire cell is not destroyed as is the case in most other types of programmed cell death. The keratohyalin granules contain proteins (*fillagin* and *tricohyalin*) that are important in the aggregation and bundling of the large number of cytoplasmic keratin filaments; the bundled filaments are often referred to as *tonofilaments*. In the transition to become stratum corneum keratinocytes, cells in this layer secrete the contents of the membrane-coating granules. The granule contents are lipid-rich and coat the outer surface of the plasma membrane with lipids, thereby contributing to the water barrier established in this layer.

The stratum lucidum is found only in thick skin. It is the first anucleate cell layer of skin and is about four to six cell layers thick. It stains poorly with most stains, which makes it look clear—hence its name (Fig. 9-5).

The stratum corneum is the most superficial layer of skin. Like the stratum spinosum, it exhibits a wide range of thickness in different regions of the body. It may be only five to ten cell layers thick on the eyelids and inner surface of the wrist. In contrast, it may be dozens of cell layers thick on the palmar and plantar surfaces. The stratum corneum is the most mature or differentiated layer of skin. Its cells are polygonal, plate-like, keratin-filled, flattened, squamous epithelial cells ("squames") that become desquamated. In addition to the contents and appearance of the squames, their plasma membrane becomes thickened and covalently cross-linked by enzymes that are expressed as they complete their differentiation and migration from the underlying cells of the stratum granulosum.

Specialized Cells

Melanocytes are found distributed among the cells in the stratum basale; depending on the part of the body examined, their abundance ranges from one in four to one in ten basal

IMMUNOLOGY & PATHOLOGY

Role of Dendritic Cells in Viral Infections

Certain epidermal regions of the male and female genitalia are particularly rich in dendritic cells of the immune system. The epidermis has a significant population of Langerhans cells. The stratified squamous epithelia of the male and female genitalia not only have a typical complement of Langerhans cells but also a significant population of dendritic cells lacking Birbeck granules. Hence, they are non-Langerhans dendritic cells. Because of their role in the immune system, epidermal dendritic cells (Langerhans and non-Langerhans types) are highly receptive to viral invasion and infection, particularly to HIV. The virus replicates in the dendritic cells, and the infected dendritic cells migrate from the epidermis to lymph nodes. HIV-infected dendritic cells interact with T lymphocytes in the lymph nodes, passing the virus to these cells. Of particular significance is the infection of T lymphocytes carrying the CD4+ marker. Infection of these T lymphocytes with HIV results in a reduction in this population of T lymphocytes. This may be the mechanism that initiates one of the hallmarks of HIV infection, namely, pathologically low CD4+ T lymphocyte counts.

cells; they extend cytoplasmic processes up into the stratum spinosum. They synthesize and secrete melanin, the dark brown pigment that colors the epidermis. Melanin granules are released from the melanocytes and are taken up by the keratinocytes of the stratum basale and spinosum. Some forms of melanin are dark brown and some are yellowish-brown. Humans all have about the same number of epidermal melanocytes (ca. 3% of epidermal cells); consequently, differences in skin color are due primarily to the nature and amount of melanin synthesized by the melanocytes (Fig. 9-6).

Langerhans cells are derived from bone marrow stem cells and are part of the peripheral immune system; they are distributed in the stratum spinosum and stratum basale of the epidermis (Fig. 9-7). These cells have a stellate or dendritic morphology, and they detect and take up microbial protein antigens; they account for 4% or less of epidermal cells but as much as 25% of the cell surface area of the epidermis. The Langerhans cells process the material they take up and then migrate to lymph nodes. Once there, they pass, or "present," the antigens to naïve T cells; hence, Langerhans cells are called antigen-presenting cells (APCs). In most cases, Langerhans cells undergo programmed cell death after reaching lymph nodes and interacting with T cells.

Merkel cells function as cutaneous sensory receptors; they are most abundant in the lips and fingertips and account for less than 1% of epidermal cells in these locations. They are associated with the expanded terminal bulb of certain myelinated nerve fibers. They are difficult to recognize in conventional stains but can be visualized by immunofluorescence staining using an antibody to an actin-bundling protein called espin (Fig. 9-8). This protein is found in many sensory cells and has served as a useful marker for such cells.

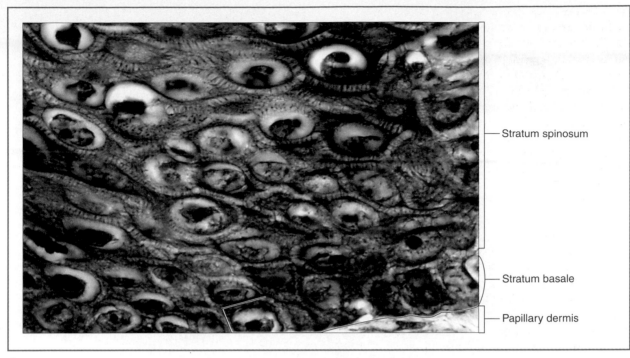

A

Stratum spinosum

Stratum basale

Papillary dermis

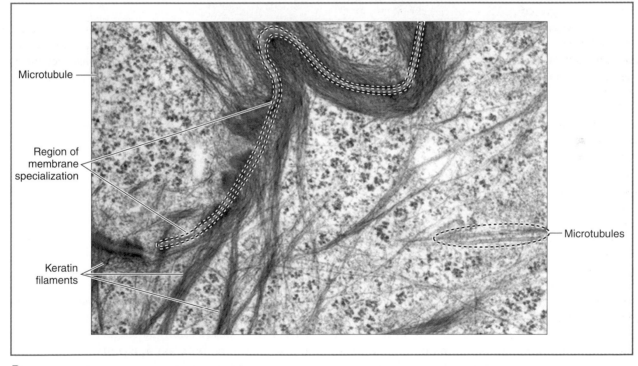

B

Microtubule

Region of
membrane
specialization

Keratin
filaments

Microtubules

Figure 9-4. **A,** High magnification of the stratum spinosum from the specimen in Figure 9-1B (900×). Most of the field is filled with the cells of the spinosum with a few basal cells and a small amount of papillary dermis. The desmosomes (spines) connecting the keratinocytes are seen clearly. **B,** Electron micrograph of desmosomes in the stratum spinosum of skin. The keratin filaments associated with the desmosomes are sectioned in various planes; nonetheless, the membrane specializations in the regions of cell-cell contact are clearly seen. Many cytoplasmic ribosomes are seen in the cytoplasm of the adjacent cells. (Courtesy of Kathleen Green.)

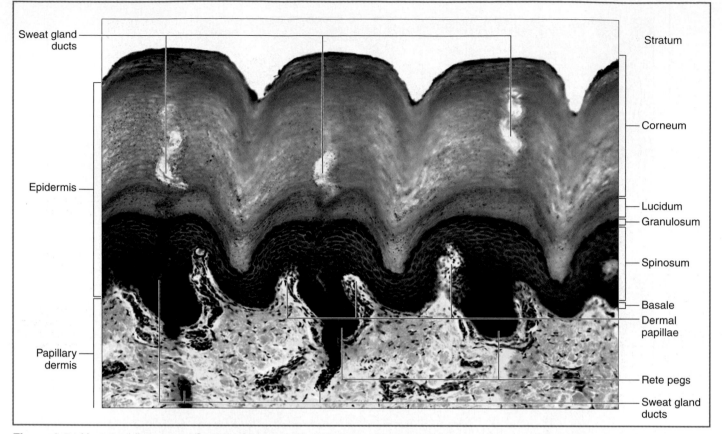

Figure 9-5. Hematoxylin–orange G stain of plantar skin (80×). The five layers of the epidermis of thick skin and other features of the integument are visible.

Figures 9-6 through 9-9 show examples of these specialized cells.

Dermis and Hypodermis

Dermis

The dermis is a layer of connective tissue directly under the epidermis and is thicker than the epidermis (see Fig. 9-1). The dermis is composed mostly of collagen and elastin fibers. An extensive network of blood vessels in the dermis provides nourishment to the epidermis, which (like other epithelial tissues) lacks blood vessels. The dermis also contains many sweat glands, nerves and nerve endings, lymphatic vessels, hair shafts, and specialized oil-secreting glands called sebaceous glands.

The dermis has two layers. The upper layer, called the papillary dermis, forms the interface with the epidermis and accounts for about one fifth of the dermal thickness; it is a good example of loose connective tissue. In a section of skin, the papillary dermis appears to consist of an irregular set of interdigitating structures, somewhat like interlocking fingers of clasped hands. The downward projections from the epidermis are called rete pegs, and those that project upward from the papillary dermis are called dermal papillae. In three dimensions, the pegs and dermal papillae actually are a series of interdigitating ridges and grooves, but they were originally named based on their appearance in tissue sections. The papillary dermis has many capillaries and small caliber arterioles and venules. Certain regions of the integument (e.g., fingertips) have large numbers of sensory receptors. They are called Meissner's corpuscles and are nerve endings of unmyelinated nerves; they function as fine touch receptors (Fig. 9-10). Sweat gland ducts and hair shafts are seen in this layer.

The deeper and thicker layer of the dermis is called the reticular dermis. Fibers within this layer are thicker, more densely packed than those in the papillary dermis, and irregularly arranged to form a tough, flexible meshwork. The reticular dermis is a good example of dense irregular connective tissue (see Figs. 9-1B and 9-6B). This layer is also highly vascular and may contain large arterioles and venules, nerve bundles, sweat glands and their ducts, and hair follicles with their associated sebaceous glands.

Hypodermis

In anatomic and some histologic nomenclature, the hypodermis is often not considered part of the skin and is called superficial fascia. However, from a histologic point of view, the hypodermis can be considered part of the integument, since it contains the secretory portions of sweat

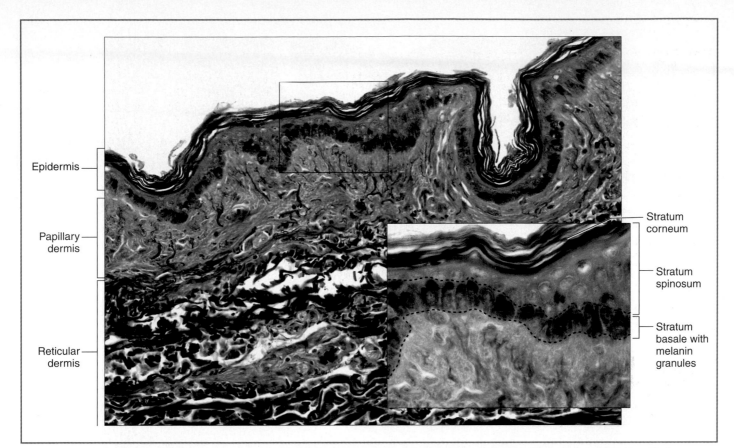

Figure 9-6. Trichrome stain of thin skin from an individual with a pigmented epidermis (200×). The stratum basale cells have many melanin granules, which are seen more clearly in the inset (1250×). The papillary and reticular dermis show large amounts of collagen (green-blue) and elastin (magenta) fibers.

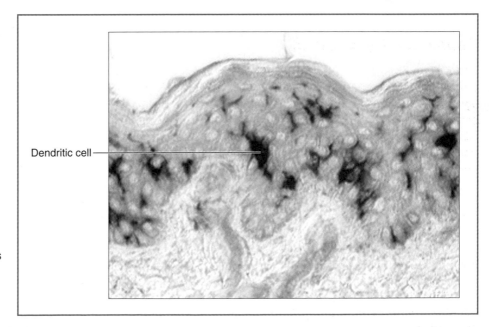

Figure 9-7. Immunostain of Langerhans cells in the epidermis. (From Abbas AK, Lichtman AH. *Cellular and Molecular Immunology,* 5th ed. Philadelphia, WB Saunders, 2005, p 87.)

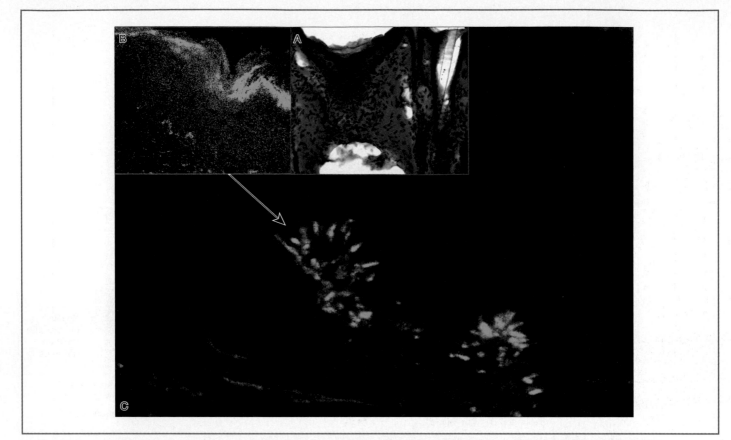

Figure 9-8. A, H&E stain of mouse epidermis (130×). **B,** Confocal immunofluorescence image of the same section of two Merkel's cells in the basal layer of the epidermis stained with an antibody to espin, an actin bundling protein. **C,** Higher magnification of part B (about 500×.) (Courtesy of Gabriella Sekerkova and James R. Bartles.)

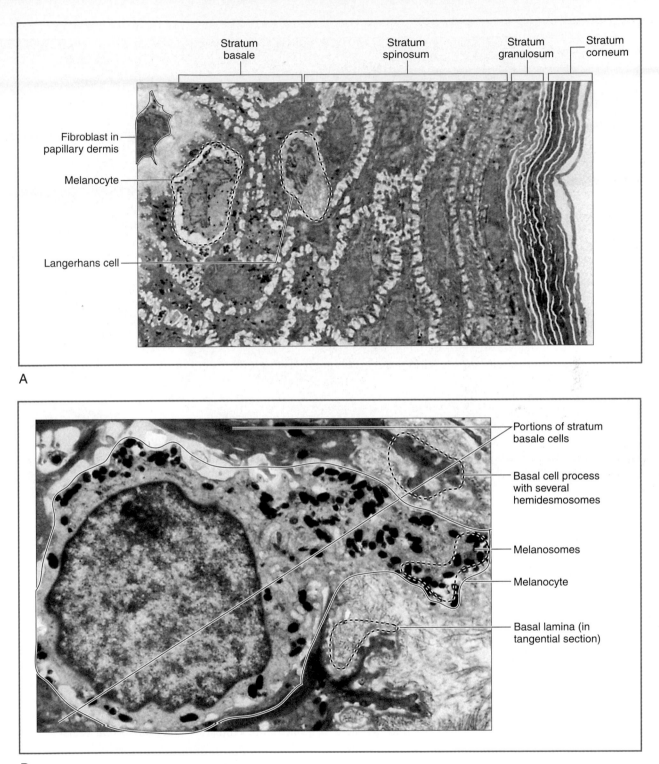

Figure 9-9. Pair of electron micrographs of the epidermis. **A,** Section of a region of thin epidermis in which a melanocyte and a Langerhans cell can be seen (1800×). **B,** Higher magnification of a different melanocyte in which the abundance of melanosomes can be seen (10,000×). (Courtesy of Judith Taggert Rhodin.)

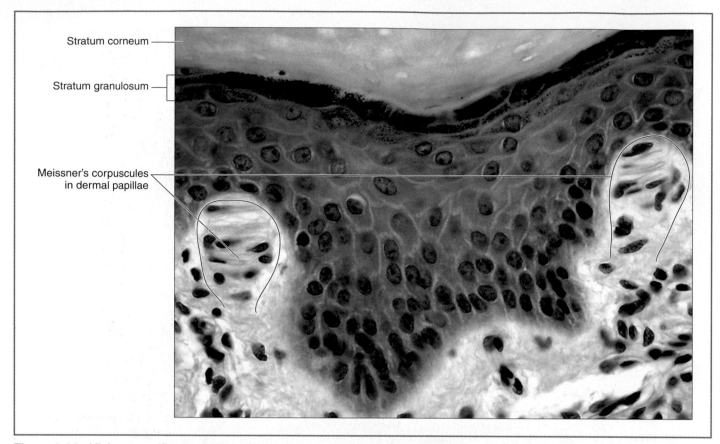

Stratum corneum

Stratum granulosum

Meissner's corpuscules
in dermal papillae

Figure 9-10. Higher magnification (360×) of the micrograph in Figure 9-2B. A Meissner corpuscle is seen in each of two of the dermal papillae, their typical location, and some layers of the epidermis are seen more clearly.

glands and the base (bulbs) of hair follicles. It consists of loose, fatty connective tissue and long strands of dermis-like connective tissue that help anchor it to the deep fascia (Fig. 9-11; see also Fig. 9-1B). The reticular dermis and hypodermis may have specialized nerve endings called pacinian corpuscles (see Innervation of the Integument).

●●● GLANDS OF THE INTEGUMENT

Sweat Glands

Humans have two kinds of sweat glands: eccrine and apocrine. Both are exocrine glands and secrete by the merocrine mechanism. The secretory portions of both are surrounded by myoepithelial cells.

Eccrine sweat glands are the most abundant and are found throughout the entire integument except the lips and parts of the external genitalia. The secretions of eccrine sweat glands are watery, slightly salty (hypotonic), and odor-free. They are simple coiled tubular glands with a tightly coiled secretory portion and a long, slightly wavy duct that opens onto the surface of the epidermis via pores. The secretory cells are tall cuboidal and have a light-staining cytoplasm; the ducts may have two layers of cuboidal cells and stain more darkly than the secretory cells. The secretory segments are mainly

found in the deep reticular dermis or the upper hypodermis (Fig. 9-12).

Apocrine sweat glands are found in the axilla (armpits and groin) and in the perianal areas of the body. They are larger than eccrine sweat glands, have a much larger lumen, and are also coiled tubular glands (Fig. 9-13). Their secretory products are stored in the apical part of the cell. The secretions have protein and lipid components; these products are odorless at the time of secretion but are acted upon by bacteria on the surface of the skin, resulting in an odor characteristic of the specific location of the glands. The suggestion that apocrine secretions are a source of one or more human pheromones has been the subject of study for several years.

Sebaceous Glands

Sebaceous glands are almost always found in association with hair follicles. Their secretions empty into the emerging hair shaft through a duct called the *pilosebaceous* duct. The glands have a tubuloalveolar shape and secrete by the holocrine mechanism. This means the cell undergoes a process of programmed cell death, which in this case results in production of a protein- and lipid-rich material called sebum, which is derived from the entire cell. The oily sebum is a lubricant for hair and skin (Fig. 9-14).

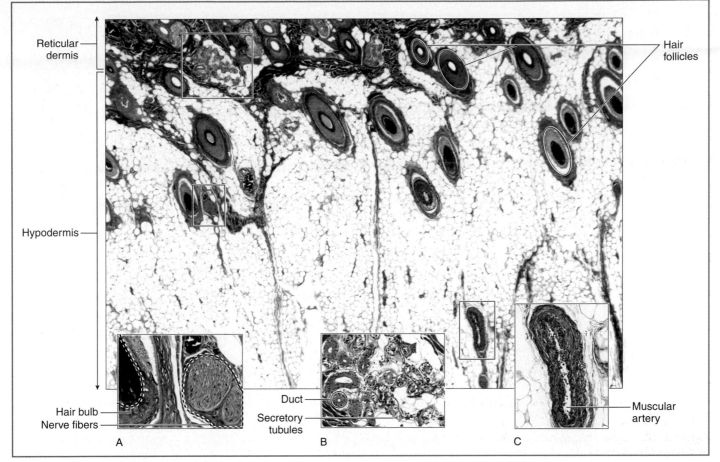

Figure 9-11. Low-magnification image of the hypodermis (Mallory's trichrome stain, 15×). A small amount of reticular dermis is seen at the upper part of the field. Many slightly oblique sections of hair follicles appear in the upper half of the field. The majority of the hypodermis is filled with adipose tissue with some long strands of collagen fibers that anchor it to the underlying tissue. There are many small blood vessels in the hypodermis. **A,** Higher magnification (210×) of part of a hair bulb, a small artery, and a nerve fiber bundle. **B,** Higher magnification (140×) of a sweat gland at the dermal-hypodermal interface. **C,** Higher magnification (125×) of a small muscular artery in the middle of the hypodermis.

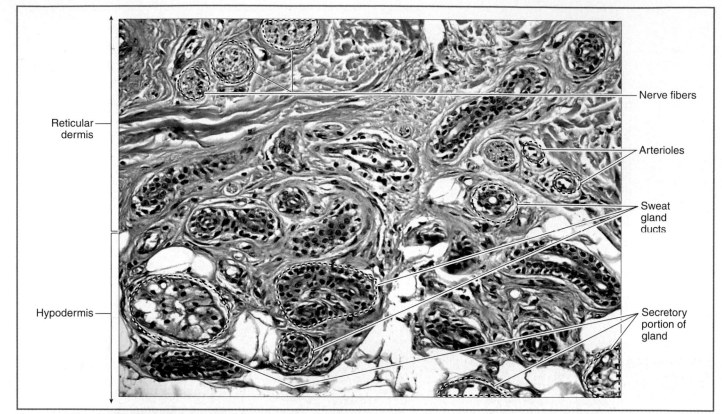

Figure 9-12. H&E stained section of eccrine sweat glands at the dermal/hypodermal boundary of the integument (140×). There are several profiles of the secretory tubules of the coiled glands and many more sweat gland ducts than secretory portions in this field of view. The secretory portions have a dense magenta-pink stained outline; these are the myoepithelial cells of this part of the gland.

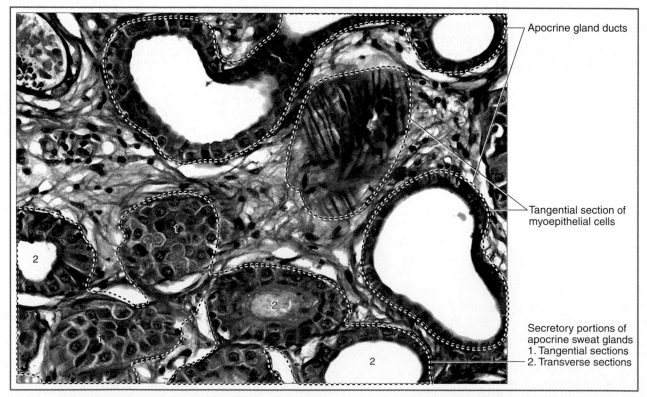

Figure 9-13. H&E stained section of apocrine sweat glands in the hypodermis (200×). Several sections of the secretory portions of the glands are seen at lower left. Some of the tubules are sectioned tangentially (1) and some are sectioned transversely (2). Note the dark-staining secretory contents stored at the apical end of the cells of the transversely sectioned tubules. A tangential section of the myoepithelial cells of a secretory portion of a gland is seen in the upper right central part of the field.

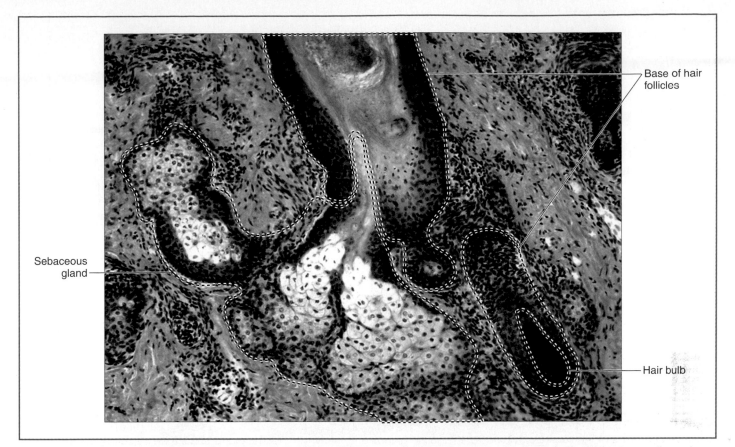

Figure 9-14. Hematoxylin–orange G stain of a hair follicle and its associated sebaceous gland (80×). The secretory cells and their duct entering the hair follicle are clearly seen.

●●● HAIR AND NAILS

Hair is a complex structure. Each individual hair originates in a hair follicle whose most active living cellular components are found deep in the dermis, or more commonly, the hypodermis. Hair has most of the same epithelial and connective tissue components as the rest of the integument; however, there are no stratum granulosum or stratum corneum components. Furthermore, the keratinized plates of hair do not desquamate as does the epidermis. The bottom of a follicle is called the hair bulb and has a small basal invagination of vascular connective tissue called a dermal papilla. The growing portion of a hair follicle has about 10 layers depending on where along the length of the growing hair shaft a section is taken. The hair itself is a long, tapering cylinder of flattened cells filled with keratin, which is commonly called hard keratin. In general terms, hair is described as having a medulla, a cortex, and a cuticle (Fig. 9-15).

Unlike the epidermis, of which hair is a derivative, not all hair grows continuously throughout life. An actively growing hair follicle is referred to as being in *anagen*. A follicle may become quiescent, at which time it is said to be in *catagen*.

Many follicles typically cycle between anagen and catagen. Quiescent follicles may undergo a long rest period followed by follicular atrophy at which time they enter a phase called *telogen*. It is this progression that leads to baldness, since follicles in telogen do not reenter the anagen phase. While these three phases are characteristic of all hair follicles, the telogen phase is most prevalent on the scalp. Males have a much larger proportion of follicles in telogen than females; consequently, they may exhibit extensive baldness. Females do not usually become bald, but their hair may thin substantially as they age.

Structures Associated with Hair

Two major structures are associated with hair follicles: *sebaceous glands* (described previously in this chapter) and *arrector pili* muscles.

Most individual hairs are connected to a small slip of smooth muscle called the arrector pili muscle; it is found in the reticular dermis at an acute angle to the hair. Most body hair is oriented at an acute angle to the epidermis. One end of the arrector pili muscle is connected to the connective

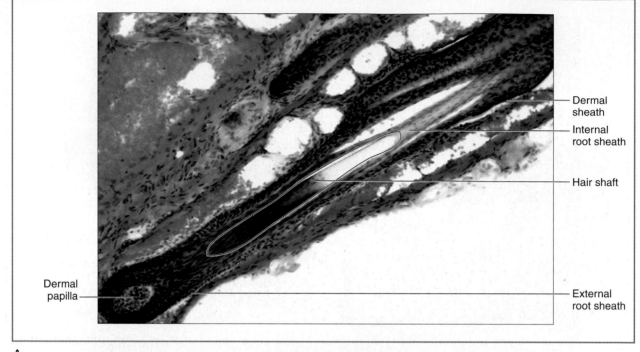

Dermal
sheath

Internal
root sheath

Hair shaft

Dermal
papilla

External
root sheath

A

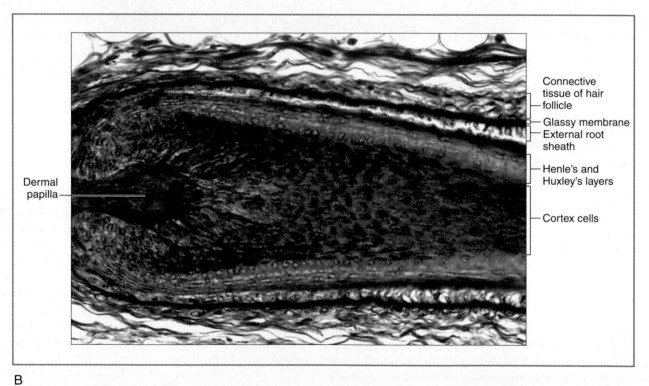

Connective
tissue of hair
follicle

Glassy membrane
External root
sheath

Henle's and
Huxley's layers

Cortex cells

Dermal
papilla

B

Figure 9-15. A, H&E stain of a hair bulb, follicle, and shaft of mouse epidermis (100×). These structures are sectioned in a longitudinal plane somewhat away from the diameter of the overall cylinder. Part of the dermal papilla is seen. **B,** H&E stain of a longitudinal section of a hair bulb (180×). Most of the individual layers of the generative region of a growing hair can be seen in this section. The cells of the cortex are those that form the lasting keratinized substance of the hair seen protruding from the epidermis. The other cells become keratinized but are shed from the hair shaft as it grows toward the free surface of the skin. Note the pigmented cortex cells near the dermal papilla.

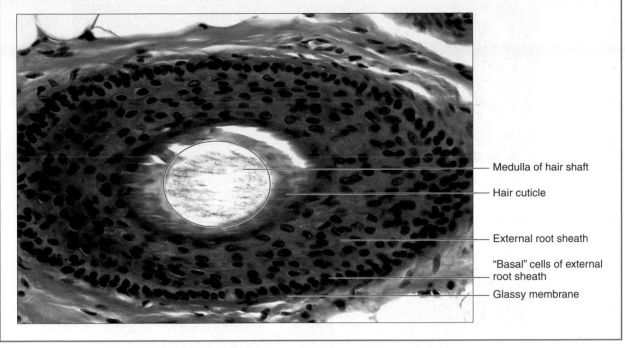

C

Figure 9-15 cont'd. C, Transverse section of a hair follicle in the reticular dermis (H&E, 250×). This section is slightly oblique. Since it is well above the dermal papilla seen in the preceding figure, there are fewer cellular layers than are seen in part B. There is a thick layer of stratified cells of the external root sheath; these will keratinize but desquamate before the hair emerges from the epidermis.

tissue sheath of the hair, and the other end is connected to the papillary dermis. During times of stress (cold, fear, excitement) hair may "stand on end" or the skin may feel like it has "goose bumps." This appearance or feeling is due to the contraction of the arrector pili muscles. When they contract, the surface of the epidermis is slightly depressed and the hairs are pulled to an angle more perpendicular to the epidermis. Figure 9-16 shows a longitudinal section and two cross-sections of hair follicles and their associated structures.

Nails

Like hair, the fingernails and toenails (nail plates) are composed of hard keratin. The proximal part of the nail, the nail root, is firmly embedded in the epidermis at the base of the nail and along its lateral margins. The keratin matrix of the nail is produced by cells that are equivalent to the stratum basale and spinosum; a stratum granulosum and a stratum corneum are lacking. As the nail grows, it is pushed along the nail bed, where the flattened keratinocytes become drier, flatter, and somewhat more translucent. This allows the underlying vasculature to be seen through the nail plate, giving it a pinkish color. A white crescent-shaped area, the lunula, near the nail root is a region of more hydrated (less mature) flattened keratinocytes; hence, they are less transparent than the mature keratinocytes (Figs. 9-17 and 9-18).

●●● INNERVATION OF THE INTEGUMENT

Several specialized nerve endings are associated with the integument. A few are encapsulated, and some are described as being "free nerve endings," since they lack a connective tissue or Schwann cell sheath. It is common to see numerous profiles of sectioned nerves in the dermis and hypodermis.

The dermal papillae of the fingertips and lips contain receptors that respond to delicate touch; these are called Meissner's corpuscles (see Fig. 9-7). Pacinian corpuscles are found deep in the dermis and in the hypodermis. These receptors are responsive to vibration and to deep pressure. Each of these structures is in a connective tissue space and is surrounded by a delicate connective tissue capsule; both can readily be seen in light micrographs (Fig. 9-19).

There are also some receptors that are visualized only with special stains or the electron microscope. Two kinds are free nerve endings that terminate in the epidermis. One appears to contact keratinocytes directly, and the other interacts with Merkel cells. A third is a very small (about 1 to 2 μm) encapsulated body called Ruffini's corpuscle; it is found in the dermis. It is thought to be responsive to sustained or mechanical stress of the fibers in the dermis.

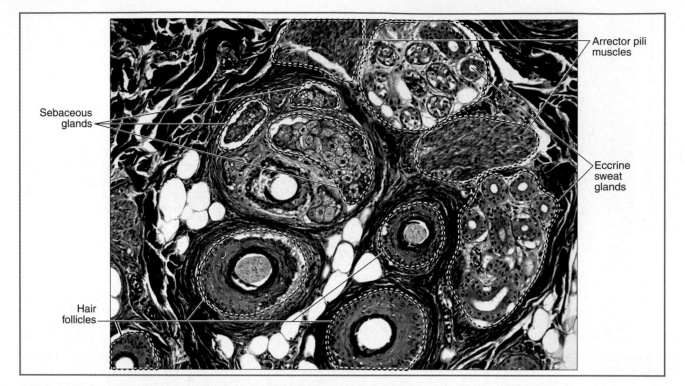

Figure 9-16. Section of the scalp in a plane parallel to the epidermis just about at the level of the interface of the reticular dermis and the hypodermis (Mallory's trichrome, 80×). The presence of hair follicles, a sebaceous gland, sweat glands, and arrector pili muscles illustrates the intimate structural and functional relationship of these components. The structures that occupy the large circular area in the center of the field appear to be a functional unit of scalp hair.

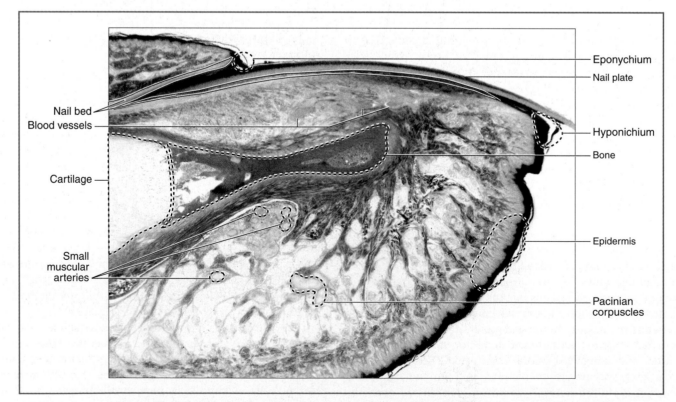

Figure 9-17. Longitudinal section of the fingertip of an infant (Milligan's trichrome stain, 8.5×). The major characteristics of a fingertip are seen—the eponychium, the hyponychium, nail bed and nail plate, the highly vascular nature of the connective tissue under the nail, and most of the other features of the integument.

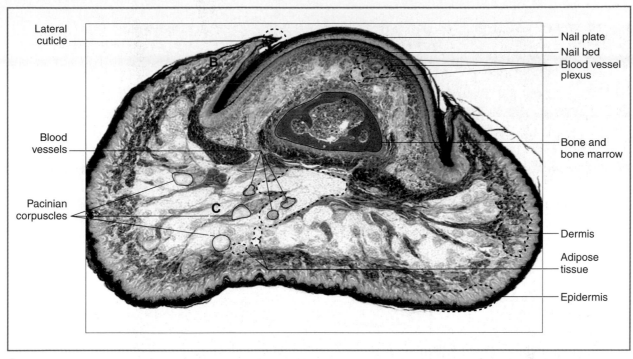

A

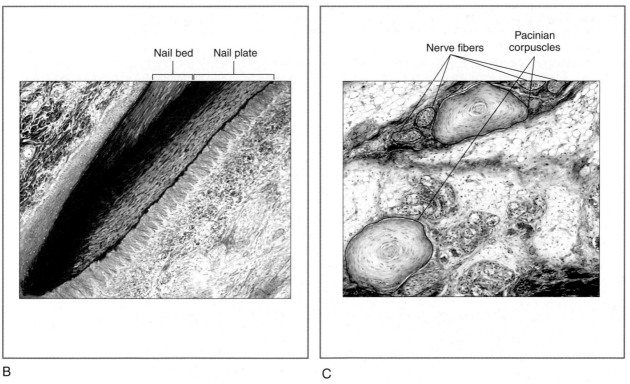

B   C

Figure 9-18. A, Transverse section of a similar fingertip as in Figure 9-17 (8×). The keratin of the curved nail plate is stained bright red. Many blood vessels are seen just underneath the nail plate, and although they are difficult to discern at this low magnification, there are four pacinian corpuscles in the hypodermis. **B,** Insertion of the nail plate into the lateral fold of the adjacent skin (80×). There is a layer of columnar cells that lie under the nail bed and another layer of stratum basale and stratum spinosum cells above it; these cells actively produce the nail matrix of the nail plate. **C,** Two pacinian corpuscles at higher magnification and several sweat glands (90×).

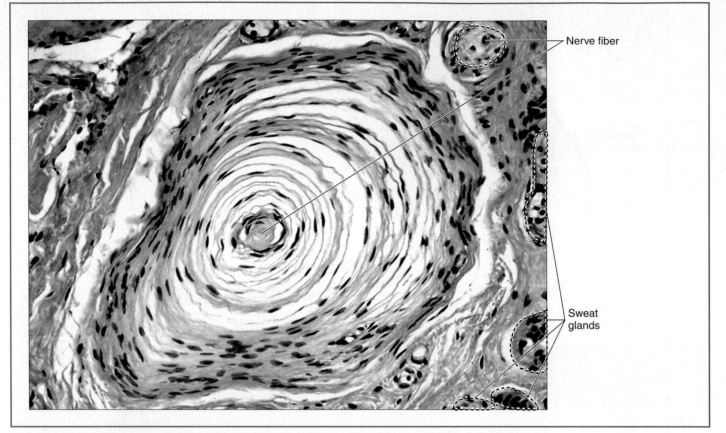

Nerve fiber

Sweat glands

Figure 9-19. Section of a pacinian corpuscle from deep in the reticular dermis of a fingertip (H&E, 170×). The nerve is at the center of the spirally wrapped fibroblast-like supporting cells of the corpuscle. In the living state, the empty spaces are filled with fluid. A somewhat more dense connective tissue sheath surrounds the entire structure. A small nerve fiber, possibly associated with this corpuscle, is seen in the upper right corner of the field; portions of a few sweat gland tubular glands are seen at the right edge of the field.

Endocrine Organs

10

The task of describing the endocrine organs histologically has become more daunting in recent years because the boundaries of the endocrine system have enlarged. In the past, the endocrine system was defined as a discrete number of organs that secrete biologically active molecules—hormones—into the bloodstream to affect the function of other organs. By this definition, however, the endocrine system has expanded enormously. It is now known that many tissues and organs secrete hormones. Many examples come to mind: fat cells secrete leptin, a hormone that regulates adiposity; cardiac muscle cells secrete atrial natriuretic peptide, which regulates water balance in the body; the kidney secretes erythropoietin, which regulates red blood cell production; and so on. What saves us from examining the endocrine roles of almost all tissues and organs in the body is that they have a nonendocrine primary function. Thus, we can focus our attention on those organs having a primary function of secreting hormones that traditionally have represented the endocrine system.

●●● PITUITARY GLAND

The pituitary gland has two main divisions: an anterior lobe, derived from epithelial cells of the buccal ectoderm of the embryo (Rathke's pouch), and a posterior (neural) lobe, derived from a down-growth of the neural tube of the embryo (infundibulum) (Fig. 10-1).

The long history of study of the pituitary gland by histologists has led to a rather complex nomenclature for this organ. It is also known by a term originating from the Greek (hypophysis) and thus can be divided into an anterior adenohypophysis (pars distalis) and a posterior neurohypophysis (pars nervosa). The portion of the anterior pituitary that wraps around the neural infundibular stalk that descends from the brain is called the pars tuberalis.

Anterior Pituitary

The anterior pituitary is formed mainly by masses of endocrine epithelial cells plus small amounts of connective tissue and an abundant vasculature dominated by fenestrated capillaries. Two types of hormone-secreting cells are detectable:

ANATOMY & EMBRYOLOGY

The Pituitary

Creation of the two outgrowths of pituitary tissue is under the control of a number of transcription-regulating proteins (homeotic proteins) that become expressed in the early stages of embryogenesis. One of these proteins, called Ptx1, also seems to be involved in the creation of outgrowths from the brain that become the eyes. Another homeotic protein, called Lhx3, is more specific to the pituitary and is required for the creation of Rathke's pouch and the differentiation of hormone-secreting cells of the pituitary. The unusual developmental process that creates the pituitary from the union of two different types of tissues leaves behind some traces that can have functional consequences for the adult. For example, a small scrap of pituitary tissue—the pharyngeal hypophysis—can be found beneath the periosteum overlying the junction between the sphenoid and vomer bones of the nasal cavity. It is much smaller than the pituitary proper but does contain some endocrine cells. Additional rests of tissue between the nasal cavity and the pituitary persist after embryogenesis and, in some circumstances, form tumors called craniopharyngiomas that can enlarge and compress the pituitary. Pituitary tumors in general represent almost 10% of all intracranial tumors; about 75% of these tumors secrete hormones.

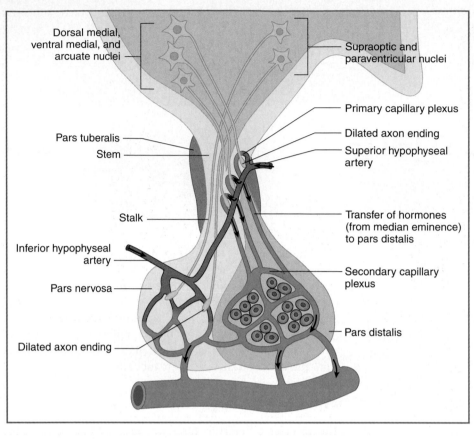

Figure 10-1. Diagram of the anatomy of the pituitary gland.

Labels (clockwise):
Dorsal medial, ventral medial, and arcuate nuclei
Supraoptic and paraventricular nuclei
Primary capillary plexus
Dilated axon ending
Superior hypophyseal artery
Transfer of hormones (from median eminence) to pars distalis
Secondary capillary plexus
Pars distalis
Dilated axon ending
Pars nervosa
Inferior hypophyseal artery
Stalk
Stem
Pars tuberalis

acidophil cells that have a cytoplasm brightly stained by acid dyes such as eosin, and basophil cells with a basophilic cytoplasm that stains with hematoxylin (Fig. 10-2). The basis for this differential staining pattern of the two cell types is different from that underlying the staining of most cell types.

In other tissues, cells with a basophilic cytoplasm (such as plasma cells) contain large amounts of rough endoplasmic reticulum (rER), which is basophilic owing to ribonucleic acid content. In the pituitary, cytoplasmic basophilia arises not from rER but from the staining properties of hormone-containing secretion granules.

Hormones secreted from basophils have a common feature: their polypeptide chains are highly glycosylated (the proteins are 27% carbohydrate by weight). Moreover, the carbohydrate groups are sialic acid rich. It is the acid nature of the carbohydrate groups that makes them basophilic. In fact, however, this cytoplasmic basophilia is not always a reliable way to distinguish basophils from acidophils. Preferable ways of identifying pituitary basophils include the periodic acid–Schiff (PAS) stain for carbohydrates, or an immunocytochemical method for the specific hormones produced by basophils (Fig. 10-3).

Basophil cells account for 15% to 25% of the cells of the anterior pituitary and are named according to the hormones they secrete. Gonadotrope cells secrete follicle-stimulating hormone (FSH) or luteinizing hormone (LH); about 70% of gonadotropes secrete both hormones, which control the gonads. Thyrotrope cells secrete thyroid-stimulating hormone (TSH) but also commonly secrete either LH or FSH as well.

Another cell type classifiable as a basophil, because of its content of glycosylated hormones, is a cell that produces a long, glycosylated, precursor protein called pro-opiomelanocortin (POMC). POMC can be cleaved into a number of molecules, including α-melanocyte-stimulating hormone (α-MSH), β-endorphin, and adrenocorticotropic hormone (ACTH). In the human pituitary, which lacks a discrete intermediate lobe, basophils of the anterior lobe secrete all three molecules. ACTH stimulates the human adrenal cortex to synthesize cortisol, whereas MSH stimulates melanin production by skin cells and β-endorphin reduces the reactivity of nerves to painful stimuli.

Curiously, the pituitary is not the only source of POMC peptides in the body—keratinocyte cells of the skin also produce these peptides. When damaged by sunlight, keratinocytes release α-MSH, which stimulates melanocytes and causes the skin to darken for protection against ultraviolet light. Also, in furry mammals, production of ACTH by skin cells stimulates sebaceous glands to secrete an oily substance that helps hairs shed water during a rainfall. Since cells in both the anterior pituitary and skin are ectodermal epithelial cells, it may not be so surprising that they share the ability to make these hormones.

The acidophils of the anterior pituitary, which account for at least two thirds of the total cells, secrete either growth

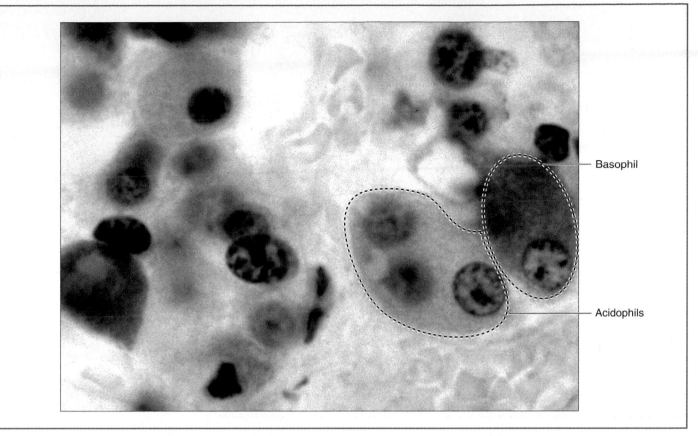

Figure 10-2. Human anterior pituitary, stained with H&E. Darker staining basophils often possess a more prominent Golgi apparatus than do acidophils, probably because of the extensive glycosylation of basophil hormones that is conducted within the Golgi. The pale area near the nucleus in the basophil cell probably represents the Golgi apparatus.

hormone or prolactin, protein hormones that are not glycosylated. Growth hormone (GH) stimulates growth of muscles and other soft tissues as well as the epiphyseal growth plates of long bones. However, GH accomplishes this indirectly, by stimulating the synthesis of insulin-like growth factor 1 (IGF-1) by peripheral tissues such as bones, muscles, and liver. Excessive secretion of growth hormone before puberty can cause excessive height (gigantism). When this occurs after puberty and the closure of epiphyseal growth cartilage plates, growth hormone can no longer affect overall height, but it may cause an overgrowth of hands and feet and of soft tissues of the face (acromegaly).

Prolactin has a stimulatory effect on milk synthesis by the mammary glands. However, prolactin also appears to have a potent stimulatory effect on cells of the immune system. Consequently, elevated blood levels of prolactin are now thought to play a role in the development of autoimmune diseases such as systemic lupus erythematosus.

All the cell types of the anterior pituitary can be specifically stained by antibodies against the hormones they secrete with immunocytochemical methods. This is the preferred technique of microscopic examination of the pituitary. Another way to distinguish one cell type from another is via transmission electron microscopy. High

magnification views of the anterior pituitary show that the secretory granules of each cell type have distinctive sizes and staining characteristics (e.g., the secretory vesicles found in cells that synthesize prolactin are larger than the vesicles found in cells that make growth hormone). This is not the only example of a correlation between the *content* of a secretory granule and the *size* of a secretory granule (e.g., mast cells that secrete histamine have very large secretory granules, whereas salivary gland cells that secrete amylase have smaller granules).

Regulation of Anterior Pituitary Function

Anterior pituitary cells are regulated by small peptides (releasing hormones) that are synthesized by neurons of the hypothalamus and released into portal capillaries that carry these peptides from the brain to the pituitary. Isolation and identification of these small and scarce peptides required heroic efforts by their discoverers, Andrew Schally and Roger Guillemin, who were awarded the Nobel Prize for their work. For example, originally, 50 tons of sheep hypothalami had to be processed to yield only 1 mg of the first releasing hormone to be characterized: thyrotropin-releasing hormone (TRH). Since then additional stimulatory peptides (corticotropin-releasing hormone, growth hormone–releasing hormone,

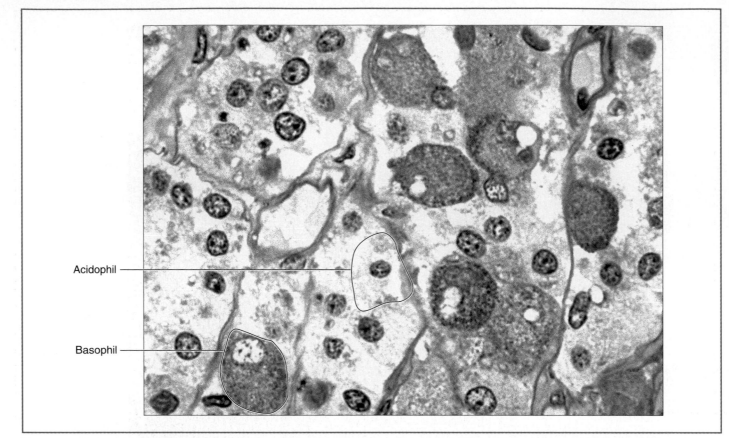

Figure 10-3. Anterior pituitary, stained with the PAS procedure for carbohydrates and counterstained with toluidine blue. The basophil cells have cytoplasmic granules that stain intensely pink after exposure to PAS reagent. This allows their identification as cells that produce the glycosylated hormones FSH, LH, or TSH. The paler staining cells are acidophils, which produce growth hormone or prolactin. Note that the PAS reaction also stains the basal laminae surrounding capillaries; this is due to the high carbohydrate content of basal laminae.

gonadotropin-releasing hormone, and prolactin-releasing hormone) and inhibitory peptides (somatostatin) have been found. Gonadotropin-releasing hormone, presently known as LHRH but also known as GnRH, is some 15-fold more effective in causing the release of LH than of FSH; this has led some to speculate that a yet undiscovered FSH-releasing hormone may exist.

If the portal capillaries leading from the hypothalamus are severed or blocked, most anterior pituitary hormones show a decreased rate of secretion, except for prolactin. Control of prolactin secretion thus has some unique features; experiments suggest that prolactin secretion is primarily inhibited by the hypothalamus rather than stimulated. Furthermore, the inhibitory agent produced by the hypothalamus (in the arcuate nucleus) is the neurotransmitter dopamine, a catecholamine and not a peptide (Fig. 10-4). In addition, another peptide produced by pituitary cells, endothelin, has an inhibitory effect on prolactin secretion.

Production of all these hypothalamic releasing hormones is controlled by negative feedback. Most anterior pituitary hormones exert their effects by stimulating the production of secondary hormones in peripheral organs (e.g., ACTH stimulates cortisol production; TSH stimulates thyroxine production; GH stimulates IGF-1 production; LH stimulates testosterone production; FSH stimulates the production of a protein hormone, inhibin, by the gonads). All these secondary hormones "feed back" on both the hypothalamus and pituitary to regulate anterior pituitary hormone production. Thus, secretion of pituitary hormones is a self-regulating system. However, it does not imply that all pituitary hormones are secreted at the same rates throughout life. In fact, it appears that a decrease in inhibitory negative feedback of sex steroids on LH and FSH secretion is responsible for the stimulation of the gonads that occurs at puberty. The causes of this peripubertal change in anterior pituitary function are incompletely understood but may involve an effect of rising levels of the adipocyte hormone, leptin, that are seen as physical maturity progresses.

Posterior Pituitary

The posterior pituitary is composed of bundles of axons that originate in the hypothalamus plus associated support cells called pituicytes that resemble CNS astrocytes (Fig. 10-5). The

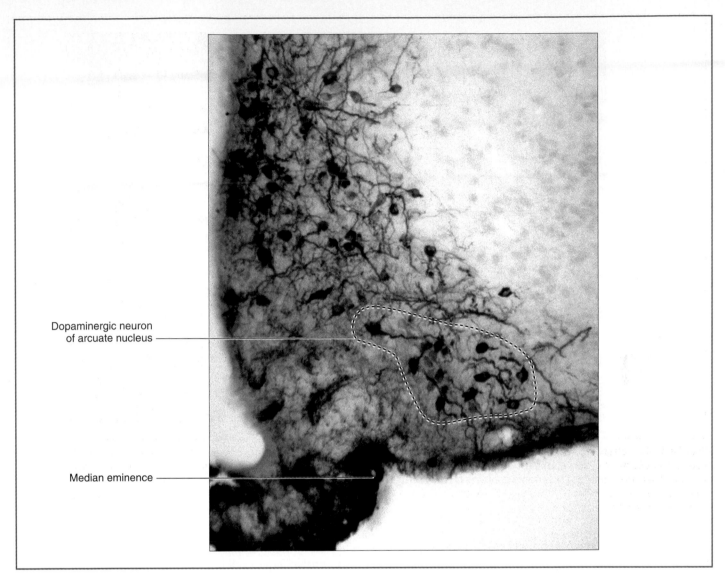

Dopaminergic neuron
of arcuate nucleus

Median eminence

Figure 10-4. Hypothalamus of a rat. This micrograph shows a cluster of neurons that have been stained for tyrosine hydroxylase with an immunocytochemical method. These neurons produce the neurotransmitter dopamine. They are located in a collection of neurons called the arcuate nucleus, and they project to fiber pathways in the median eminence. Dopamine is released into capillaries in the median eminence, a structure that connects the pituitary to the hypothalamus. Dopamine that is carried to the anterior pituitary inhibits the release of prolactin.

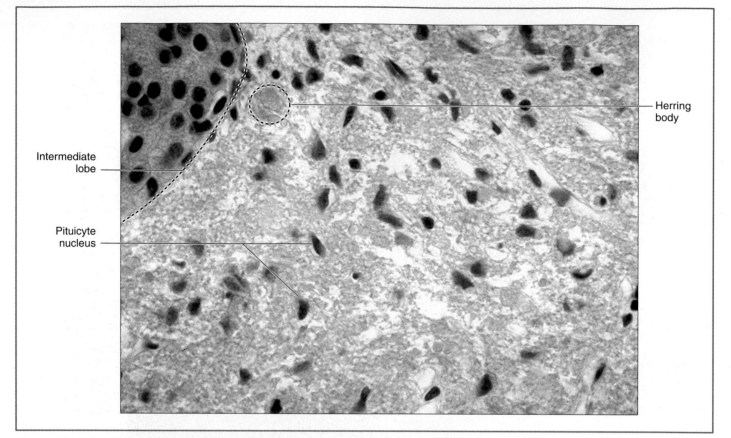

Intermediate lobe

Pituicyte nucleus

Herring body

Figure 10-5. Posterior pituitary, stained with H&E. This image of the monkey pituitary shows cells that belong to the intermediate lobe of the pituitary, which is absent as a discrete structure in humans. The posterior lobe cells are pituicytes. The pale pink–staining structure is a hormone-containing axon terminus termed a Herring body.

PATHOLOGY

The Posterior Pituitary

The endocrine function of the posterior pituitary was discovered by Alfred Frank, a German physician. Frank examined a patient with a gunshot wound to the head. The patient had largely recovered from his injury but complained of a need to urinate frequently and constant thirst. These symptoms arose from a bullet that lodged in the posterior pituitary and prevented the secretion of vasopressin. The resultant constant water loss in the urine (diabetes insipidus) provoked excessive thirst and consumption of large volumes of water. Less dramatic forms of posterior pituitary dysfunction result in a similar condition that is occasionally seen in clinical practice.

axons originate in two clusters of large, dark-staining, magnocellular hypothalamic neurons called the paraventricular and supraoptic nuclei. Neurons in these nuclei synthesize either vasopressin (antidiuretic hormone, ADH) or oxytocin. Both hormones are small peptides (9 amino acids in length) that originally were part of a larger protein that becomes cleaved into the hormone and a carrier protein, neurophysin, which is transported along an axon with the hormone. Along the course of the axon, masses of hormone-containing secretory granules accumulate within axonal swellings called Herring bodies. These can sometimes be visualized with special stains such as aldehyde thionin, but in routine preparations of the posterior pituitary, they are difficult to perceive (Figs. 10-6 and 10-7).

Vasopressin is a hormone that is released during dehydration or osmotic stress, and it elevates blood pressure by acting on the kidneys to inhibit water loss in the urine. This function seems primarily mediated by neurons in the supraoptic nucleus, which are substantially more sensitive to osmotic stimuli than those in the paraventricular nucleus.

Oxytocin stimulates contraction of myoepithelial cells of the mammary glands and thus promotes milk ejection during nursing. Oxytocin can also stimulate contraction of uterine smooth muscle and so can be used clinically to accelerate labor. Viewpoints about this action of pituitary oxytocin have undergone a substantial revision in recent years. Originally, oxytocin was viewed as essential for labor and delivery, but studies in mice genetically manipulated to lack oxytocin have shown that these mice have no deficits in parturition, whereas they do have difficulty in suckling their offspring. Thus, the

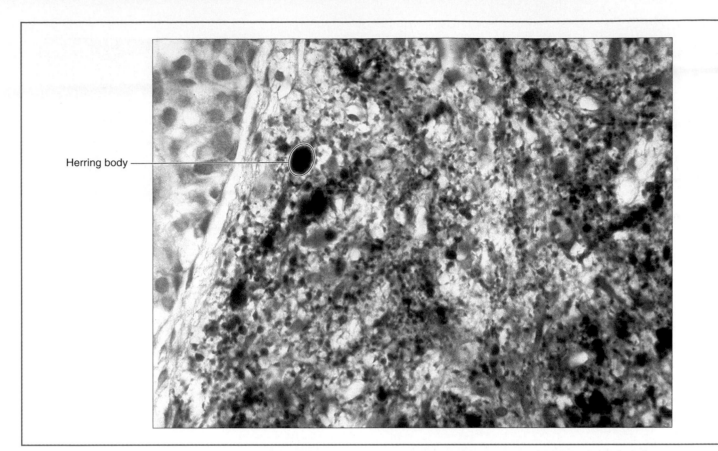

Herring body

Figure 10-6. Posterior pituitary stained with aldehyde thionin, to demonstrate neurosecretory material, plus a fast green counterstain, to demonstrate cell nuclei. As in Figure 10-5, the cells of the intermediate lobe and pituicyte cells of the posterior lobe are visible. This preparation clearly shows accumulations of hormone (oxytocin and vasopressin) within Herring bodies.

precise role of oxytocin in reproduction is not completely clear. Recent studies have shown that oxytocin also exerts effects on the brain and enhances cooperative social behavior and parenting behavior in rodents. Finally, oxytocin is also produced in extrapituitary sites such as the uterine endometrium and the heart and appears to have an important influence on heart development and cardiovascular function. This may not be so surprising in view of the substantial sequence homology of oxytocin with vasopressin, another cardiovascular hormone.

●●● ADRENAL GLAND

The adrenal gland has a distinct cortex, derived from mesoderm, and medulla, derived from neuroectoderm. Unlike the pituitary, the cortical portion of the adrenal gland forms first and then is invaded by neural crest cells that burrow into it to form small islands of medullary tissue that eventually coalesce into a discrete medulla. The exact mechanisms underlying this mixing of two previously separate tissues to form an adult organ are not completely understood. However, some details of the development of the adrenal gland have emerged.

The adrenal gland forms from tissue located on the ventral surface of the embryonic kidney (mesonephros), termed the genital ridge. Early in development, this tissue splits into two masses. One mass of mesodermal cells migrates cranially to form the adrenal gland; the other mass migrates caudally to form the gonad. Subsequently, a protein called steroidogenic factor-1 accumulates in both the adrenal and gonadal cells and promotes their further differentiation. An experimental disruption of this protein results in mice born without adrenals or gonads.

When neural crest cells settle within the adrenal, they acquire a new transcription regulating protein (homeotic protein) called Phox2B. This protein binds to the promoter region of a gene for tyrosine hydroxylase, an enzyme critical for the synthesis of catecholamines. Henceforth, the neural crest cells are transformed into chromaffin cells that make catecholamines such as norepinephrine and epinephrine. These adult cells acquired their name when it was found that exposure to an ingredient in a fixative, potassium dichromate, caused a brown precipitate to form within them. This was due to an affinity, or reactivity, of catecholamines with dichromate. Thus, adult adrenal glands possess both medullary chromaffin cells that synthesize catecholamines

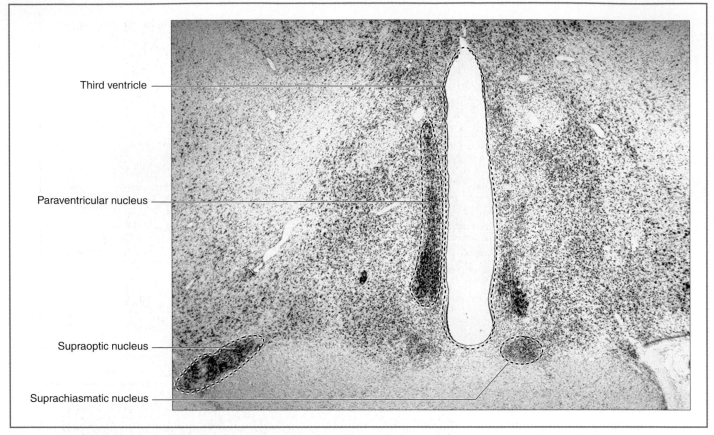

Third ventricle

Paraventricular nucleus

Supraoptic nucleus

Suprachiasmatic nucleus

Figure 10-7. Hypothalamus. This overview of a monkey hypothalamus shows the sites where posterior pituitary hormones are synthesized. Neurons of the supraoptic nucleus are visible just dorsal to the optic tracts. Another collection of large, dark-staining neurons is called the paraventricular nucleus owing to its proximity to the third ventricle. The nearby suprachiasmatic nucleus regulates circadian (24-hour) rhythms of hormone secretion.

and also cortical cells with a completely different appearance that synthesize steroid hormones.

Adrenal Cortex

The adrenal cortex is composed of steroid-secreting cells located beneath a capsule of dense, irregular connective tissue. The cells have a morphology dominated by structures required for steroid synthesis. They have round, euchromatic nuclei, consistent with the transcription of large numbers of genes required for the many steps of steroid synthesis. They possess many cytoplasmic lipid droplets that store cholesterol, a precursor molecule for steroids. Since lipid is extracted from cells by organic solvents such as alcohol and xylene, which are commonly used to prepare tissue for embedding and sectioning, these lipid droplets appear empty in sections of the adrenal cortex and so cortical cell cytoplasm is very lightly stained.

While adrenal cortical cells all basically have a similar morphology, they are arranged in three different patterns that correspond to three different zones within the cortex. In the outermost zone, cells are organized into roughly spherical arrangements, so this zone is named the zona glomerulosa after Latin *glomus*, "small ball" (Fig. 10-8). Cells in this outermost region of the cortex mainly synthesize the steroid aldosterone, which regulates sodium retention by the kidney. The activity of zona glomerulosa cells is controlled by a circulating protein hormone called angiotensin II. Angiotensin II is produced in response to fluctuations in water and sodium levels in the body.

In the next zone of the cortex, the zona fasciculata, cells are organized into long rows, or fascicles, by numerous fenestrated capillaries that traverse the cortex on their way to the medulla (see Fig. 10-8). These cortical cells have abundant smooth endoplasmic reticulum (sER) and mitochondria with distinctive tubular cristae. These organelles are the sites where many of the enzymes required for steroid synthesis are found (see Fig. 10-8). Cells in the zona fasciculata primarily secrete cortisol, a steroid hormone that (1) stimulates the release of glucose from the liver, (2) promotes the breakdown of cellular proteins and their transformation into glucose (catabolism), and (3) suppresses the activity of the immune system. These effects of cortisol and similar steroids would be harmful in the long term but, in short-term situations of injury or stress, they provide the energy to run away from a harmful environment and temporarily suppress swelling or other immune responses that could interfere with escape. Cells of the zona fasciculata are controlled by the

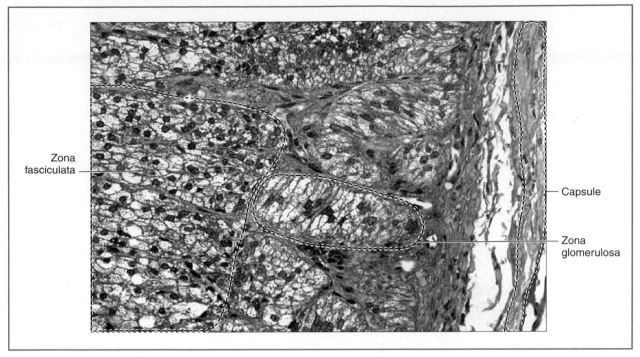

Zona
fasciculata

Capsule

Zona
glomerulosa

A

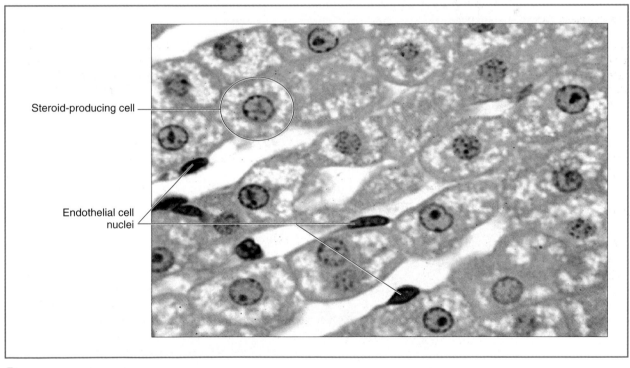

Steroid-producing cell

Endothelial cell
nuclei

B

Figure 10-8. Adrenal gland. **A,** The outermost connective tissue capsule of the gland is visible. Beneath the capsule, more or less spherical arrangements of aldosterone-secreting cells of the zona glomerulosa are seen. **B,** The long rows of cortisol-secreting cells of the zona fasciculata, plus fenestrated sinusoidal capillaries that carry hormone into the bloodstream, are visible.

Continued

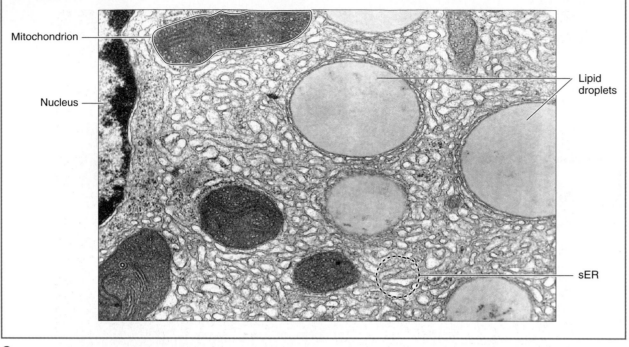

Mitochondrion

Nucleus

Lipid droplets

sER

C

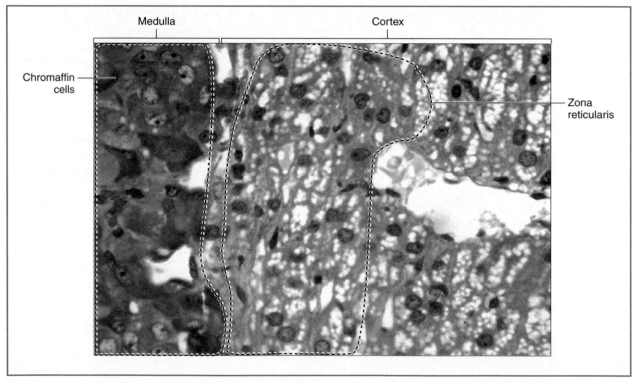

Medulla

Cortex

Chromaffin cells

Zona reticularis

D

Figure 10-8 cont'd. C, Transmission electron micrograph of an adrenal cortical cell showing several mitochondria with tubular cristae, lipid droplets, and extensive sER. (Courtesy of Don Fawcett.) **D,** This view shows the junction between the adrenal medulla and cortex. Some cells in the medulla have secretory granules that stain darkly and contain norepinephrine. Other more lightly stained cells probably contain epinephrine. Both cell types are called chromaffin cells. An endothelial cell of a sinusoidal capillary is visible in the zona reticularis.

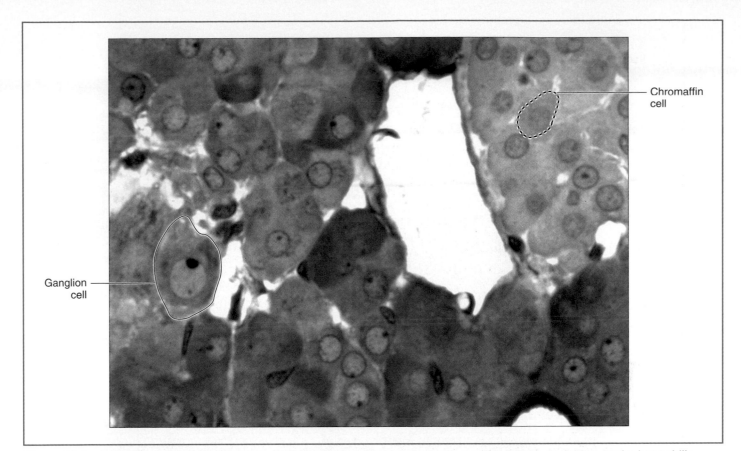

Ganglion cell

Chromaffin cell

Figure 10-9. Adrenal medulla. The ganglion cell has a large, euchromatic nucleus, a prominent nucleolus, and a basophilic cytoplasm, all characteristics of neuronal cells. These cells are quite rare in the medulla. Other nearby cells are chromaffin cells.

pituitary hormone, ACTH, which is secreted in response to stress.

Cells of the innermost zone of the adrenal cortex are organized into a network-like arrangement, hence this zone is called the zona reticularis (see Fig. 10-8). Cells of this region secrete steroids such as dehydroepiandrosterone that are readily transformed into androgens and estrogens.

Adrenal Medulla

Chromaffin cells of the adrenal medulla lack lipid droplets in their cytoplasm and thus stain distinctively darker than cortical cells. Chromaffin cells form clusters around the large venules that dominate the vasculature of the medulla. Fixatives such as glutaraldehyde enhance staining differences between two classes of chromaffin cells. After glutaraldehyde fixation, secretory granules containing norepinephrine tend to stain more darkly than those containing epinephrine, allowing differentiation between epinephrine-containing chromaffin cells (about 80% of the total) from norepinephrine-containing cells (Fig. 10-9).

Chromaffin cells also contain a peptide called enkephalin. Like pituitary β-endorphin, enkephalin binds to opiate receptors in the nervous system and can diminish the sensation of pain, although enkephalin's effects typically are

more transient than those of β-endorphin. An additional peptide called chromogranin was also originally discovered in cultures of chromaffin cells. Chromogranin peptides are now known to be found within secretory granules of many endocrine cells (e.g., anterior pituitary, pancreas). Their precise function is uncertain. The activity of chromaffin cells is controlled by axons of neurons located in the inter-mediolateral column of the thoracic spinal cord (sympathetic division of the autonomic nervous system). Once again, the secretory products of chromaffin cells, by increasing heart rate and blood pressure and by decreasing the sensation of pain, can be helpful in escaping from stress or injury.

An additional cell type found in the adrenal medulla is the ganglion cell. These large, rare cells have the enlarged nucleus and basophilic cytoplasm typical of neurons and may represent a small fraction of neural crest cells that failed to differentiate into smaller, mature chromaffin cells (see Fig. 10-9).

●●● THYROID GLAND

The thyroid gland is composed of masses of simple cuboidal epithelial cells that are arranged to form hundreds of small, spherical, fluid-filled structures called follicles (Fig. 10-10; see also Fig. 1-5). Thyroid follicle cells are responsible for

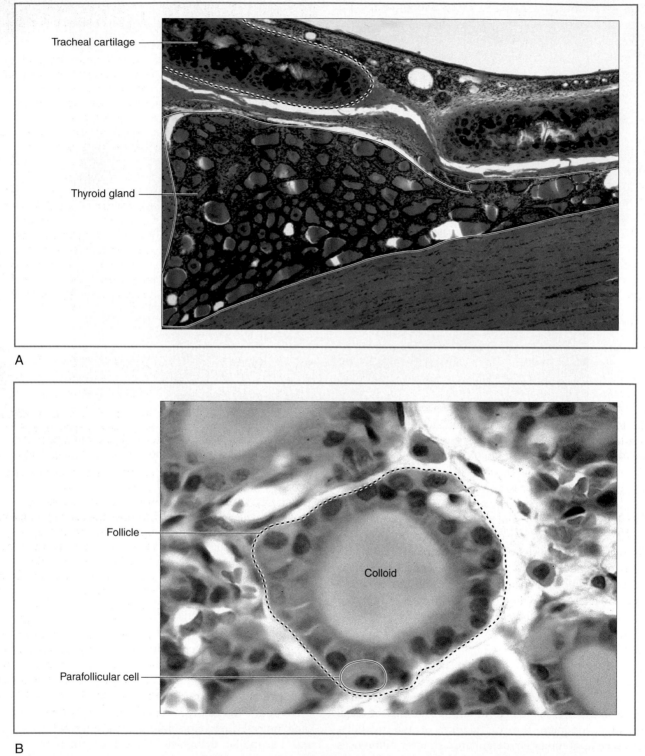

Tracheal cartilage

Thyroid gland

A

Follicle

Colloid

Parafollicular cell

B

Figure 10-10. Thyroid gland. **A,** This overview of the thyroid shows its relationship to surrounding structures. Also visible are tracheal rings composed of hyaline cartilage tissue. **B,** This detailed view of a thyroid follicle displays a variety of cell types. The viscous fluid within a follicle, called colloid, contains the protein thyroglobulin. Larger, lighter staining cells that do not touch the interior of a follicle are called parafollicular cells and produce calcitonin. Mast cells and fibroblasts are also visible.

secreting two major thyroid hormones, triiodothyronine (T_3) and tetraiodothyronine (T_4, thyroxine). These hormones are derivatives of the amino acid tyrosine; they are synthesized and secreted in a unique manner.

Thyroid Follicle Cells

The basolateral surfaces of thyroid follicular cells possess an intrinsic membrane protein called the Na^+/I^- symporter, which efficiently exchanges Na^+ ions for I^- ions across the membrane. This transporter protein, which is similar to a glucose transporter protein found in the gut, allows follicle cells to extract iodide from interstitial fluid and transport it against a concentration gradient across the cell. Ultimately, the iodide is released from the apical surface of the cell into the lumen of the follicle and can reach very high concentrations within follicular fluid (called colloid). A few other tissues, such as salivary glands and the stomach mucosa, have smaller amounts of this Na^+/I^- symporter protein and can also accumulate some iodide but to a much lesser degree than the thyroid gland.

Thyroid follicular cells secrete a large protein called thyroglobulin into the follicular lumen along with the enzyme peroxidase. Thyroglobulin is a very large, glycosylated protein that possesses some 140 tyrosine residues in its polypeptide chain. Thyroperoxidase alters the structure of some of these tyrosine residues; one or two atoms of iodine are added to each residue, and if two tyrosine residues are near each other, the peroxidase also causes some of the iodinated tyrosine residues to become covalently attached to each other. The most frequently targeted tyrosines lie close to the N-terminal end of the protein. While in the colloid, thyroglobulin is merely a large, iodinated protein and is not a hormone; it must be converted to thyroxine within follicle cells.

Thyroxine, when finally released from follicle cells, has a commanding stimulatory influence on the overall metabolic rate. A deficiency in thyroxine slows the metabolic rate and can have particularly damaging effects if it occurs in newborns. The development of brain structures is dependent on the proper level of circulating thyroxine, so that neonatal thyroid deficiency causes a diminished brain and intellectual development in a condition known as *cretinism*. Neonatal thyroxine deficiency occurs in about 1 in 4000 births. Newborns are routinely screened for this condition and can be easily treated with thyroxine to prevent permanent brain impairment.

Thyroid Parafollicular Cells

In addition to follicular cells, capillaries, and traces of connective tissue, the thyroid contains endocrine cells that lie alongside the follicles. These parafollicular cells, which are derived from neural crest cells that invade the thyroid, secrete another hormone—calcitonin. Calcitonin decreases circulating levels of Ca^{++} by stimulating the activity of osteoblasts and thus causing the deposition of Ca^{++} into bone.

BIOCHEMISTRY

Thyroid Hormones

To produce hormones, follicle cells endocytose thyroglobulin from the follicular lumen and digest it in lysosomes. Most of the amino acids thus liberated from thyroglobulin are transported into the cytoplasm from lysosomes and reutilized.

The altered, iodinated tyrosine residues, now called triiodothyronine (T_3 or thyroxine) or tetraiodothyronine (T_4), are transported out of the follicular cells where they serve as circulating hormones. This process is stimulated by thyroid-stimulating hormone (TSH), which is secreted by anterior pituitary basophils. T_3 and T_4 are transported across the cell membrane of target cells through transporter proteins that can also transport amino acids such as leucine or tryptophan. Once inside cells, thyroid hormones bind to cytoplasmic receptor proteins that are then transported into the nucleus. These proteins have structural similarities to steroid hormone receptor proteins. Like steroids, thyroxine acts via these receptors to alter DNA transcription and other aspects of cell function.

ANATOMY & EMBRYOLOGY

The Thyroid Gland

Thyroxine production is an unorthodox process that is due to the developmental and evolutionary history of the thyroid.

In ancient fishes, 350 million years ago, the thyroid developed from a ventral outgrowth of the pharynx called the endostyle. When fishes left the ancient seas for fresh water, which is relatively depleted in iodine atoms, it was advantageous for the endostyle to develop an ability to concentrate iodine and store it for later use. During evolution, this primitive thyroid gland lost its connecting duct to the pharynx and became converted into an endocrine organ that delivers an iodinated peptide throughout the body. This evolutionary history is repeated by the embryologic formation of the thyroid gland from an epithelial structure associated with the oral cavity. The process is guided by transcription regulating proteins (homeotic proteins) called TTF-1 and PAX-8. One clinical consequence of thyroid embryology in humans is the occasional appearance of remnants of thyroid tissue at the back of the tongue, which is the site of origin of the thyroglossal duct that once connected the thyroid with the oral cavity. More common is the appearance of a thyroglossal duct cyst along the route of migration of the thyroid primordium.

●●● PARATHYROID GLAND

The parathyroid glands are difficult to detect, since they lie on the dorsal surface of the thyroid between the thyroid and the trachea (Fig. 10-11). They generally number four in humans and are composed mainly of masses of endocrine cells called chief cells. Chief cells synthesize and store parathyroid

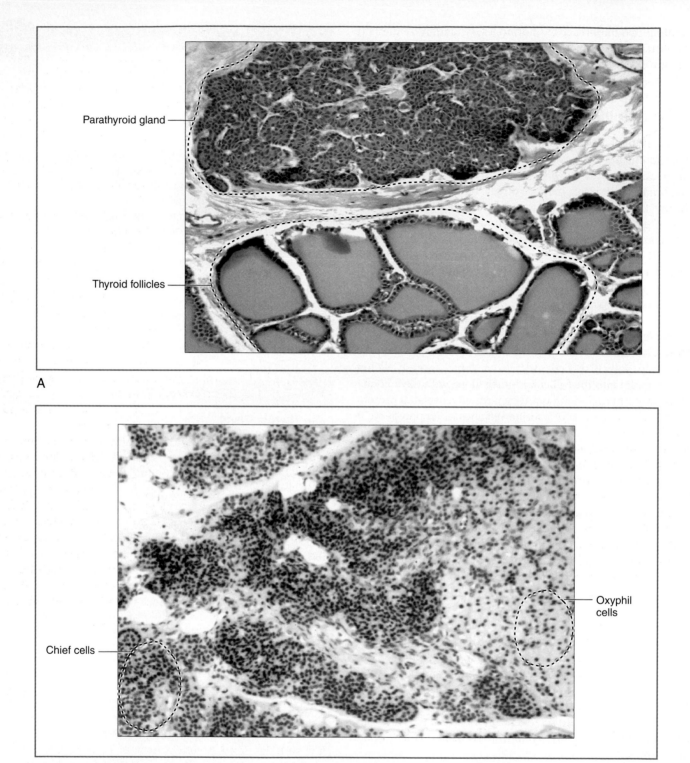

A

B

Figure 10-11. Parathyroid gland. **A,** Overview of the dorsal border of the thyroid shows an adjacent parathyroid gland embedded in a thin capsule of connective tissue. Typical thyroid follicles are also visible. **B,** Higher magnification view of the parathyroid shows a variety of cell types. The most abundant are the chief cells. Parathyroids from aged individuals also have clusters of enlarged, eosinophilic oxyphil cells, which have no apparent endocrine function. Interspersed among the endocrine cells are connective tissue elements, such as fibroblasts and white adipose cells.

hormone (PTH) in secretory vesicles and release it into the circulation whenever blood levels of Ca^{++} fall below 1 to 3 mmol/L. These cells are able to sense changes in circulating Ca^{++} because they possess an unusual receptor protein in the plasma membrane that binds and reacts to Ca^{++}. The only other cell in the body that possesses this receptor is the parafollicular cell, which is also regulated by Ca^{++}.

PTH adjusts blood Ca^{++} levels by altering the activity of bone-forming and bone-degrading cells. One effect of PTH is to inhibit the production of a protein called osteoprotegerin by osteoblast cells. Since osteoprotegerin tonically suppresses the activity of neighboring osteoclasts, PTH can reverse the inactivity of these cells and stimulate bone turnover. This is the mechanism that explains the destructive effects on bone that are seen when large doses of PTH are suddenly administered to animals, or when parathyroid tumors secrete excessive amounts of PTH.

In contrast, slow administration of small doses of PTH actually has an anabolic (i.e., stimulatory) effect on bone formation via mechanisms that are still uncertain. Small doses of PTH, in fact, may protect against the bone loss seen in osteoporosis. Thus, the role of normal levels of PTH in bone metabolism may be more complicated than previously thought.

One unusual feature of parathyroid glands taken from older individuals is the appearance of oxyphil cells. These cells appear to derive from chief cells that have lost their ability to secrete hormone. The cytoplasm of these cells is densely packed with masses of mitochondria. Experiments have shown that this odd cellular transformation is related to suppression of parathyroid function: when parathyroid glands are incubated in media with excessive amounts of Ca^{++}, oxyphil cells appear. In life, the presence of oxyphil cells in older individuals probably reflects the relative stabilization of Ca^{++} metabolism as bone growth and turnover slacken with age.

A still unresolved question about oxyphil cells is why they become filled with mitochondria. Evidently, the mechanisms governing mitochondrial replication and number have become damaged in these cells. Mitochondrial number and activity appear to be governed by a protein called mitochondrial transcription factor A (mtTFA), which activates mitochondrial genes. Levels of mtTFA, in turn, are governed by cellular energy needs. Understanding why these relatively inactive cells would generate more mitochondria may help elucidate how cells regulate total amounts of other organelles such as rER, Golgi, or cilia.

Finally, it should be mentioned that the parathyroid glands are critical for life: the accidental surgical removal of the glands during thyroid surgery led, in past decades, to drastic declines in blood levels of Ca^{++}. This event, in turn, caused a hyperexcitability of neuromuscular junctions known as *tetany*, which, if unchecked, was fatal. Tetany after total parathyroidectomy appears due to an activation of Ca^{++}-sensitive potassium channels of nerve cells.

●●● PINEAL GLAND

The pineal gland represents an outgrowth of the top of the neural tube that has become an endocrine rather than a neural structure. Its main cell type—pinealocytes—represent diminutive nerve cells that are surrounded by glial cells. The main function of pinealocytes is to secrete the hormone melatonin, which is derived from serotonin. In furry mammals, melatonin substantially depresses the activity of skin melanocytes and causes the appearance of white or light-colored fur, which allows animals to blend in against a snowy background.

This adjustment of coat color to match the season by the pineal gland is possible because the activity of the pineal gland is regulated by the number of hours that an animal is exposed to light. The short days and long nights of winter excite the pineal gland to produce more melatonin. This is possible because the pineal gland is innervated by sympathetic nerve fibers that, in turn, receive information about ambient lighting from cells in the suprachiasmatic nucleus of the hypothalamus. The origin of this information is ganglion cells in the retina. These cells possess a primitive form of visual pigment, called melanopsin, and they apparently function simply to keep track of whether it is day or night. All these cells function together to keep track of seasonal changes in lighting and hence the time of year.

While the function of the pineal in furry animals seems to be clear, its importance in humans is less evident. Infusions of melatonin during the early evening enhance sleepiness, and so melatonin may have a role in the regulation of sleep. One peculiar aspect of the pineal gland in older individuals is that masses of Ca^{++} crystals gradually form within pinealocytes and finally kill the cells, leaving calcified granules, called concretions, in their place. These seem to have little functional significance but are of considerable aid to radiologists, since they form dark spots on radiographs of the head and thus are an excellent landmark for the midline of the brain.

PATHOLOGY

Parathyroid Hormone

A similar protein to PTH, PTH-related peptide (PTHrP), is chronically secreted in small amounts by cells in other locations (e.g., skin, atrial heart muscle, epiphyseal cartilage, mammary glands, bone marrow). The physiologic significance of the peptide in normal circumstances seems to be relatively small. When tissues become cancerous, they often secrete excessive amounts of PTHrP that severely damage the skeleton. This so-called malignant hypercalcemia can be found in as many as 20% of cancer patients and is a serious complication of cancer.

Digestive System

11

CONTENTS

●●● UPPER DIGESTIVE SYSTEM

Oral Cavity and Associated Structures

The oral cavity commences at the margins of the lips, where the covering epithelium of the skin (keratinized stratified squamous epithelium, with hair follicles and sebaceous glands) is abruptly replaced by the covering epithelium of the oral mucosa (thick but nonkeratinized stratified squamous epithelium) (Fig. 11-1). This transition from one type of epithelium to the other makes functional sense, since the moist interior of the mouth does not require the protection from desiccation that a keratinized epithelium provides. The signaling molecules that are responsible for this transformation are, however, not known at present. It is known that the stratified squamous epithelial cells of the mouth and esophagus synthesize molecules that are not found elsewhere (e.g., intermediate filaments formed of type 4 keratin).

As the oral epithelium continues into the mouth, it is supported by an underlying connective tissue (lamina propria) that is analogous to the dermis of the skin. Beneath this layer, skeletal muscle fibers of the orbicularis oris muscle can be found along with occasional minor salivary glands. As the epithelium of the lips encounters the margins of the teeth it becomes the gingiva, and its superficial layers acquire

unusually large amounts of keratin (this condition is termed parakeratinization).

At birth, cells at what will become the area of the gingiva form a continuous epithelium that subsequently is torn open by the eruption of teeth. This area of the mouth is, in fact, one of the few regions of the body where an epithelium protecting the body's tissues from the external environment is completely interrupted. For this region, good dental hygiene is important to minimize the entry of oral bacteria at this vulnerable site. Poor gingival health is a major factor in the development of diseases such as endocarditis, which can be provoked by the entry of bacteria into the body via the oral cavity.

Teeth

Adult teeth are highly mineralized structures composed of enamel, dentin, and an inner pulp tissue containing loose connective tissue, nerves, and vessels (Fig. 11-2). The crown of each tooth, composed of enamel, dentin, and pulp, can have one cutting surface (cusp) or multiple surfaces, depending on whether the tooth is an incisor, canine, or molariform. The root of the tooth, composed of dentin and pulp, is surrounded by a bone-like material called cementum. Cementum, in turn, is attached to surrounding alveolar bone by a specialized dense, regular connective tissue called the periodontal ligament.

Densely packed crystals of a form of calcium phosphate (hydroxyapatite crystals) form 96% of mature enamel; the remaining 4% is composed of two proteins (amelogenin and enamelin) and water. The mineralized, crystalline nature of enamel, organized into long structures called enamel rods, makes enamel harder than steel. This allows dentists to use steel dental tools to scrape plaque off tooth surfaces without scratching the enamel. The chemical nature of enamel also makes it extremely durable and more resistant to damage than bone, which has a composition of only 50% hydroxyapatite crystal. As a result, after death, teeth tend to persist long after the remainder of the body deteriorates. This has significant consequences for the science of paleontology: quite a few species of small mammals have delicate skeletons that fail to fossilize, so these species are known only by the fossil teeth they left behind.

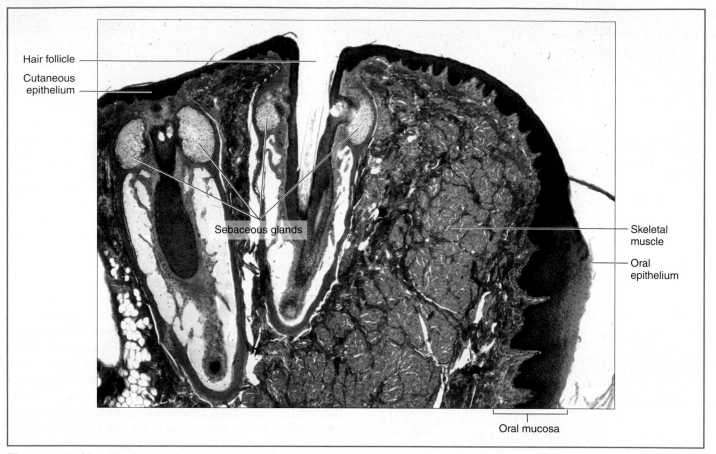

Hair follicle

Cutaneous epithelium

Sebaceous glands

Skeletal muscle

Oral epithelium

Oral mucosa

Figure 11-1. Lip, showing the thicker oral epithelium and the thinner cutaneous epithelium, which has hair follicles.

The dentin that underlies the enamel is less dense (70% mineralized), contains collagen rather than amelogenin, and is penetrated by numerous, tiny hollow tubules that in life are occupied by the thin processes of the cells that synthesize dentin (odontoblasts). These structural differences are evident in ground sections of a mineralized tooth. In such sections, enamel appears dense and dark brown, with stripes (striae) that mark incremental lines of enamel deposition. Dentin, in contrast, appears lighter and shows finer lines resulting from the presence of dentinal tubules (Fig. 11-3). The cementum that surrounds the dentin on the root of the tooth rather resembles bone and contains osteocyte-like cementocytes that occupy lacunae and have fine cell processes that radiate out from the central portion of each cell (Fig. 11-4).

Formation

Teeth are extremely hard structures. Milk teeth are formed before birth, and permanent teeth during childhood, by epithelial structures termed tooth buds and, later during development, enamel organs. These are formed when the overlying oral epithelium grows down into the ectomesenchyme (mesenchyme) below and expands into a cap-like structure, with an outer enamel epithelium forming the "outside" of the cap and an inner enamel epithelium in contact with mesenchymal cells "inside" the tooth bud (Fig. 11-5).

Between these two superficial layers of epithelia, the remaining epithelial cells proliferate to form a large structure called the stellate reticulum (Fig. 11-6; also see Fig. 11-5). The epithelial cells of the stellate reticulum secrete large amounts of a proteoglycan called perlecan, which is highly anionic and binds a large amount of water. As a consequence, large, watery extracellular spaces form among the epithelial cells, which take on a star-shaped or stellate appearance. The exact function of this stellate reticulum, which eventually collapses, is not known for certain; the large spaces within the stellate reticulum do provide for the ready diffusion of nutrients inward from capillaries outside of the enamel organ, which like most capillaries does penetrate directly into epithelial tissue. Some of the cells of the stellate reticulum condense onto the surface of the inner enamel epithelium to form a layer called the stratum intermedium (see Fig. 11-6).

A variety of signaling molecules produced by the inner enamel epithelium induce changes in the underlying mesenchymal cells, which form the dental papilla. Mesenchymal cells of the dental papilla line up against the basal lamina beneath the inner enamel epithelium to form an epithelium-

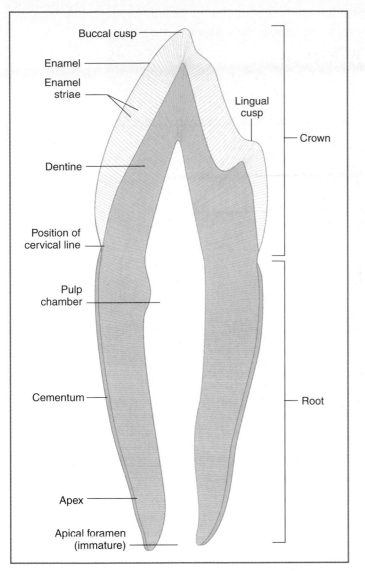

Figure 11-2. Ground section of a permanent lower first premolar tooth sectioned in the longitudinal plane. The enamel striae are incremental lines of enamel growth. (Redrawn from Standring S. *Gray's Anatomy*, 39th ed. Philadelphia, Churchill-Livingstone, 2005, p 595.)

Labels in figure: Buccal cusp, Enamel, Enamel striae, Dentine, Position of cervical line, Pulp chamber, Cementum, Apex, Apical foramen (immature), Lingual cusp, Crown, Root

dentin, like bone, retains thin cell processes (Tomes' fibers) from the odontoblasts that are contained within dentinal tubules, rather like the processes of osteocytes within canaliculi. The matrix of dentin does not completely mineralize when it is first secreted from the cell, so that a lighter stained region of predentin is discernable close to the odontoblasts. Enamel, in contrast, is an acellular, crystalline mass that mineralizes almost completely upon secretion and is contacted by ameloblasts only at the tips of temporary thin cell processes (Tomes' processes) that touch the outer surface of enamel (see Fig. 11-7). When sufficient layers of enamel and dentin have been deposited, the mature tooth erupts through the oral epithelium. The surface ameloblasts are eroded through abrasion, leaving the odontoblasts and connective tissue elements of the pulp cavity as the only remaining living inhabitants of the tooth.

Lingual Papillae and Taste Buds

The other prominent structure in the oral cavity is the tongue, a mass of skeletal muscle fibers (intrinsic muscles plus extrinsic ones such as the genioglossus and hyoglossus) covered by nonkeratinized epithelium on its ventral surface and by keratinized epithelium on its dorsal surface (Fig. 11-8). The ventral epithelium is unremarkable and resembles the lining mucosa present elsewhere in the mouth, but the dorsal epithelium possesses four distinctive types of epithelial protuberances, termed papillae. Each type of papilla has a different shape that dictates its name. Slender, pointed filiform papillae are numerous, are located all over the dorsal surface of the tongue, and appear to function as miniature rasps that roughen the tongue and enhance its ability to manipulate food (Fig. 11-9; also see Fig. 11-8). Less numerous, mushroom-shaped fungiform papillae are found in many places, and the larger vallate (or circumvallate) papillae are located mainly along a V-shaped line (the sulcus) at the back of the tongue (humans have about 12 to 15 vallate papillae). Fungiform and vallate papillae contain taste buds, the taste organs of the tongue. Finally, a few peg-shaped foliate papillae, which also bear taste buds, can be found at the lateral edges of the posterior aspect of the tongue, but these are much fewer in number in humans than in most other mammals and have little functional significance.

The large vallate papillae are particularly striking in histologic section, since they are surrounded by a cleft or trench that is continuously washed by the secretions of associated serous salivary glands called von Ebner's glands (Figs. 11-10 and 11-11). The epithelial surfaces lining this trench contain numerous taste buds, onion-shaped structures that are composed of specialized epithelial cells oriented *perpendicularly* to the orientation of most of the cells in the epithelium (Fig. 11-12). Taste bud cells, unlike their neighboring epithelial cells, contain an unusual type of keratin (keratin 8) and also possess apical microvilli that project into the fluid within the trench at the taste pore. The ability of taste bud cells to provide the sensation of taste is dependent on specialized taste receptor proteins present in the plasma membranes of taste cell microvilli.

like layer of cells, which become dentin-forming cells (odontoblasts). The odontoblasts, in turn, induce the inner enamel epithelium to take on the identity of enamel-forming ameloblasts. Ameloblasts and odontoblasts then secrete mineralizable matrix proteins from their basal surfaces and gradually become pushed apart by the steady production of enamel and dentin.

The anatomic appearance of ameloblasts and odontoblasts reflects their different origins: the epithelial ameloblasts form an extremely regular layer of tall columnar epithelial cells, whereas the odontoblasts, which are of mesenchymal origin, form a more disorderly layer of cells that resemble the osteoblast covering of bone (Fig. 11-7). Indeed, the composition of dentin resembles that of bone. Furthermore,

Text continued on page 304

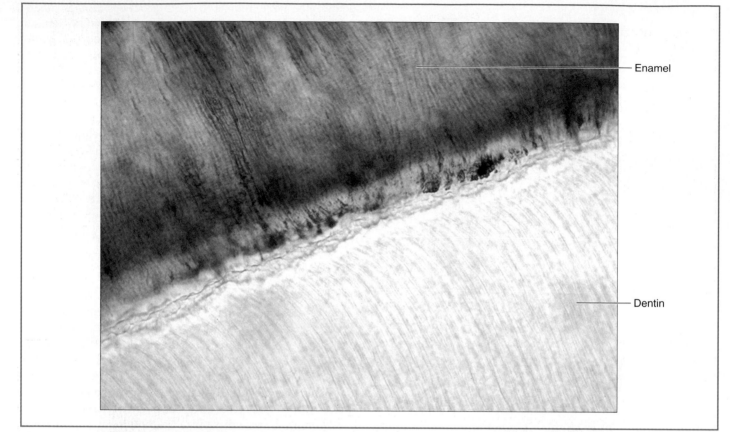

Figure 11-3. High-magnification view of a ground section of a tooth showing dense enamel (*brown*) and the less dense dentin, which contains dentinal tubules (fine lines within the white area).

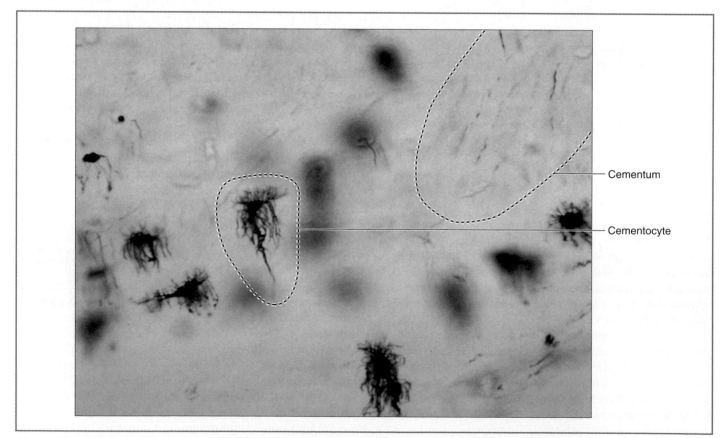

Figure 11-4. Ground section of cementum showing the dark cavities formerly occupied by cementocytes.

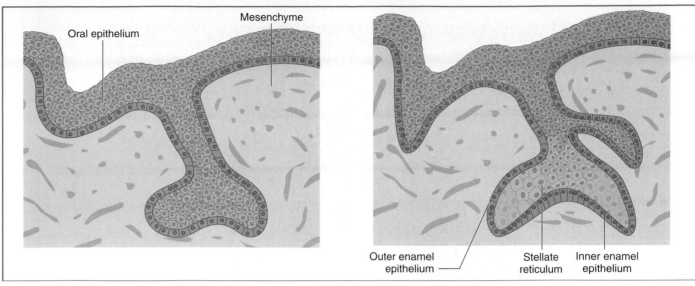

Figure 11-5. Diagram of tooth development showing two stages of the development of a tooth bud.

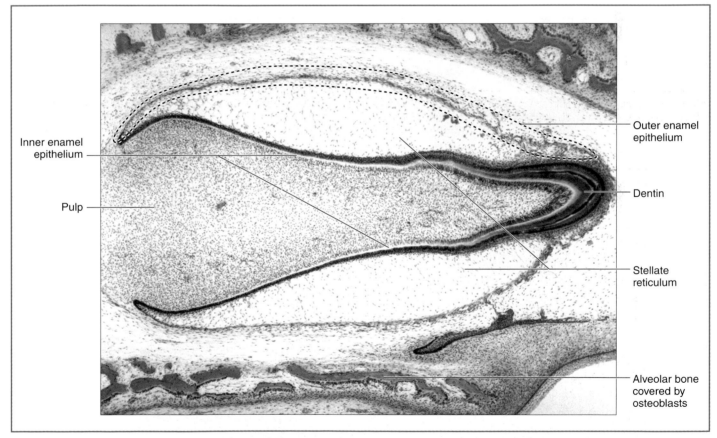

Figure 11-6. Low-magnification view of a developing tooth showing alveolar bone, the pulp cavity, the stellate reticulum, the outer enamel epithelium, the inner enamel epithelium, pink dentin, and dark purple enamel.

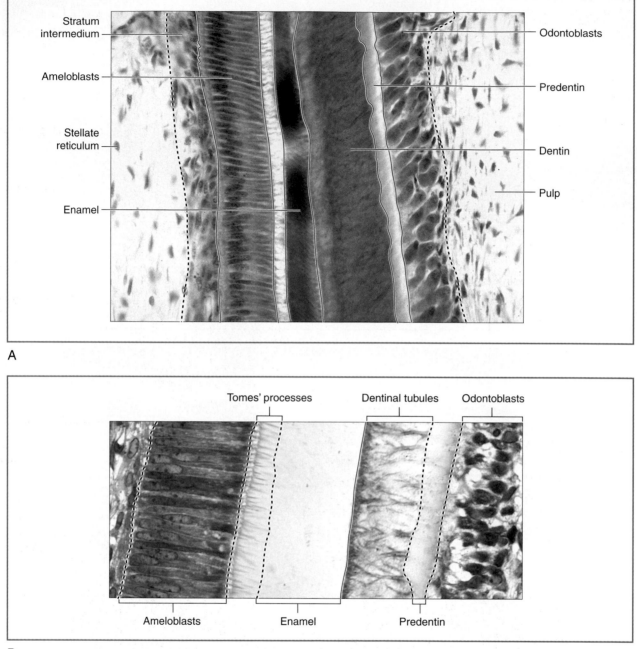

Figure 11-7. A, Paraffin section of a developing tooth at intermediate magnification showing the stellate reticulum, stratum intermedium, ameloblasts, enamel, dentin, predentin, odontoblasts, and the pulp cavity. **B,** Methacrylate section of developing tooth at high magnification showing ameloblasts, Tomes' processes, enamel, dentin and dentinal tubules, predentin, and odontoblasts.

Figure 11-8. Dorsal surface of the tongue showing the locations of vallate, fungiform, and foliate papillae.

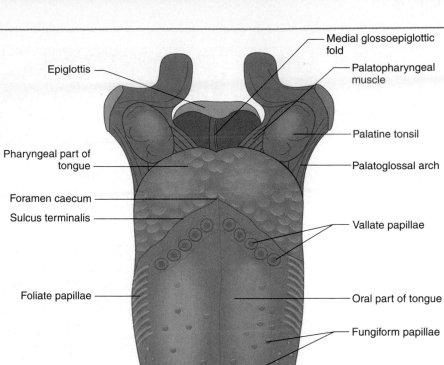

Medial glossoepiglottic fold

Epiglottis

Palatopharyngeal muscle

Pharyngeal part of tongue

Palatine tonsil

Foramen caecum

Palatoglossal arch

Sulcus terminalis

Vallate papillae

Foliate papillae

Oral part of tongue

Fungiform papillae

Filiform papillae

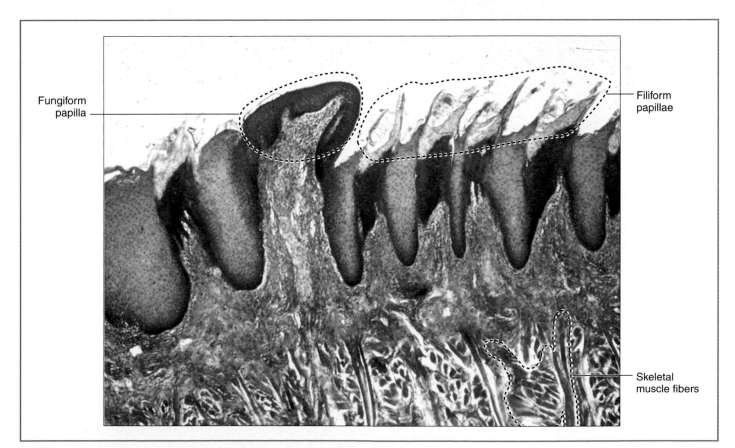

Fungiform papilla

Filiform papillae

Skeletal muscle fibers

Figure 11-9. Fungiform and filiform papillae found on the dorsal surface of the tongue.

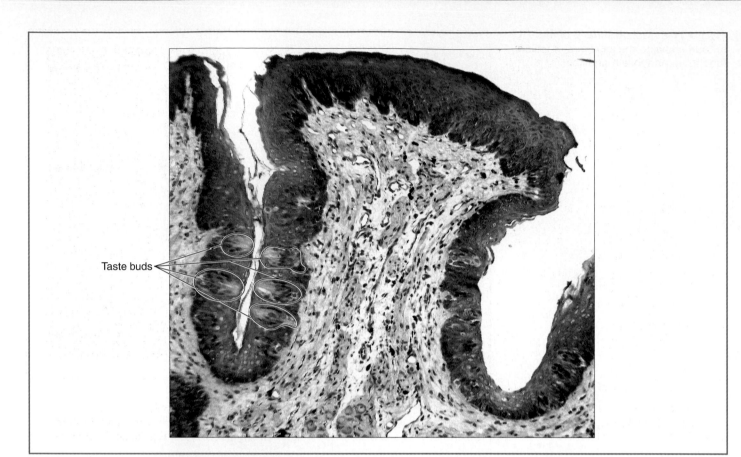

Figure 11-10. Circumvallate papilla of the tongue showing the location of taste buds.

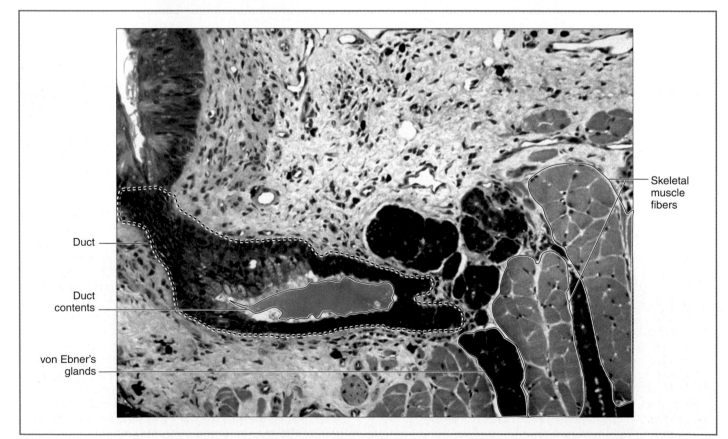

Figure 11-11. Base of the cleft around a circumvallate papilla showing a duct leading to serous von Ebner's glands that are located between skeletal muscle fibers of the tongue.

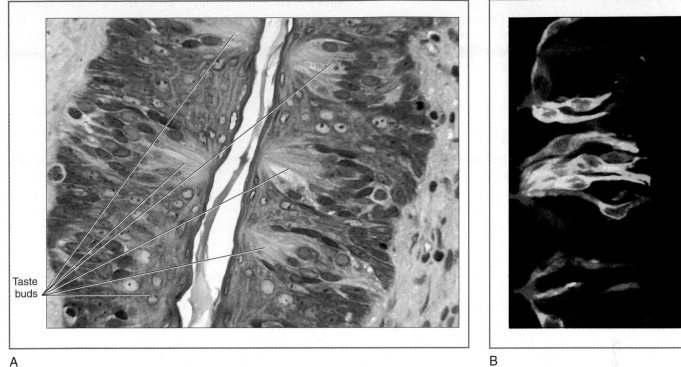

A

B

Figure 11-12. A, High-magnification view of a circumvallate papilla showing taste buds. **B,** Taste bud cells illustrated by fluorescence immunocytochemistry. The red dye labels espin, an actin-binding protein that is abundant in the microvilli at the taste pore. The green dye labels α-gustducin, a G protein specific to taste cells. (Courtesy of James R. Bartles and Gabriella Sekerkova.)

PHYSIOLOGY

Taste

Humans are believed to sense five basic taste modalities: salty, sour, sweet, bitter, and an additional savory flavor produced by monosodium glutamate that takes its name from the Japanese word *umami*.

Many diverse substances interact with receptor proteins of taste bud cells to produce the complex sensations of flavor.

- Salty tastes are produced when high concentrations of sodium affect the function of ion channels in taste cells. The specific ion channels have not been identified with precision.
- Sour tastes likewise seem to be mediated by ion channels that are influenced by extracellular concentrations of acid (H ions).
- Sweet tastes are elicited by sugars, alcohols, and some amino acids. These substances bind to integral membrane proteins called T1Rs. Three types of these sweet-sensitive receptors exist; they are found in about 30% of all taste bud cells, and all generally tend to be present at the same time in a given cell.
- Bitter tastes are elicited by a wide range of chemically dissimilar substances such as strychnine and cycloheximide. These substances bind to T2R proteins, which show a corresponding diversity of structure (24 types of these proteins have been found in humans). It makes functional sense to possess many types of bitter-sensitive proteins, since bitter-tasting molecules frequently are alkaloid poisons produced by plants that should be avoided. Bitter-sensitive T2R proteins are found only in circumvallate papillae and never in the same cell as sweet-sensitive T1R proteins. If mice are genetically engineered so that normally sweet-sensitive cells acquire bitter-sensitive receptors, the mice show a preference for bitter solutions and will drink them avidly.
- *Umami* flavor is detected by a so-called metabotropic glutamate receptor.

All these receptor proteins interact with a membrane-associated G protein that is specific to taste buds (gustducin). When activated by taste-receptor proteins, gustducin sets in motion the intracellular pathways that activate the cell. Some bitter flavorings, such as quinine and caffeine, bypass taste receptors, permeate the cell membrane, and directly affect the function of gustducin to produce a taste sensation.

Salivary Glands

Salivary glands develop from infoldings and expansions of the mucosal epithelium. There are three major salivary glands: the parotid, submandibular, and sublingual glands. These major glands form separate, identifiable organs located beneath the skin of the face that send ducts into the oral cavity and that can be dissected free of the face. In addition, dozens of smaller, minor salivary glands form smaller clumps of secretory tissue that are embedded in the mucosal and submucosal connective tissues of the oral cavity.

The generalized features of all salivary glands can be summarized in a diagram (Fig. 11-13). The cells that synthesize saliva form secretory units. Each unit is covered by contractile myoepithelial cells that exert pressure on the acini, thereby expressing the secretions into a series of ducts of increasing diameter that connect to the oral cavity. The ducts directly connected to an acinus are called intercalated ducts and possess a simple cuboidal epithelium. They connect to intralobular (striated) ducts with a simple columnar epithelium and to larger interlobular ducts surrounded by abundant connective tissue and possessing a stratified cuboidal or stratified columnar epithelium. Striated ducts are named for the thin longitudinal lines that are visible in light micrographs of the cytoplasm of duct cells (Fig. 11-14). These striations correspond to accumulations of mitochondria within basal infoldings of the plasma membrane of these duct cells. Such mitochondrial accumulations are typical of cells specialized for the large-scale transport of ions across the cell cytoplasm; in striated ducts, large amounts of sodium and chloride are transported out of the saliva to render it hypo-osmotic relative to blood plasma.

Two basic types of salivary units exist. One type is a serous acinus, containing cells with round nuclei and cytoplasms that are highly stained owing to the presence of many secretory vesicles containing serous proteins. Typical serous acini can be found in von Ebner's glands, near the circumvallate papillae (Figs. 11-15 and 11-16). The parotid gland is one of three major salivary glands and is composed entirely of serous acini (Fig. 11-17). The sublingual gland, in contrast, contains mainly mucous tubules, composed of cells with more flattened, basally located nuclei and lightly stained cytoplasms owing to the presence of mucous proteins within secretory vesicles that

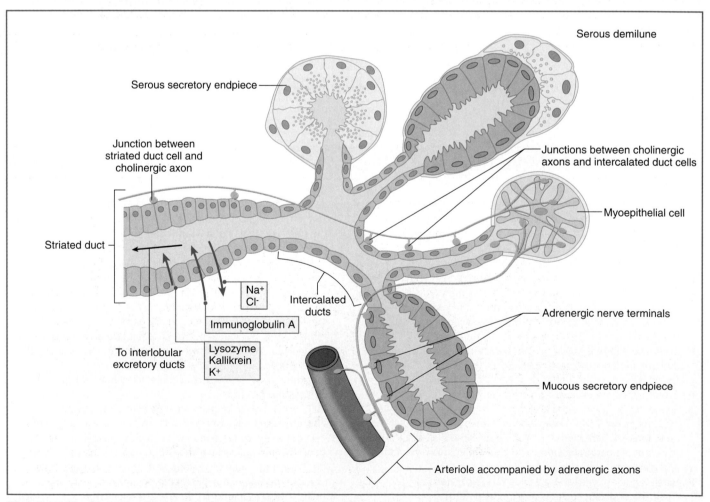

Figure 11-13. Diagram of the two types of secretory units (mucous tubules and serous acini) found in salivary glands.

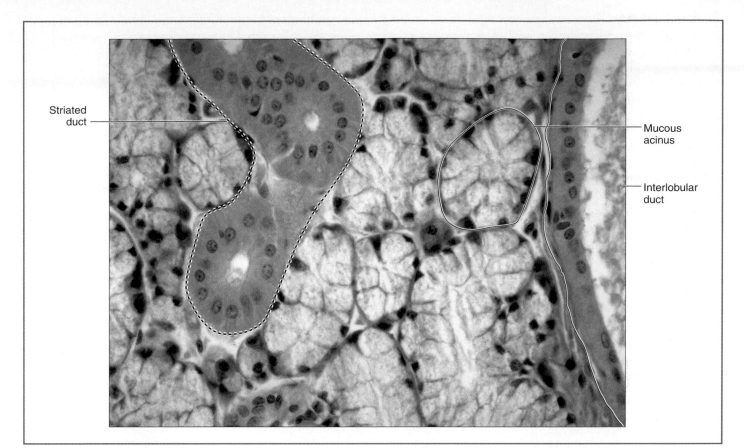

Striated duct

Mucous acinus

Interlobular duct

Figure 11-14. View of mucous acini of the sublingual gland showing striated ducts and a larger interlobular duct.

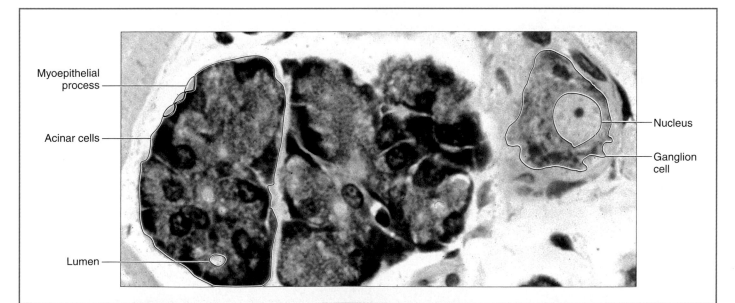

Myoepithelial process

Acinar cells

Lumen

Nucleus

Ganglion cell

Figure 11-15. View of serous secretory acini of the minor salivary von Ebner's glands. A small lumen is visible in one of the acini; the scalloped appearance of the margin of one acinus is due to the presence of lighter staining processes of myoepithelial cells. A parasympathetic ganglion cell that innervates these glands is also visible.

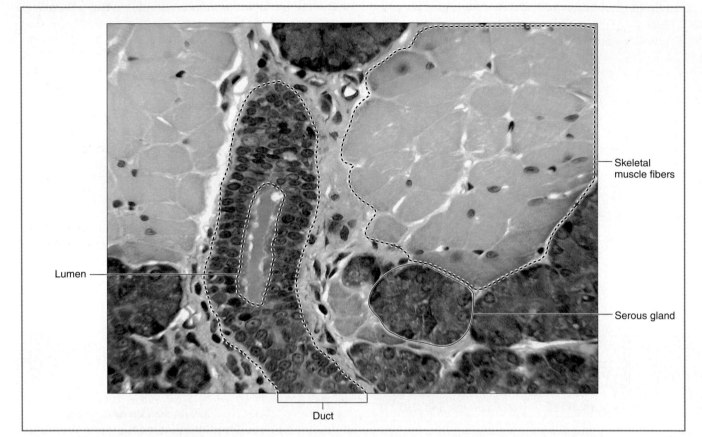

Skeletal muscle fibers

Lumen

Serous gland

Duct

Figure 11-16. Stratified columnar epithelium of a duct conveying secretory material from a von Ebner's gland.

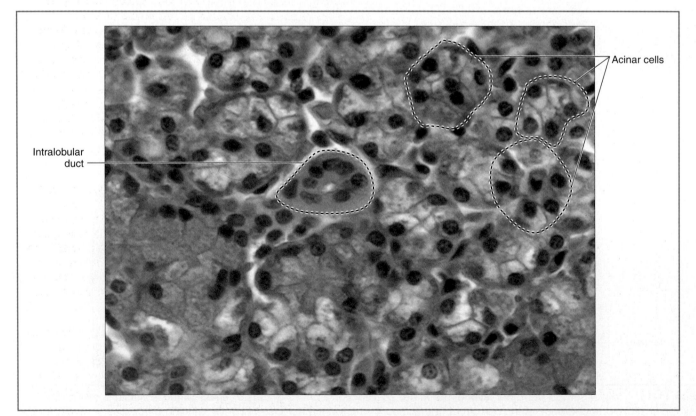

Acinar cells

Intralobular duct

Figure 11-17. View of the serous acini of the parotid gland with an intercalated duct.

fail to stain well with common histologic stains (see Fig. 11-14). Finally, the submandibular gland is another mixed gland, containing mostly serous but also a few mucous acini (Fig. 11-18). Not infrequently, accumulations of parasympathetic ganglion cells that innervate salivary acini can be found in close association with acinar cells (see Fig. 11-15).

Often, in mixed glands, serous cells form a semicircular "cap" at the distal end of a mucous acinus (Fig. 11-19). Because of the crescent moon shape of these serous accumulations, they are termed serous demilunes, and they often appear completely separated from the lumen of the acinus. A recent study suggests that this "demilune" structure may in part be due to swelling of mucous cells when they contact aqueous fixatives. If mixed acini are preserved by rapid freezing and freeze substitution, mucous cells appear smaller and serous cells do not show this compression into demilunes.

All of these complicated structures—teeth, lingual papillae, and salivary glands—originate as outgrowths from the oral epithelium. The embryology of these structures begins with localized accumulations of signaling molecules. Why these signaling molecules come to be located where they are is not completely understood, but the identity of some important signals is at least becoming clear.

●●● HOLLOW ORGANS OF THE DIGESTIVE SYSTEM

Esophagus

The esophagus is a muscular tube lined with nonkeratinized, stratified squamous epithelium. The wall of the esophagus,

---

PHYSIOLOGY

Salivation

Salivary glands deliver about 1 L of saliva per day into the oral cavity and digestive tract. Autonomic nerves terminating upon acini stimulate this secretion; cholinergic fibers particularly increase the transport of water and sodium chloride into saliva, whereas adrenergic fibers stimulate acini to produce a protein-rich saliva. About 300 distinct proteins can be detected in saliva. However, the bulk of salivary proteins fall into a few categories:

- Secretion from mucous glands is enriched in mucin proteins. Eleven human mucin proteins are known and are synthesized by salivary glands and by goblet cells of the respiratory and digestive tracts. Some mucins, such as salivary mucins, are readily soluble in water, whereas others form a thick gel upon epithelial surfaces. All mucin proteins contain large numbers of carbohydrate molecules (mucin is 80% carbohydrate by weight). Since the carbohydrate molecules are highly charged, they repel each other, forcing the polypeptide chain of a mucin into a rigid, rod-like configuration. As a result, in solution, mucin proteins behave like a mass of logs floating in a river, getting tangled up with each other and causing mucus to be very viscous. Mucin proteins also have antibacterial properties.
- Secretion from serous glands like the parotid gland is enriched in amylase and proline-rich proteins, which seem to regulate the interaction between the surfaces of teeth and bacteria. Another serous protein, statherin, helps maintain high levels of calcium in saliva. An impaired secretion of these salivary proteins, due to nerve damage or as a side effect of radiation therapy of facial tumors, can have a catastrophic effect on dental health and lead to severe dental caries (cavities). In solution, globular serous proteins readily roll over each other, much like beach balls tossed into a pool, so that serous saliva is not so viscous as mucous saliva.

EMBRYOLOGY

Specialized Oral Structures

Teeth

Tooth buds initially form in epithelium that synthesizes a molecule called Wnt. This protein derives its name from a similar developmental protein that was first found in fruit flies (wingless). Under the influence of Wnt, epithelial cells secrete an unknown factor that induces the underlying mesenchyme to form a dental papilla. Mesenchymal cells, in turn, express the *PAX9* transcription factor that is required for further development; mutations in this factor in humans result in the agenesis of molar teeth. Mesenchymal cells expressing a homeotic protein called Dlx induce the epithelium to produce molar teeth, whereas the expression of another factor, activin, induces the appearance of canine and incisor teeth. In all teeth, the appearance of a protein called SP3 induces the transcription of most ameloblast genes. These are only a few examples of molecules that have been found to guide the complex process of tooth development.

Lingual papillae and taste buds

Recent work has shown that the production of brain-derived neurotrophic factor (BDNF) by epithelial cells of the growing circumvallate papilla has a crucial effect on its development. BDNF attracts the ingrowth of nerves, which secrete unknown trophic factors that induce the appearance of taste buds in the epithelium. If nerves to the tongue are severed in developing or even adult animals, taste buds disappear and the taste bud epithelium reverts to its previous undifferentiated appearance.

Salivary glands

Recent studies have shown that the development and epithelial branching of salivary glands from an initial epithelial bud is strongly dependent on the production of fibroblast growth factor 10 (FGF10) by the underlying mesenchyme. FGF10 is one of 22 related molecules that influence the development of many epithelial structures throughout the body.

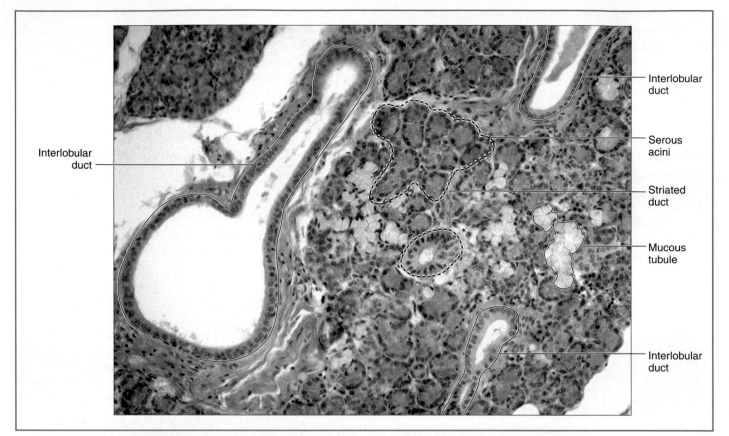

Figure 11-18. View of the mixed serous and mucous acini of the submandibular gland. A small striated duct and a larger interlobular duct, surrounded by connective tissue, are visible.

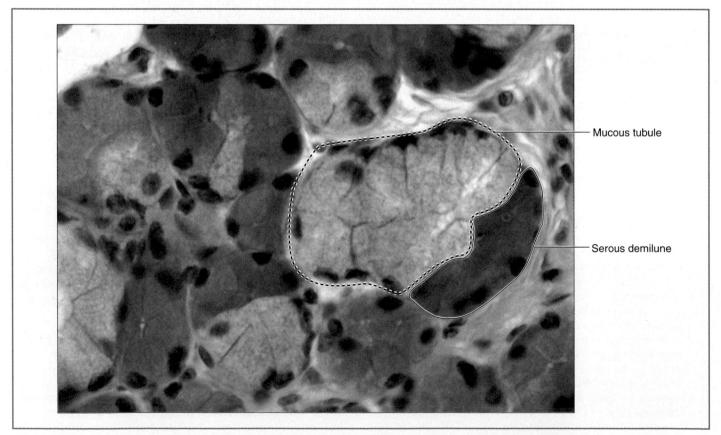

Figure 11-19. A mixed acinus of the sublingual gland showing mucous cells capped by a darker staining serous demilune.

and indeed the remainder of the digestive system, is organized into four specific layers (see Fig. 2-11):

Layer 1—Mucosa
    A. Mucosal epithelium
    B. Lamina propria
    C. Muscularis mucosae
Layer 2—Submucosa
Layer 3—Muscularis externa
Layer 4—Adventitia or serosa

When this outermost layer of connective tissue is covered by a simple squamous epithelium (mesothelium), this outer layer is termed a serosa; when it lacks a mesothelial covering (as in certain portions of the esophagus and duodenum), it is called an adventitia. All these structures can be observed in an overall view of a section of the esophagus from a small mammal (rat), which shows each layer clearly (Fig. 11-20). The muscularis externa and submucosal layers both contain a number of structures that can best be described in the context of the intestine. The following sections focus on the specialized features of the mucosa of the esophagus and stomach, which is quite different in these organs from that of the intestines.

Just beneath the mucosa of the esophagus, irregular clusters of smooth muscle constituting the muscularis mucosae are present (Fig. 11-21). In addition, a number of glands can be found beneath the epithelium of the esophagus. In the regions closest to the oral cavity, the lamina propria possesses clusters of mucous glands called cardiac esophageal glands. These produce a lubricating mucus. More distally in the esophagus, mixed serous and mucous glands are found in the submucosal layer that secrete lysozyme. Other than these features, the structure of the esophagus is quite simple, in keeping with its simple task of conveying food and fluid to the stomach.

Stomach

The mucosal epithelium of the stomach forms a lining surface that possesses tubular infoldings, termed gastric pits (foveolae), that in turn lead to tubular structures termed gastric glands (Fig. 11-22). In two portions of the stomach (the fundic stomach closest to the esophagus and the pyloric stomach closest to the small intestine), the lining epithelium is mainly occupied by mucus-secreting epithelial cells. However, the main portion of the stomach (the corpus or fundus) possesses five types of epithelial cells, each having distinctive functions.

The most superficial cells are simple columnar epithelial cells called surface mucous cells; these cells secrete a bicarbonate-rich mucus that protects the gastric tissues from stomach acid. As the epithelium dives down into the gastric pits, another type of cell, the mucous neck cell, is

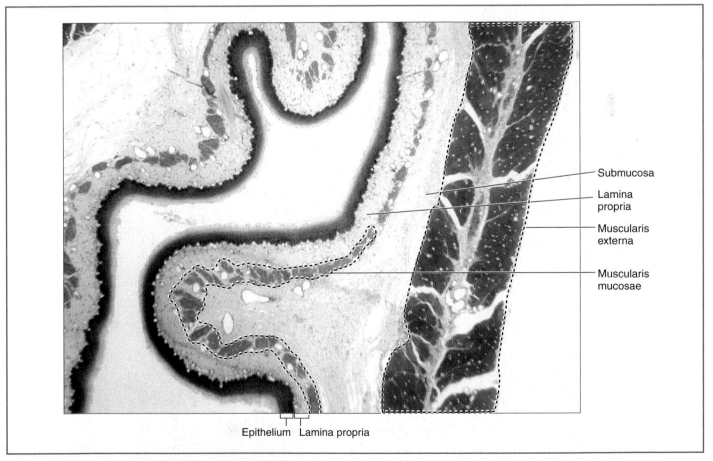

Submucosa

Lamina propria

Muscularis externa

Muscularis mucosae

Epithelium   Lamina propria

Figure 11-20. Low-magnification view of the esophagus of a rat showing the lining epithelium, lamina propria, muscularis mucosae, submucosa, and muscularis externa layers.

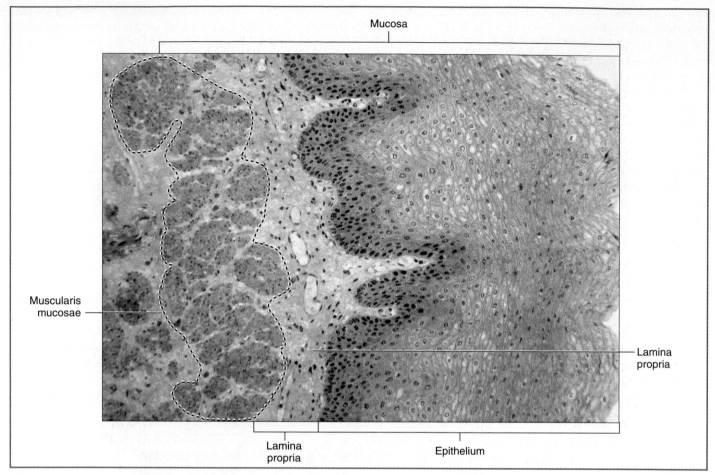

Figure 11-21. High-magnification view of the human esophagus showing the mucosa, nonkeratinized stratified squamous epithelium, lamina propria, and muscularis mucosae.

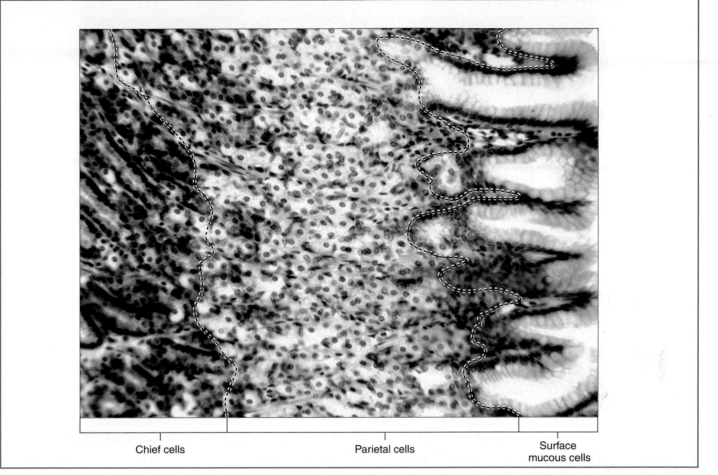

Figure 11-22. Low magnification view of the stomach showing the three main regions of the mucosa that are dominated by, respectively, surface mucous cells, parietal cells, and chief cells at the bottom of each gastric pit.

encountered. These cells produce another variant of mucous and also to serve as stem cells that replace the other types of epithelial cells in the gastric mucosa.

A third type of gastric epithelial cell is called the parietal cell. Parietal cells have a centrally located nucleus, a brightly staining, eosinophilic cytoplasm, and a distinctive round shape (Figs. 11-23 and 11-24). A diagram of the ultrastructure of these cells shows the unusual features that explain the staining characteristics of their cytoplasms (Fig. 11-25). Parietal cells bear deep cytoplasmic invaginations called canaliculi that are decorated with long, flexible microvilli; in addition, numerous long vesicles and mitochondria fill the remaining cytoplasm. The abundance of mitochondria and integral membrane proteins within all these membranous structures is what makes the cytoplasm of parietal cells so eosinophilic.

Parietal Cell Function

Membranes of the parietal cell canaliculi contain an integral protein termed H^+/K^+-ATPase, which functions as a hydrogen transporter. These proteins, relying on a steady supply of ATP from nearby mitochondria, allow the cell to export large amounts of H^+ ions and thereby secrete a fluid rich in acid (hydrochloric acid). If the hydrogen transporter proteins are deleted from parietal cells by genetic engineering, the cells show a dramatic loss in canalicular features, so these proteins themselves must somehow stimulate the rearrangement of the membranes and cytoskeleton of the parietal cell to produce its unusual ultrastructure.

The production of a highly acidic fluid from parietal cells is what permits the initial stages of the breakdown of food in the stomach. This acid would be harmful to mucosal cells except for the protective coating of bicarbonate-rich mucus produced by mucous neck cells. These cells actually acquire bicarbonate from the parietal cells, which utilize an enzyme (carbonic anhydrase) to split carbonic acid into bicarbonate and H^+ ions. The H^+ ions are exported at the apical end of the parietal cell into the stomach lumen, and the bicarbonate is exported at the basal end to travel within the lamina propria of the stomach up to the mucous neck cells, which incorporate it into mucus. Spare hydrogen transporter proteins are stored within the membranes of cytoplasmic vesicles of parietal cells until needed. When parietal cells are stimulated to secrete acid, by acetylcholine from nerve terminals or by

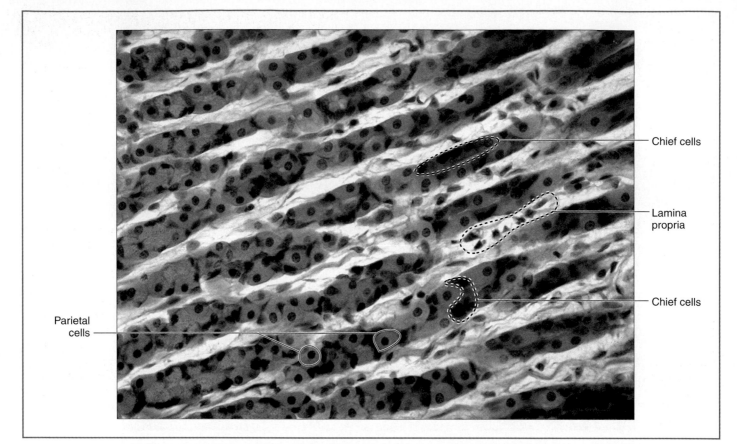

Figure 11-23. Mid-portion of a gastric gland showing rows of eosinophilic parietal cells covering over a sparse lamina propria.

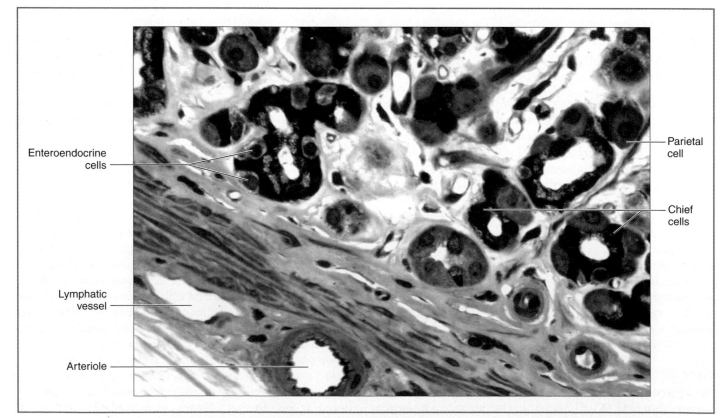

Figure 11-24. Bottom of a gastric pit showing parietal cells, dark-staining chief cells, and small, light-staining enteroendocrine cells. An arteriole and lymphatic capillary are visible in the submucosa, just beneath the thin muscularis mucosae.

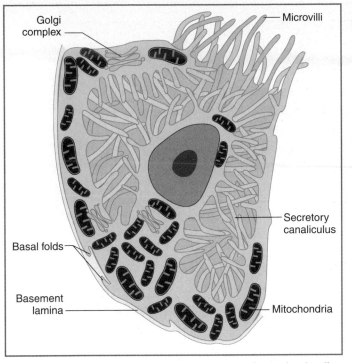

Figure 11-25. Diagram of the ultrastructure of a parietal cell showing abundant mitochondria and canaliculi lined by microvilli.

Labels: Golgi complex, Microvilli, Secretory canaliculus, Basal folds, Basement lamina, Mitochondria

MICROBIOLOGY

Stomach Ulcers

Stomach ulcers arise when damage to the epithelium exposes the underlying lamina propria to acid, causing damage and bleeding. For many years, a psychogenic cause of ulcers was proposed, in which psychological stress had a major role in enhancing vagal stimulation of acid secretion by the stomach. In spite of the failure of this approach to satisfactorily treat ulcers, it was stubbornly adhered to, until the 1980s. At that time, a completely novel explanation for ulcers was proposed by two Australian researchers, Barry Marshall and Robin Warren.

- Most ulcer patients were experiencing infection of the digestive system due to a gram-negative bacterium called *Helicobacter pylori* that damages the mucosal epithelium and allows damage by stomach acid.
- To convince skeptics of their proposal, Marshall deliberately infected himself with the bacterium to show that it could cause acute gastric illness. Marshall and Warren were awarded the Nobel Prize for medicine in 2005 for their work.
- These bacteria can be killed by administration of the antibiotic clarithromycin in the presence of an inhibitor of the hydrogen transporter such as omeprazole. These treatments kill the bacteria and lower the acidity of the stomach, leading to a cure for ulcers.

histamine from mast cells, the vesicles move and fuse with the plasma membrane, adding their transporter proteins to the membrane and enhancing the export of acid. This structural solution to the problem of how to increase the transport of a substance across a cell membrane—by fusing transporter-rich vesicles to the membrane—is used by many cells in many situations (glucose transport, water transport, etc) and will be encountered again in this book.

Another vital function of the parietal cells is the production of a protein called gastric intrinsic factor. This protein binds ingested vitamin B_{12} (cobalamin). Cobalamin bound to gastric intrinsic factor is carried down the digestive tract to the small intestine (ileum), where lining cells possess a receptor that binds it, allowing uptake of vitamin B_{12} by these cells. A deficiency of vitamin B_{12} interferes with the production of red blood cells (RBCs) in bone marrow, causing pernicious anemia.

Two other cell types are found within the epithelium of gastric pits (see Figs. 11-22 and 11-24). One type, most abundant at the bottom of each pit, has a basophilic cytoplasm and is called the chief cell. Chief cells secrete enzymes, such as pepsin and rennin, which help digest food proteins. The other type, the enteroendocrine cell (diffuse neuroendocrine system cell, or DNES cell), usually has a light-staining cytoplasm and produces peptide hormones that are secreted basally into capillaries or the lamina propria rather than apically into the gastric lumen. These hormones include gastrin, which stimulates acid secretion by parietal cells, and a more recently discovered hormone called ghrelin that is produced by about 20% of the enteroendocrine cells in the stomach and has important modulatory effects on the hypothalamus and the growth hormone–producing cells of the anterior pituitary.

Intestines

The intestines are lined by a simple columnar epithelium that, as in the stomach, is also highly folded (Fig. 11-26). Tubular invaginations of the epithelium of the intestines are called intestinal glands (or, in an older nomenclature, crypts of Lieberkühn). In addition to these intestinal glands, the mucosa of the small intestines (but *not* of the large intestines) possesses finger-shaped epithelial projections termed villi. The villi provide for an expanded surface area that enhances the absorption of nutrients from the lumen. The simple columnar epithelium of each villus covers a highly cellular lamina propria containing masses of fibroblasts, macrophages, plasma cells, and smooth muscle cells. While all portions of the small intestine have much in common, distinct changes in anatomy and function that occur along the length of the small intestine allow it to be divided into three named regions: duodenum, jejunum, and ileum.

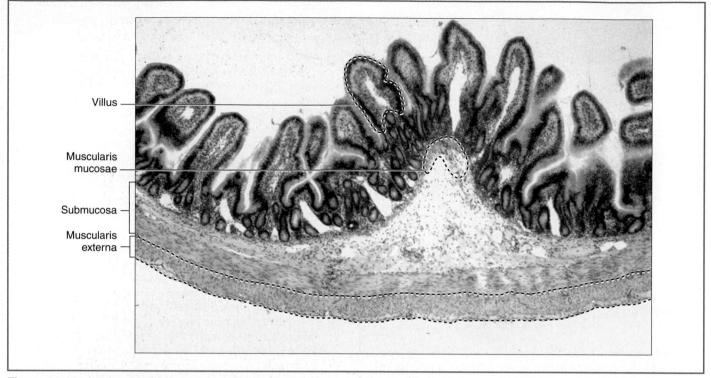

Figure 11-26. Low-magnification view of the small intestine (jejunum) showing villi, the muscularis mucosae, the submucosa, and the muscularis externa.

PATHOLOGY & CLINICAL MEDICINE

Surgical Treatment for Acid Reflux

Barrett's esophagus may arise when the lower esophageal sphincter between the esophagus and stomach fails to function properly, allowing stomach acid to enter and irritate the mucosa of the esophagus. Barrett's esophagus results from the replacement of the normal squamous epithelium of the esophagus by columnar epithelium as a consequence of long-standing reflux esophagitis. This condition can also result from a hiatal hernia that allows the stomach to move up into the thorax via an enlarged opening in the diaphragm. Acid reflux that is refractory to medical management may be treated with a *fundoplasty*, in which a portion of the fundic stomach is gathered together, passed behind the esophagus, and sutured to the anterior surface of the stomach to form a muscular loop encircling the esophagus.

Duodenum

The duodenum is a relatively short portion of the small intestine that borders the lower margin of the stomach. Duodenal villi are relatively broader compared with villi of the rest of the small intestine, and in the submucosa of the duodenum, masses of mucous glands called Brunner's glands

can be found (Figs. 11-27 and 11-28). These glands secrete an alkaline mucus that neutralizes the acid entering the gut from the stomach.

Jejunum

The jejunum possesses taller and narrower villi and lacks Brunner's glands. As in the duodenum, most of the cells covering the villi are surface absorptive cells (enterocytes) (Figs. 11-29 to 11-31). The apical surface of these surface absorptive cells is decorated with a brush border composed of microvilli, organelles that are specialized for increasing the surface area to facilitate the absorption of nutrient molecules (Fig. 11-32). The plasma membranes of these microvilli anchor enzymes required for the breakdown of complex sugars such as sucrose and lactose into smaller, simple sugars such as glucose, fructose, and galactose that can be transported across the plasma membrane via integral membrane sugar carrier proteins. Other frequently encountered cells that can be found adjacent to absorptive cells are mucus-producing goblet cells (see Figs. 11-31 and 11-32) and intraepithelial lymphocytes (see Figs. 11-30 and 11-32).

Absorption of lipids by intestinal cells poses a particularly severe problem: high-molecular-weight lipid molecules such as triacylglycerides cannot readily be transported across the plasma membrane. This problem is solved in several stages: (1) lipases and bile salts secreted into the intestinal lumen

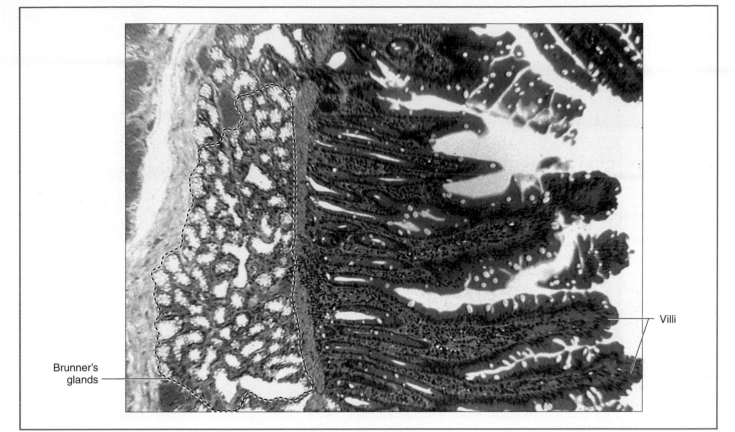

Figure 11-27. Low-magnification view of the duodenum showing villi and Brunner's glands in the submucosa.

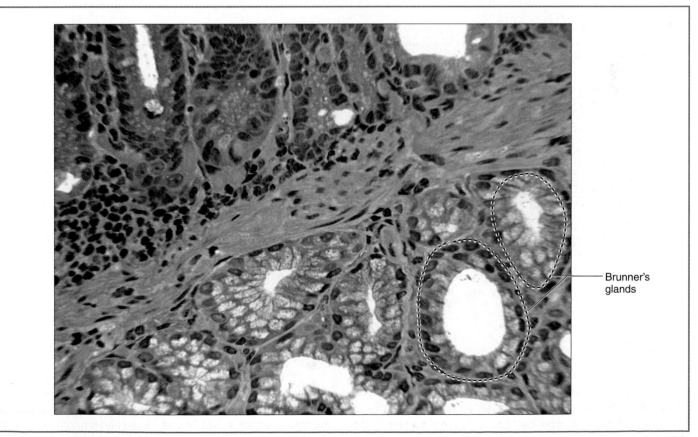

Figure 11-28. Higher magnification view of the small intestine showing the crypts of Lieberkühn, muscularis mucosae, and light-staining, mucus-producing cells of Brunner's glands.

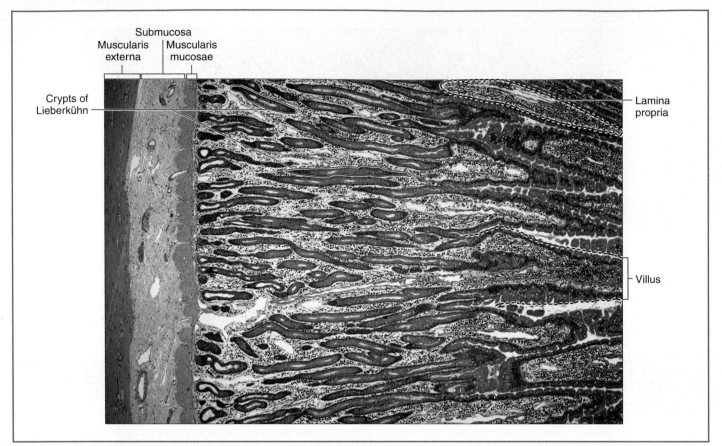

Figure 11-29. Low-magnification view of the jejunum showing villi, crypts of Lieberkühn, the muscularis mucosae, the submucosa, and the muscularis externa.

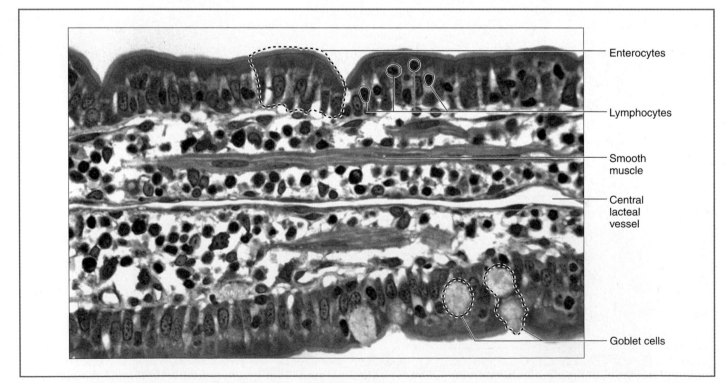

Figure 11-30. Longitudinal section through a villus showing a central lacteal vessel, loose connective tissue, smooth muscle cells, intraepithelial lymphocytes, and simple columnar epithelium.

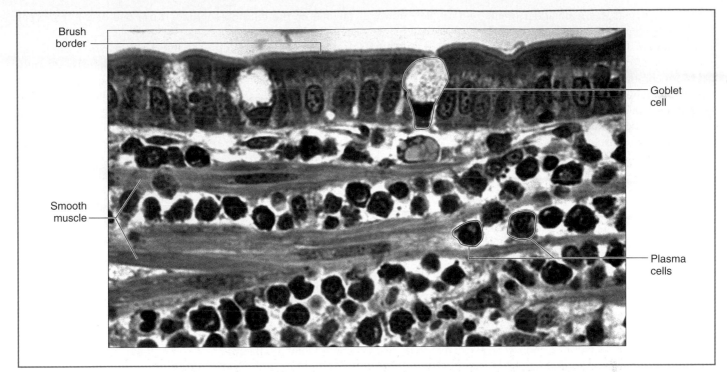

Figure 11-31. High-magnification view of a villus showing plasma cells in the connective tissue, smooth muscle cells, a simple columnar epithelium bearing a brush border of microvilli, and a goblet cell. The light-staining supranuclear regions in the epithelial cells probably correspond to Golgi stacks.

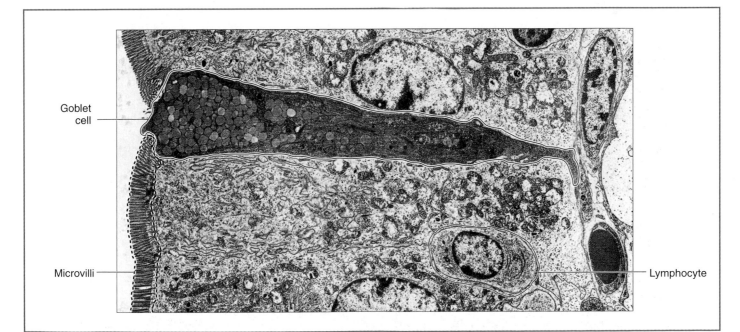

Figure 11-32. Transmission electron micrograph of columnar absorptive cells (enterocytes) covering a villus in the small intestine. Note the apical microvilli present on the absorptive cells. An intraepithelial lymphocyte and a goblet cell, containing secretory vesicles filled with mucin protein, are also visible. (From Standring S. *Gray's Anatomy*, 39th ed. Philadelphia, Churchill-Livingstone, 2005, p 1160.)

from the pancreas and gallbladder break lipid droplets down into tiny aggregations called micelles, (2) fatty acids derived from micelles are bound by enterocyte fatty acid–binding proteins and are taken up into the cell cytoplasm, (3) fatty acids are combined with glycerol to re-form triacylglycerides that are combined with apolipoproteins and are known as chylomicra, and (4) chylomicra are packaged in membrane-bounded vesicles and are transported across the cell cytoplasm for secretion at the basal surface of the cell. Ultimately, chylomicra are transported into specialized lymph capillaries of the villi called central lacteals (see Fig. 11-30), which convey a lipid-rich fluid away from the small intestine to the liver.

Deeper into the wall of the small intestine, at the base of the intestinal glands, additional cell types can be found. Pale-staining enteroendocrine cells, similar in appearance to those in the stomach (see Fig. 11-24), secrete hormones such as cholecystokinin and secretin, which influence the function of the pancreas and gallbladder. Other simple columnar epithelial cells in the intestinal glands show rapid rates of mitosis and function as stem cells. These cells are responsible for the production of about 70 billion cells per day that arise within the digestive epithelium. This rapid rate of cell proliferation is required to offset the continual damage that epithelial cells encounter during exposure to stomach acids, food molecules, and intestinal bacteria. Proliferating cells migrate up the villi to eventually form one of the two types of cells there.

A final cell type within the intestinal glands is called the Paneth cell (Fig. 11-33). These cells possess strongly eosinophilic apical secretory granules and are particularly abundant in the jejunum. The secretory granules of Paneth cells contain at least three types of molecules: tumor necrosis factor (TNF), lysozyme, and defensins (also called cryptidins). TNF has a modulatory effect on lymphocytes present in the intestine, and lysozyme can break down the polysaccharides of the cell walls surrounding bacteria. Defensins belong to a family of small peptides with at least 16 members that are produced both by Paneth cells and by leukocytes. These proteins can render the plasma membranes of bacteria or other target cells permeable to water, so that the cells swell and burst. All these molecules point to a role for Paneth cells in controlling the bacterial population of the gut.

Ileum

The main distinguishing feature of the ileum is the presence of unusually prominent masses of lymphocytes, macrophages, and dendritic cells in the submucosa called Peyer's patches (Fig. 11-34). The presence of these structures in the ileum is unquestionably linked to the increase in the total mass of intraluminal microorganisms along the length of the gut. In

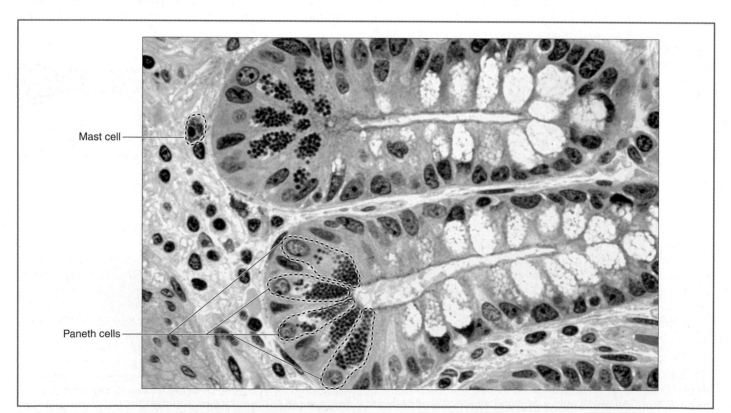

Figure 11-33. Paneth cells, possessing eosinophilic, apical secretion granules, are shown at the bottom of a crypt of Lieberkühn. In the adjacent lamina propria composed of loose connective tissue, fibroblasts and a mast cell can be seen.

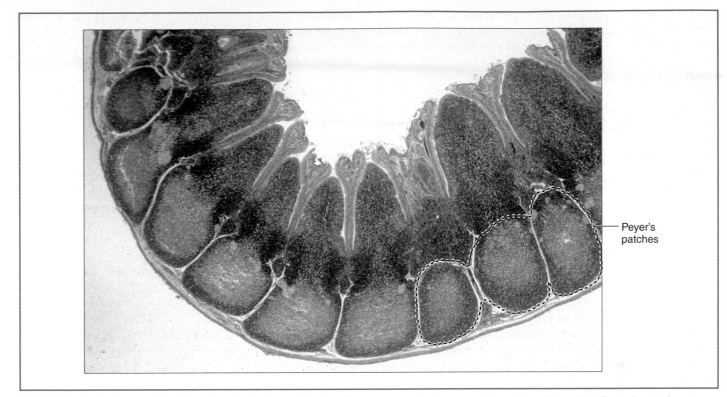

Figure 11-34. Low-magnification view of the ileum showing the masses of submucosal lymphocytes called Peyer's patches.

fact, if mice are raised in a germ-free environment that limits the growth of intestinal bacteria, Peyer's patches decrease in volume by eight-fold. Thus, the structure of lymphoid aggregations within the intestine reflects the continuing hostile, but restrained, interaction between the host epithelium and the bacteria resident in the gut.

In addition to containing lymphoid cells, Peyer's patches are covered by epithelial cells termed M cells. These cells, which in light microscopy simply resemble clusters of lymphocytes enclosed by a thin rim of M-cell cytoplasm, envelop lymphocytes and macrophages and pass on to them whole, intact proteins recovered via transcytosis from the gut lumen. This method of antigen presentation of whole, undigested proteins is not found anywhere else in the immune system. In addition, the subset of lymphocytes (T cells) found within the epithelium of the villi is quite different from the T cells circulating in the blood: they possess cell surface proteins such as CD8$\alpha\alpha$, which are absent from T cells elsewhere. Finally, yet another subset of T cells in the gut, called regulatory T cells, possesses receptor proteins called Toll-like receptors that react to bacterial antigens by firmly suppressing an immune attack on gut bacteria. Immunosuppression occurs through both the death (apoptosis) of reactive lymphocytes and through the inhibition of lymphocyte activity. All these special immune properties are required to permit the existence of vast numbers of bacteria in the gut, which in other hollow organs would present an enormous potential for infection that could be very harmful.

In addition to these complex features of the gut mucosa, the anatomy and function of the underlying layers of the gut

MICROBIOLOGY

Intestinal Lumen

The gastrointestinal tract has been estimated to contain some 100 trillion bacteria. Dozens, if not hundreds, of bacterial species are detectable within the intestines and fall into several major groups.

Four major genera (*Bacteroides, Peptostreptococcus, Bifidobacterium,* and *Eubacterium*) account for the majority of nonpathogenic (commensal) bacteria.

Less abundant species include *Escherichia coli,* streptococci, lactobacilli, and clostridia.

In addition to nonharmful bacteria, about 5% to 10% of stool samples from the United States population shows evidence of the presence of protozoa, such as *Giardia* or amebae, or roundworms, such as *Ascaris.*

Bacteria resident in the gut perform many useful, symbiotic functions for humans. They partially digest long-chain polysaccharides using enzymes that human cells lack; the resulting molecules can then be absorbed by the gut and utilized. They compete with and resist invasion of the gut by other, potentially harmful microorganisms. Finally, intestinal bacteria stimulate the development of gut-associated lymphoid tissue (GALT) such as Peyer's patches.

are not without interest. The submucosa of the entire digestive system contains dense, irregular connective tissue and large numbers of neurons (the submucosal plexus of Meissner) grouped into numerous ganglia (Fig. 11-35). These ganglia are frequently adjacent to the numerous blood vessels and lymphatic vessels of the submucosa that participate in the transport of nutrients away from the gut to the liver and to the rest of the body. Other nerve ganglia can be found between the two layers of smooth muscle of the muscularis externa (the inner layer of muscle is arranged in a circular fashion, whereas the outer layer runs longitudinally along the gut, so that in a cross-section of the gut, these outer smooth muscle cells are cut in cross-section) (Fig. 11-36). The ganglia between these two muscle layers make up the myenteric plexus of Auerbach. These masses of nerve cells constitute a significant enteric nervous system that has been relatively overlooked until recently.

It has been estimated that the entire human digestive system contains some 300 million neurons, more than the total number of neurons in the spinal cord. Many of these neurons utilize serotonin as a neurotransmitter (there is 100-fold more serotonin in the gut than in the brain). The neurochemical properties of these neurons have important implications for patients taking drugs that affect serotonin metabolism (e.g., antidepressants that interfere with the reuptake of serotonin). Such drugs may have helpful effects on the "brain of the head" but have harmful effects on the "brain of the gut" and can cause nausea and gastrointestinal problems. Submucosal plexus neurons seem to regulate the secretion of mucus, water, and NaCl by the gut mucosa, whereas the neurons of the myenteric plexus control the regular contractions of the gut wall (peristalsis), which moves material along the gut. The enteric nervous system can regulate peristalsis perfectly well on its own, so that severing the vagus nerve and other connections with the central nervous system does not preclude a normal reflex functioning of the digestive system.

Large Intestine (Colon)

The histologic features of the large intestine resemble those of the small intestine, with two notable exceptions: the mucosa of the large intestine possesses intestinal glands but *lacks* villi, and the percentage of goblet cells within the lining epithelium is much higher in the large intestine than in the small intestine (Fig. 11-37). The reason for this second special

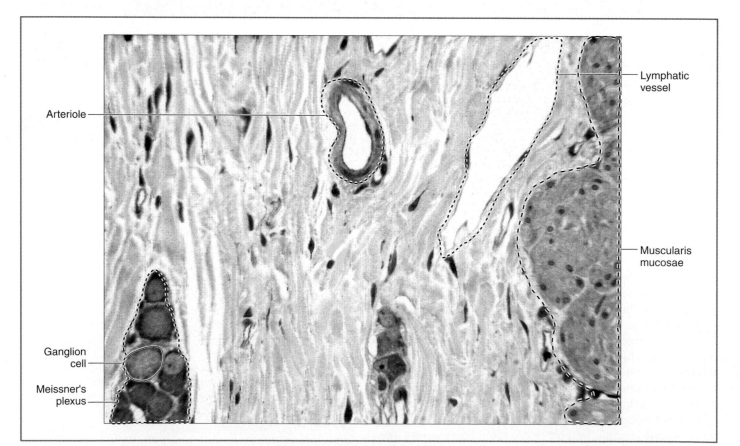

Figure 11-35. High-magnification view of the smooth muscle of the muscularis mucosae and the dense, irregular connective tissue of the submucosa of the jejunum. Note the presence of an arteriole and a lymphatic vessel in the highly vascular submucosa. Ganglion cells of the submucosal plexus of Meissner also are present.

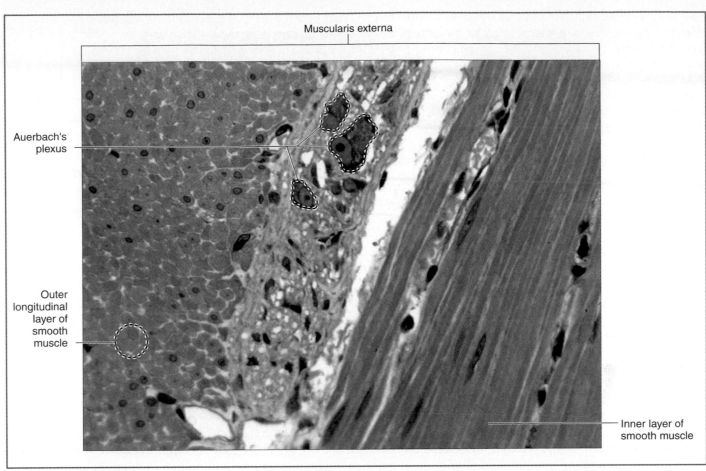

Muscularis externa

Auerbach's plexus

Outer longitudinal layer of smooth muscle

Inner layer of smooth muscle

Figure 11-36. High-magnification view of the muscularis externa of the jejunum. The inner (circular) layer of smooth muscle is cut in longitudinal section, whereas the outer layer of smooth muscle is cut in cross-section. Note the presence of a ganglion cell between these two layers that represents a portion of the myenteric plexus of Auerbach.

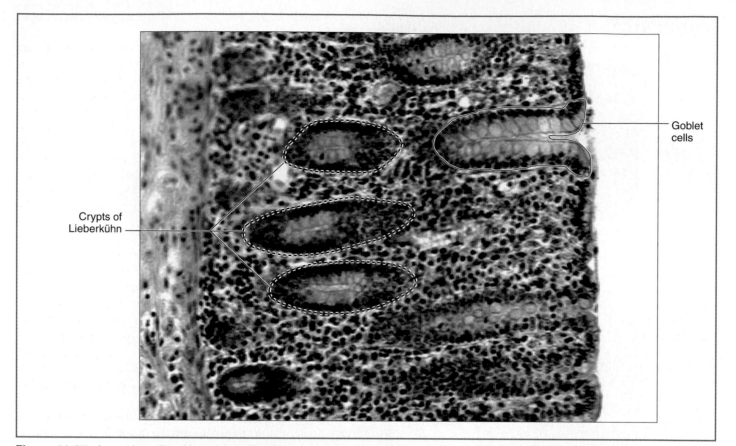

Crypts of Lieberkühn

Goblet cells

Figure 11-37. Large intestine. Note the abundance of goblet cells and the lack of villi between crypts of Lieberkühn.

feature of the large intestine is directly related to the remarkable absorptive ability of the intestine; although almost 9 L of fluid enters the gut daily, the vast majority of this fluid is reabsorbed, so that only 100 mL of fluid eventually leaves the body in the stool. As a consequence, the gut contents steadily become less liquid and more solid and exert more friction on the lining epithelium. To counteract this, the numerous goblet cells of the large intestine secrete more lubricating mucus.

●●● ACCESSORY ORGANS OF THE DIGESTIVE SYSTEM

Liver

The liver functions as gatekeeper or filter interposed between the gut and the remainder of the body. Large blood vessels convey nutrients and other molecules from the gut to the liver, where they are processed, stored, or released into the body. To carry out this function, the liver receives almost a third of the total cardiac output of blood, making it, like the kidney, an extraordinarily well-vascularized organ.

The blood vessels of the liver exert an organizing influence on the distribution of the cells of the liver. The liver receives blood from two sources—the hepatic portal vein, originating from the gut (70% of total blood flow), and the hepatic artery, originating directly from the aorta (30% of blood flow). Branches from these blood vessels travel adjacent to each other within the liver; they deliver mixed arterial and venous blood into thin channels, hepatic sinusoids, which eventually drain into branches of the hepatic vein, the route of exit of blood from the liver. The parenchymal cells of the liver are arranged in narrow rows that follow the courses of the sinusoids.

In histologic sections, branches of the portal vein and hepatic artery are usually accompanied by profiles of tubular structures—bile ducts—that typically possess a simple cuboidal epithelium. Clusters of these three structures are therefore termed *portal triads*. Imaginary lines can be drawn between portal triads in the liver to form the boundaries of a mass of cells centered on a branch of the hepatic vein (central vein). This roughly hexagonal mass of cells is termed a central or classical liver lobule. In some animals, such as pigs, these central lobules are differentiated from one another by thin sheets of connective tissue, but in humans, the borders of a central lobule cannot be visualized, so imaginary lines are used.

A second, higher magnification diagram of one of the rows of cells between a portal triad and a central vein shows the

EMBRYOLOGY

The Gut

Most of the digestive system is formed from the hollow, tubular structure of the embryo named the endoderm. Region-specific signaling molecules that control embryogenesis of specialized regions of the gut are gradually coming to be understood.

The development of the stratified squamous epithelium of the esophagus seems dependent on a transcription factor called p63. If mice are genetically engineered to lack this factor, the esophagus develops a ciliated columnar epithelium.

The continued division of simple columnar epithelial stem cells within intestinal villi results from the action of the same protein (Wnt) that stimulates the formation of simple columnar epithelia within developing teeth. Another protein, called Notch, stimulates the differentiation of absorptive cells, whereas a factor called Math1 guides the development of goblet cells.

In the stomach region, mesenchymal cells produce a homeotic protein called Barx1. Cells possessing this protein secrete Wnt-antagonizing proteins into their environment that cause epithelial cells to form the specialized cells of the gastric mucosa. If these antagonizing proteins are blocked experimentally, the stomach epithelium follows a default pathway and forms cells normally found in the intestine.

Neurons of the gut are formed from neural crest cells that migrate from the region of the developing medulla oblongata all along the length of the developing gut. These cells dive into the wall of the gut at specific places and take up residence as mature neurons.

In Hirschsprung's disease, which affects about 1 in 5000 newborns, the program for the neural network of the colon is not completed and colonic ganglia do not form. As a result, portions of the colon do not contract and the colon becomes overfilled with material, a painful and debilitating condition called megacolon. The cause now appears to be improper function of a number of proteins: glial-derived neurotrophic factor (GDNF) and its receptor, a protein called RET, and endothelin-3 and its receptor.

cells present in the liver. Hepatocytes are cuboidal epithelial cells with a round, euchromatic nuclei and eosinophilic cytoplasms. Each hepatocyte possesses at least one surface with a groove-like indentation. These grooves in adjacent hepatocytes line up to form bile canaliculi (extracellular spaces) that convey bile to a bile duct. The opposite surfaces of hepatocytes contact the endothelial cells of sinusoids, which are specialized blood vessels that lack a continuous basal lamina and have a discontinuous endothelium.

A third liver cell type—the Küpffer cell—anchors itself to the interior of the sinusoid. These cells are derived from monocytes and have a phagocytic function. Finally, a fourth cell type—the stellate cell of Ito—inhabits the space between hepatocytes and endothelial cells, which is called the space of Disse. These stellate cells constitute the connective tissue elements of the liver and can synthesize collagen. They also store large amounts of vitamin A within cytoplasmic lipid droplets.

Low-magnification micrographs of the liver show the characteristic arrangement of hepatocytes within a classical lobule: the cells appear to radiate away in long rows from the central vein (Fig. 11-38). Higher magnification views show the distinctive appearances of portal veins, hepatic arteries, and bile ducts, which all differ in overall diameter, wall thickness, and epithelial type (Fig. 11-39). Some of the larger bile ducts in human livers have increased amounts of connective tissue surrounding them and possess a simple columnar epithelium (Fig. 11-40). The appearance of the thin-walled sinusoids can most easily be appreciated in the vicinity of the central vein (Fig. 11-41).

Each individual hepatocyte has a characteristic appearance that distinguishes it from smaller Küpffer cells or stellate cells (Fig. 11-42). A hepatocyte has a round, euchromatic nucleus and a mainly eosinophilic cytoplasm with patches of basophilia because of the presence of rough endoplasmic reticulum. The highly euchromatic nucleus indicates that these simple-appearing cells are engaged in a multiplicity of highly complex functions: large amounts of dispersed nuclear chromatin point to the transcription of a large variety of genes. These are needed for the extraordinarily large number of tasks performed by the hepatocyte.

One subset of tasks, termed the endocrine function of the hepatocyte, involves monitoring the blood levels of various molecules and either importing them or exporting them to maintain overall nutrient homeostasis. For example, hepatocytes store glucose ingested during a meal as cytoplasmic glycogen; later, when blood glucose levels fall between meals or during a fast, the liver breaks down the glycogen and releases glucose into the bloodstream to provide fuel for the brain and other organs. The high glycogen content of hepatocytes can be illustrated by use of the periodic acid–Schiff (PAS) reaction, which stains carbohydrate molecules a bright magenta color (Fig. 11-43).

Glucose Regulation

Cells require integral membrane proteins, termed glucose transporter proteins, to move glucose across the plasma membrane. Twelve types of hexose transporter proteins, found in specific cell types, are known to exist. Some of these, such as the one utilized by intestinal absorptive cells, require the co-transport of sodium with glucose for their function. Another glucose transporter protein, called GLUT2, is found in the plasma membranes of glucose-sensing cells such as hepatocytes (Fig. 11-44). These transporters have a high capacity for glucose transport but a low affinity for glucose, so that they allow glucose import into hepatocytes only when circulating levels of glucose are elevated. This avoids brain-damaging hypoglycemia between meals.

Analogous transporters allow hepatocytes to import amino acids when blood levels of these molecules are elevated following a meal. Amino acids are broken down within hepatocytes and reutilized to make other molecules such as glucose via gluconeogenesis. An initial step in this process is

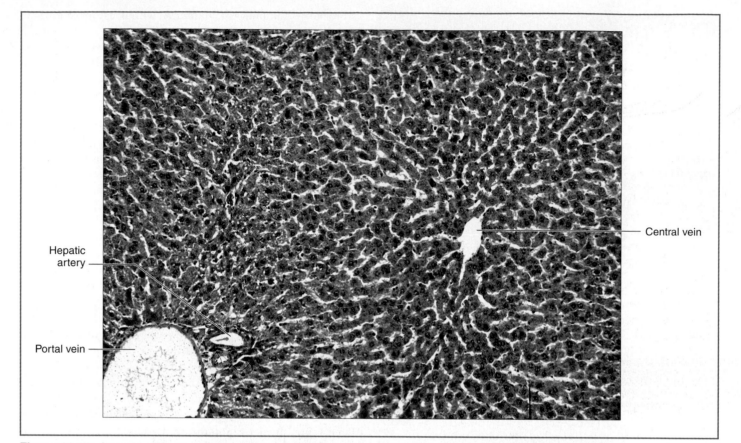

Hepatic artery

Portal vein

Central vein

Figure 11-38. Low-magnification view of a liver lobule showing a central vein, rows of hepatocytes, and a portal triad.

the removal of amino groups from the amino acids. This forms ammonia, a highly toxic chemical that would be harmful if liver cells released it into the bloodstream. Instead, hepatocytes convert the ammonia to urea, a less harmful molecule that eventually is excreted from the body by the kidneys. If this vital function is interrupted by liver injury, high levels of ammonia appear in the bloodstream. This ammonia is particularly damaging to the brain, provoking hepatic encephalopathy.

Lipid metabolism is another activity that falls into the category of the endocrine function of the liver. For example, although most cells have some capacity to oxidize lipids, in fact, more than half of all the lipid oxidation in the body occurs in the liver. Hepatocytes also synthesize lipids in addition to oxidizing them: most of the cholesterol in the body is synthesized by the liver and is transported to the remaining tissues in association with low-density lipoproteins that are also synthesized by the liver to carry the insoluble lipid in the bloodstream. In addition to lipoproteins, the liver synthesizes many other blood proteins such as albumin, insulin-like growth factor, and many blood-clotting proteins.

These endocrine functions of hepatocytes require a high capacity to transport molecules between the cell and the bloodstream. This transport function is assisted by the abundant microvilli found on the sinusoidal surfaces of

hepatocytes (Fig. 11-45). These microvilli increase the surface area available for transport across cell membranes.

The exocrine functions of hepatocytes are performed at the opposite surfaces of the hepatocytes, where bile canaliculi are found (Fig. 11-46; see also Fig. 11-42). A considerable number of substances are transported into the bile for eventual excretion into the lumen of the duodenum and release from the body.

In routine histologic preparations, hepatocytes all look alike and show no signs of specialization. Nevertheless, the activity of hepatocytes varies considerably, depending on how close the cells are to the sources of oxygen and nutrition (portal triads). Cells in these areas are much more metabolically active and show higher turnover (lability) of cytoplasmic glycogen. Consequently, during a prolonged fast, glycogen is more likely to be withdrawn from periportal cells than from cells surrounding the central vein (Fig. 11-47). These demonstrable metabolic differences between liver cells in different locations have led to the development of an alternative way of viewing the histologic organization of the liver. Rather than emphasizing the arrangement of cells surrounding a central vein (central lobule), this viewpoint organizes cells of similar metabolic activities into periportal liver acini (Fig. 11-48). In the human liver, neither viewpoint has a clearly discernable anatomic advantage, but the acinar

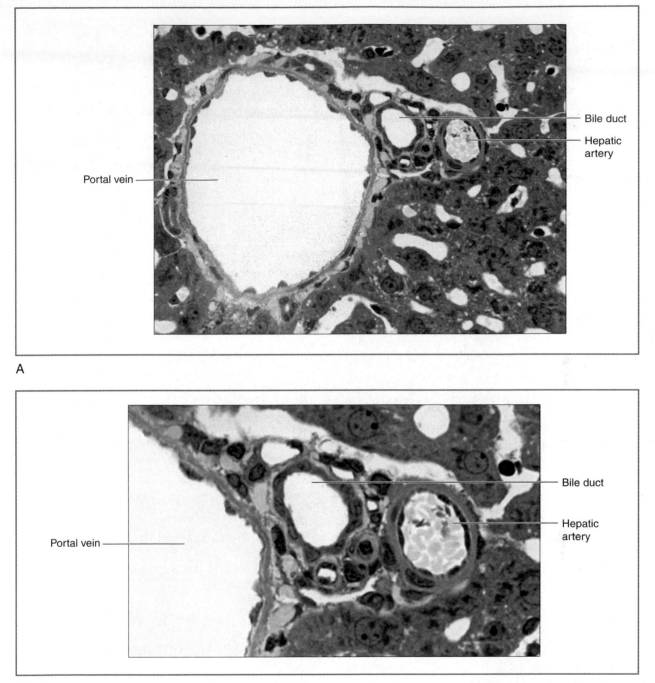

A

B

Figure 11-39. **A,** Intermediate-magnification view of a portal triad showing branches of the portal vein, bile duct, and hepatic artery. **B,** Higher magnification view showing the bile duct (simple cuboidal epithelium), hepatic artery, and part of the portal vein.

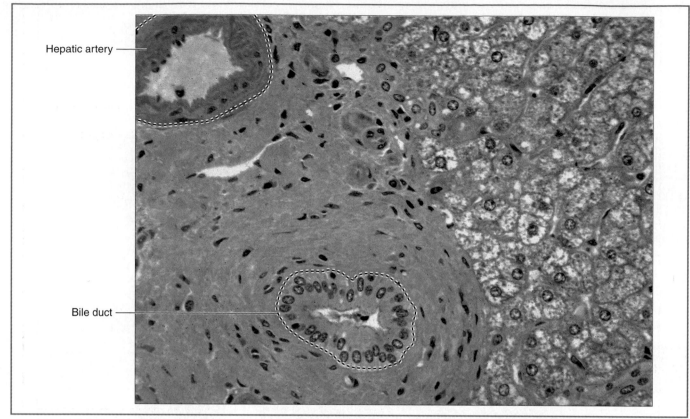

Hepatic artery

Bile duct

Figure 11-40. Human liver tissue showing a large bile duct with a simple columnar epithelium and a branch of the hepatic artery.

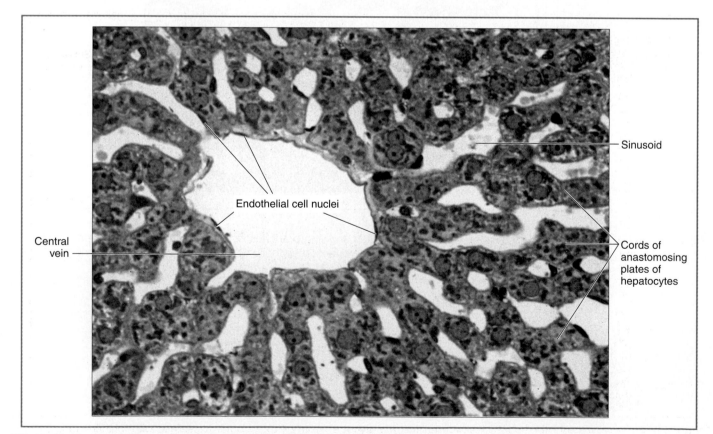

Sinusoid

Endothelial cell nuclei

Central vein

Cords of anastomosing plates of hepatocytes

Figure 11-41. A central vein, which receives blood from surrounding sinusoids.

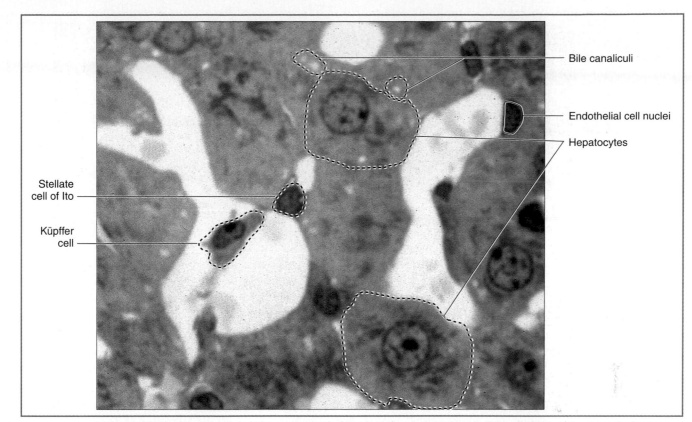

Figure 11-42. High-magnification view of the liver showing hepatocytes, cross-sections of tiny bile canaliculi, a Küpffer cell within a sinusoid, and a stellate cell of Ito.

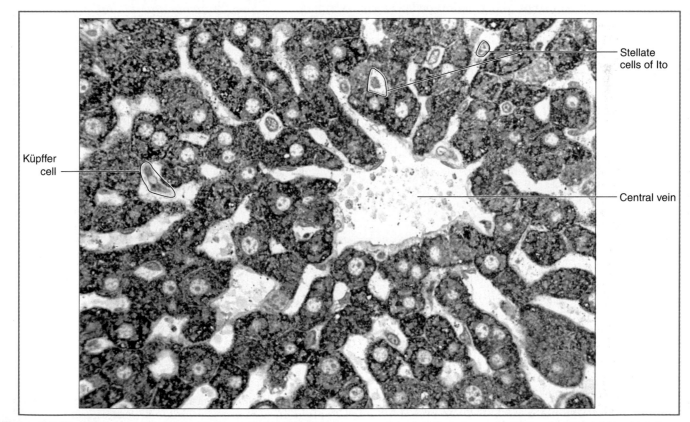

Figure 11-43. Liver stained with the PAS reaction to illustrate glycogen (magenta) and counter-stained with toluidine blue to demonstrate cell nuclei (blue). The smaller cells that lack glycogen are stellate cells of Ito.

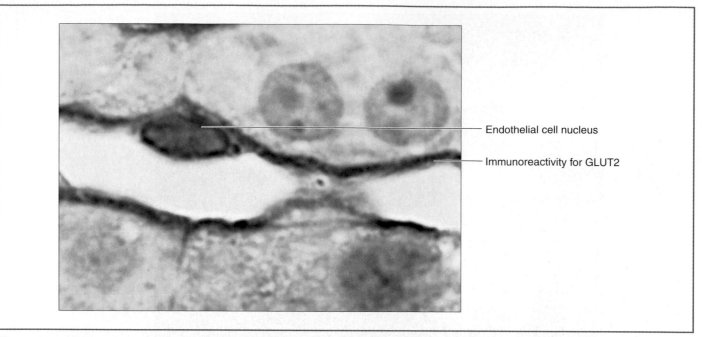

— Endothelial cell nucleus

— Immunoreactivity for GLUT2

Figure 11-44. View of two hepatocytes stained with immunocytochemical method to illustrate the presence of GLUT2-type glucose transporter proteins (brown line at sinusoidal surface of the hepatocytes). Note that this protein is absent from the endothelial cell and from the surfaces between the hepatocytes themselves.

model of the liver does more closely conform to functional divisions of the liver parenchyma. For example, ingestion of toxic chemicals such as carbon tetrachloride preferentially damages specific regions of liver tissue.

Another means of illustrating functional differences between liver cells is the application of Perls' test for iron, which shows that cells near the central vein contain much more iron than do periportal cells (Fig. 11-49). This iron distribution may partly reflect the distribution of some types of heme-containing enzymes called cytochrome P-450 enzymes. This procedure also shows numerous, intensely stained loci that correspond to the locations of phagocytic Küpffer cells, which become filled with iron subsequent to ingesting worn-out RBCs.

Gallbladder

The histology of the gallbladder is simple. The gallbladder is lined by a tall columnar epithelium and has only three additional layers: the lamina propria of loose connective tissue, a muscularis formed by smooth muscle, and an adventitia composed of dense, irregular connective tissue (Fig. 11-50). It receives bile from the liver via the hepatic ducts, which empty into the cystic duct entering the gallbladder. The epithelial cells transport water from the bile so that it becomes up to 10-fold more concentrated than when first secreted from the liver. Bile stored in the gallbladder is released into the duodenum via the cystic duct leading from the gallbladder, which unites with the common hepatic duct from the liver to form the bile duct. Bile enters

BIOCHEMISTRY

Bile Formation

The bile salts form a major component of bile. Bile salts are synthesized by combining a form of cholesterol (cholic acid) with an amino acid such as glycine or taurine. These compounds function in the lumen of the duodenum as detergents, emulsifying lipids into small lipid droplets that can be more easily digested. About 94% of bile salts are reabsorbed by enterocytes, transferred to the bloodstream, and taken up again by hepatocytes for reuse. Cholesterol is also secreted into the bile.

Heme-containing compounds (porphyrins) are secreted into the bile. Failure to accomplish this leads to excessive blood levels of porphyrins (porphyria), damage to the brain, and behavioral abnormalities.

A poorly soluble breakdown product of heme metabolism, bilirubin, is also taken up from the bloodstream by hepatocytes for secretion into the bile. Pure bilirubin is conjugated to glucuronic acid (a modified form of glucose) within liver cells to make it more soluble, and then this compound is secreted into the bile. Failure to accomplish this leads to excessive blood levels of bilirubin, a yellowish tinge to the skin and eyeballs (called *jaundice*), and injury to the brain. Bilirubin and similar compounds are responsible for the color of feces.

Copper is transported into the bile via a plasma membrane copper-transporting protein of hepatocytes (ATPase 7B). Dysfunction of this protein causes Wilson's disease, a widespread tissue accumulation of copper that, once again, is particularly damaging to the brain (hepatolenticular degeneration).

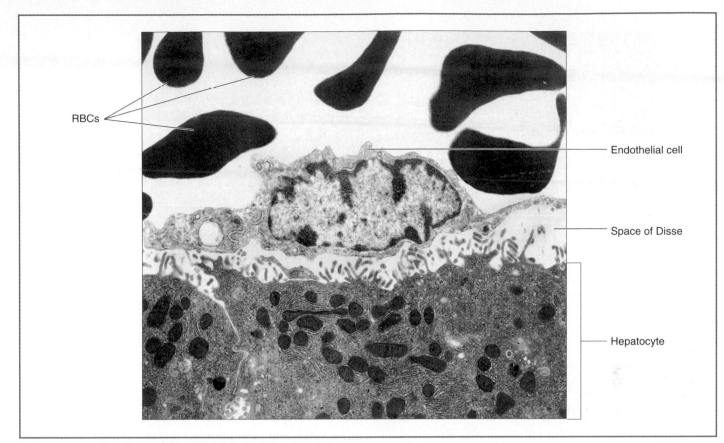

Figure 11-45. Transmission electron micrograph of the sinusoidal surface of a hepatocyte showing hepatocyte microvilli, the space of Disse, an endothelial cell of a sinusoid, and RBCs. (From Standring S. *Gray's Anatomy*, 39th ed. Philadelphia, Churchill-Livingstone, 2005, p 1224.)

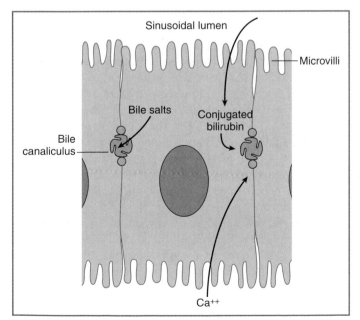

Figure 11-46. Diagram of bile formation by a hepatocyte. Bile salts (glycocholic acid) are formed within the hepatocyte and transported into a bile canaliculus. Other components of bile (e.g., bilirubin or copper) are taken up from the sinusoidal circulation for excretion into the bile.

the duodenum from the bile duct when the smooth muscle of the gallbladder contracts.

Pancreas

Another major gland associated with the gut is the pancreas. About 4% of the cells of the pancreas are endocrine cells and form small clusters called islets of Langerhans. The majority of pancreatic cells have an exocrine function and secrete into ducts. The typical arrangement of pancreatic exocrine cells (acinar cells) is illustrated in Figure 11-51.

Pancreatic acinar cells are highly polarized; at their basal portions, nuclei and large amounts of rough endoplasmic reticulum are found, whereas the apical portion of each cell is killed by many large secretory granules. This ultrastructural polarization causes the basal portion of each cell to be highly basophilic and the apical portion to be very eosinophilic (Fig. 11-52). The histologic appearance of the pancreas somewhat resembles that of the parotid gland except that (1) striated ducts are absent from the pancreas, (2) the secretory acini of the pancreas lack the myoepithelial cells that are present in most other serous glands, and (3) islets of Langerhans are present scattered throughout the pancreas.

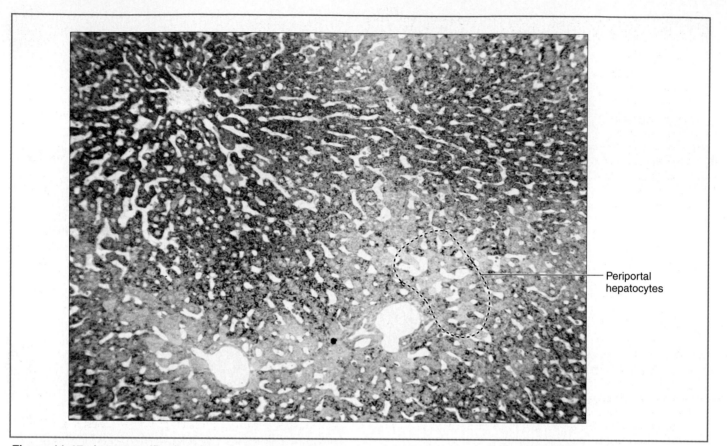

Figure 11-47. Low-magnification view of a liver from a fasted rat, stained for glycogen with the PAS reaction. Glycogen is preferentially depleted from more metabolically active hepatocytes near portal triads and far from central veins.

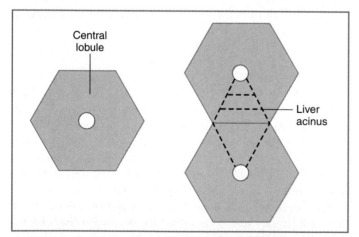

Figure 11-48. Two organizational schemes of liver cells representing two different concepts of liver function. Central lobules emphasize the endocrine functions of liver cells that deliver molecules into the central vein. Acinar lobules emphasize the metabolic heterogeneity of liver cells, which are more active when they are in close proximity to portal triads.

Histologic Differences

Striated ducts in salivary glands function to add water to the saliva and make it hypotonic relative to blood plasma. Pancreatic secretions need not be so watery, so striated ducts are not found in the pancreas. Instead, most ducts, called intercalated ducts, are composed of a low cuboidal epithelium and simply convey secretions toward the intestine (Fig. 11-53; see also Figs. 11-51 and 11-52). The initial segments of these ducts protrude into the lumen of a secretory acinus; these initial duct cells are called centroacinar cells (see Figs. 11-51 and 11-53). Intercalated ducts converge on large, infrequent ducts (interlobular ducts) that possess a simple columnar or stratified columnar epithelium.

Notable is the absence of myoepithelial cells in the pancreas. They have a required function in other glands but are absent from the pancreas perhaps because of the anatomy of pancreatic acini. Studies of serial sections of the pancreas, carried out in the 1990s, revealed an unexpected feature of the pancreas: instead of being composed of blind-ended pockets, many secretory acini of the pancreas are in fact tubular in shape, with openings to ducts at both ends. This

Liver Toxicity

A primary function of the liver is the breaking down of potentially harmful chemicals that enter the body via the digestive tract. Liver cells contain many enzymes, which are associated physically with the smooth endoplasmic reticulum, to accomplish this.

- Humans synthesize 57 different members of a family of enzymes called cytochrome P-450 enzymes. These proteins took their name originally from the absorption spectrum of a solution of these enzymes, which showed a major band at a wavelength of 450 nm. These enzymes catalyze dozens of chemical reactions that can modify thousands of different chemicals.
- Another liver enzyme, alcohol dehydrogenase, can be greatly increased in the liver by chronic consumption of large amounts of alcohol (e.g., more than three cocktails per day). These elevated enzymes create toxic levels of a chemical, acetaldehyde, which causes liver damage and cirrhosis of the liver. In this condition, stellate cells overproduce collagen, which accumulates around vessels and impairs circulation of blood through the liver.
- Another potent liver toxin is acetaminophen, a common ingredient in pain-killing medicines. Overconsumption of acetaminophen, or consumption by persons with alcoholism, leads to a high level of acetaldehyde, which is responsible for 42% of liver failure cases currently seen in the United States.

Gallbladder Contraction

Gallbladder contraction is tightly controlled by signals emanating from the small intestine. One of these signals is the hormone cholecystokinin (CCK), which is secreted from enteroendocrine cells of the gut. CCK receptors on smooth muscle cells prompt smooth muscle contraction.

Another signal controlling gallbladder contraction arises from neurons in ganglia surrounding the gallbladder. Many of these neurons, which utilize a variety of peptides as neurotransmitters, are in turn controlled by direct connections from the myenteric plexus of the small intestine. Inhibitory neurons of these ganglia are stimulated by CCK to cause relaxation of the sphincter of Oddi surrounding the bile duct, so that, when the gallbladder contracts, bile is free to leave the gallbladder and enter the intestine. There is some evidence that an impaired response to CCK, causing diminished gallbladder emptying, may contribute to gallstone formation.

Gallstones

By age 60 years, 15% to 20% of the population has experienced clinically significant gallstones. Gallstones often necessitate gallbladder excision, which is one of the most common surgical procedures.

Gallstones are principally composed of cholesterol. The reasons why gallstones form are uncertain; there is some evidence that intestinal bacteria, invading the gallbladder via the common bile duct, may convert cholic acid into the less soluble deoxycholic acid, which may form an insoluble nucleus for gallstones.

---

allows for a freer exit of secretory material from acini and perhaps explains the absence of contractile myoepithelial cells.

The apical secretory granules of pancreatic acinar cells are called zymogen granules because they contain inactive forms of digestive enzymes (termed zymogens). It is essential that these powerful enzymes (trypsin, carboxypeptidase) be secreted as inactive forms because otherwise they would digest the proteins of the pancreas itself (such pancreatic damage can indeed occur if pancreatic duct dysfunction allows the activated enzymes back up into the pancreas).

Intestinal Digestive Enzyme Activation

Intestinal absorptive cells of the duodenum possess an integral membrane protein called enteropeptidase (this protein is sometimes called an enterokinase, a term that erroneously suggests that its function is to add phosphate groups to proteins). This enteropeptidase cleaves off an initial portion of the precursor to trypsin, which activates it. Trypsin, in turn, activates the other peptidases secreted by the pancreas into the intestinal lumen. In addition, other pancreatic enzymes (amylase, lipase, DNAse, RNAse) contribute to the digestion of the nonprotein components of food.

Exocrine secretion from the pancreas is under both hormonal and neural control. Enteroendocrine cells of the gut produce cholecystokinin (CCK), which stimulates the release of zymogen enzymes from acinar cells, and secretin, which stimulates the duct cells to secrete water and bicarbonate ions into the duodenum. Nerves also terminate on acinar cells (see Fig. 11-52). These nerves can derive either from the vagus, which has a stimulatory influence on pancreatic secretion, or can be branches that arise from the myenteric plexus of the small intestine.

The endocrine portion of the pancreas consists of spherical islets of Langerhans, wherein four main cell types exist, each one of which primarily secretes one major peptide hormone (Fig. 11-54):

- α-Cells of pancreatic islets mainly secrete glucagon, which stimulates the liver to release glucose into the

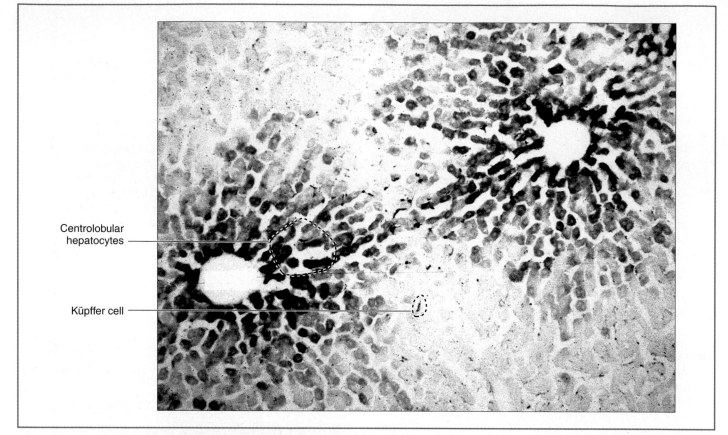

Centrolobular
hepatocytes

Küpffer cell

Figure 11-49. Perls' stain for iron (intensified by diaminobenzidine) illustrates biochemical differences between centrolobular and periportal hepatocytes. Small dots intensely stained for iron correspond to the locations of Küpffer cells, which have phagocytosed iron-rich red blood cells.

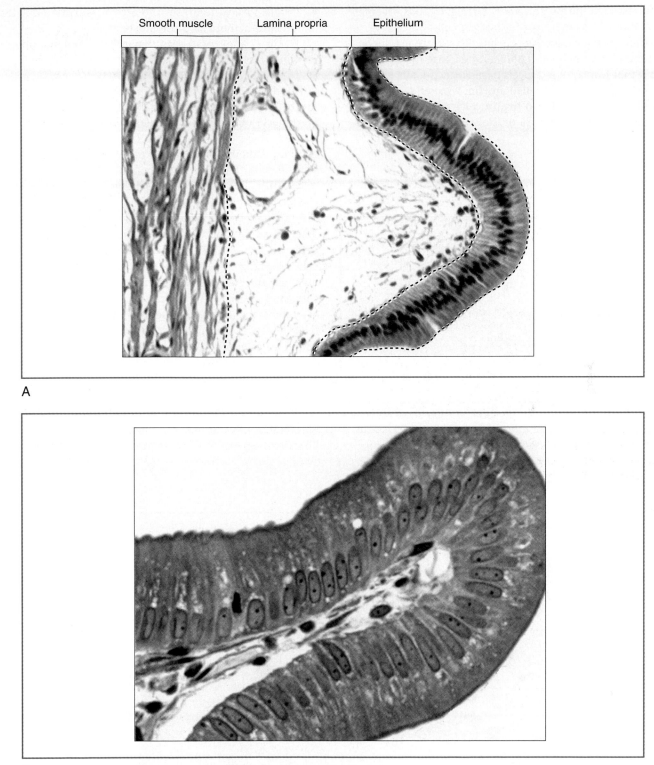

Smooth muscle   Lamina propria   Epithelium

A

B

Figure 11-50. A, Low-magnification view of the gallbladder showing the epithelium, loose connective tissue of the lamina propria, and smooth muscle. **B,** Higher magnification view of the lining epithelium of the gallbladder showing the characteristically tall, simple columnar epithelial cells.

bloodstream during periods of fasting. α-Cells account for about 10% to 15% of total islet cells.

- β-Cells of pancreatic islets primarily secrete insulin, a hormone that enhances uptake of glucose by most cells and that lowers blood levels of glucose. β-Cells also synthesize a peptide called amylin, which has an amino acid sequence similar to that of calcitonin. β-Cells account for 70% to 80% of islet cells.

- δ-Cells (5% of total) secrete gastrin, which modulates stomach activity, and somatostatin.
- F cells (2% of total) secrete pancreatic polypeptide, which blocks the stimulatory effects of CCK on pancreatic secretion.

The distribution of these four cells types is not random: the α-, δ-, and F cells typically are found at the margins (periphery) of an islet while the β-cells occupy the center of an islet. These cell types cannot be distinguished from one another, although with most routine stains toluidine blue stains δ-cells metachromatically (pink). The most reliable way to identify the specific islet cell types is by immunocytochemical techniques.

The arrangement of cells within an islet appears to be determined by the cells themselves. When islet cells are detached from each other by enzyme treatments in vitro, the cells rearrange themselves into renewed islets and still maintain the peripheral distribution of δ-cells on the outer surface of an islet. This appears to be due to the presence of an adhesion molecule—neural cell adhesion molecule (NCAM)—on δ-cells that allows them to recognize and adhere to each other.

β-Cells secrete insulin in response to an elevation in blood glucose; secreted insulin causes the excess blood glucose to be transported into muscle, liver, and fat cells. If insulin secretion were not regulated in this way, it could be secreted at inappropriate times and provoke a dangerous hypoglycemia. To avoid this, β-cells utilize the same type of

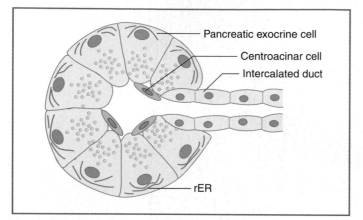

Figure 11-51. Diagram of a pancreatic acinus showing acinar cells with basal rER, apical zymogen granules, centroacinar cells, and an intercalated duct.

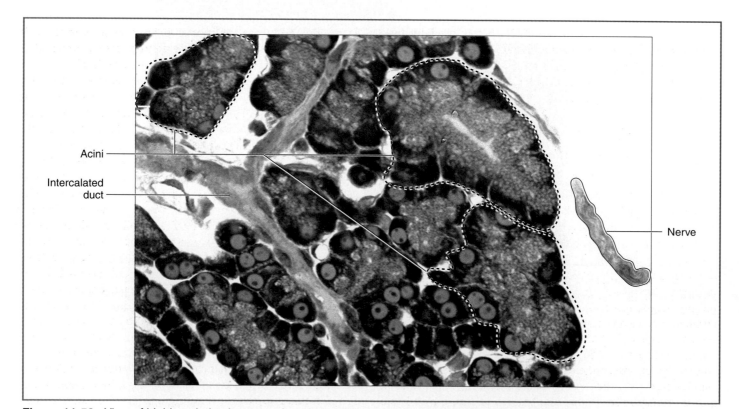

Figure 11-52. View of highly polarized pancreatic acinar cells plus several intercalated ducts and a nerve.

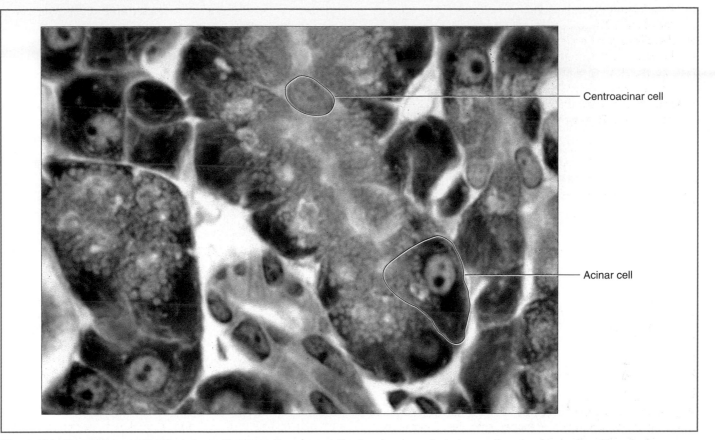

Figure 11-53. High-magnification view of pancreatic acinar cells showing a centroacinar cell and acinar cells with apical secretion granules.

glucose transporter protein (GLUT2) that is used by liver cells as part of a glucose-sensing mechanism (see Fig. 11-44). These transporters only allow glucose import when extracellular levels of glucose are quite high. Once within a β-cell, glucose is metabolized, yielding high amounts of ATP that cause ATP-sensitive potassium channels to open, depolarizing the β-cell. The result is the release of insulin.

Insulin Stimulation of Tissues and Glucose Uptake

Insulin provokes a molecular rearrangement of membrane structures within target cells. It does this by first binding to a plasma membrane receptor protein (Fig. 11-55). Unlike receptors for many protein hormones, the insulin receptor does *not* stimulate the production of intracellular cyclic AMP to exert its effects on cell function. Instead, the activated receptor phosphorylates another protein called the insulin receptor substrate (IRS). The IRS protein, in turn, activates a number of different intracellular signaling systems. One system causes a migration of cytoplasmic vesicles toward the plasma membrane. These vesicles contain extra, unused glucose transporter proteins (GLUT4 transporters). When the vesicles fuse with the plasma membrane, they add the extra glucose transporters to the membrane, increasing by 10-fold the ability of a cell to import glucose. This movement of

intracellular, glucose transporter–bearing vesicles to the cell membrane is another example of a common mechanism that cells utilize to alter their permeability to a molecule.

An unusual anatomic aspect of the pancreas that has considerable functional importance is the fact that clusters of endocrine cells (islets) are scattered throughout the exocrine pancreas and carry with them the blood vessels that supply them. This arrangement of endocrine cells is found in no other endocrine organ. Approximately 85% of blood entering the pancreas first passes through capillaries in the islets and then enters capillaries surrounding acinar cells. As a result, acinar cells are exposed to higher concentrations of insulin than all other cells in the body. The insulin stimulates acinar cells to synthesize amylase, which facilitates the digestion of a carbohydrate-rich diet. If an animal is fed a high-protein, carbohydrate-poor diet, circulating levels of insulin fall and the pancreas adapts by not synthesizing much amylase, which is no longer necessary. Thus, the blood supply of the pancreas, by establishing a functional communication between endocrine and exocrine cells, helps coordinate their activity and provides for a more efficient use of the exocrine and endocrine products of the pancreas. Not all animals enjoy the benefits of this dispersion of islets among acinar tissue; some fish, for example, form a pure aggregation of endocrine cells on one side of the pancreas called a Brockmann body.

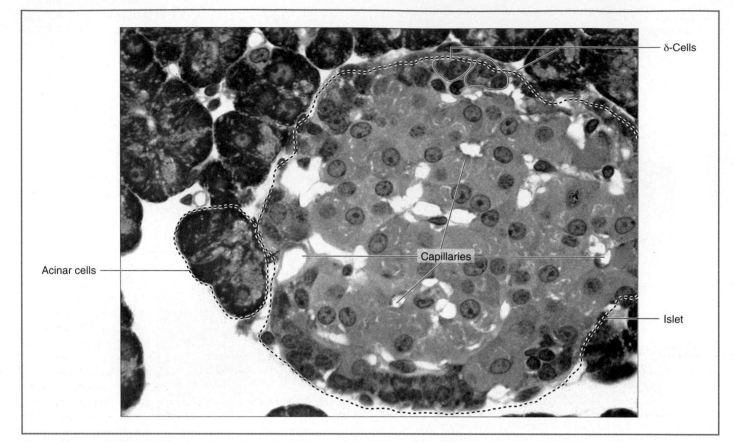

Figure 11-54. High-magnification view of an islet of Langerhans. Most of the cells in each islet are either capillary endothelial cells or insulin-secreting β-cells. The toluidine blue stain employed in this preparation stains δ-cells metachromatically (deep magenta-pink), so that a few of these peripherally located cells can be discerned.

Diabetes Mellitus

Diabetes mellitus is a condition in which insulin fails to control adequately tissue uptake of glucose and blood levels of glucose. Improper maintenance of glucose homeostasis by glucose-sensing cells of the endocrine pancreas, liver, and hypothalamus appears to be present in diabetes mellitus. It is estimated that 30 million people worldwide currently have this condition. Its incidence is increasing, probably owing to the increasing incidence of obesity, which exacerbates diabetes mellitus. Some statisticians predict that, as world populations become more obese, about 1 in 3 people born in 2000 may develop this disorder. Since diabetes causes many debilitating conditions (heart disease, kidney disease, blindness, poor circulation, etc.), the prospect of a continual increase in this disorder is extremely serious.

EMBRYOLOGY

Liver and Pancreas

The accessory organs of the digestive system originate as outgrowths from the gut endoderm. Distinct signals provoke the differentiation of each organ.

Fibroblast growth factors secreted from mesenchyme induce the hepatic gene program in endodermal cells destined to become the liver and also suppress the pancreatic genes.

Transcription factors called Hex and hepatocyte nuclear factor-4 promote the differentiation of hepatocytes. During development, the liver transiently acquires the ability to promote blood cell formation and at that time constructs the sinusoids found in other blood-forming organs (spleen, bone marrow). These sinusoids persist, but the blood-forming ability of the liver wanes after birth.

Development of the pancreas is dependent on unidentified signaling molecules from mesenchyme. Growth of the early pancreatic bud requires a homeotic protein called IPF-1; if this gene is inactivated, the pancreas fails to develop. Endocrine cells form before exocrine cells; all pancreatic cells show some growth after birth, and islet cells require a transcription factor called *PAX4* for cell division and renewal.

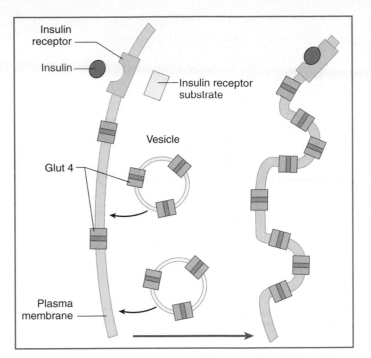

Figure 11-55. Diagram of the mechanism of insulin's action on cellular glucose uptake. Upon the binding of insulin to its receptor in the cell membrane, a cytoplasmic protein called the insulin receptor substrate is activated. As a consequence, cytoplasmic vesicles move to the plasma membrane. These vesicles possess extra GLUT4-type glucose transporter proteins. Movement of these vesicles to the plasma membrane of a cell permits a 10-fold increase in glucose import by the cell.

PATHOLOGY

Diabetes Mellitus

Type I (juvenile-onset) diabetes mellitus accounts for about 10% of all cases and results from an outright insufficiency of insulin. This is due to an autoimmune attack of unknown origin on islet cells and to a failure of the remaining islet cells to proliferate and replenish the needed amount of insulin. Recent data suggest that a defect in the *PAX4* transcription factor that drives β-cell regeneration may be present in this type of diabetes.

Type II (adult-onset) diabetes accounts for 90% of all cases and results from generalized resistance to the effects of insulin and from gradual exhaustion of β-cells, which attempt to compensate for insulin resistance by secreting ever-increasing amounts of insulin. Defects in the ATP-sensitive potassium channel of β-cells, in hepatocyte nuclear factor 4, and in mitochondria are currently suspected to contribute to this disorder. The arcuate nucleus of the hypothalamus also may have a role in diabetes. Neurons in this brain region, acting via the autonomic nervous system, have a potent influence on glucose release from the liver and on overall responsiveness to insulin. Arcuate astrocytes possess the same GLUT2 proteins as do liver cells and β-cells and presumably play a role in glucose sensing by the hypothalamus. Recent studies have shown that if the abnormal function of arcuate neurons in genetically obese mice is corrected by genetic engineering, all abnormalities in glucose homeostasis in these obese mice are quickly corrected.

Respiratory System 12

CONTENTS

The nasal cavities, pharynx, larynx, trachea, main bronchi, and lungs form the respiratory system. Within the lungs, the two main bronchi branch repeatedly, forming first a succession of smaller bronchi and then a series of bronchioles. The airways finally end blindly as millions of thin-walled alveoli. It is primarily in the alveoli that gas exchange between the blood and the inspired air occurs. The alveoli-containing structures (respiratory bronchioles, alveolar ducts, and alveolar sacs) are thus often referred to as the *respiratory portion* of the respiratory system, while the nonalveolar structures are referred to as the *conducting portion* of the respiratory system. It is important to keep in mind that the conducting airways carry out a number of important functions, the most crucial of which is conditioning the air to minimize possible damage to the delicate alveoli.

●●● RESPIRATORY MUCOSA

Most of the extrapulmonary parts of the respiratory tract are lined by a mucosa consisting of a pseudostratified, ciliated columnar epithelium with goblet cells and an underlying lamina propria; the latter is a connective tissue layer containing many blood vessels, mixed serous and mucous glands, and a rich elastin fiber network (Figs. 12-1 and 12-2). Immune cells are common and may accumulate as mucosal-associated (or bronchial-associated) lymphoid tissue (MALT or BALT). Some authors refer to the deeper layers of the mucosa as a submucosa, but there is no distinct morphologic boundary between the lamina propria and the submucosa, as is seen in the digestive tract.

The free surface of the mucosa is covered by a layer of mucus that floats on a watery layer adjacent to the cells (see Fig. 12-1). As air passes over the respiratory mucosa, it is warmed by the blood in the blood vessels and is humidified by the wet mucus. At least some microorganisms and particles of dust present in the air stick to the wet mucus and thus are prevented from entering the lungs. Water-soluble airborne pollutants are absorbed by the mucus as well.

The major cell types in the epithelium are

- Ciliated cells
- Goblet cells
- Neuroendocrine cells (PNECs)
- Basal or stem cells

The ciliated cells are arranged so that all cilia beat toward the pharynx; those in the nasal cavity carry the mucus posteriorly and those in the larynx, trachea, and lungs carry the mucus upward. Thus, they transport the mucus, and any adhering dirt particles, pollutants, and microorganisms, to the pharynx; from there it enters the esophagus and is swallowed, removing it from the respiratory tract altogether. This mechanism of clearing particulate matter from the respiratory tract is sometimes referred to as the *mucociliary escalator*. In addition to moving mucus, the ciliated cells transport chloride ions across their apical membranes into the lumen. Water follows osmotically, and this fluid helps hydrate the mucus and contributes to the watery layer that the mucus floats on. Only the tips of the cilia contact the mucus, allowing them to beat freely within the watery layer close to the cells (see Fig. 12-1).

The goblet cells secrete mucins, both constitutively and in response to irritants. When the mucin secretion granules are released by exocytosis, the mucins become hydrated and rapidly expand. Goblet cell hyperplasia is a common response to a variety of irritants and is characteristic of several respiratory diseases.

Neuroendocrine cells (often called pulmonary neuroendocrine cells or PNECs, even when found in the upper respiratory tract) occur singly or in clusters in the epithelium

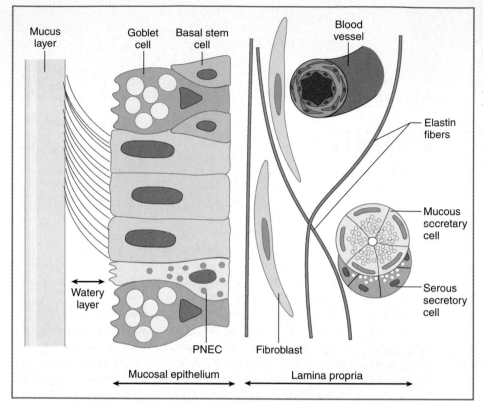

Mucus layer

Goblet cell

Basal stem cell

Blood vessel

Elastin fibers

Mucous secretary cell

Serous secretory cell

Watery layer

PNEC

Fibroblast

Mucosal epithelium

Lamina propria

Figure 12-1. Diagram of the respiratory mucosa. The goblet and mucous gland cells secrete mucus onto the surface of the epithelium. The mucus floats on a watery layer formed by secretions of the serous gland cells and water, which follows osmotically when the ciliated cells transport ions into the lumen. The cilia all beat toward the pharynx, where the mucus, along with adsorbed pollutants, is swallowed. PNEC, (pulmonary) neuroendocrine cell.

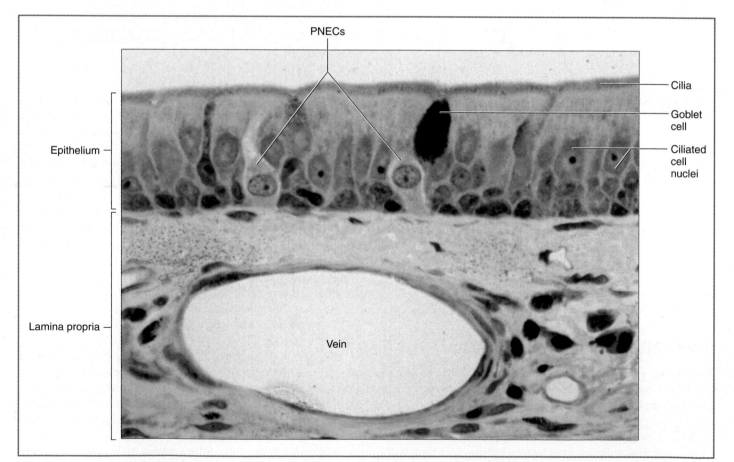

PNECs

Cilia

Goblet cell

Ciliated cell nuclei

Epithelium

Lamina propria

Vein

Figure 12-2. This plastic section of the respiratory mucosa from the trachea was stained with toluidine blue and basic fuchsin. Although not visible in many preparations, the PNECs here are distinguished as pale cells that may be basal or extend to the lumen.

throughout the respiratory tract (see Figs. 12-1 and 12-2). They secrete basally a variety of peptide factors, which may have endocrine (via the bloodstream) or paracrine (via local diffusion) effects. These cells are sensitive to hypoxia and affect both airway and vascular muscle tone. They also stimulate growth and development in the immature lung and likely stimulate repair in the adult lung. Nicotine stimulates PNEC hyperplasia, and these cells are believed to be the source of small cell lung cancer.

Basal cells in the epithelium are stem cells that replace all other cell types (see Figs. 12-1 and 12-2). There is evidence that some duct cells in the glands also act as stem cells. The airway epithelium is in a high-risk location for damage from microorganisms and pollutants, and stem cells are needed for normal cell turnover and to replace damaged cells in the epithelium.

The mucous secretory cells in the mucosal or submucosal glands contribute to the mucus layer covering the free surface of the epithelium. The serous cells secrete a watery fluid that hydrates the mucus and contributes to the watery layer that the mucus floats on. The serous cells also secrete antibacterial lysozyme and transport IgA into the lumen by transcytosis, so they play an important role in immune defense in the respiratory tract.

The respiratory mucosa has a similar structure in all extrapulmonary organs and continues into the lungs in the bronchi. In the bronchioles it is modified (as described later in the chapter). In some regions, the pseudostratified columnar epithelium normally is replaced by a stratified squamous epithelium. These regions are the nasal mucosa near the anterior nares, the oropharynx, the laryngopharynx, the upper part of the larynx, and the true vocal folds. The presence of stratified squamous epithelium in other regions is generally a sign of pathology.

●●● NASAL CAVITY

The surface area of the nasal cavity is increased by the bony nasal conchae in the lateral wall. The conchae also cause turbulence in the air, ensuring that the air makes extensive contact with the warm, moist, and sticky surface of the nasal mucosa. The lamina propria of the middle and inferior conchae is richly supplied with blood vessels, mostly veins (Fig. 12-3). These are referred to as *nasal swell bodies* and resemble erectile tissue. Mixed mucous and serous glands are

abundant in the mucosa and submucosa. Damage to the nasal mucosa from inflammation or trauma can lead to significant bleeding (*epistaxis*) because of its rich vascularity.

Paranasal Sinuses

The paranasal sinuses are hollow cavities in several of the bones surrounding the nasal cavity. These drain into the nasal cavity and are lined by a respiratory mucosa and so can be considered extensions of the nasal cavity.

Olfactory Mucosa

The pseudostratified columnar epithelium covering the superior nasal concha is unusual in that a major cell type in the epithelium is a bipolar sensory neuron (Fig. 12-4). The apical dendrite expands at the free surface and sprouts about a dozen atypical, nonmotile cilia. These olfactory cilia have a normal 9 + 2 arrangement of microtubules extending out of the cell for about 1 μm; then the number of microtubules decreases, and the cilia lie flat along the surface. Odor receptors reside in the ciliary plasma membranes. The unmyelinated axons extend upward through the lamina propria and the cribriform plate to synapse in the olfactory bulbs. Another unusual feature of this epithelium is that

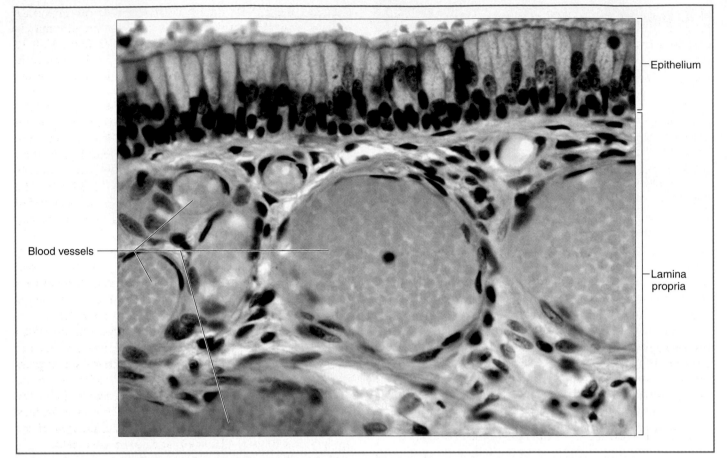

Figure 12-3. Nasal mucosa from the inferior concha. Note the abundant blood vessels in the lamina propria, which resembles erectile tissue. The epithelium here contains many goblet cells.

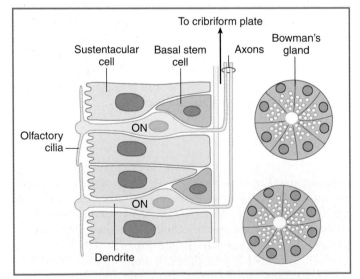

Figure 12-4. Diagram of the olfactory mucosa. Olfactory neurons (ONs) are present in the epithelium. The odor receptors are membrane proteins on the atypical olfactory cilia. The cilia are covered with serous secretions from Bowman's glands.

olfactory neurons are replaced every 1 to 2 months with new neurons developing from stem cells within the epithelium.

A second cell type in the olfactory epithelium is the columnar sustentacular cell, which has apical microvilli rather than cilia. The sustentacular cells express high levels of cytochrome P-450 enzymes and are believed to metabolize some of the toxic molecules in the inspired air that would otherwise damage the neural cells. In addition, the sustentacular cells phagocytose dying olfactory neurons. The basal stem cells replace both the olfactory neurons and the sustentacular cells. In the lamina propria of the olfactory mucosa are serous Bowman's glands (see Fig. 12-4). These secrete a watery fluid in which soluble odor molecules are dissolved.

●●● LARYNX

The larynx is the organ of sound production and also acts as a valve that closes during swallowing to prevent food from entering the lower respiratory tract. Sound is produced when the space between the vocal cords is narrowed, causing vibrations in the air passing through it. The larynx (Fig. 12-5) is supported by the hyoid bone and hyaline (thyroid, cricoid)

PHYSIOLOGY

Olfactory Receptors

There are approximately 1000 odor receptor genes, and each olfactory neuron expresses only one of these. The receptors are linked to G proteins, which in turn activate adenylyl cyclase. The cAMP binds directly to ion channels, causing depolarization of the olfactory neuron membrane. The perception of a given odor depends on which combination of receptors bind odorant ligands. The physiology of odor detection is complex, with some odorant ligands stimulating the G protein–linked receptors and others being inhibitory.

and elastic (epiglottis, arytenoid) cartilages. These support tissues are extensively interconnected by the intrinsic (skeletal) muscles of the larynx. The mucosa is lined by stratified squamous epithelium near the laryngeal entrance and over the vocal folds (see Fig. 12-5C) but is typical respiratory mucosa elsewhere in the larynx (see Fig. 12-5B). The vocal cords consist of bands of elastin fibers that stretch between the arytenoid and thyroid cartilages. The connective tissue of the vestibular (false vocal) folds is richly supplied with mixed mucous and serous glands.

●●● TRACHEA AND MAIN BRONCHI

The trachea is held open by a series of 15 to 20 C-shaped hyaline cartilages and is lined by typical respiratory mucosa (Figs. 12-6 and 12-7). The opening of the C is oriented posteriorly, and the gap is filled with the trachealis (smooth) muscle. The cartilage rings are interconnected with dense fibrous tissue, which blends with the perichondrium of the cartilages. This arrangement of separate, but connected, cartilage rings allows the trachea to stretch and contract as is required when the larynx is raised during swallowing (like an accordion). It also allows the trachea to be flexible and bend during neck movements while maintaining its patency. The lamina propria of the trachea is particularly well supplied with elastin fibers, which accommodate the tracheal stretching (see Fig. 12-7). Contraction of the trachealis muscle narrows the tracheal diameter, thereby causing air to pass though more rapidly. This occurs, for example, during coughing and sneezing.

In the mediastinum, the trachea bifurcates into the two main bronchi that enter the lungs. The main bronchi are similar to the trachea in structure, except they are supported by several incomplete curved cartilage plates instead of C-shaped cartilage rings.

●●● LUNGS

Bronchial Tree

After entering the lungs, the primary bronchi branch repeatedly, with each successive branch becoming smaller in diameter and thinner walled. The incomplete cartilage rings become irregular cartilage plates and the smooth muscle increases to form complete encircling bands (Figs. 12-8 to 12-10; see also Fig. 12-6). The mucosal and submucosal glands and epithelial goblet cells decrease in number in the more distal branches.

Eventually the smallest bronchi give rise to bronchioles (see Fig. 12-8), which in turn branch successively and give rise to smaller and smaller bronchioles. Bronchioles are characterized as having no glands and no cartilage in their walls, but they do have a complete layer of smooth muscle supporting the mucosa (Figs. 12-11 and 12-12). The epithelium in the proximal bronchioles is pseudostratified ciliated columnar, then simple columnar, and eventually simple cuboidal in terminal (distal) bronchioles. Initially, there are a few goblet cells, but soon these are replaced by another type of nonciliated cell, the Clara cell. The fact that the ciliated cells extend farther down the respiratory airways than the mucus-secreting cells ensures that mucus is efficiently cleared from the airways in the normal lung.

Clara cells have an apical dome that bulges into the lumen of the bronchiole (see Fig. 12-12). They secrete surfactant lipoproteins (see Alveoli and Alveolar Septum) and express cytochrome P-450 enzymes, which are believed to be important in removing hydrophobic toxicants from the inspired air. Clara cells also act as bronchiolar stem cells; they will undergo mitosis and repopulate a damaged area of the epithelium with new Clara cells and new ciliated cells.

The walls of the smallest bronchioles are interrupted periodically by thin-walled sacs, the alveoli. These bronchioles are called respiratory bronchioles (Fig. 12-13; see also Fig. 12-8), since some gas exchange occurs within them. The respiratory bronchioles branch into several alveolar ducts, whose walls are composed of many alveoli. The blind ends of the alveolar ducts are called alveolar sacs (see Fig. 12-8). The branching pattern of the respiratory bronchioles and alveolar ducts is extensive, allowing all the free space within the lung (i.e., all space not occupied by larger airways or blood vessels) to be filled with alveoli (see Figs. 12-11 and 12-13).

The abundant elastin fibers present in the lamina propria of the respiratory mucosa continue into bronchioles, forming a network around the bronchioles and then extending to cover

Text continued on page 351

PATHOLOGY

Asthma

Patients with asthma have two different pathologic processes that make breathing difficult. First, there is inappropriate constriction of airway smooth muscle. This affects primarily the bronchioles, which have no cartilage to keep them open. Inhaled smooth muscle relaxants are used to treat this symptom. Second is swelling of the mucosa and hypersecretion of mucus. This affects all the respiratory airways and can be treated with inhaled corticosteroids.

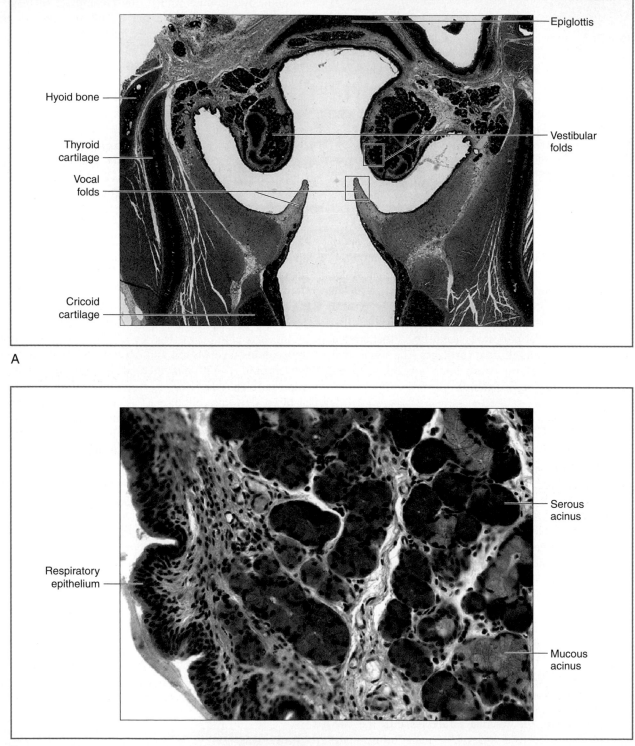

A

B

Figure 12-5. A, Low-power image showing a coronal section of the larynx. The hyoid bone and the cartilages that form the skeleton of the larynx are interconnected by the intrinsic (skeletal) muscles of the larynx. Mixed mucous and serous glands are present in the mucosa and submucosa and are particularly abundant in the vestibular (false vocal) folds. **B,** Enlargement of the mucosa of a vestibular fold showing mixed glands and the typical respiratory epithelium.

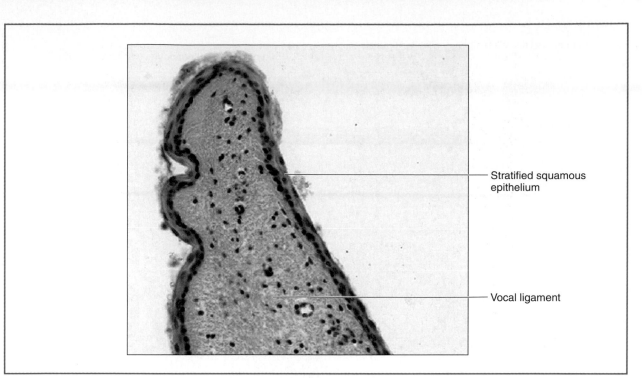

C

Figure 12-5, cont'd. C, Enlargement of a vocal fold, which is covered with a thin stratified squamous epithelium and contains the cross-sectioned vocal (elastic) ligament.

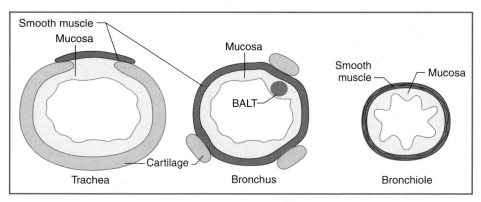

Figure 12-6. Diagram comparing the structure of the trachea, an intrapulmonary bronchus, and a bronchiole. The trachea is supported by 15 to 20 C-shaped cartilages. The gap in the cartilages is oriented posteriorly and is filled by the trachealis (smooth) muscle. In the bronchus, the smooth muscle forms complete rings and the cartilage is in the form of irregular plates. In the bronchiole, the smooth muscle layer is relatively thick and there is no cartilage. All three structures are lined by a respiratory mucosa, but in the bronchioles the mucosa is modified. Accumulations of lymphoid cells referred to as BALT or MALT, shown in the bronchus, may be found anywhere in the respiratory tract.

Pseudostratified cilated columnar epithelium   Elastin fibers cut in cross-section   Mixed glands   Perichondrium   Hyaline cartilage

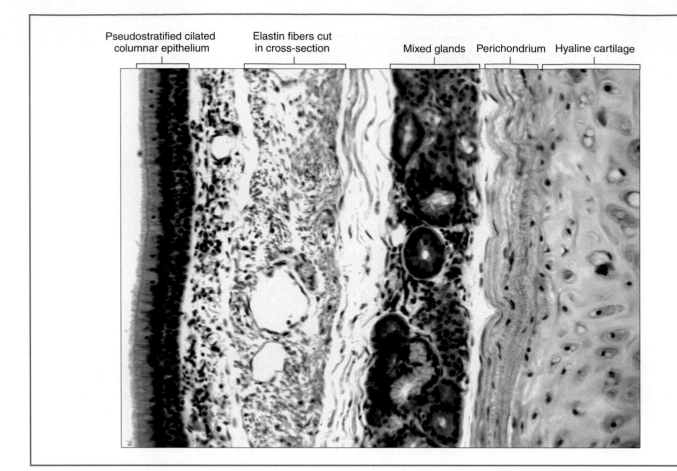

Figure 12-7. The wall of the trachea.

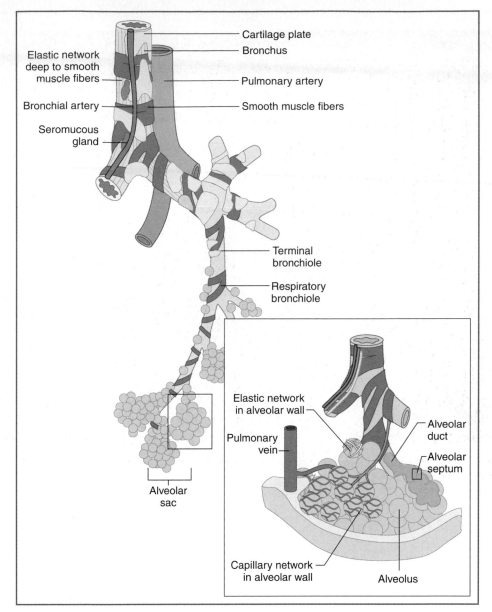

Figure 12-8. Diagram of the distal respiratory tree and its accompanying blood vessels. Note that the pulmonary artery branches closely follow the airways while the pulmonary veins run in adjacent connective tissue septa. The bronchial vessels are part of the systemic circulation and supply the walls of the bronchi, the larger bronchioles, and the pulmonary vessels.

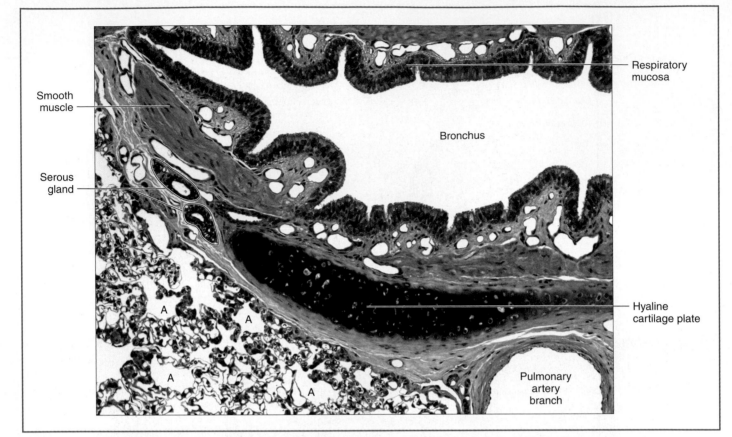

Smooth muscle

Serous gland

Respiratory mucosa

Bronchus

Hyaline cartilage plate

Pulmonary artery branch

A

A

A

A

Figure 12-9. Low-power image of the lung with a bronchus, recognized by the presence of cartilage in its wall, and an accompanying branch of the pulmonary artery. Clear dots in the connective tissue of the lamina propria are cross-sectioned elastin fibers. A, alveoli in the surrounding lung tissue.

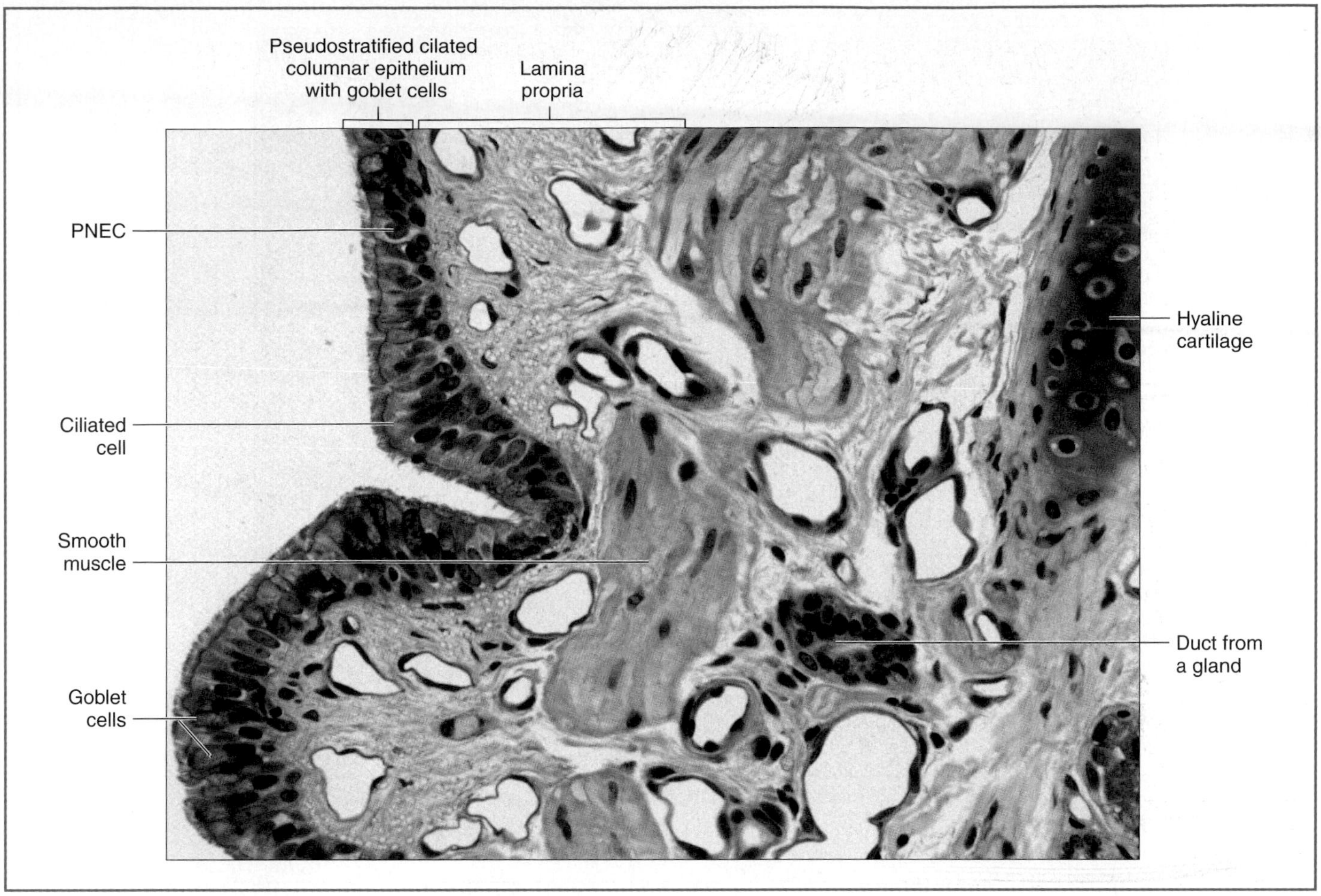

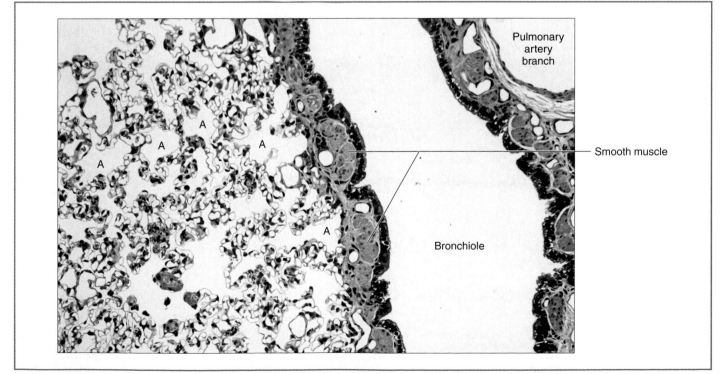

Figure 12-10. Detail of the wall structure of a bronchus.

Figure 12-11. Low-power image of the lung showing a bronchiole surrounded by many alveoli (A). The epithelium of this bronchiole is simple low columnar to cuboid, and no goblet cells are present.

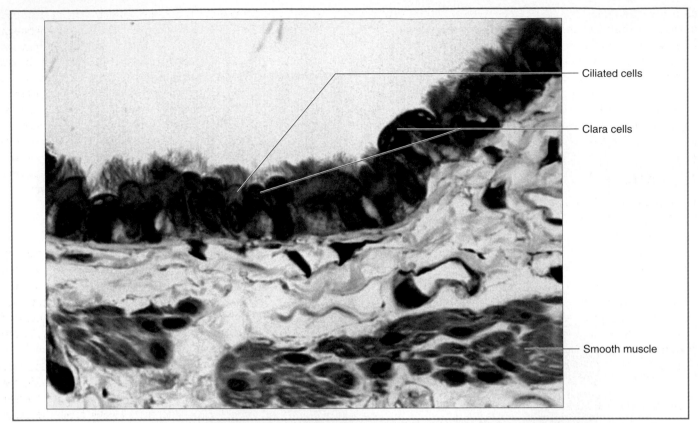

Ciliated cells

Clara cells

Smooth muscle

Figure 12-12. Detail of the wall of a bronchiole. The simple epithelium has ciliated cells and Clara cells but no goblet cells. Cartilage plates and glands are absent as well.

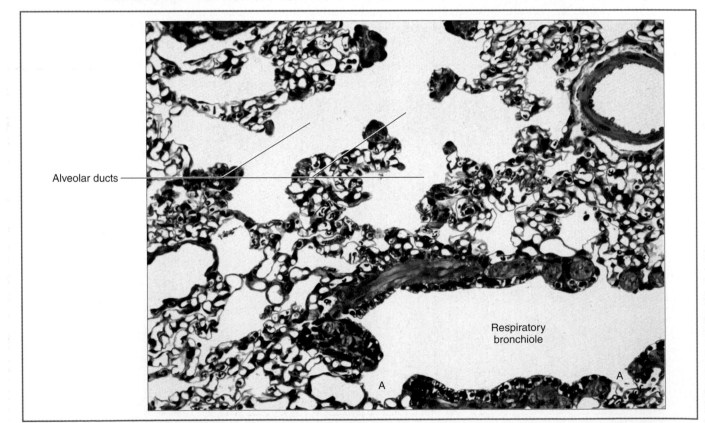

Alveolar ducts

Respiratory bronchiole

A

A

Figure 12-13. Low-power image of the lung showing a respiratory bronchiole with two alveoli (A) in its wall and alveolar ducts. The epithelium of the bronchiole is composed mostly of Clara cells at this level.

each alveolus (see Fig. 12-8). These elastin fibers contract during expiration, compressing the alveoli and small bronchioles and forcing air out of the lungs. While the force for inspiration is provided by the diaphragm and intercostal muscles, expiration is largely due to passive elastic recoil of tissues in the lungs and thoracic wall. While these elastin fibers are often not visible in histologic preparations, it is important to keep them in mind, since they are critical for proper lung function.

Terminology

A *terminal bronchiole* is the last purely conducting bronchiole (see Fig. 12-8). Usually, it is not possible to determine which bronchioles are terminal bronchioles in histologic sections.

A *pulmonary lobule* (often called a secondary lobule) is a small region of lung tissue surrounded by connective tissue septa. It is supplied by three to five terminal bronchioles and is visible in high-resolution CT scans.

A *pulmonary acinus* is a respiratory bronchiole and all its branches. While these are important functional units of the lung, it normally is not possible to identify them in histologic sections.

Pulmonary Vessels

The pulmonary arteries and veins enter and leave the lungs along with the main bronchi and have a similar branching pattern. The pulmonary arteries closely follow the airways (bronchi and bronchioles), but the smaller branches of the pulmonary vein run in connective tissue septa between pulmonary lobules (see Figs. 12-8 and 12-9). This information is useful in distinguishing these vessels; since the blood pressure in the pulmonary circulation is much lower than that in the systemic circulation, the distinction between arteries and veins is much less marked than in the systemic vessels. At the level of the respiratory bronchioles, the pulmonary arterioles break up into capillaries, with a network of continuous capillaries surrounding each alveolus (Figs. 12-14 and 12-15; see also Fig. 12-8). Here the blood is oxygenated and then is returned to the heart via the pulmonary veins.

Alveoli and Alveolar Septum

Since alveoli fill all the space in the lung not occupied by larger airways or blood vessels, each alveolus is surrounded by other alveoli. The common wall between two alveoli is the alveolar septum (see Fig. 12-15). It is within the alveolar septum that the capillary bed is found. Small amounts of connective tissue with elastin fibers and collagen type III are present as well.

A very thin, simple squamous epithelium covers most of the surface of the sac-like alveoli (Figs. 12-16 to 12-18; see also Fig. 12-15). The cells of the epithelium are alveolar (pneumocyte) type I cells. The type I cells form the main interface between the air and the tissues of the lung. Their thinness allows for rapid exchange of gases between the air and the blood in the underlying capillaries.

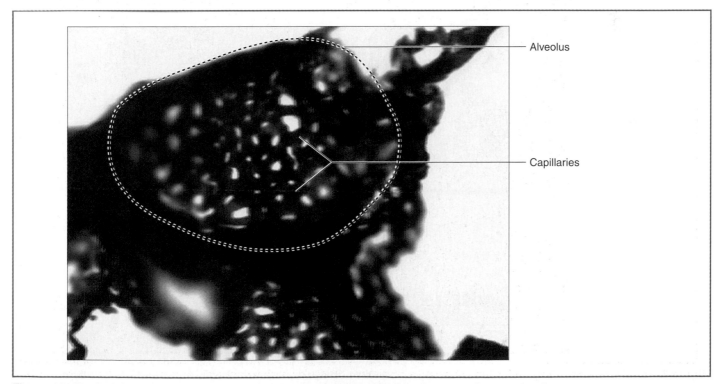

Figure 12-14. An injected lung preparation showing the dense capillary bed surrounding an alveolus.

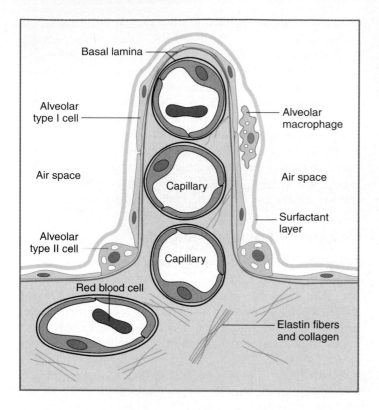

Basal lamina

Alveolar type I cell

Air space

Capillary

Alveolar type II cell

Capillary

Red blood cell

Alveolar macrophage

Air space

Surfactant layer

Elastin fibers and collagen

Figure 12-15. Diagram of an alveolar septum separating two alveoli (see Figure 12-8). Note that in many areas the basal laminae that underlie the alveolar epithelium and surround the capillaries are frequently fused into a single structure. In these areas the blood-air barrier is extremely thin, allowing for rapid exchange of O_2 and CO_2.

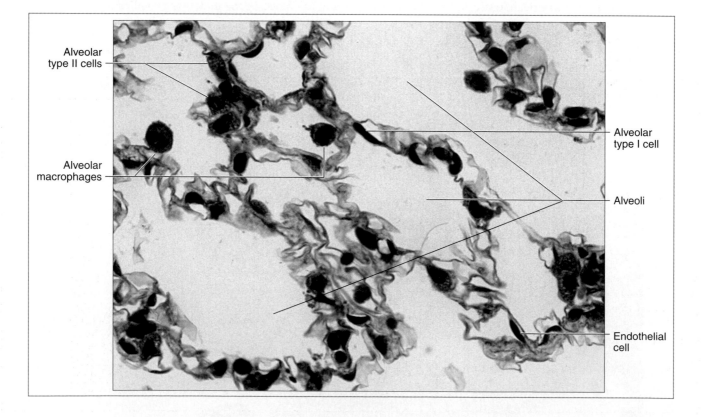

Alveolar type II cells

Alveolar macrophages

Alveolar type I cell

Alveoli

Endothelial cell

Figure 12-16. Section through several alveoli showing alveolar type I cells, alveolar type II cells, endothelial cells of the alveolar capillaries, and alveolar macrophages. At this resolution, it is often difficult to distinguish between the endothelial cells and the type I cells.

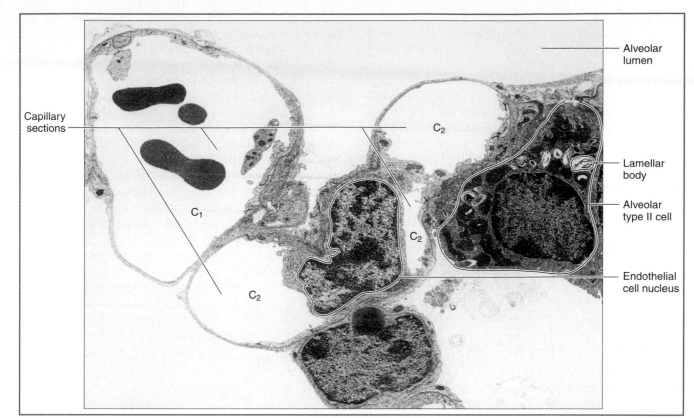

Figure 12-17. Low-power electron micrograph of an alveolar septum showing parts of three alveoli and sections of two capillaries. C_1 and C_2, sections through two different capillaries (C_2 is sectioned several times). (From Young B, et al. *Wheater's Functional Histology: A Text and Color Atlas,* 5th ed. Philadelphia, Churchill-Livingstone, 2006, p 243.)

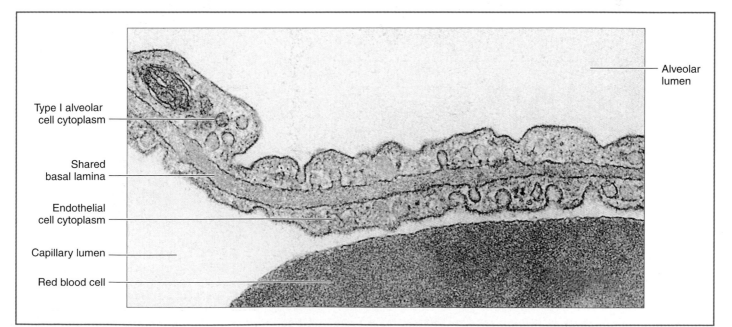

Figure 12-18. Detail of the blood-air barrier. Visible are the cytoplasm of a type I alveolar cell, the cytoplasm of an endothelial cell, a shared basal lamina, and a red blood cell in the capillary. (From Young B, et al. *Wheater's Functional Histology: A Text and Color Atlas,* 5th ed. Philadelphia, Churchill-Livingstone, 2006, p 245.)

Occupying a smaller area of the surface of the alveoli are the rounded alveolar (pneumocyte) type II cells. The alveolar type II cells (Fig. 12-19; see also Figs. 12-16 and 12-17) secrete a complex mixture of lipid (mostly phospholipid) and protein, which is called surfactant. Surfactant is stored in secretion granules (lamellar bodies), which have a characteristic appearance of stacked membranes because of their high content of phospholipid. Surfactant covers the free surface of the alveoli (see Fig. 12-15) and has several important functions. It lowers surface tension in the alveoli and thus greatly reduces the force needed to expand them during inspiration. Proteins in surfactant bind to microorganisms present on the surface of the alveoli; this protein coat facilitates their removal by phagocytosis. Finally, the moist, oily layer helps prevent desiccation of the alveolar epithelial cells. Alveolar type II cells are capable of division and act as stem cells in the alveoli, forming both new alveolar type II cells and new alveolar type I cells.

Alveolar macrophages are present on the free (air) surface of the alveoli (see Figs. 12-15 and 12-16). These cells crawl around within the surfactant layer, keeping it clean and sterile. While many dust particles and microorganisms are removed from the inspired air by adhering to the mucus layer higher up in the respiratory tract, some reach the alveoli and are then phagocytosed by the alveolar macrophages. When stimulated by infectious agents, alveolar macrophages will initiate an immune response, secreting chemoattractants for leukocytes, particularly neutrophils. These then invade the alveolus and join the attack on the foreign organisms. The alveolar macrophages also phagocytose surfactant and thus are important in its turnover. Some debris-laden alveolar macrophages migrate to the bronchioles and are carried out of the lung by cilia.

Within the alveolar septum are numerous continuous capillaries, which are closely apposed to the epithelial cells. Frequently, a basal lamina is shared by the alveolar epithelial

PATHOLOGY

Respiratory Distress Syndrome (RDS)

Alveolar type II cells begin to function at about 26 weeks of gestation and become fully functional at about 35 weeks. Infants born prematurely often have inadequate surfactant production, making breathing difficult and putting them at risk of developing RDS, a pathologic condition which makes breathing even more difficult. Such infants have a poor chance of survival. Prenatal corticosteroids, which increase surfactant production, and postnatal exogenous surfactant treatments have contributed to improving the survival of premature infants.

PATHOLOGY

Emphysema

In the normal lung, stimulated alveolar macrophages secrete chemoattractants for neutrophils. Neutrophils secrete proteases, including an elastase, which is inhibited by the α_1-antitrypsin present in the blood. With persistent stimulation (e.g., smoking), however, neutrophil elastase secretion increases and may not be completely neutralized by the α_1-antitrypsin. The elastase damages the elastin fibers surrounding the alveoli, and the alveoli become enlarged and do not contract on expiration.

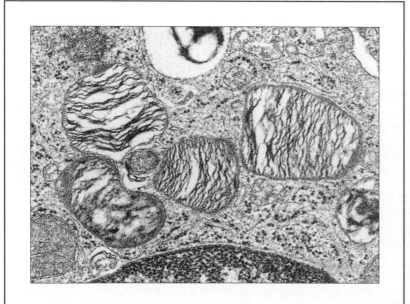

Figure 12-19. Detail of an alveolar type II cell showing its unusual secretion granules, the lamellar bodies, which contain lipid and protein components of surfactant. (From Young B, et al. *Wheater's Functional Histology: A Text and Color Atlas,* 5th ed. Philadelphia, Churchill-Livingstone, 2006, p 244.)

cell on one side and the endothelial cell on the other. In these areas, the blood-air barrier (the distance traveled by gases moving from the air to the blood) is 0.2 μm or less (see Fig. 12-18). Since there are hundreds of millions of alveoli in the lungs and numerous capillaries in each alveolar septum, the area for gas exchange is enormous, reportedly the size of a tennis court.

Many alveolar septa have permanent holes, the pores of Kohn. These epithelium-lined pores interconnect adjacent alveoli, even alveoli derived from different terminal bronchioles. They function to equalize air pressure among the alveoli and allow for collateral circulation. They also provide a path for the migration of alveolar macrophages and possibly the spread of infection among alveoli.

Urinary System

CONTENTS

The organs of the urinary system—the kidneys, ureter, urinary bladder, and urethra—have an exocrine function of extraordinary importance and an endocrine function that is only slightly less vital. The exocrine function consists of producing urine and conveying it out of the body, in just the right quantity and quality so as to ensure that the blood-stream becomes purified of metabolic end products and potentially harmful molecules. At the same time, the blood must retain as much of the metabolically useful molecules as possible during this process of purification so that the body does not waste or become depleted of them. The kidneys also monitor the composition of the blood and function as an endocrine organ, secreting proteins (renin, erythropoietin) into the bloodstream that affect blood pressure and blood cell development. All these complex tasks are carried out by highly specialized cells that display a considerable variety in appearance and function.

●●● KIDNEYS

The kidney is a bean-shaped solid organ covered by a capsule of dense connective tissue and indented at the hilum, a medial structure that admits blood vessels, efferent lymphatics, and nerves. The hilum is also pierced by the ureter, which conveys urine away from the kidney to the urinary bladder. Blood enters the kidney via the renal artery, which promptly divides into a complex hierarchy of smaller arteries—interlobar arteries, arcuate arteries, and interlobular arteries—that provide blood to nephrons, the basic functional units of the kidney.

The kidney is an extremely well vascularized organ, a fact that is consistent with its function of purifying the blood. The kidneys collectively receive as much as 20% of total cardiac output. Thus, in many histologic sections of the kidney, blood vessels are prominent. Most of the rest of the kidney is composed of tubular epithelial structures that make up the nephrons, the main functional unit of the kidney.

Each human kidney typically contains about 1.5 to 2 million nephrons. Each portion of a nephron (Fig. 13-1) is specialized for a different function and contains epithelial cells whose structure varies considerably from one portion to another. Most parts of a nephron are located in the cortex of the kidney and tend to stain intensely with common stains. Other portions of nephrons, located in the innermost medulla, stain less intensely, leaving the medulla with a lighter stained appearance.

A nephron begins at the renal corpuscle, where blood plasma is filtered to produce a provisional urine. The provisional urine is then conveyed into the proximal convoluted tubule, which occupies most of the space near the renal corpuscle in the renal cortex. The proximal tubule turns toward the medulla as the descending (straight) thick portion of the proximal tubule (Fig. 13-2). In the medulla, the proximal tubule becomes a thin epithelial tube that forms a hairpin loop (loop of Henle) and that continues back up to the cortex to form the distal convoluted tubule, the terminal portion of a nephron. The distal tubule delivers urine to collecting ducts that again leave the cortex and convey urine toward the medulla.

Masses of collecting tubules and loops of Henle form large, cone-shaped medullary structures called renal pyramids. At the tip of each renal pyramid, called a renal papilla, urine is released into a small, hollow space called a minor calyx, which is lined on one surface by transitional epithelium (Fig. 13-3). Minor calyces lead into larger collecting spaces called major calyces, which in turn lead to a cavity at the beginning of the ureter called the renal pelvis.

All these portions of the kidney process a prodigious amount of fluid: about 125 mL/min (ca. 120 L/day) of initial, unmodified fluid is formed by nephrons of the kidney. If all of

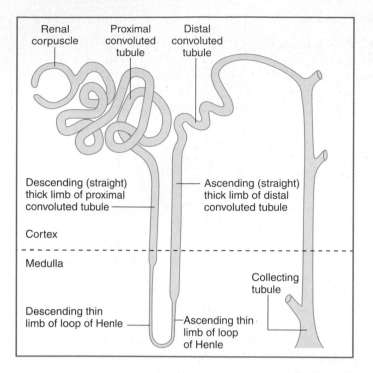

Renal corpuscle Proximal convoluted tubule Distal convoluted tubule

Descending (straight) thick limb of proximal convoluted tubule

Ascending (straight) thick limb of distal convoluted tubule

Cortex

Medulla

Collecting tubule

Descending thin limb of loop of Henle

Ascending thin limb of loop of Henle

Figure 13-1. Diagram of a nephron showing the renal corpuscle, the proximal convoluted tubule (cortex of the kidney), the descending (straight) portion of the proximal tubule, the loop of Henle, the distal convoluted tubule, and a collecting tubule (medulla of the kidney).

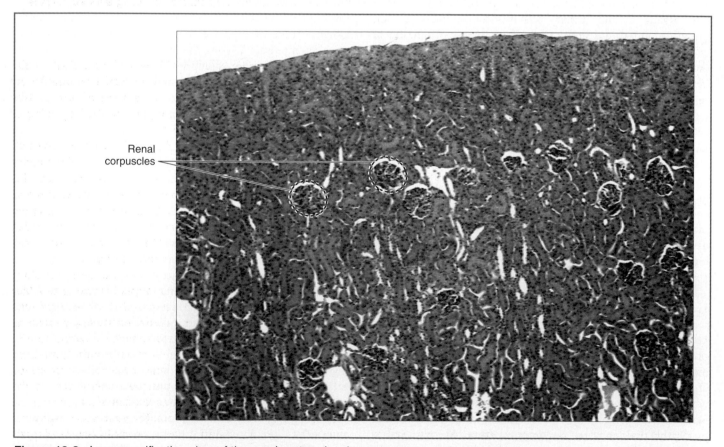

Renal corpuscles

Figure 13-2. Low-magnification view of the renal cortex showing numerous renal corpuscles.

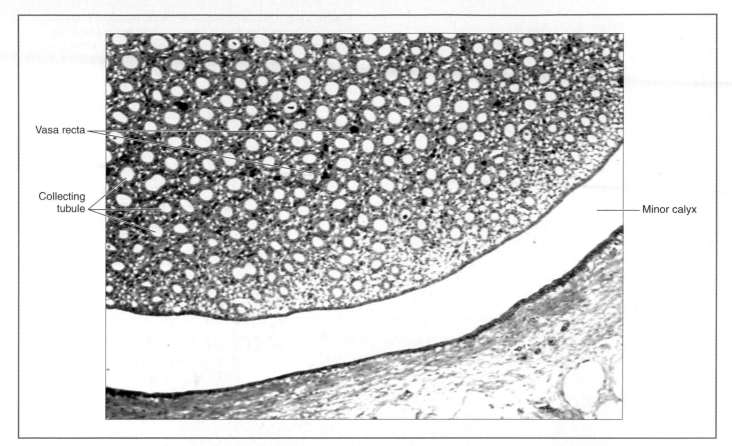

Figure 13-3. Low-magnification view of the renal medulla, which is composed mainly of collecting tubules, thin segments of the loop of Henle, and capillaries called vasa recta (dark, blood-filled structures). The transitional epithelium lining a minor calyx is also visible.

this fluid, not to mention essential substances such as Na⁺, proteins, and nutrient molecules, were to be lost from the body as urine, the result would be quickly fatal. A major challenge for each nephron, therefore, is not only the filtration of blood but also the rapid recovery of about 99% of the water and other molecules that would otherwise be lost in the urine.

Renal Corpuscle

The process of urine formation begins at the renal corpuscle, which is composed of two basic parts, Bowman's capsule and a tuft of capillaries called a glomerulus. During development, the renal corpuscle initially takes the form of a hollow ball, which gradually becomes indented on one side by a mass of glomerular capillaries. This event divides the epithelium of Bowman's capsule into a portion in direct contact with the capillaries (visceral layer of Bowman's capsule) and the parietal layer of Bowman's capsule. The fluid-filled space between the two layers is called the urinary space (Fig. 13-4). Blood flows into the glomerular capillaries from an afferent arteriole and then leaves the renal corpuscle via an efferent arteriole that exits at the vascular pole of a renal corpuscle.

The visceral layer of Bowman's capsule is composed of epithelial cells called podocytes that tightly adhere to the surface of glomerular capillaries. These cells participate in the filtration of plasma in the glomerular capillaries that forms the initial provisional urine. This initial form of urine leaves the renal corpuscle at the urinary pole via the beginning of the proximal tubule (see Fig. 13-4).

A light microscopic picture of a renal corpuscle shows all of these features (Fig. 13-5). In addition to capillary endothelial cells and podocytes, a glomerulus also contains numerous pericyte-like cells that adhere to the capillaries. These cells, which do *not* filter blood to produce urine, are thought to be contractile and phagocytic and are called mesangial cells. These cells are difficult to distinguish from capillary endothelial cells by light microscopy.

A diagram of a podocyte shows its remarkable morphology (Fig. 13-6). These cells wrap themselves around a capillary like an octopus and extend numerous cell processes, called foot processes, away from the portion of the cell containing the nucleus (podocytes derive their name from Latin, "foot"). Foot processes of one podocyte interdigitate with those from another, forming small, slit-like spaces between them called filtration slits that permit the passage of fluid out of the capillaries. The filtration slits are covered by a thin membrane containing a protein called nephrin. The glomerular capillaries themselves are also unusual: they possess hundreds of open fenestrations. This is the only place in the body that has open

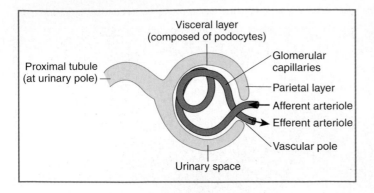

Figure 13-4. Diagram of a renal corpuscle showing the parietal layer of Bowman's capsule, the visceral layer of Bowman's capsule (formed by podocytes), the afferent and efferent arterioles at the vascular pole of the renal corpuscle, and the initial portion of the proximal tubule.

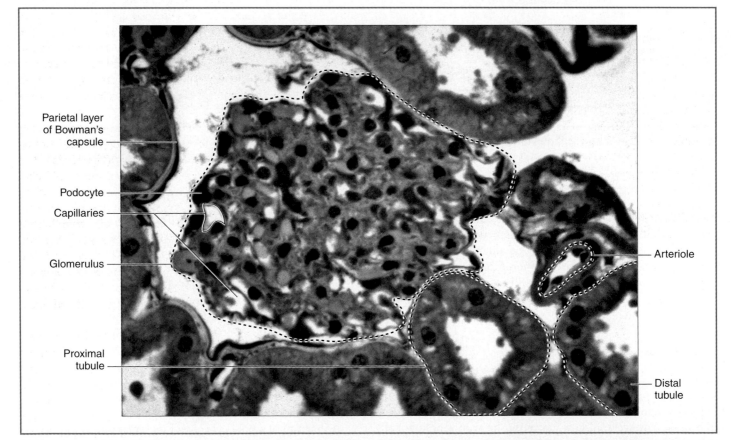

Figure 13-5. Light micrograph of a renal corpuscle showing the parietal layer of Bowman's capsule, the visceral layer of Bowman's capsule (formed by podocytes), glomerular capillaries plus mesangial cells, an arteriole, and numerous proximal tubules surrounding the renal corpuscle.

Figure 13-6. Diagram of a podocyte showing foot processes that wrap around the endothelial cells of a capillary.

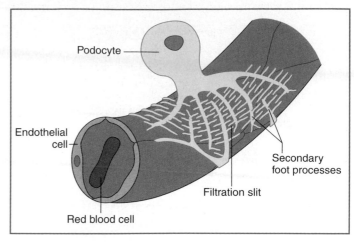

fenestrated capillaries. The open structure of the fenestrae makes these capillaries more porous than any other capillaries and permits a rapid efflux of fluid from the capillaries. The best way to visualize the complex anatomy of podocytes is via scanning electron microscopy (Fig. 13-7).

All the details of how podocytes acquire their peculiar anatomic features are not known, but it has been established that a particular protein is important for podocyte morphogenesis. This protein, called podocalyxin, is an integral membrane protein found at the basal surface of each podocyte. Podocalyxin regulates the adherence of each podocyte to underlying capillaries and also interacts, via its cytoplasmic domain, with the actin cytoskeleton of the podocyte. If podocalyxin is deleted from a podocyte, the cell loses its ability to form foot processes.

Transmission electron micrographs of podocytes show the details of the filtration barrier between the blood and the urine (Figs. 13-8 and 13-9). Fluid containing most small molecules with a molecular weight below 5000 kDa leaves the blood by passing through the endothelial fenestrae, across the basal lamina between the endothelium and podocytes, and then between foot processes. The barrier between podocytes and endothelia, termed the glomerular basement membrane, arises from the fusion of basal laminae produced by both podocytes and capillary endothelial cells. Cells and large proteins (with molecular weights above 40,000 kDa) cannot pass through these small spaces and so are retained within the blood. Smaller, negatively charged proteins are repelled by the negative charges on glycosaminoglycan molecules present in the basal lamina and also cannot pass into the urine. The main challenge for the remainder of the nephron, therefore, is to reabsorb small molecules that do manage to pass through the filtration barrier.

Proximal Tubule

At the urinary pole of a renal corpuscle, the simple squamous epithelium of the parietal layer of Bowman's capsule undergoes an abrupt change to become the tall cuboidal epithelium of the proximal tubule (Fig. 13-10). Proximal tubules are six-fold longer than distal tubules and so make up the majority (ca. 75%) of tubular profiles visible in the cortex of the kidney (see Fig. 13-5). The large cells of the proximal tubules display an irregular luminal surface owing to the presence of many apical microvilli; in some proximal tubules, the lumen may appear to be almost completely occluded by these microvilli.

A diagram of the ultrastructure of proximal tubule cells shows the three-dimensional appearance of proximal tubule cells, which interdigitate in complex ways (Fig. 13-11). The shape of these cells is different from that of most epithelial cells, which typically form smooth borders with each other, much like round or hexagonal paving stones of a street. Proximal tubule cells, in contrast, interlock like complicated puzzle pieces and have an overall shape only slightly less odd than that of podocytes. The peculiar shapes of the epithelial cells of the nephron may be related to their developmental origin as embryonic connective tissue cells, which commonly do not form epithelial sheets with the regularity of most epithelia (see later in the chapter).

Another explanation for the elaborate basolateral interdigitations of proximal tubule cells may be the role of these cells in resorbing about 80% of the volume of the provisional urine and essentially all the organic macromolecules, amino acids, vitamins, hormones, glucose, etc. The interdigitations account for a substantial expansion of the basolateral surface area of these cells. Figure 13-11 also shows both apical microvilli and abundant amounts of mitochondria that are located within infoldings of the basal plasma membrane of proximal tubule cells.

These ultrastructural features are recognizable hallmarks of cells devoted to the transcellular transport of molecules; microvilli increase the surface area available for absorption, and the many mitochondria provide the required energy. However, these ultrastructural features alone cannot explain the prodigious ability of proximal tubule cells to transport molecules, since the lipid bilayer of the cell membrane is impermeable to most substances. Transcellular transport also

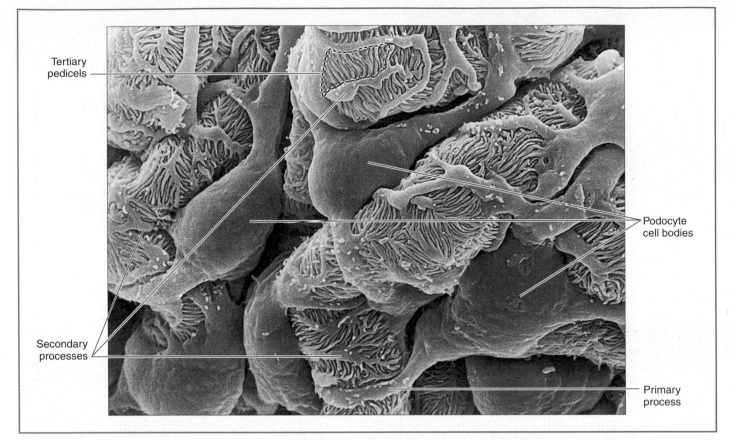

Tertiary
pedicels

Podocyte
cell bodies

Secondary
processes

Primary
process

Figure 13-7. Scanning electron micrograph of podocytes showing cell bodies and processes that branch into foot processes (pedicels). (Standring S. *Gray's Anatomy,* 39th ed. Philadelphia, Churchill-Livingstone, 2005, p 1281.)

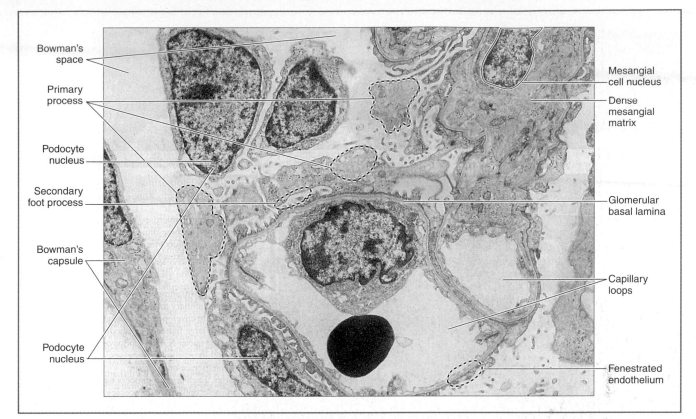

Bowman's
space

Primary
process

Podocyte
nucleus

Secondary
foot process

Bowman's
capsule

Podocyte
nucleus

Mesangial
cell nucleus

Dense
mesangial
matrix

Glomerular
basal lamina

Capillary
loops

Fenestrated
endothelium

Figure 13-8. Transmission electron micrograph showing podocytes, capillary endothelial cells, and a mesangial cell. (Standring S. *Gray's Anatomy,* 39th ed. Philadelphia, Churchill-Livingstone, 2005, p 1281.)

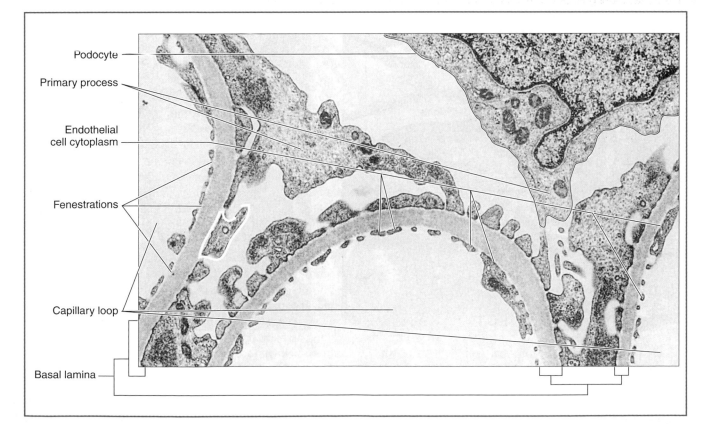

Podocyte

Primary process

Endothelial
cell cytoplasm

Fenestrations

Capillary loop

Basal lamina

Figure 13-9. High-magnification transmission electron micrograph showing podocyte foot processes, endothelial cells of fenestrated capillaries, and the thick basal lamina interposed between them. (Standring S. *Gray's Anatomy,* 39th ed. Philadelphia, Churchill-Livingstone, 2005, p 1282.)

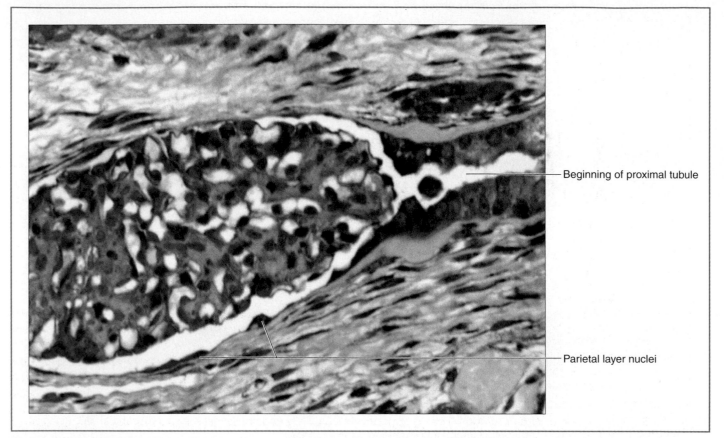

Beginning of proximal tubule

Parietal layer nuclei

Figure 13-10. View of a renal corpuscle cut in a section that illustrates the transition between the parietal layer of Bowman's capsule and a proximal tubule.

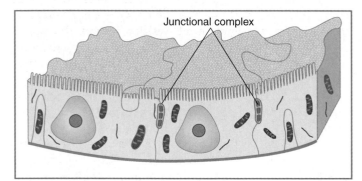

Junctional complex

Figure 13-11. Diagram of the ultrastructure of proximal tubule cells showing long apical microvilli, abundant mitochondria located basally in the cells, and the unusual, interdigitating shape of the cells in three dimensions.

requires the presence of many types of transporter proteins within the plasma membranes of these cells.

In addition to reabsorbing small molecules, proximal tubule cells have a major role in the endocytosis and digestion of small proteins and peptides to form amino acids, which are returned to the blood for reuse. This process is particularly important for carrier proteins such as transferrin, retinol-binding protein, and vitamin D–binding protein. These proteins are recognized by huge integral membrane proteins of proximal tubule cells called megalin and cubilin, which bind proteins to their large extracellular domains and stimulate their endocytosis. Once inside a cell, the bound proteins are shuttled to lysosomes and digested.

It is important to note that not all molecules in the urine are reabsorbed by the proximal tubule. Urea, for example, is only poorly reabsorbed via the three types of urea transporters that have been identified in various portions of the kidney. Another substance that is neither reabsorbed nor secreted by cells of the nephron is a carbohydrate molecule called inulin that can be introduced into the body by clinicians to study renal function. The rate of appearance of inulin in the urine can therefore be used to estimate the fraction of blood fluid that is filtered by renal glomeruli. Another compound, *para*-aminohippuric acid (PAH), is almost completely secreted into the urine by proximal tubule cells (via organic ion transporter proteins) in addition to being passively filtered into the urine in the glomerulus. The rate of appearance of PAH in the urine can be used to estimate the total amount of blood passing through the glomeruli.

One final function of the proximal tubule is the hydroxylation of vitamin D to create its more active form, 1,25-dihydroxyvitamin D_3. This is accomplished by yet another member of the cytochrome P-450 family of enzymes (see

Reabsorption by the Proximal Tubule

Water is reabsorbed across the plasma membrane via transport proteins called aquaporins. Each aquaporin protein has six membrane-spanning domains that are clustered together to form a barrel-shaped pore. Seven varieties of aquaporins exist within the kidney. Aquaporins-1 and -7 are utilized by proximal tubule microvilli to import water from the tubular fluid.

Glucose is reabsorbed from the tubular fluid via the same type of high-capacity glucose transporter (GLUT2) that is utilized for glucose sensing by hepatocytes and pancreatic β-cells (see Chapter 11). Lower capacity GLUT1 transporters export glucose from the basal compartment of proximal tubule cells. When urinary glucose concentrations are too high to permit recovery of all of the glucose, as in diabetes mellitus, glucose as well as water is lost in the urine.

About 60% to 70% of sodium and chloride ions present in the urine are recovered by the proximal tubule. A chloride transporter called ClC-5 seems particularly important for this, since disruption of the gene for this protein has the most severe functional effects on the proximal tubule.

Amino acids are reabsorbed by four different types of transporters (excitatory amino acid transporter 3, heteromeric rBAT/b^0 amino transporter, proton-dependent amino transporter, and B^0 amino transporter 1). These different transporters distinguish between glutamate, proline, and the remaining amino acids of differing charges (positive, negative, or neutral). These same transporters are also present in the microvilli of absorptive cells of the intestine. A defect in one type of transporter seems to lead to Hartnup disease, in which neutral amino acids are lost in the urine.

Chapter 11) called CYP27A1. This enzyme is attached to the inner mitochondrial membrane within proximal tubule cells and is 40 to 50 times more abundant in the kidney than in other organs such as the skin.

Loop of Henle

As urine progresses through the thick descending (straight) portion of the proximal tubule, it enters the medulla and a thin epithelial tube of simple squamous epithelium called the loop of Henle (Fig. 13-12). The loop of Henle then makes a hairpin turn and moves up toward the cortex. The simple squamous epithelial cells of this region have an unusual ability—they actively recover about 30% of the remaining Na$^+$ and Cl$^-$ from the urine but fail to transport water along with the Na$^+$ and Cl$^-$. Na$^+$ reabsorption is accomplished by two proteins working in tandem: one protein, the Na$^+$/K$^+$/Cl$^-$ co-transporter, imports all three ions into the cytoplasm, while another, the so-called ROMK1 channel, selectively recycles K$^+$ back into the urine, so that there is a net reabsorption of Na$^+$ and Cl$^-$ but not of K$^+$. Since this portion of the nephron lacks aquaporin protein channels, no water is recovered to dilute the Na$^+$ and Cl$^-$, so a region near the tip of the loop of Henle acquires a highly concentrated level of extracellular Na$^+$. This phenomenon, generated by a counter-current mechanism that partly depends on the flow of urine in opposite directions in the descending and ascending portions of the loop of Henle, has important functional consequences for adjacent collecting tubules, as will be discussed next.

Collecting Tubule

Collecting tubules are composed of a simple cuboidal epithelium containing two distinct cell types: principal (light) cells and intercalated (dark) cells. The collecting ducts are distinguished by unusually clear, sharp cell boundaries (Fig. 13-13; see also Fig. 13-12). They are surrounded on all sides by thin segments of the loop of Henle and also by blood-filled capillaries derived from the efferent arterioles of juxtamedullary glomeruli; these capillaries are called vasa recta. The Na$^+$-rich environment surrounding the collecting tubules tends to draw water from them via osmosis, a process that can recover still more water from the urine and that can permit the excretion of a highly concentrated urine. This additional recovery of water does not, however, take place at all times, but in fact is regulated by a hormone called antidiuretic hormone (ADH or vasopressin) that is secreted from the posterior pituitary (see Chapter 10). ADH has the remarkable and reversible ability to make collecting tubules permeable to water. How this process is accomplished is diagrammed in Figure 13-14.

Principal cells of collecting tubules possess receptors for ADH on their basolateral plasma membranes. When ADH binds to these receptors, intracellular signals are generated that provoke a migration of vesicles toward the apical plasma membrane. These vesicles possess aquaporin-2 water transporter proteins; when they fuse with the apical plasma membrane, they add water transporters to it that permit the entry of water into the cell. Water traverses the cell and exits via aquaporin-3 and aquaporin-4 water transporters on the basolateral surface of the cell. In the absence of ADH, this process is reversed and cells once again become incapable of withdrawing water from the urine. An inability to produce ADH provokes a condition called diabetes insipidus, in which excessive amounts of dilute urine are excreted (see Chapter 10).

Any agent interfering with the accumulation of Na$^+$ around the collecting tubules necessarily also interferes with the production of concentrated urine. Furosemide (Lasix) is a widely used drug; it is actively transported into the urine via organic ion transporters of proximal tubule cells and, by promoting the production of dilute urine, causes diuresis (loss of water from the body). Other drugs that block Na$^+$ transport in the distal tubule are the thiazide diuretics.

About 90% of collecting tubule cells are called principal (light) cells, and the remaining 10% of cells are called intercalated (dark) cells. The principal cells possess microvilli and a single apical cilium (a *primary cilium*) that has a probable sensory function.

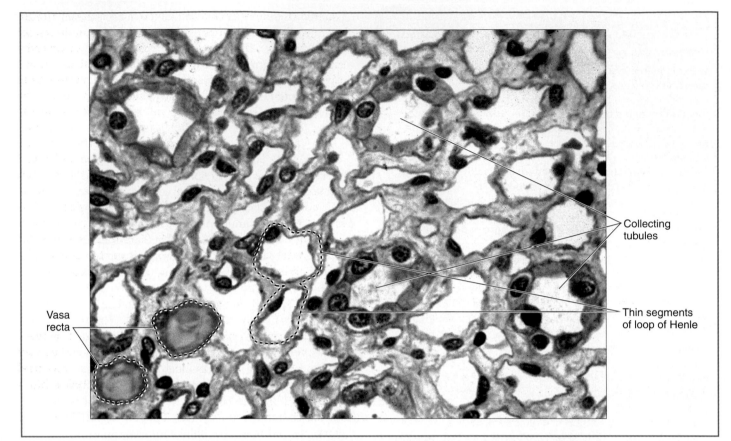

Figure 13-12. View of the renal medulla that shows collecting tubules, thin sections of the loop of Henle, and blood-filled vasa recta.

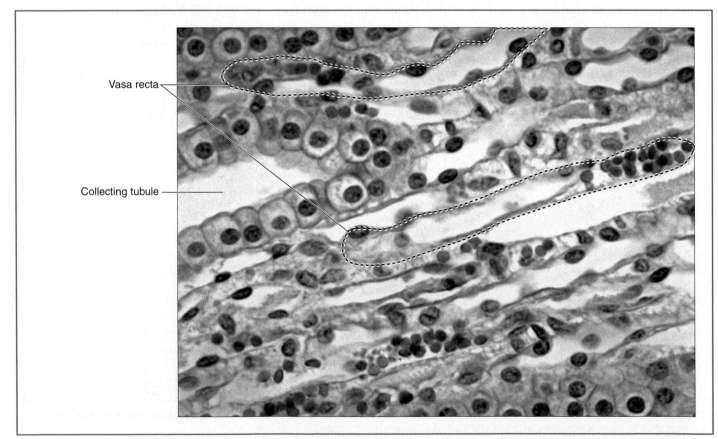

Figure 13-13. Section of the medulla that shows longitudinal sections through collecting tubules and blood-filled vasa recta.

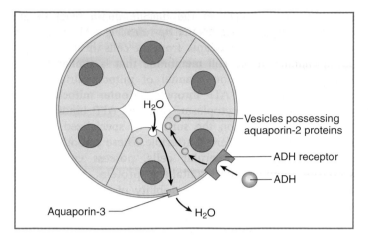

Figure 13-14. Diagram of the induction of permeability to water in a collecting tubule. When antidiuretic hormone (ADH) binds to basal receptors of collecting tubule cells, it triggers the movement of cytoplasmic vesicles to the cell surface. These vesicles, containing aquaporin-2 water transporters, allow the entry of water, which then exits the cell at its basolateral surface via aquaporin-3 and -4 channels.

Intercalated cells have more abundant cytoplasmic mitochondria. These cells adjust urinary pH by secreting either H^+ ions or bicarbonate ions. These cells are also noteworthy because they synthesize a peptide called atrial natriuretic peptide (ANP) (Fig. 13-15). (The name of ANP derives from Latin, *natrium*, "sodium.") This peptide, also produced by atrial muscle cells of the heart, has potent effects on the kidney. ANP causes contractile mesangial cells and smooth muscle cells of the afferent arteriole to relax. This increases the amount of blood flowing through each glomerulus and thus increases the glomerular filtration rate and the amount of urine produced. In addition, ANP prevents the reabsorption of Na^+ by cells of the collecting ducts, thus promoting diuresis of Na^+. Although collecting ducts account for only about 2% of the Na^+ reabsorbed from the urine, this small proportion nevertheless adds up over the course of a day and can substantially affect Na^+ loss from the body.

Distal Tubule

Distal tubules are relatively less abundant and prominent compared with other elements of the renal cortex, but they nevertheless can easily be distinguished from proximal tubules because they possess smaller cells that lack a brush

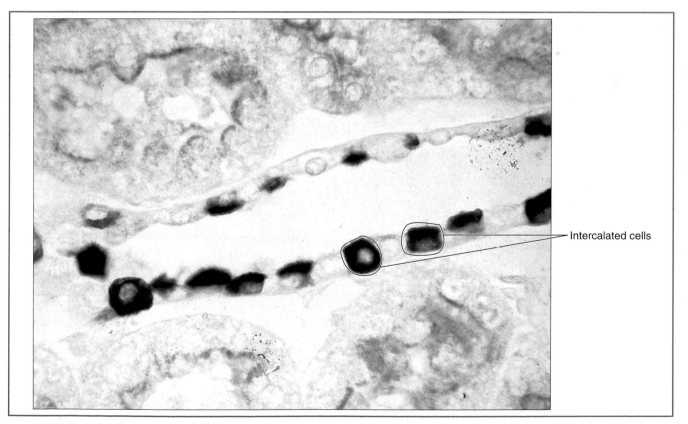

Figure 13-15. Longitudinal section through a collecting tubule, stained to demonstrate atrial natriuretic peptide (ANP) in intercalated (*dark*) cells of the tubule. (Courtesy of Dr. James McKenzie.)

Hypertension

Almost one fifth of the adult population is likely to develop hypertension at some period in life. Hypertension is a serious disease and increases the likelihood of heart disease and stroke.

In 90% of cases (primary or essential hypertension), the cause is not known. Primary hypertension can be aggravated in certain individuals by a salt-rich diet.

A recent study showed that adults with primary hypertension possess half the normal number of renal glomeruli. These results have led to speculation that an impairment in nephron development in the embryo, perhaps due to maternal undernutrition, could be a factor predisposing to hypertension.

The causes of rare, heritable forms of hypertension are becoming known. For example, a mutation in the ENaC Na^+ channel of the distal nephron impairs Na^+ retrieval from the plasma membrane. This leads to increased salt resorption and hypertension in a disorder named Liddle syndrome.

produced by capillary endothelial cells of the lung. The final form of angiotensinogen is angiotensin II (AII). This biologically active peptide elevates blood pressure and body Na^+ levels by causing a generalized constriction of blood vessels and by stimulating the release of aldosterone from the adrenal cortex. AII is the most potent natural vasoconstrictor.

Aldosterone, as noted above, enhances the reabsorption of Na^+ by the distal tubule. Thus, signals emanating from the macula densa to the juxtaglomerular cells to the adrenal gland and then to the distal tubule constitute a complicated negative feedback loop whereby the distal tubule regulates its own Na^+ conserving function, a mechanism of considerable biological utility.

When high environmental temperatures cause water and Na^+ loss due to sweating, urinary levels of Na^+ fall and the macula densa releases its inhibition on renin release. Release of renin then stimulates the production of AII, which conserves body stores of Na^+ and which prevents the development of low blood pressure and circulatory collapse. The juxtaglomerular system can also be manipulated to decrease blood pressure instead of increasing it. For example, a class of drugs called ACE inhibitors prevent the creation of AII from AI and are commonly used to treat hypertension (high blood pressure).

Another important endocrine function of the kidney is the production of a glycoprotein hormone, erythropoietin, which stimulates the production of red blood cells in the bone marrow. The source of erythropoietin appears to be interstitial fibroblasts in the peritubular renal cortex. The synthesis of erythropoietin by these cells is tightly linked to O_2 tension in the blood—more RBCs are needed only if the O_2-carrying capacity of the blood declines. In the kidney, O_2 directly regulates the stability of a protein called the hypoxia-inducible factor. This transcription-regulating protein governs the translation of at least 40 different cellular proteins that respond to hypoxia. Erythropoietin is one of these proteins. Recently, injections of erythropoietin have been used to combat the anemia that often is provoked by anticancer drugs and renal dialysis machines.

●●● URETER

Urine produced by the kidney is conveyed to the urinary bladder via a small muscular tube, the ureter (Fig. 13-20). The ureter is lined by transitional epithelium, which overlies a lamina propria of loose connective tissue and a muscularis layer of smooth muscle. The surrounding adventitial layer commonly contains abundant adipocytes.

●●● URINARY BLADDER

The urinary bladder has a histologic structure similar to that of the urethra, with similar layers (Fig. 13-21). Functionally, however, the urinary bladder must respond to a substantially greater physiologic challenge than does the ureter. The empty bladder contains less than 10 mL of urine, but as it fills, it must expand to contain 300 to 400 mL of urine before increasing intraluminal pressure stimulates the reflex of urination (micturition). To do this, the layering and shape of the epithelial cells that line the bladder must be rapidly readjusted. This creates certain difficulties for the epithelium.

When the transitional epithelium lining the bladder stretches out to accommodate a larger volume of urine, the superficial, rounded cells of the epithelium must change their shape from round to flat (Fig. 13-22). This involves a drastic change in the surface-to-volume ratio, since geometrically, a sphere has a much smaller surface area than a flat disk of the same volume. Thus, extra plasma membrane is needed to cover the cell surface when the epithelial cell flattens out.

Transitional epithelial cells solve this problem by fusing membranous cytoplasmic vesicles to the plasma membrane as the cells flatten. As a result, the plasma membrane of a bladder cell is a patchwork of numerous plaques that are joined together when cytoplasmic vesicles fuse with the plasma membrane. These plaques, rich in a bladder-specific protein called uroplakin, give the outlines of a superficial bladder cell an irregular, scalloped appearance (Fig. 13-23).

●●● URETHRA

The urethra is a muscular tube that carries urine from the bladder to the exterior of the body. In males, it passes through the prostate gland and penis (see Figs. 14-12 and 14-15). The prostatic urethra is lined by a transitional epithelium, but the penile urethra acquires a pseudostratified columnar epithelium. In females, the shorter urethra is mainly lined by transitional epithelium. In both sexes, the terminal portions of the urethra acquire a stratified squamous epithelium similar to that of skin.

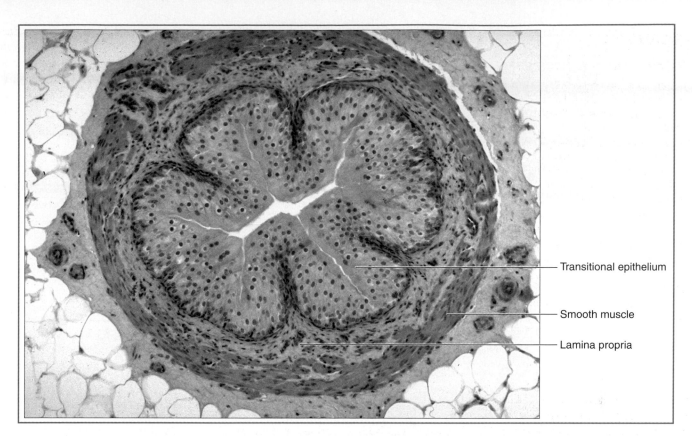

Figure 13-20. Light micrograph of a cross-section of the ureter showing the lining transitional epithelium, lamina propria, smooth muscle of the muscularis portion, and surrounding adipose-rich adventitia.

EMBRYOLOGY

The Urinary System

At least 30 signaling molecules that participate in kidney formation have been identified so far, but the complete story is still unknown. Key participants in several main events, at least, are becoming clear.

Initially, masses of embryonic connective tissue cells (mesenchymal cells) condense around the tips of the growing ureter (ureteric bud). These cells secrete glial-derived neurotrophic factor (GDNF), which stimulates the ureteric bud to branch.

The ureteric bud secretes a protein called leukemia inhibitory factor that stimulates the mesenchymal cells to form tubules; these tubules eventually become most portions of a nephron. Branches of the ureteric bud, which have a typical epithelial phenotype, become collecting tubules. This may partly explain why collecting tubule cells resemble most other epithelial cells, whereas the mesenchymal cells of the proximal tubule and glomeruli acquire a peculiar morphology not normally found in epithelia.

Mesenchymal cells express a transcription factor, WT1, that seems responsible for turning on many podocyte genes and for maintaining the unusual morphology of podocytes. An abnormality in this protein provokes Wilms' tumor of the kidney, which occurs mainly in children at a low incidence (1 in 200,000 children).

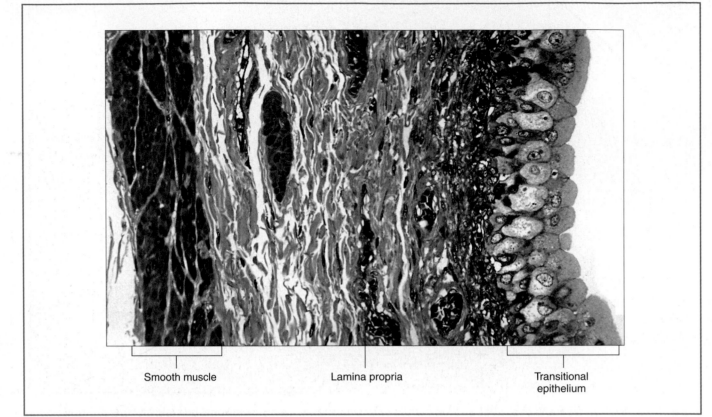

Smooth muscle	Lamina propria	Transitional epithelium

Figure 13-21. Low-magnification micrograph of the urinary bladder showing transitional epithelium, connective tissue of the lamina propria, and smooth muscle.

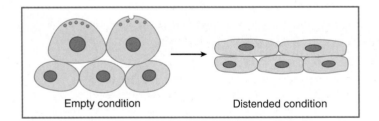

Empty condition   Distended condition

Figure 13-22. Diagram of the transitional epithelium of the urinary bladder showing the changes in cell shape and the fusion of vesicles with the plasma membrane that occur when an empty bladder becomes distended with urine.

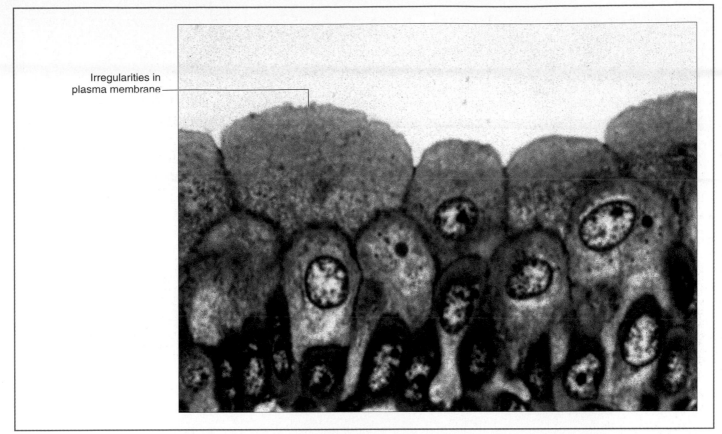

Irregularities in
plasma membrane

Figure 13-23. High-magnification view of the superficial cells of the bladder epithelium. The irregular contours of the plasma membrane result from the insertion of relatively rigid vesicles into the membrane.

Reproductive Systems 14

●●● MALE REPRODUCTIVE SYSTEM

The most important components of reproductive systems are the gonads (testes or ovaries). These comparatively small organs are the source of germ cells, which when combined form a new organism (a baby), and of sex hormones, which direct the function of many other organs toward the goal of reproduction. The gonads also have a critical influence on the embryogenesis of the reproductive system as a whole.

The adult testis is an ovoid organ enclosed within a tough connective tissue covering called the tunica albuginea (Fig. 14-1). Within the testis, separated from each other by trabeculae of connective tissue, are many interconnected tubules. The bulk of the tubules are seminiferous tubules in which germ cells (spermatozoa) are formed. Spermatozoa are conveyed from these tubules out of the testis via a series of hollow structures: straight tubules (tubuli recti), the rete testis, and efferent ductules (ductuli efferentes). These structures drain into a single, highly coiled tubule called the epididymis, which in turn is connected to the ductus (vas) deferens. The microanatomy of all of these structures will be described individually.

Seminiferous Tubules of the Testis

Sertoli Cells

The wall of a seminiferous tubule is formed by epithelial cells called Sertoli cells (Figs. 14-2 to 14-4). The irregular boundaries of each Sertoli cell are difficult to distinguish because the Sertoli cell plasma membranes adhere tightly to developing germ cells, but these cells can nevertheless be identified in histologic sections by virtue of their elongated, euchromatic nuclei containing prominent nucleoli. The appearance of each Sertoli cell nucleus suggests that these cells are actively transcribing many genes for many tasks, and this is indeed the case. Some of the many functions of Sertoli cells can be listed as follows:

1. Sertoli cells establish the blood-testis barrier. Abundant, highly specialized, tight junctions between Sertoli cells prevent the passage of blood-borne molecules into the lumen of the seminiferous tubule. The main function of this barrier is thought to be the protection of germ cells from cells and molecules of the immune system. This protection is required because of the timing of instructions to the immune system that prevent it from damaging normal body structures ("self"-antigens). During development, cell surface molecules from muscle cells, fat cells, fibroblasts, etc, are shed into the blood and are carried to the developing thymus. Any lymphocytes within the thymus that react to these self-antigens are identified and destroyed, so that when the immune system is mature, it will not attack normal body constituents. This process, however, cannot protect spermatozoa, since newborn baby boys do not produce these cells and will not until puberty. Hence, the developing thymus is never exposed to spermatozoa-specific proteins and is never "trained" to ignore spermatozoa. These cells therefore need to be protected from the immune system, which does not recognize them as self-antigens.

2. If Sertoli cells erect a barrier between germ cells and the bloodstream, how are germ cells nourished? This is the same problem encountered by astrocytes of the CNS, which establish a barrier between the blood and the brain.

EMBRYOLOGY

The Gonads

The gonads first develop as a ventral thickening (genital ridge) of the mesonephros (see Chapter 10). They are formed under the influence of a protein called steroidogenic factor–1 (SF-1), which is essential for their development. Curiously, the only other site in the body where SF-1 regulates development is in the ventromedial nucleus of the hypothalamus, just dorsal to the arcuate nucleus (see Chapter 10). In experimental animals (and probably in humans), this mass of neurons is known to respond to sex steroids by facilitating the stereotyped display of female sexual behavior and is essential for reproduction. Without SF-1, both the gonads and this brain nucleus fail to develop. It is remarkable that this same protein operates in two widely separated parts of the body to make reproductive function possible.

The mesenchyme of newly formed gonads is rapidly covered by a mesothelial epithelium, which penetrates the connective tissue as epithelial strands called sex cords. Initially, male and female gonads are structurally identical. Then, in the male, the central (medullary) sex cords enlarge to form seminiferous tubules and associated structures. This occurs because of a transcription regulating protein, testis-determining factor, that is coded for by the *SRY* gene present on the Y chromosome.

This protein blocks the action of another protein called DAX1, which would otherwise suppress the activity of a variety of maleness-associated genes.

Two tubular structures form alongside the gonads. One, the mesonephric duct, originally conveyed urine from the primitive kidney. In males, a portion of this duct becomes adapted to carry seminal fluid from the testis and acquires new names: the epididymis and ductus deferens.

The other duct, called the müllerian duct, has the potential to form the uterus and uterine tube. It regresses and disappears in male embryos under the influence of a protein, mullerian-inhibiting factor, which is secreted from the epithelial cells of the seminiferous tubules (Sertoli cells).

An important cellular component of the testis—the germ cells—do not originate in the testis at all. These cells are formed separately in the embryonic yolk sac and must actively migrate into the peritoneal cavity to come to rest within the testis. They are guided in their journey by a chemoattractant, stromal cell–derived factor–1, which is secreted by the testis.

The testis does not retain its intra-abdominal position but migrates caudally, through the muscles of the abdominal wall (inguinal canal), and into the scrotal sac. It is tugged in this direction by an attached cord of mesenchymal tissue called the gubernaculum, which undergoes relative and absolute shortening to draw the testis into the scrotal sac.

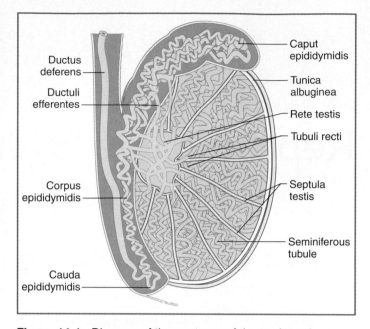

Figure 14-1. Diagram of the anatomy of the testis and associated ducts.

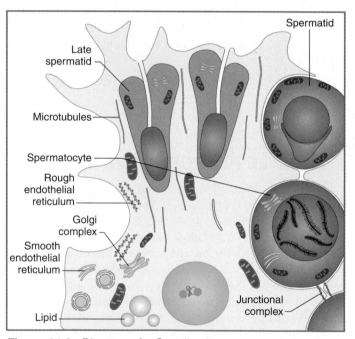

Figure 14-2. Diagram of a Sertoli cell and associated germ cells.

Sertoli cells, like astrocytes, take up nutrients from the blood and export them to germ cells. For example, Sertoli cells metabolize glucose into lactate and transport lactate to germ cells. Sertoli cells make transferrin so that they can carry iron to germ cells, and they also synthesize a lipid-transporting protein called clusterin. Finally, Sertoli cells synthesize an androgen-binding protein so that they can secrete bound steroid hormone into the lumen of the seminiferous tubules.

3. Sertoli cells have an endocrine function and secrete inhibin, which is carried to the anterior pituitary to suppress the secretion of FSH. This function of Sertoli cells is actively modified by germ cells, which secrete an uncharacterized substance that influences inhibin production.

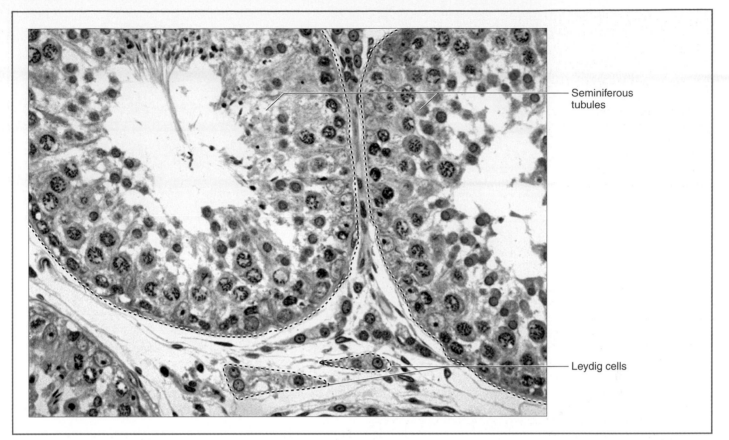

Figure 14-3. Low-magnification view of seminiferous tubules and interstitial Leydig cells.

When germ cell activity and cell division are sufficient, Sertoli cells release inhibin to prevent overstimulation of the testis by FSH.

4. Sertoli cells stimulate cell division and differentiation of germ cells. This task requires cell-cell contact between the germ cells and Sertoli cells. When the cell membranes of the two cell types meet, this brings into contact an integral membrane protein of Sertoli cells (stem cell factor) and an integral membrane receptor protein of germ cells (c-kit). The binding of stem cell factor by c-kit stimulates intracellular processes that lead to the differentiation of germ cells. Mutations in either of these proteins that lead to an overactivity of this pathway can provoke germ cell tumors, which are the most common type of cancer in males between the ages of 15 and 40 years.

5. A poorly understood function of Sertoli cells is their ability to facilitate the movement of germ cells from the basal region of the epithelium toward the apical region without a simultaneous disruption of the blood-testis barrier. What is known so far is that some modifications of cell junctions must be carried out to allow this. Sertoli cells attach to germ cells via a specialized type of adherens junction. These apical junctions contain a type of integrin that, in other cells, is restricted to basal junctions between the cell and extracellular matrix. Clearly, the attachment of Sertoli cells to germ cells is unique and malleable.

Germ Cells

When primordial germ cells colonize the testis during embryogenesis, they take up residence at the basal surfaces of Sertoli cells within seminiferous tubules and are termed spermatogonia and divide via mitosis. Spermatogonia function as stem cells that constantly replenish the germ cell population as cells are shed into the lumen. This is necessary, since a male human can produce as many as 100 million fully differentiated sperm cells each day! Recent studies suggest that spermatogonia may also function as stem cells for other tissues after removal from the testis and culturing in appropriate nutritive media. As they differentiate and divide via meiosis, spermatogonia move apically and are termed spermatocytes (this entire process is called spermatogenesis). Each spermatocyte passes through two meiotic divisions that result in the formation of haploid cells called spermatids. Finally, each spermatid undergoes dramatic morphologic changes, a process called spermiogenesis, to become anatomically mature spermatozoa that are shed into the lumen. Before reviewing the structures of these cells, a brief discussion of meiosis is in order.

Meiosis

The cell division procedure called meiosis utilizes many of the same structures and proteins active in mitosis, but instead of producing two cells with a diploid complement of DNA,

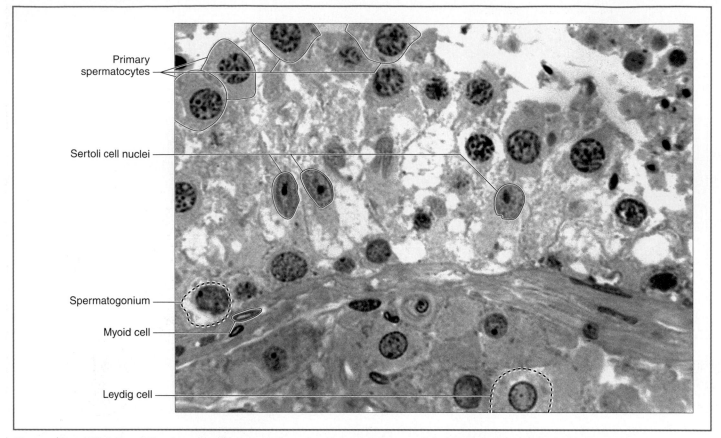

Figure 14-4. High-magnification view of a seminiferous tubule showing nuclei of Sertoli cells, spermatogonia, primary spermatocytes, and spermatids. Myoid cells and Leydig cells are visible at the external surface of the tubule.

meiosis produces four cells with half the full complement of DNA (haploid cells). This is achieved by undergoing one round of DNA synthesis followed by two rounds of cell division rather than one. This process is diagrammed in Figure 14-5, which, for simplicity, follows the fate of only the two copies (maternal and paternal) of chromosome 21 that are present in all cells.

The DNA of each chromosome is first duplicated, forming two chromatids that are attached to each other at the centromere (S phase of the cell cycle). Then, germ cells either simply enter mitosis or, alternatively, begin meiosis. The trigger for this decision is not precisely known but may involve the activation of a germ cell–specific RNA polymerase called Gld-2 or an integral membrane signaling protein called Notch.

Once a cell has entered prophase of meiotic division 1, the two versions of chromosome 21 (homologous chromosomes) become attached to each other longitudinally in a process called synapsis. Subsequently, the strand of DNA that forms one of the two chromatids of each copy of chromosome 21 develops breaks at multiple sites, and at these places, the DNA strand crosses over (e.g., from the paternal to the maternal homolog) and fuses with the DNA of the opposite chromosome. This process is called meiotic recombination.

Meiosis I is terminated when these remodeled, homologous chromosomes are pulled away from each other during metaphase, anaphase, and telophase. Meiosis II completes the process by separating the chromatids from each other, producing four haploid cells with versions of chromosome 21 that are different from either the original maternal or paternal chromosome. Meiosis, in this way, generates haploid cells with a genetic composition that is different from those of either parent.

The complicated processes of the first meiotic prophase require about 10 days to complete in male germ cells. Four stages of the first meiotic prophase can be discerned. In the first stage, chromosomes have just begun to condense into thin ribbons, so this stage is termed leptotene (the Greek root for "thin" in this word is also used to name the obesity-fighting, fat cell hormone leptin). At the second stage, zygotene, homologous chromosomes begin to be linked together to form a structure called the synaptonemal complex (the Greek word for "yoke" or "link" also forms part of the word for the zygomatic bone that is part of the cheek). In the third stage, pachytene, completely paired homologous chromosomes form a thick structure (remember the thick skin of a pachyderm). This structure is held together by units of a protein, the synaptonemal protein, which can bind both

Figure 14-5. Diagram of meiosis.

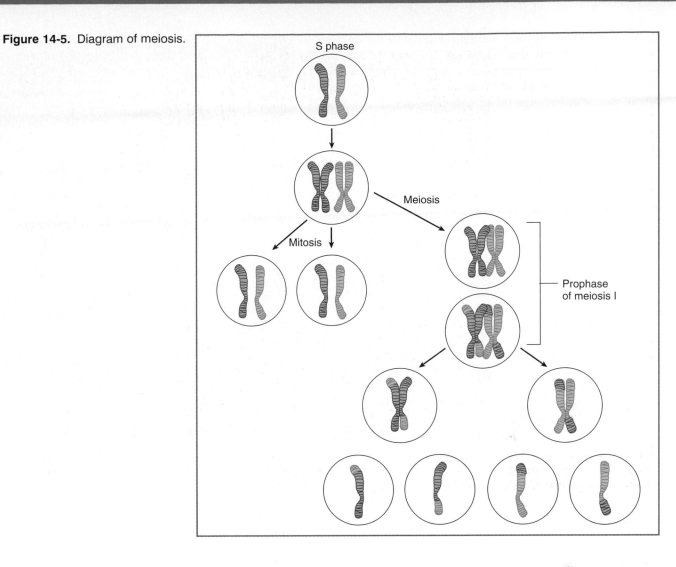

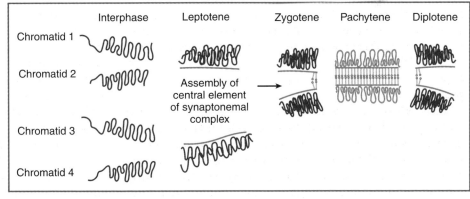

Figure 14-6. Diagram of the synaptonemal complex between chromosomes that forms during the four phases of the first meiotic prophase.

to DNA and to itself to form a zipper-like structure. Finally, in diplotene, the synaptonemal complex has relaxed somewhat and chromosomes are held together only at chiasmata, the places where DNA strands have crossed over and been exchanged (Fig. 14-6).

This description of meiosis is deceptively simple. It ignores many fundamental and poorly understood questions. For example, in meiosis I, why does the paternal copy of chromosome 21 pair up only with the maternal homologous chromosome 21? How does one homolog "find" the other, and what prevents paternal chromosome 21 from promiscuously pairing up with any other maternal or paternal chromosome? One good guess relates to stretches of repetitive DNA sequences near chromosome telomeres that do not code for any protein. It seems likely that some sort of protein can recognize these sequences on chromosome 21 and bind to them to bring both copies of chromosome 21 together, but the specifics for this procedure are not known.

Another puzzle is how chromosomes become so well aligned longitudinally that telomeres pair only with homologous telomeres and centromeres with centromeres. This problem seems to be solved during meiosis by the attachment of all the telomere tips of all chromosomes to one small region on the inner surface of the nuclear envelope. This forces the chromosomes to form a bundle of long loops tethered at their ends in one spot. This bundle of meiotic chromosomes, termed a bouquet, serves to both bring homologous chromosomes nearer to each other and to make sure that synapsis begins at the chromosome tips and proceeds in an orderly fashion along the length of the chromosome.

A further problem relates to the process of recombination that is seen in prophase of meiosis I. Chromosomal DNA can be broken and recombined in this manner partly owing to a recombinase called Rad51. This unusual enzyme is particularly abundant in the testis and ovary. It is also found in lymphoid organs, where the DNA of lymphocytes is physically cut and spliced to generate the myriad types of cell surface receptors that are needed by T lymphocytes to recognize millions of different types of antigens.

All these steps are governed by cell division proteins called cyclin-dependent kinases. These proteins, by phosphorylating histones, nuclear lamins, and other proteins, regulate the structure of the chromosomes and the nuclear envelope and initiate the various stages of mitosis and meiosis. Somehow, the activities of these kinases are adjusted so that the S phase of DNA synthesis that normally intervenes between cell divisions is eliminated during meiosis.

Spermatocyte cells that are undergoing meiosis are readily distinguishable in the testis by their large, round nuclei and condensed, paired chromosomes (see Fig. 14-4). As noted, the first meiotic division lasts a long time, but the second meiotic division requires only a few hours. Thus, primary spermatocytes undergoing the first meiotic division are prominent and numerous in the testis, but secondary spermatocytes undergoing the second division have a fleeting existence and are difficult to detect.

Spermiogenesis

Following meiosis, the haploid spermatid cells have an undistinguished appearance, with a simple, spherical shape and round nucleus. To form mature spermatozoa, these cells must undergo drastic anatomic changes in a process called spermiogenesis. All of the organelles within the cell are dramatically transformed to produce a streamlined, tapering, motile cell with a small nucleus.

The changes in the cell nucleus of a spermatid are arguably the most remarkable: spermatid nuclear volume shrinks to only about 1/40th the size of a content somatic cell nucleus. Even allowing for a 50% reduction in nuclear DNA, it is still quite a feat to pack all this DNA into such a small volume. To accomplish this, the DNA of a spermatid is completely reconfigured and condensed. The histone proteins that normally organize the DNA into nucleosomes are removed and replaced by a smaller peptide called protamine. This allows the DNA to be reordered into a much smaller, con-

GENETICS

Defects In Meiosis

Failure of chromosomes to segregate properly in meiosis results in germ cells (gametes) with an improper number of chromosomes. When such sperm or egg cells fuse during fertilization, an embryo formed from this fertilized egg may thus retain an extra chromosome or lack a specific chromosome in each cell. This condition is termed aneuploidy. About 5% of all sperm cells show a type of aneuploidy, and it has been estimated that as many as 20% of all oocytes contain an improper number of chromosomes. In most cases, possession of an extra chromosome introduces a 50% increase in gene copy number for so many genes that the embryo is not viable and perishes. However, aneuploidy of small chromosomes increases the copy number of only a relatively small set of genes. (Chromosome 21, for example, contains only 225 transcribed genes.) These embryos can survive to term as viable fetuses.

About 20% of fetuses born with meiotic abnormalities possess three copies of the autosomal (non-sex) chromosome 21. This condition is called trisomy 21, or Down syndrome.

Transcription of the extra genes on Chromosome 21 results in impaired brain functioning and abnormalities in facial anatomy. In addition, a number of patients with Down syndrome develop Alzheimer's disease at a much earlier age than normal, probably because the gene for amyloid precursor protein is located on Chromosome 21. The frequency of Down syndrome births increases with the age of the mother (1 in 5000 births at a maternal age of 20, but 25 in 5000 births at a maternal age of 45). The maternal age effect has been well documented but remains poorly understood. In addition, alterations in meiotic recombination appear to be associated with chromosome nondisjunction, but again, the precise mechanism remains hidden.

More commonly, sex chromosomes may be gained or lost during meiosis. The XXY condition, occurring in about 1 of 700 births, is called Klinefelter's syndrome and results in increased height and some learning abnormalities.

The 45,X (Chromosome 45,X monosomy) condition, Turner's syndrome, often is toxic to embryos and results in a spontaneous abortion. Fetuses that survive fail to develop normal ovaries, so that women with this syndrome are infertile and require estrogen administration to elicit pubertal changes in overall anatomy and physiology.

densed form. It also means that DNA is no longer accessible for transcription, so that no new proteins can be made by a mature spermatozoon.

In addition to shrinking, the nucleus of a spermatid must be reshaped to create the streamlined and elongated form seen in the spermatozoon. This is accomplished by a number of mechanisms. First, spermatids acquire a testis-specific form of lamin protein. These lamins have the capacity to reshape the nucleus; if they are introduced into ordinary somatic cells, the nuclei of these cells will also become torpedo-shaped. Second, a rigid perinuclear ring containing keratin is assembled in the cytoplasm. This ring becomes attached to long, parallel rows of microtubules that comprise an unusual organelle called the manchette. As the spermatid develops, the perinuclear ring migrates along the manchette from the apical portion of the nucleus toward the distal portion, compressing it as it goes along. This is another crucial step in transforming an ordinary-appearing nucleus into the condensed, streamlined nucleus of a spermatozoon.

Other organelles within the spermatid are utilized in extraordinary ways. The Golgi apparatus begins to secrete vesicles containing hydrolytic (lysosomal) enzymes. However, instead of directing these vesicles toward the cell membrane as usual, the microtubules of spermatids send them in the opposite direction, toward the anterior pole of the nucleus. There, they accumulate on the surface of the acroplaxome, a keratin-rich plate that becomes anchored to the nucleus. The vesicles merge to eventually form an enzyme-rich, membrane-bound compartment covering the anterior pole of the nucleus called the acrosome (Fig. 14-7). Release of these enzymes from a spermatozoon will aid in penetrating the barriers between sperm and egg during fertilization.

At precisely the opposite pole of the nucleus, other remarkable developments occur. The spermatid centrioles migrate toward the nucleus, and one of the pair of centrioles becomes attached to the nucleus at the implantation fossa. This centriole becomes greatly enlarged and elongated and forms the core of a growing flagellum. Simultaneously, this growing centriole somehow stimulates all the mitochondria in the cell to wrap around its proximal portion to fill the cytoplasm of the mid-piece of the flagellum (see Fig. 14-7). These mitochondria provide the ATP needed for microtubule sliding within the axoneme.

Mitochondria are not the only structures that cluster around the axoneme of the flagellum. Just beneath the mitochondria, nine long filaments termed outer dense fibers form. These are composed of at least 14 different proteins; one of them, termed Odf2 protein, can bind to both microtubules and to itself and probably plays a role in the assembly of the outer dense fibers. Curiously, Odf2 protein is not restricted to sperm cells but is a common component of the centrosome in most cells that has simply been produced to a much greater extent in sperm cells than in other cells. Outer dense fibers probably help strengthen the flagellum and modulate the whipping motion produced when ATP activates microtubule sliding in the central axoneme.

A cross-section of the sperm flagellum through its more distal portion (the principal piece) shows an absence of mitochondria. Moreover, the outer dense fibers have diminished in number to seven and have been enclosed within a tough covering called the fibrous sheath. A number of proteins have been isolated from the fibrous sheath; surprisingly, many seem to be enzymes or enzyme-binding proteins (e.g., protein kinase A binding protein) that may regulate glycolysis and other metabolic pathways within sperm.

One noteworthy feature of spermatogenesis is that it takes place simultaneously in numerous spermatocytes that are all linked together by small cytoplasmic bridges. Unlike other cells, spermatocytes do not fully complete cytokinesis after each cell division, so that the daughter cells all have a certain continuity of their cytoplasm as they differentiate and all ascend apically toward the lumen of a seminiferous tubule.

The specialized proteins and structures seen in spermatids are undoubtedly not the only factors that transform a simple-appearing spermatid into a highly specialized spermatozoon. Recent studies suggest that 1600 genes become activated in the testis during this process and that as many as 350 genes are expressed in no other organ.

Leydig Cells

Small masses of highly vascular connective tissue can be found just external to the seminiferous tubules, in the interstices between tubules. Specialized cells called the interstitial cells of Leydig are located in this connective tissue. These cells have an endocrine function: they secrete testosterone

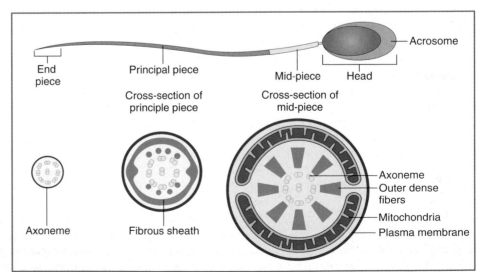

Figure 14-7. Diagram of the structure of a mature spermatozoon.

and their own specific isoform of insulin called insulin-3. A Leydig cell has a round, euchromatic nucleus and a large, eosinophilic cytoplasm dominated by lipid droplets, mitochondria, and smooth endoplasmic reticulum, much like other steroid-producing cells (see Fig. 14-4).

Testosterone is responsible for the growth of sex organs such as the penis, prostate, and seminal vesicles; for the sexual dimorphisms in overall body size, muscle strength, and hair distribution that are visible in humans; and for the sexual dimorphisms in the function and structure of hypothalamic nuclei that regulate male sexual behavior and aggressive behavior. Testosterone production is under the control of pituitary luteinizing hormone (LH).

One curious aspect of Leydig cell function is that it is substantially depressed with age, arguably to a greater extent than the age-related decline seen in other organ systems. Plasma testosterone concentrations peak in men at about 500 ng/mL (age 20 years) and gradually decline to 300 ng/mL by age 60. This decline has deleterious effects on overall strength, health, and sexual behavior. Why should aging provoke these changes? Experimental evidence in rats suggests that simple aging of Leydig cells alone cannot be responsible for the age-related decline in testosterone production, since the body has the capacity to replace them with new, vigorous Leydig cells in the right circumstances.

The other endocrine product of Leydig cells, insulin-3, was discovered recently. Mice genetically engineered to lack insulin-3 display *cryptorchid* testicles, i.e., testes that fail to leave the abdominal cavity and descend to the scrotal sac. Apparently, insulin-3 critically influences the function of the gubernaculum and is required for testicular descent.

PATHOLOGY

Aging and Reproductive Senescence

Are other explanations for the effects of aging available?

A recent study has shown that an accumulation of oxidative stress in mitochondria may underlie aging. When an enzyme that repairs oxidative damage to mitochondrial DNA in mice was blocked, the mice developed all the signs of premature aging: reduced body weight, lower muscle mass, hair loss, and testicular atrophy.

Since the release of certain molecules from mitochondria can stimulate cell death (apoptosis), these mice also show increased apoptosis of cells in muscle and in seminiferous tubules. This did not appear to extend, however, to Leydig cells.

It seems likely that a major site of age-related damage may be the hypothalamus, which does not regulate LH properly in aged animals and humans. It may not be coincidental that the hypothalamus contains peculiar astrocytes (Gomori-positive astrocytes) that undergo age-related damage to their mitochondria. Thus, aging-related damage to mitochondria may lead to some of the neuroendocrine changes seen in aging.

Cryptorchidism in both mice and humans leads to sterility owing to an unusual feature of male germ cells: the elevated body temperature seen in the abdominal cavity provokes apoptosis in germ cells but not in other cells of the testis. The reason for this is unknown, but it necessitates the migration of the testes to the cooler scrotal sacs.

The unexplained temperature sensitivity of mammalian male germ cells is not only puzzling but also leads to questions about the reproductive abilities of other animals. Male birds possess intra-abdominal testicles that are exposed to even higher temperatures ($41°C$) than those seen in mammals because of the higher metabolic rate of birds. Nevertheless, avian testes produce fertile gametes with no apparent difficulty. A possible reason is that avian testicles produce unusually high levels of heat-shock proteins that protect cellular structures from the effects of elevated temperature.

Myoid Cells

Myoid cells (myofibroblasts), found at the outermost margins of seminiferous tubules, are modified fibroblasts with contractile properties. These appear to exert a gentle pressure on seminiferous tubules to promote the movement of seminal fluid and cells into tubules that exit the testis.

Straight Tubules, Rete Testis, and Efferent Ductules

Straight tubules (tubuli recti) are seminiferous tubules lined by cells resembling Sertoli cells that lack intraepithelial germ cells. These structures are short and are difficult to detect in routine sections of the testis. The more prominent rete testis is a mass of hollow tubules found in the midline (mediastinum) of the testis (Fig. 14-8). Rete testis tubules are the only testicular structures lined with a simple cuboidal epithelium. They carry spermatozoa out of the testis toward efferent ductules (ductuli efferentes). In humans, these are a bundle of about 12 tubules that connect the testis to the epididymis. They have a distinctive appearance in cross-section being composed of alternating tall ciliated columnar epithelial cells and short epithelial cells bearing microvilli. The varying heights of these cells produce an irregular-appearing epithelium that does not fit into standard classifications of epithelia (Fig. 14-9). It is believed that the cells of the ductuli efferentes absorb much of the luminal fluid produced by the Sertoli cells.

Epididymis and Vas Deferens

The epididymis is a single highly coiled tube that collects seminal fluid from the testis. It is divisible into three regions: the head (caput), the body (corpus), and a tail region (cauda) that is closest to the vas deferens. Epithelial cell height diminishes from the caput to cauda regions. The epithelium lining the epididymis has traditionally been classified as pseudostratified columnar. Two abundant cell types—tall columnar principal cells and rounded basal cells—do indeed contact the basal lamina. However, a third cell type, called an apical cell, can occasionally be seen in this epithelium

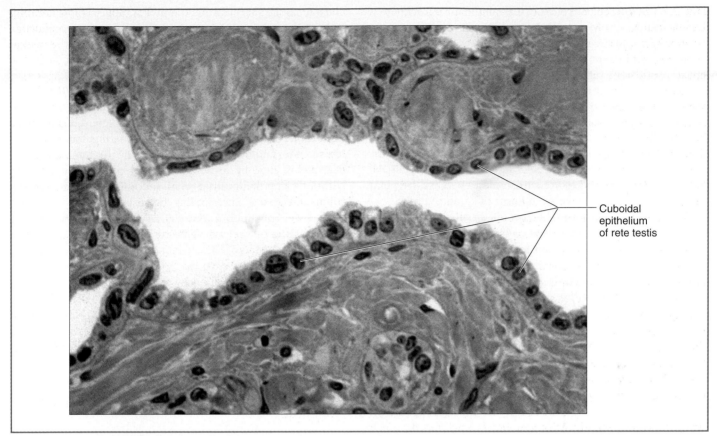

Figure 14-8. Simple cuboidal epithelium of the rete testis.

Cuboidal
epithelium
of rete testis

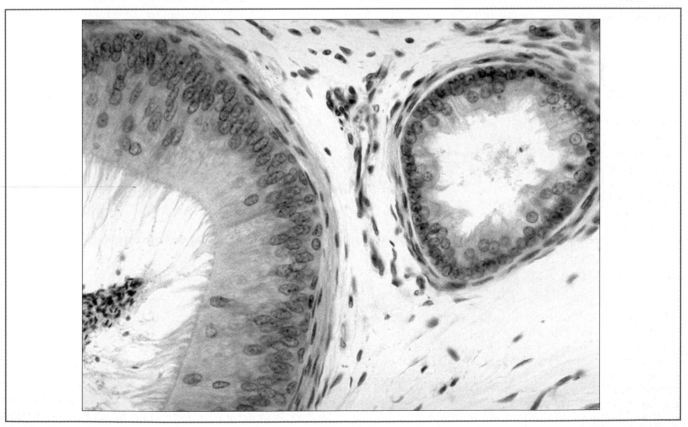

Figure 14-9. Cross-sections of an efferent ductule (*right*) and the epididymis (*left*).

(Fig. 14-10). The apical cells possess abundant mitochondria and transport proteins called H^+-ATPases, and appear to secrete acid into the epididymal lumen.

The tall columnar principal cells possess unusually long apical protrusions termed stereocilia. Like microvilli in other epithelia, these probably assist in the transport of water and ions, since almost 90% of the water in fluid exiting the testis is absorbed by the epididymis. Another function of the principal cells is the transport of chloride ions. The function of the basal cells is uncertain although they may serve as stem cells regenerating themselves and the principal cells. All these epithelial cell types are surrounded by dense, irregular connective tissue plus a small amount of smooth muscle.

One important process that occurs in the epididymis is sperm maturation. Spermatozoa collected from the rete testis appear structurally mature but are immotile. They gradually acquire the ability to move as they pass through the epididymis from the head to the tail, but they are restrained from attaining full motility by uncharacterized factors present in epididymal fluid. If seminal fluid containing sperm is recovered from the epididymis and then diluted by buffer, this appears to restore complete motility to sperm. Sperm capacitation (the ability of the spermatozoa to fertilize an egg) is prohibited by glycerophosphocholine, a glycoprotein secreted by the principal cells. Capacitation does not take place until the sperm enters the uterus. Sperm capacitation is still poorly understood, but seems to involve the modification of surface glycoproteins present on sperm by enzymes secreted by cells lining the male reproductive tract.

Vas Deferens, Ejaculatory Ducts, and Seminal Vesicles

Seminal fluid leaving the epididymis is conveyed out of the scrotum, via the vas deferens, through the inguinal canal and toward the midline prostate gland. The lumen of the vas deferens is lined by a pseudostratified columnar epithelium with long microvilli plus a small amount of dense, irregular connective tissue. Surrounding these layers is an unusually thick layer of smooth muscle, which is a distinguishing characteristic of the vas deferens (Fig. 14-11). This smooth muscle is activated during ejaculation to propel the contents of the vas deferens to exit the body via the penile urethra.

At the point where each vas deferens penetrates the prostate gland, the coat of smooth muscle greatly diminishes and the tubules acquire a new name—the ejaculatory ducts. These move toward the midline and fuse with the prostatic urethra, which is lined with the transitional epithelium typical of the urinary system. As the ejaculatory ducts pass through the masses of secretory acini (alveoli) of the prostate gland, they acquire dense coverings of connective tissue and

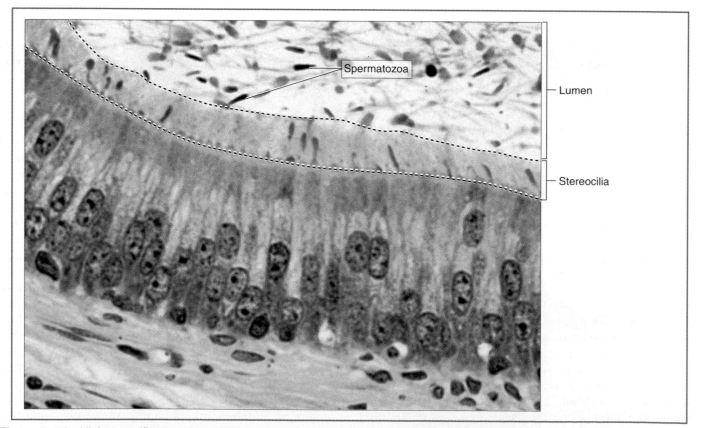

Figure 14-10. High-magnification view of the epithelium of the epididymis. Note the small volume of the spermatozoon nucleus in comparison with the nuclei of the epithelium.

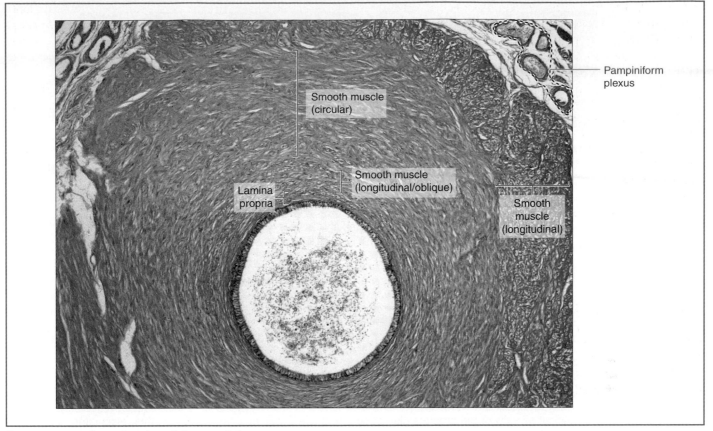

Figure 14-11. Cross-section of the vas deferens.

pass by an additional hollow structure called the prostatic utricle. This vestigial structure is all that remains of the müllerian duct in the male; without suppression by müllerian-inhibiting substance and androgens, it would have enlarged to form the uterus and oviducts. The prostatic utricle is a reminder that the reproductive system begins its existence with the potential to form either female or male structures (Fig. 14-12).

Before the vas deferens enters the interior of the prostate gland, it expands into a highly irregular, branched evagination called the seminal vesicle (Fig. 14-13). This hollow structure is lined by an epithelium that can vary from simple columnar to pseudostratified columnar; the remainder of its wall is composed of subepithelial dense connective tissue covered by a layer of smooth muscle. The epithelial cells of this organ produce over half of the volume of seminal fluid. Molecules secreted into this fluid include fructose, as a nutrient fuel, and prostaglandins. In addition, the seminal vesicles secrete proteins called semenogelins, which bind to each other to create high-molecular-weight complexes. These complexes make seminal fluid more viscous and enhance the coagulation of seminal fluid after ejaculation. In rodents and many other mammals, a copulatory plug of coagulated seminal fluid forms within the female reproductive tract after sexual intercourse that blocks the entry of sperm from other males. It is believed that in species in which copulation with multiple partners is frequent, these coagulating proteins of semen are functionally important to ensure that sperm from only one male fertilizes an ovum.

Prostate Gland

The prostate is a midline gland that secretes a protein-rich fluid from many secretory acini into the prostatic urethra. Secretory acini are composed of a pseudostratified columnar epithelium surrounded by loose connective tissue and smooth muscle fibers. Some of the most abundant proteins in prostatic secretions are trypsin-like proteases that, in contrast to seminal vesicle proteins, tend to liquefy seminal fluid (make it less viscous). One such enzyme, termed prostate-specific antigen (PSA), is secreted in high quantities by the prostate, although other tissues such as mammary epithelia can also synthesize small quantities of this protein. If the prostate gland becomes overactive (hyperplastic), the high quantities of PSA enter the bloodstream and can be detected by immunoassay blood tests. These can provide a helpful, but by no means infallible, indication of whether prostate cancer is developing.

Accumulations of calcified secretory product within the lumina of secretory acini become particularly prominent in older men. These accumulations are called prostatic concretions and represent a useful histologic characteristic of

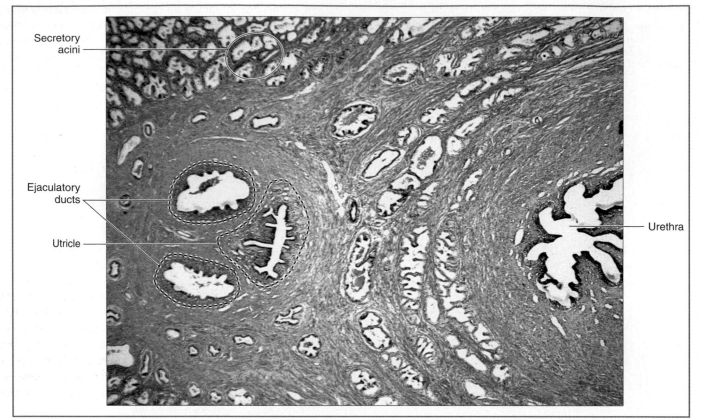

Secretory acini

Ejaculatory ducts

Utricle

Urethra

Figure 14-12. Low-magnification view of the prostate gland showing secretory acini, the prostatic urethra, ejaculatory ducts, and the prostatic utricle.

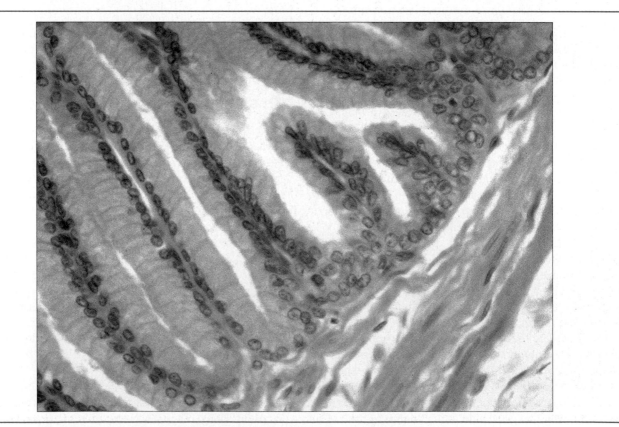

Figure 14-13. High-magnification view of the epithelium lining the seminal vesicles.

the prostate gland that distinguishes it from other glandular organs (Fig. 14-14).

Penis

The penis is a cylindrical extension of the skin that encloses three highly vascular masses of tissue: two corpora cavernosa that occupy the dorsal half of the penis and a single corpus spongiosum, containing the penile urethra, that is found in the ventral half of the penis (Fig. 14-15). Skeletal muscle fibers of the ischiocavernosus and bulbospongiosus muscles insert into these structures. The erectile tissues of the penis contain large numbers of venous sinuses that become filled with blood during penile erection (Fig. 14-16). The expansion of these sinuses during sexual intercourse compresses adjacent veins, hindering exit of blood from the penis and thereby provoking an enlargement and stiffening of this organ. This process is under the control of a number of CNS structures.

Studies of rodents and primates show that sexually arousing stimuli (olfactory, auditory, visual, and tactile) seem to converge on a cluster of neurons in the anterior hypothalamus termed the sexually dimorphic nucleus. This nucleus is several times larger in males than in females owing to a developmental influence of androgen.

Projections from the hypothalamus excite testosterone-sensitive neurons in the lumbar region of the spinal cord that innervate penile muscles such as the ischiocavernosus. Studies in rodents show that this collection of neurons is also sexually dimorphic (larger in males). Spinal cord neurons that provide autonomic innervation to the vasculature of the penis are also activated. The neural mechanisms that operate at the level of the penis to facilitate penile erection are briefly summarized in Figure 14-17.

●●● FEMALE REPRODUCTIVE SYSTEM

Ovaries

The ovaries of a fetus form when, under the influence of the X chromosomes, the cortical sex cords of the developing gonads predominate. This leads to an accumulation of primordial germ cells, now called oocytes, in the outermost cortical region of the ovary. Each small oocyte becomes enclosed in a single layer of simple squamous cells derived from the surrounding ovarian connective tissue (stroma). The combination of an oocyte plus its surrounding cells is called a primordial follicle. This cortical region of an ovary is covered by (1) a layer of dense connective tissue called the tunica

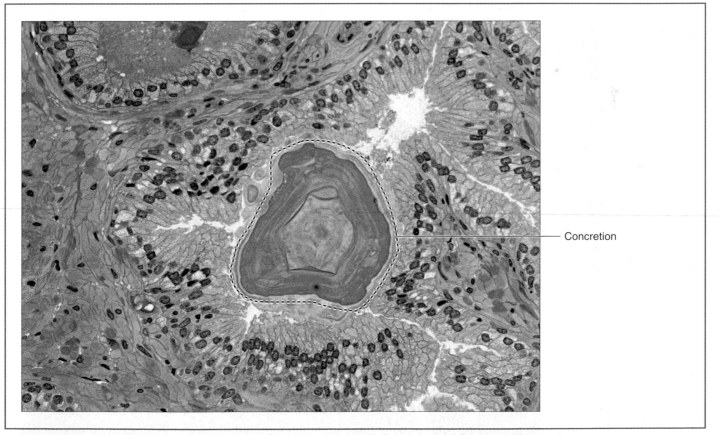

Concretion

Figure 14-14. High-magnification view of a prostatic acinus, containing a prostatic concretion composed of calcified secretory material.

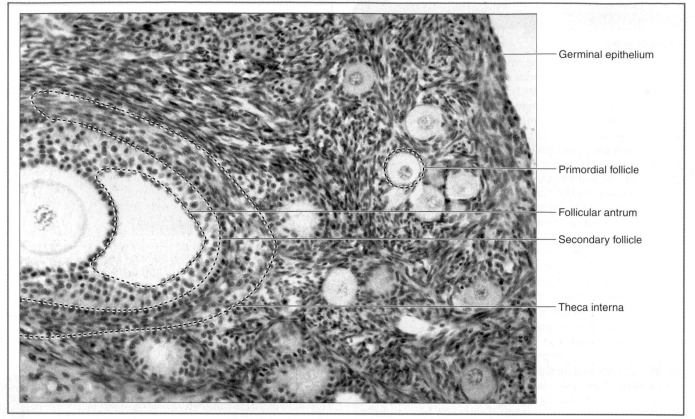

Germinal epithelium

Primordial follicle

Follicular antrum

Secondary follicle

Theca interna

Figure 14-18. Low-magnification view of the cortex of the ovary showing a secondary follicle with an antrum and a prominent theca interna, primordial follicles, and the overlying germinal epithelium.

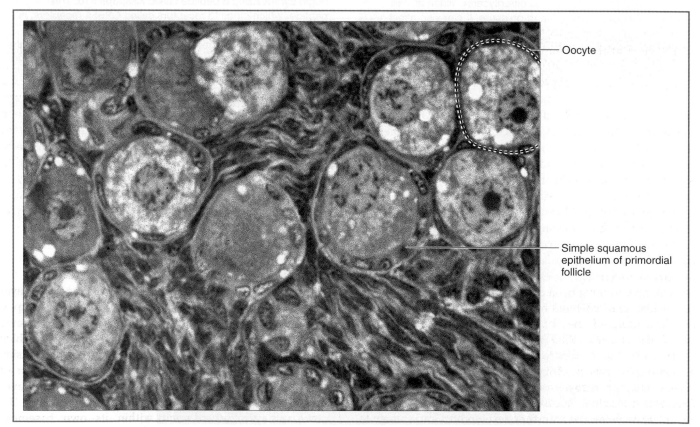

Oocyte

Simple squamous epithelium of primordial follicle

Figure 14-19. Primordial follicles, consisting of oocytes enclosed by a simple squamous epithelium.

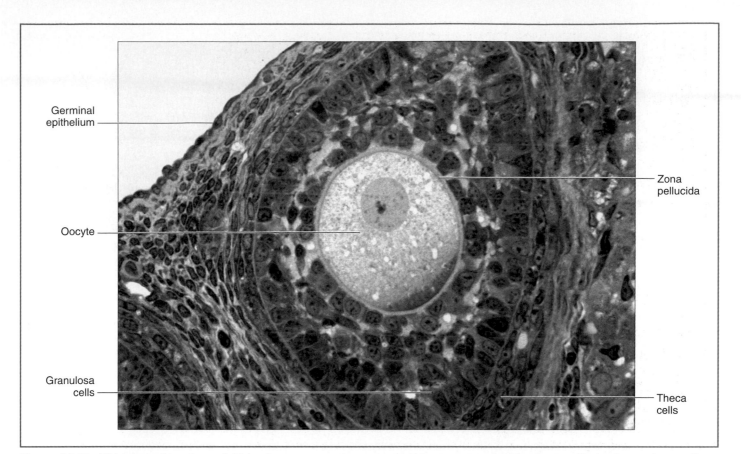

Germinal epithelium

Oocyte

Granulosa cells

Zona pellucida

Theca cells

Figure 14-20. This view of a primary follicle shows an oocyte surrounded by a zona pellucida, theca cells, and granulosa cells. The ovarian stroma and germinal epithelium are also visible.

membrane is another layer of specialized stromal cells called the theca layer. This layer can be separated into an inner theca interna layer that is well vascularized and contains cells with ovoid nuclei and an outer theca externa layer composed of more flattened cells that blends into the surrounding stoma. The large number of capillaries seen in the theca layer is required for the enormous growth of the follicle. These capillaries are stimulated to develop by angiogenic factors (e.g., vascular endothelial growth factor) that are secreted by granulosa cells.

The dramatic transition from a primordial to a primary follicle seems to be governed by the oocyte itself, as indicated by the following experiment: if enlarged, mature oocytes are transferred from a donor ovary to a host ovary in a mouse, the enlarged oocytes cause the cells surrounding them to form enlarged (primary and secondary) follicles. A number of proteins are secreted from the oocyte to stimulate the granulosa cells. These include a protein called growth differentiation factor–9 (GDF-9).

Many primary follicles never enlarge further, but a poorly understood selection process ensures that a fraction of primary follicles become transformed into the next stage of development called secondary follicles (Fig. 14-21). In secondary follicles, the granulosa cells secrete large amounts of a fluid called liquor folliculi that accumulates within a large space called an antrum. The antrum subdivides the granulosa cells into two populations: those in contact with the oocytes (these cells form an enclosing mass of cells called the cumulus oophorus) and those in contact with the glassy membrane (these cells are called mural granulosa cells after the Latin word for "wall"). As the antrum enlarges, the follicle becomes larger and larger until it is ready for ovulation (this very enlarged follicle is called a graafian follicle after the 17th century Dutch anatomist Regner de Graaf).

Communication between the oocyte and the granulosa cells is bidirectional: granulosa cells also exert a powerful influence on the oocyte. For example, the granulosa cells prevent the oocyte from completing the first meiotic division, which is stopped at the stage of meiotic prophase I called diplotene. This halt to meiotic progression lasts until the oocyte is ovulated, in some cases for decades between infancy and adulthood! The granulosa cells accomplish this by producing some yet-uncharacterized factor that binds to a receptor called Gpr3 on the surface of an oocyte. This receptor activates adenylate cyclase, increases intracellular levels of cAMP, and inactivates the cyclin-dependent kinases that would otherwise force a progression through meiotic metaphase, anaphase, and telophase.

This constant, mutual interaction between granulosa cells and oocyte would seem at first glance to be impossible: the

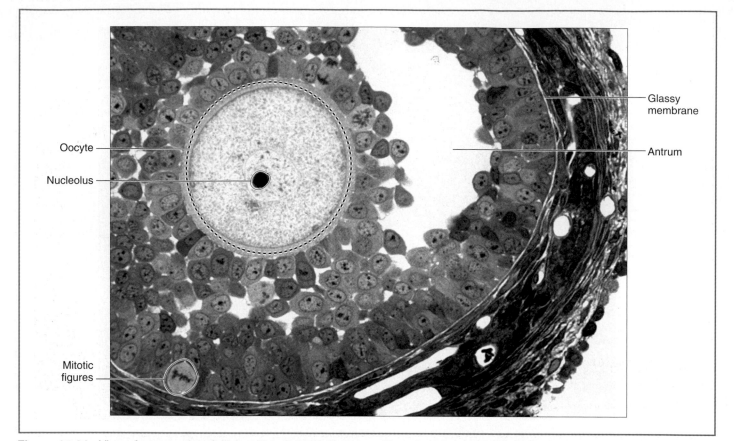

Figure 14-21. View of a secondary follicle with a fluid-filled antrum. Note the large size of the oocyte cytoplasm and the large, euchromatic nucleus with a large, prominent nucleolus. Mitotic figures are visible in the granulosa layer, which is separated from the theca layer by the glassy membrane.

two cell types are separated from each other by a thick and seemingly impenetrable zona pellucida. However, the granulosa cells extend thin cellular processes through small channels that penetrate the zona pellucida (Fig. 14-22). At the tips of these granulosa cell processes, the two cell types can make contact and even exchange small cytoplasmic molecules via gap junctions.

As the granulosa cells of a secondary follicle proliferate and enlarge, the theca cells also become activated to synthesize precursors of steroid hormones such as androstenedione. This molecule appears to cross the glassy membrane to the granulosa cells, which contain an enzyme (aromatase) that converts it to estrogen. The estrogen is then secreted into the bloodstream as a sex hormone that influences many tissues (e.g., the uterus, the bones, and the patterns of fat deposition). Estrogen also modifies brain function by influencing hypothalamic neurons responsible for libido and appetite control (ventromedial hypothalamus) and temperature regulation (preoptic area of the hypothalamus). Variations in body temperature that occur during the reproductive cycle, induced by variations in estrogen and progesterone, can be utilized to indicate the timing of ovulation. Granulosa cells also secrete inhibin, which dampens the secretion of FSH by the pituitary.

When a secondary follicle enlarges, it seems to secrete yet-uncharacterized factors that suppress the activity of neighboring follicles by making them less responsive to gonadotropins. The result is that a given ovary (in humans) tends to have only one large, preovulatory follicle at any one time. When this follicle is ovulated, the remaining follicles are released from inhibition until one grows large enough to once again suppress the others. This suppression of ovarian follicles by a single dominant follicle is an explanation for why ovulation tends to alternate between one ovary and the other each month.

Ovulation

An enlarging secondary follicle gradually secretes increasing amounts of estrogen until estrogen levels reach a critical level in the bloodstream. Then estrogen provokes a massive release of LH from the pituitary. This LH surge, which is three to four times larger in amplitude than is biologically necessary, has a transforming effect on the follicle. Granulosa cells secrete a plasminogen activator protein that converts an enzyme, plasmin, from its inactive precursor (plasminogen). Plasmin degrades the extracellular proteins that hold the follicle together, so that it weakens and bursts. Since the swollen follicle has grown so large as to approach the germinal

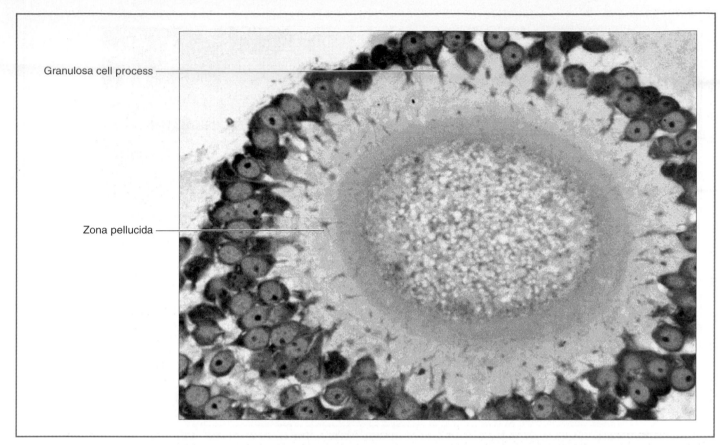

Granulosa cell process

Zona pellucida

Figure 14-22. Tangential section through an oocyte of a secondary follicle. This view shows the processes from the granulosa cells that traverse the zona pellucida to contact the oocyte cytoplasm.

epithelium covering the ovary, follicular fluid escapes from the ovary into the peritoneal cavity. The oocyte, together with an enclosing mass of granulosa cells called the corona radiata, is borne along with this fluid in the process of ovulation. In most cases the ovulated oocyte is taken up into the lumen of the closely adjacent oviduct (see Oviducts).

In addition to changing its location, the oocyte undergoes a significant functional change: it is released from inhibition by the granulosa cells, completes the first meiotic division, and proceeds through the second meiotic division until halting once again in the middle of metaphase of the second meiotic division. This is due to an LH-stimulated secretion of progesterone by the granulosa cells, which seems to close the gap junctions between the oocyte and granulosa cells and to loosen the attachments of granulosa cells to each other and to the oocyte (Fig. 14-23).

The LH surge also transforms the follicular cells that remain behind within the ovary. These cells proliferate to form a large structure called a corpus luteum. A major function of the corpus luteum is to secrete the steroid hormone progesterone (Fig. 14-24).

Until recently, this series of events has been difficult to understand. Normally, estrogen functions as a negative feedback signal from the ovary to chronically *suppress* pituitary LH secretion. Estrogen, on the correct day of the reproductive cycle of women, suddenly *stimulates* LH secretion.

Effect of Estrogen

Once an oocyte has ovulated, it completes the first meiotic division and continues its preparation for union with a spermatozoon during fertilization. In oocytes, the first meiotic division is asymmetric and unequal: the meiotic spindle migrates to one pole of the oocyte, under the direction of the same type of PAR proteins that cause epithelial cells and neurons to become polarized. A bulge develops on this side of the oocyte, allowing for an unequal division of the cytoplasm during the first meiotic division (see Fig. 14-23). Only a small portion of oocyte cytoplasm, containing one set of chromosomes, pinches off from the main portion of the cell to form the first polar body. This will eventually degenerate.

Special Features of Oocyte Cytoplasm

At this point, the oocyte, suspended in the oviduct, has acquired an enormous volume of cytoplasm and chromosomes are poised to complete the two divisions of meiosis. The oocyte cytoplasm appears unremarkable but in fact has a number of extraordinary features that require discussion.

In much of this book, the commanding influence of the cell nucleus on the cytoplasm is a recurring theme. In oocytes, however, the opposite situation is true: the cytoplasm has a unique and powerful influence on the function of the nucleus. This fact can be demonstrated during

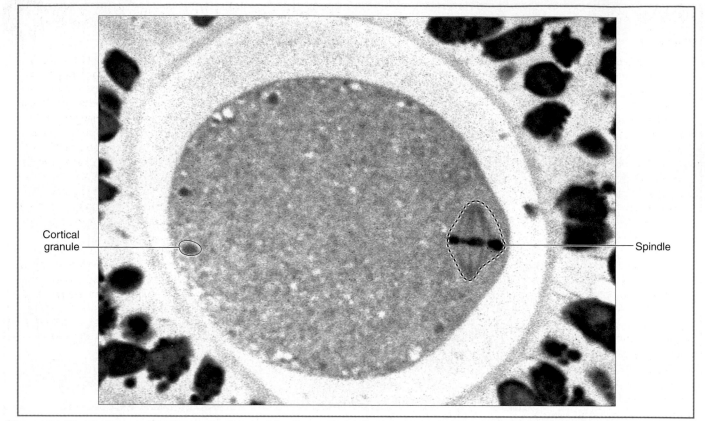

Figure 14-23. Oocyte undergoing metaphase of the first meiotic division. The meiotic spindle has moved to one pole of the oocyte, the zona pellucida has loosened its attachments to the oocyte, and the granulosa cells of the corona radiata are starting to detach. Several cortical granules are visible just beneath the oocyte plasma membrane.

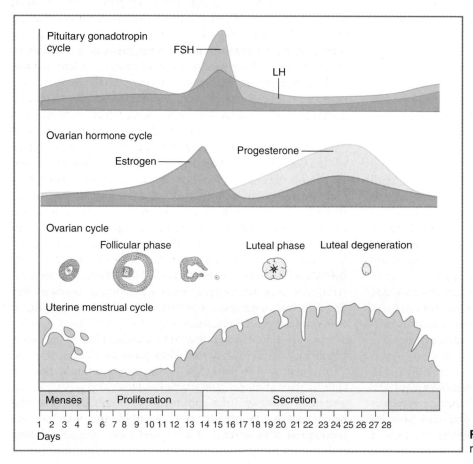

Figure 14-24. Diagram of the human reproductive cycle.

PHYSIOLOGY

The Ovarian Cycle

A novel explanation for the two opposite effects of estrogen on LH secretion over the ovarian cycle now seems at hand: estrogen acts on two separate populations of hypothalamic neurons to produce these two different effects.

Low levels of estrogen secreted during the maturation of a follicle, lasting 12 days or so (the estrogenic or follicular phase of the ovarian cycle), are detected by hypothalamic neurons that synthesize a specific form of gonadotropin-releasing hormone (GnRH-I). The activity of these cells, which are located throughout the preoptic area of the hypothalamus, is suppressed by estrogen (negative feedback suppression of LH by estrogen).

Higher levels of estrogen at the end of the follicular phase are detected by another subset of hypothalamic neurons that contain a second form of GnRH (GnRH-II). These neurons, which possess another type of estrogen receptor (the β rather than the α form), respond to estrogen with an increase in activity rather than a decrease (positive feedback stimulation of LH by estrogen). These cells are located in the paraventricular, supraoptic, and arcuate nuclei of the hypothalamus. These cells likely induce the LH surge.

The corpus luteum, created in response to the LH surge, secretes progesterone for the next 13 days or so (progestational or luteal phase of the cycle). This progesterone suppresses any further LH surges, so that no additional ovulations take place. Progesterone also prepares the uterus for a possible pregnancy. If pregnancy does not occur, the corpus luteum degenerates. The resultant fall in progesterone causes the uterine changes seen in menstruation and allows for a gradual increase in LH that re-initiates the ovarian cycle.

BIOCHEMISTRY

DNA in Reproductive Cloning

In highly differentiated cells, large stretches of DNA become methylated. Methylated DNA is bound by a repressor protein that removes acetyl groups from histones. Histones that lack acetyl groups, in turn, fail to bind RNA polymerase II and thus do not permit gene transcription. Nuclei from differentiated cells therefore can transcribe only a limited subset of genes.

When a skin cell nucleus is inserted into an oocyte, almost 75% of its nuclear proteins are removed and degraded. For example, oocyte histones replace the somatic histones. An oocyte protein called nucleoplasmin is among the many proteins that guide this process. The cell nucleus thus transits from a differentiated state with limited options to an immature state with many developmental potentials.

This influence of the oocyte cytoplasm should not be too surprising. It is also required during fertilization, when a highly condensed and specialized spermatozoon nucleus enters the oocyte, decondenses, and fuses with the haploid oocyte nucleus. The resultant cell acquires a new state of multipotential transcriptional ability.

the process of reproductive cloning. In this procedure, the oocyte nucleus is removed in vitro with a glass micropipette and is replaced with the nucleus of a donor somatic cell (often a skin cell). Then, the oocyte is induced to divide, and in the right circumstances it will produce an embryo that is genetically identical to the donor animal (this has now been accomplished with mice, rats, sheep, and dogs).

On the face of it, reproductive cloning would seem to be impossible. To be sure, skin cells can readily be induced to divide in vitro, but when they do so, they only produce more skin cells. This is because a skin cell nucleus has already gone through a process of terminal differentiation, so that skin cell genes are activated and the remaining genes are permanently turned off. However, the oocyte cytoplasm can induce a dedifferentiation of the skin cell nucleus, restoring it to a pristine condition in which it can differentiate into almost anything.

In addition to possessing special factors that influence the cell nucleus, the cytoplasm of oocytes of many species is noteworthy for possessing a hidden structure and polarity that influences subsequent cell divisions and the function of

cells in an embryo. Several model organisms possess this oocyte polarity.

In fruit flies (Drosophila melanogaster), the cytoplasm of an unfertilized oocyte contains an anteroposterior gradient of a transcription factor called bicoid, a so-called maternal effect protein, that was created by maternal cells enclosing the oocyte. After fertilization and the initiation of cell division, cells form from this cytoplasm and all contain different levels of bicoid. Anterior cells with a high level of bicoid are stimulated to produce another transcription factor, a homeotic protein called orthodenticle, which instructs the cells to form head structures. Middle cells exposed to lower levels of bicoid produce another homeotic protein called hunchback and form thoracic structures. Yet a lower level of bicoid in more posterior cells stimulates the production of a third homeotic protein called knirps and the formation of abdominal structures. Cells formed from the extreme posterior end of the oocyte are never exposed to bicoid and express a protein called oskar that causes them to form germ cells. Thus, an initial gradient in the unfertilized oocyte sets the stage for the formation of a segmented embryo. Homologous homeotic proteins can be found in humans, but they do not seem to be expressed until later stages of embryonic development.

In oocytes from frogs (Xenopus laevis), there is a similar but much less complex gradient of proteins. In the so-called vegetal pole of the oocyte, a cloudy substance called nuage forms that contains a protein called DAZ. The name of this protein, originally found in humans, originated from the words "deleted in azoospermia," a condition in which sperm production was absent. This vegetal pole protein of frog oocytes stimulates cells that enclose it to become gametes. If it is damaged or deleted during the division of the oocyte, the resultant embryos lack gametes and grow up to be sterile.

Mammalian oocytes also show some signs of polarity. These signs include the following: (1) the meiotic spindle migrates to one pole of the cytoplasm, (2) dark-staining material can sometimes be detected in portions of the cytoplasm (see Fig. 14-20), (3) nuage-like material can be detected in ultrastructural studies of rat oocytes, (4) receptors for leptin and a leptin-stimulated cytoplasmic protein seem to show a polarized distribution in oocytes, (5) DAZ protein can also be found in human oocytes and influences the embryonic production of germ cells, and (6) a number of maternal effect proteins (e.g., Mater protein) and at least six homeotic genes (Obox genes) have been found to be localized exclusively to mouse oocytes and appear to guide their later development.

On the other hand, most experimental studies of mammalian oocytes have shown that each cell of 4- or 8-cell embryos appears equally able to generate a complete and healthy embryo if allowed to develop on its own. This seems to contradict the notion that an unfertilized oocyte could contribute a specialized portion of cytoplasm to only a few daughter cells. Thus, the question of oocyte polarity in mammals is controversial and not fully resolved. It is not a totally academic question, for it is related to procedures for the cloning and generation of embryonic stem cells from early embryos that could be utilized to produce a range of adult tissues. So far the success rate for cloning is quite low: only about 1% to 5% of cloned embryos develop normally. The reasons for this low success rate are not totally understood, but if the cloning procedure were to disrupt some polarized structures in oocyte cytoplasm, this would surely have injurious results.

Fertilization

If a spermatozoon encounters an oocyte within the oviduct, it releases acrosomal enzymes that enable it to penetrate the corona radiata of granulosa cells surrounding the oocyte. Subsequently, the sperm cell binds to the zp3 protein of the oocyte zona pellucida and releases additional enzymes that penetrate the zona and allow the spermatozoon cell membrane to fuse with the oocyte cell membrane.

Fusion of the sperm with the egg cell triggers an influx of calcium into the oocyte. This has a number of consequences. First, calcium promotes the movement of vesicles called cortical granules toward the oocyte plasma membrane (see Fig. 14-23). These granules release an enzyme (a glycosidase) into the environment of the oocyte that changes the structure of the zp3 protein of the zona pellucida. As a consequence, additional sperm are unable to bind to the zona pellucida and thus cannot also fertilize the oocyte. This cortical reaction prevents the entry of extra sperm chromosomes, an event called polyspermy, that would disrupt the fusion of the male and female pronuclei and prevent normal cell division.

A second consequence of Ca++ entry during fertilization is that the blockade of the second meiotic division at metaphase II is released and the oocyte finally completes meiosis. This is due to Ca++-induced activation of a complex of anaphase-promoting proteins. These proteins tag another protein, cyclin B, for destruction. This inactivates cyclin-dependent kinase, allowing the appearance of anaphase and telophase and the re-forming of the nuclear envelope.

Postfertilization Events

Following fertilization, the oocyte initiates cleavage and cell division and starts to form an embryo and placenta. In the meantime, other events take place in the ovary. The remnants of the follicle that once contained the antrum and the ovulated oocyte collapse (Fig. 14-25). The small amount of follicular fluid is resorbed, and small cells from the theca layer invade the follicle and become theca lutein cells as a result of the influence of the LH surge. The more numerous and larger granulosa cells become transformed into granulosa lutein cells. These two cell types, plus accompanying vessels and connective tissue cells, enlarge into a structure called the corpus luteum (Figs. 14-26 and 14-27).

Normal ovarian corpora lutea primarily function to produce progesterone for about 13 days after ovulation and then begin to degenerate. The reasons for this dramatic decline are uncertain. There is evidence that it is stimulated by ovarian prostaglandins; also, an invasion of macrophages and lymphocytes into a degenerating corpus luteum almost

PATHOLOGY

Infertility

The normal union of sperm and egg does not always proceed smoothly. If a couple has had unprotected sexual intercourse for a year without the initiation of pregnancy, some degree of fertility problems can be suspected. Lowered fertility can be ascribed to a number of causes.

In about 30% of patients, the cause of infertility originates with the woman. Another 30% of cases are due to male reproductive problems. The remaining cases involve both the man and the woman or spring from uncertain causes.

Female infertility can be caused by a failure of ovulation or blockage of oviducts as a result of pelvic inflammatory disease secondary to infections. These conditions can be treated by drugs that induce ovulation or by oviduct surgery. One frequently used drug, clomiphene, is an antiestrogen that blocks negative feedback effects of estrogen on LH and thus provokes an LH surge.

Male infertility can result from many defects. Cystic fibrosis (incidence of 1 in 2500 persons) is a disease in which the chloride transporter (cystic fibrosis transmembrane conductance regulator protein, or CTFR) is dysfunctional. Since the epididymis requires this protein for chloride transport, it becomes obstructed or damaged, causing infertility. Other gene defects can also result in low sperm production (oligozoospermia), which affects 3% to 4% of all men. For example, a mutation in the DAZ protein can block the production of germ cells.

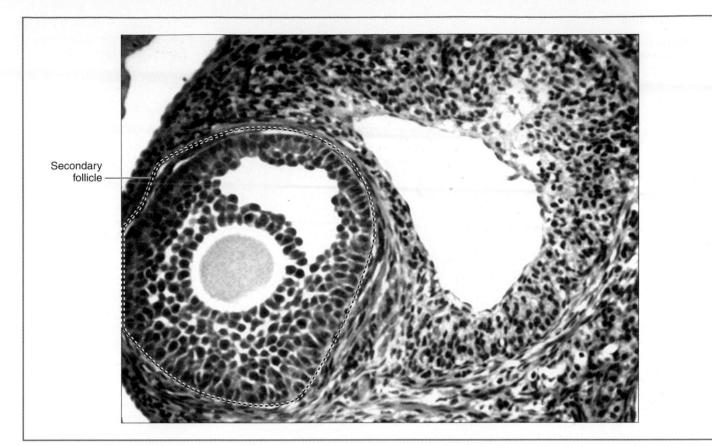

Figure 14-25. View of a secondary follicle.

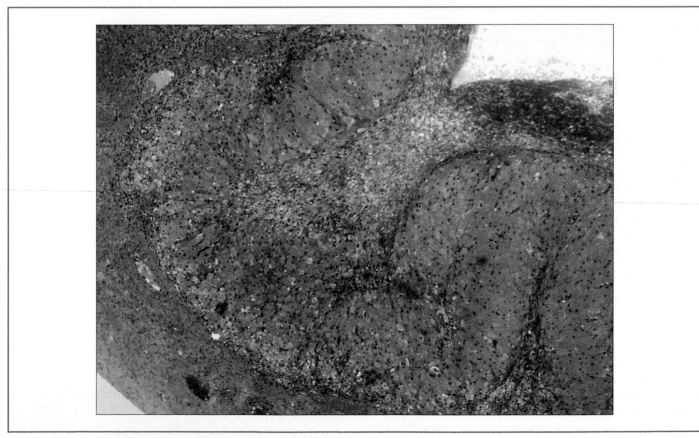

Figure 14-26. Low-magnification view of a corpus luteum.

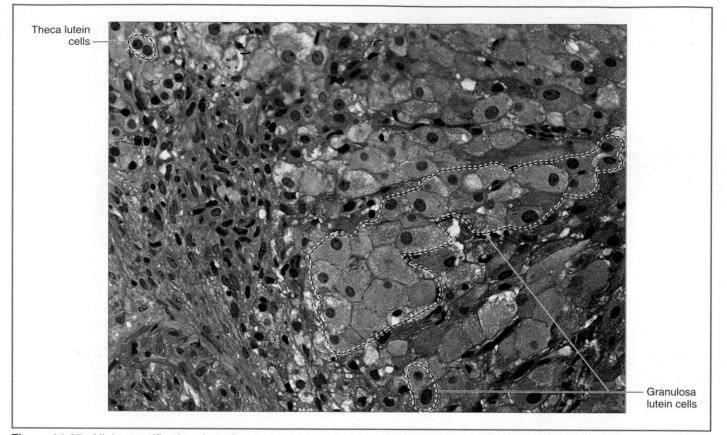

Theca lutein cells

Granulosa lutein cells

Figure 14-27. High-magnification view of a corpus luteum showing granulosa lutein cells and theca lutein cells.

suggests similarity to the rejection of "foreign" tissue by the immune system. This would not be surprising, since luteal cells represent a novel cellular phenotype that had not been present during the development of the immune system. Conceivably, unless restrained, the immune system would function to destroy corpora lutea much as it would destroy spermatozoa unprotected by the blood-testis barrier.

Only one factor can "rescue" a degenerating corpus luteum from oblivion: LH or an LH homolog produced by the developing placenta called human chorionic gonadotropin (hCG). These hormones allow a corpus luteum to grow even larger and linger on, producing more progesterone to keep the uterus in a state suitable to maintain a pregnancy. Granulosa cells of the enlarged corpus luteum of pregnancy secrete progesterone, and like most steroid-producing cells, contain abundant mitochondria, lipid droplets, and smooth endoplasmic reticulum.

In addition to progesterone, granulosa lutein cells of pregnancy also produce large amounts of a peptide hormone called relaxin that is structurally similar to insulin. Relaxin weakens the connective tissues of several sites in the reproductive system. It relaxes the ligaments of the pubic symphysis and softens the margins of the opening to the uterus, the cervix. These changes prepare the reproductive organs for the passage of a baby. Relaxin is stored in small secretion granules within the cytoplasm of granulosa lutein cells. Like Leydig cells of the testis, these cells are unusual in having the capacity to secrete both steroid and peptide hormones at the same time.

As the corpus luteum of pregnancy degenerates, its vasculature also becomes degraded, and gradually the entire structure is transformed into a poorly vascularized mass of connective tissue called a corpus albicans (Fig. 14-28).

The vast majority of ovarian follicles are destined to degenerate, since only about 400 ovulations occur within the reproductive life of a woman. It has been estimated that, from the original 10 million oocytes present in the ovary at birth, only 300,000 survive past puberty. These degenerating follicles experience massive apoptosis in a process called atresia (Fig. 14-29). In the early stages, an atretic follicle is a mass of cells surrounded by the glassy membrane and enclosing a collapsed zona pellucida; many of the cells possess shrunken, darkened nuclei that are diagnostic for apoptosis. Later on, only the collapsed zona pellucida, which is resistant to proteolysis, will remain.

The biochemical pathway for apoptosis in these cells is well understood: it involves the action of at least 14 types of enzymes that cleave proteins between *cy*steine and *asp*artate amino acids and so are called caspases. These caspases are responsible for the destruction of nuclear DNA and cytoplasmic organelles and are activated by an extracellular protein called Fas ligand and by an intracellular release of

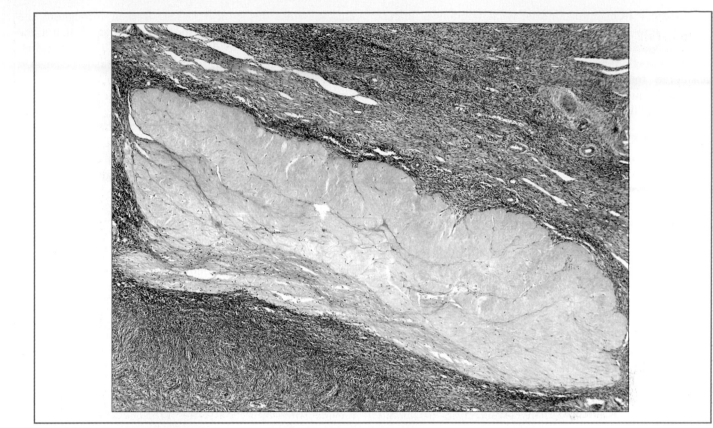

Figure 14-28. Low-magnification view of a corpus albicans.

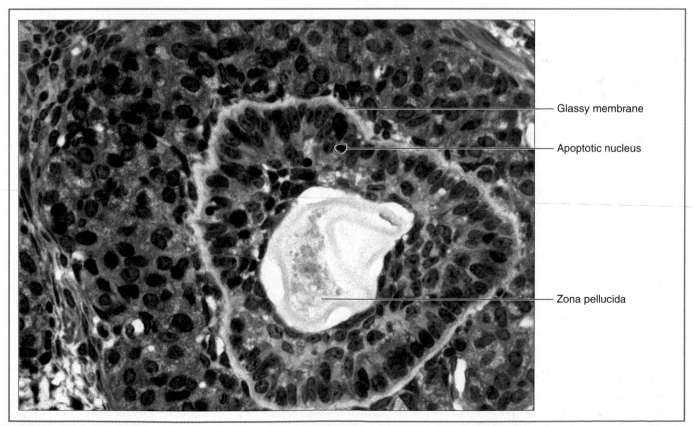

Glassy membrane

Apoptotic nucleus

Zona pellucida

Figure 14-29. Atretic follicle, containing a collapsed zona pellucida, apoptotic cell nuclei in the granulosa layer, and a collapsing glassy membrane.

cytochrome *c* from mitochondria. What is not well understood is how some follicles are chosen to escape this degenerative fate and others go through it.

The destruction of ovarian oocytes has traditionally been considered to be the cause of menopause; as oocytes decrease in number, ovulation stops and the ovarian cycle ceases at about age 50. This interpretation has been challenged by recent evidence that stem cells for oocytes seem to persist throughout life and can migrate from the bone marrow to the ovaries and form new follicles. In adult mice, hundreds of new follicles have been observed to form within 24 hours under the right conditions. If these observations are confirmed, they would seem to undermine conventional thinking about the cause of reproductive senescence in women. Perhaps, as in male senescence, an extragonadal (hypothalamic) change in function with age is the cause of menopause.

Oviducts

Ovulated oocytes that are released from the ovary are guided into adjacent tubular organs called oviducts or uterine (fallopian) tubes (Figs. 14-30 and 14-31). The lining of the oviduct is a simple columnar epithelium containing interspersed ciliated and nonciliated cells. Loose connective tissue lies beneath the epithelium and is surrounded by several layers of smooth muscle. While this basic structure is seen throughout the oviduct, it shows some variations along its length that allow the oviduct to be divided into four regions. The first region, the infundibulum, has a wide lumen and is nestled alongside the ovary to receive oocytes. Its margins are decorated with finger-like epithelial projections termed fimbriae. The next region, the ampulla, has a mucosa possessing a labyrinthine array of folds (Fig. 14-32). The isthmus of the oviduct has a much less complex and folded mucosa, and the interstitial portion of the oviduct lies within the wall of the uterus and is surrounded by masses of uterine smooth muscle.

Uterus

The uterus is a large, hollow organ divisible into three regions: a dome-shaped fundus lying above the oviducts, a main corpus (body), and a more cylindrical cervical region at the junction between the uterus and vagina. The uterus is lined by a mucosa, or endometrium, consisting of a layer of simple columnar epithelial cells covering a highly cellular connective tissue (stroma). The surface epithelium projects down into the stroma to form numerous tubular uterine glands. Beneath the endometrium is a thick layer of smooth muscle, the myometrium.

The appearance of the endometrium changes greatly during the menstrual cycle, under the influence of sex hormones.

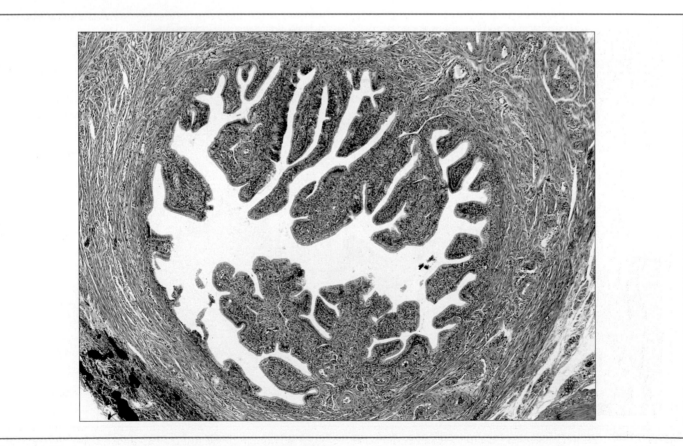

Figure 14-30. Low-magnification view of the oviduct (isthmus).

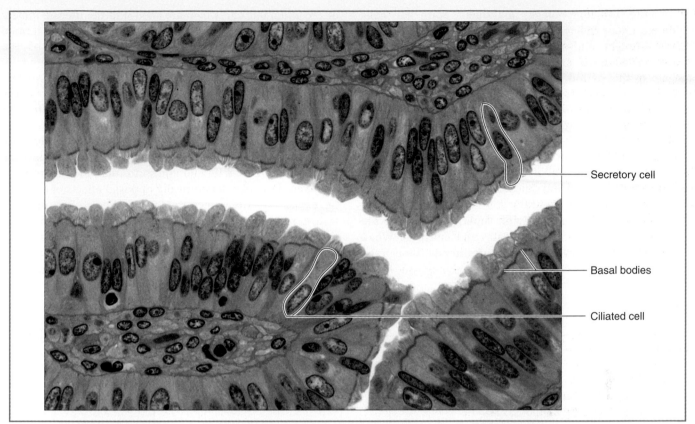

Secretory cell

Basal bodies

Ciliated cell

Figure 14-31. High-magnification view of the oviduct showing simple columnar, ciliated epithelium.

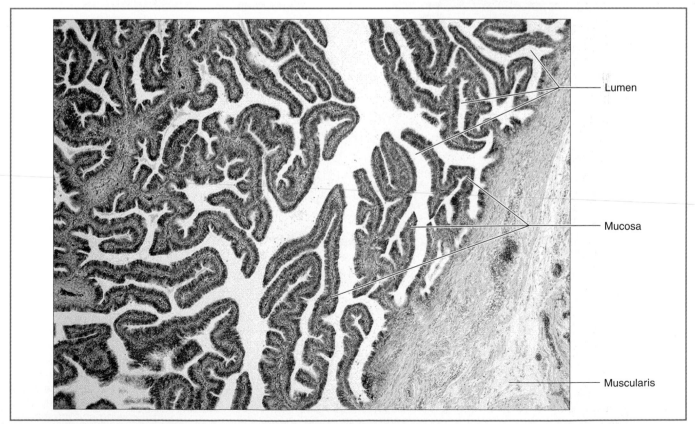

Lumen

Mucosa

Muscularis

Figure 14-32. Low-magnification view of the oviduct (ampulla region). This portion of the oviduct has an extremely convoluted mucosal lining.

During the follicular stage, glandular epithelial cells proliferate under the influence of estrogen, and the glands become straight and taller (Fig. 14-33). Accompanying arteries, called spiral arteries because of their shape, also elongate in this period. During the luteal stage, the glands stop enlarging and start secreting molecules into the uterine lumen. Glands become distended with secretory material and acquire a tortuous, irregular appearance (Fig. 14-34).

Finally, during the menstrual stage, the sudden withdrawal of progesterone has a profound effect on the endometrium. The hormone-sensitive smooth muscle of the spiral arteries, which had been relaxed and quiescent under the influence of progesterone, starts spasmodically contracting. This interrupts the blood supply to the overlying superficial layer of the endometrium, provoking cell death and necrosis. When additional blood is allowed to pass intermittently through the spiral arteries, the flow of fluid disrupts the dying tissue layers

of the endometrium, which are shed into the uterine lumen. These changes last for 5 days or so in the process termed menstruation, which eventually destroys most of the superficial layer of the endometrium. At the end of menstruation, increasing levels of estrogen again stimulate the remaining basal (functional) layer of the endometrium to heal and proliferate, and the uterine cycle begins again.

The ability of estrogen to cause epithelial proliferation in the uterus is at odds with its influence elsewhere. In the skin, for example, estrogen diminishes cell division and causes the skin of women to be thinner and softer than the skin of men. How can these two diametrically opposed effects of estrogen be explained? The same problem applies to testosterone: testosterone causes hair loss (baldness) in the scalp, but centimeters away at the jawline, causes hair growth (beards)! The diverse effects of steroids on various tissues may partly be due to tissue-specific molecules. When a steroid binds to a

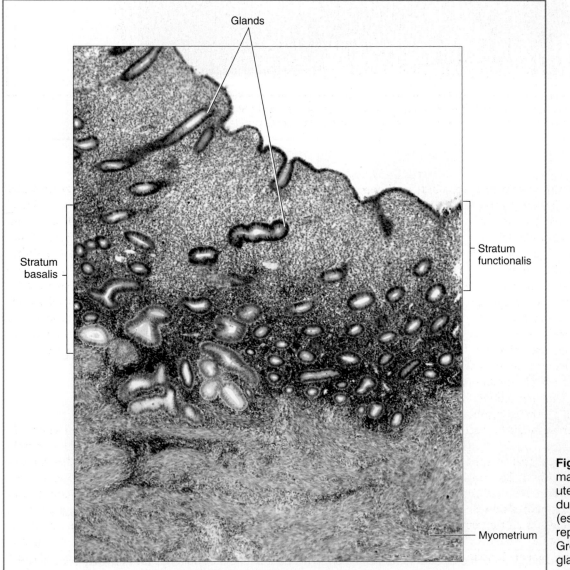

Figure 14-33. Low-magnification view of the uterine endometrium during the proliferative (estrogenic) phase of the reproductive cycle. Growing endometrial glands have straight profiles.

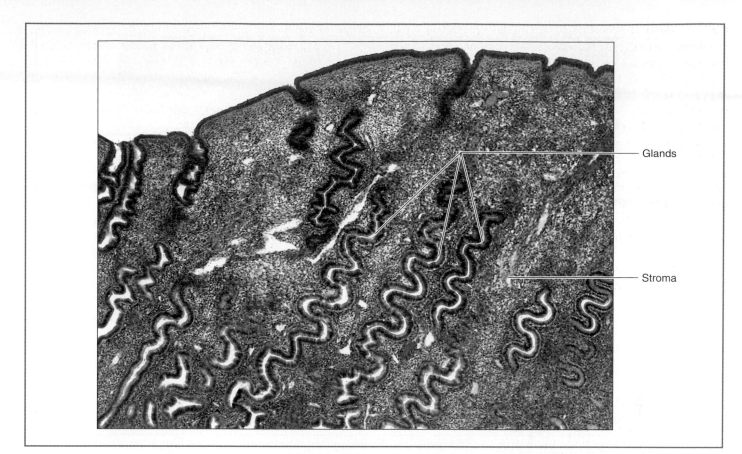

— Glands

— Stroma

Figure 14-34. Low-magnification view of the uterine endometrium during the secretory (progestational) phase of the reproductive cycle. Endometrial glands are actively secreting and have contorted profiles.

steroid receptor protein, the steroid receptor binds to other proteins called steroid co-activator proteins, which influence the ability of the steroid receptor to bind to gene sequences in DNA and initiate transcription. Different tissues appear to have different co-activator proteins, which may explain why they respond to steroids differently.

Most mammals do not experience such severe uterine changes during their reproductive cycle, and while cells can be cast off into the uterine and vaginal lumina, little blood loss occurs. Only humans and a few species of primates undergo such drastic uterine changes. In addition, the reproductive cycles of rodents are much shorter, lasting 4 to 5 days. Some mammals are reflex ovulators and ovulate only during specific seasons following mating. It is clear that the specific parameters of the female reproductive cycle have diverged during evolution to meet the ecologic requirements of each species.

It may or may not be significant that the average length of the human ovarian cycle—about 28 days—is similar to the length of time between full moons (29.5 days). However, it has been well established that ambient lighting and day length have powerful influences on the reproductive systems of many mammals, including humans. These effects are mediated by changes in pineal function and melatonin secretion (see Chapter 10).

Sex steroids induce an increased expression of at least 150 different genes in uterine tissues. Some of these induced proteins are growth factors produced by stromal cells that stimulate endometrial growth. Other proteins dampen the responses of immune cells and may be related to the ability of the uterus to tolerate the implantation of an embryo bearing foreign antigens. Still other proteins are secreted by the simple columnar epithelial cells of endometrial glands into the uterine lumen (Fig. 14-35). A few of these, such as a protein called glycodelin, have been studied and named, but the functions and forms of most uterine secretory proteins are not known at present.

Vagina

At the zone of transition between the uterus and vagina, the cervix, the lining epithelium changes from the simple columnar epithelium of the uterus to the stratified squamous epithelium of the vagina (Fig. 14-36). Cells of the vaginal epithelium contain abundant amounts of glycogen and consequently often have a pale-staining appearance with conventional stains such as hematoxylin and eosin. When these cells are shed into the vaginal lumen, the glycogen is converted to lactate by bacteria, resulting in an acid pH that helps depress the growth of foreign microorganisms. The

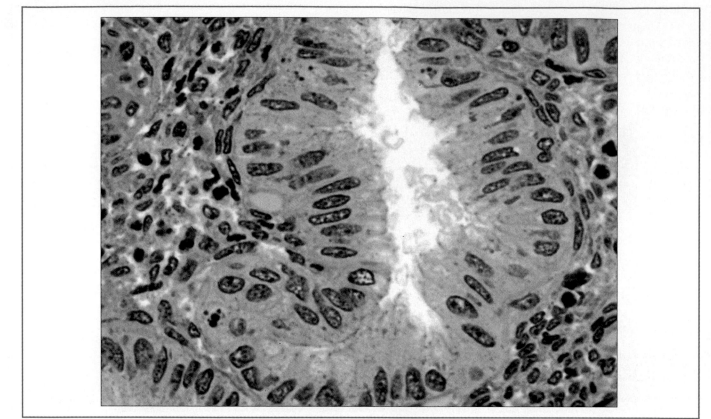

Figure 14-35. High-magnification view of an endometrial gland showing simple columnar epithelial cells surrounded by a highly cellular stroma of the endometrium.

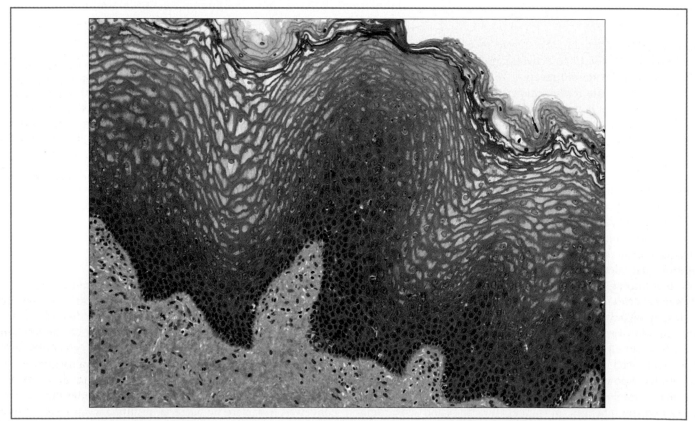

Figure 14-36. Mucosa of the vagina.

histologic appearance of the vaginal mucosa could easily be confused with the similar-appearing esophagus but for the lack of a muscularis mucosae layer in the vagina. Underlying the epithelium is a layer of connective tissue (lamina propria) and a thicker layer of smooth muscle.

Placenta

The fetal tissues that form the placenta become intimately associated with the lining of the uterus, and therefore it is appropriate to describe it in the context of the female reproductive system. Placenta formation begins when the fertilized ovum divides into two, four, and eight cells to form a compact ball called a morula. As more cell division occurs, the enlarging morula develops a fluid-filled cavity and at this point is called a blastocyst.

From the beginning, the blastocyst can be divided into two regions: the inner cell mass, which will form the embryo, and the trophoblast layer, which will form the placenta (Fig. 14-37). Both regions quickly acquire subdivisions. The inner cell mass forms the amnion, the bilaminar disc, and the yolk sac. As the bilaminar disc develops, it in turn divides into the epiblast, which will form ectodermal and mesodermal structures, and the yolk sac. As development proceeds, the entire embryo becomes surrounded by extraembryonic mesenchyme (mesoderm) that contains abundant fibroblasts and macrophages. The trophoblast region separates into an external syncytiotrophoblast and an internal cytotrophoblast that overlies the extraembryonic mesenchyme.

The syncytiotrophoblast layer is perhaps the most remarkable layer of cells in the body, for it amounts to an enormous mass of cytoplasm, filled with cell nuclei, that is undivided by any cell membranes. Thus, this tissue layer represents an unbroken barrier that surrounds and protects the fetus. A cellular layer, the cytotrophoblast, lies beneath it. This cell layer appears to function as a stem cell layer that contributes to the constantly growing syncytiotrophoblast layer. All these structures form by day 6 of pregnancy, when implantation into the endometrium begins.

As the blastocyst matures, it "hatches" from the enclosing zona pellucida and starts to secrete hCG. This hormone, in turn, causes nearby endometrial cells to synthesize a surface protein called trophinin, which helps the blastocyst adhere to the endometrium. In addition, the blastocyst acquires an outer layer of carbohydrate molecules that bind to receptor proteins such as selectin and heparin-binding growth factor, which are present at the apical surfaces of the endometrial cells. A portion of endometrial cells that bind the blastocyst undergo apoptosis, and then the syncytiotrophoblast layer secretes proteolytic enzymes such as matrix metalloproteinases that degrade the extracellular structures beneath the endometrial epithelium. This permits the blastocyst to invade the endometrium and to become implanted within the endometrial stroma.

The implanted blastocyst begins to extrude processes, called chorionic villi, from its surface (Fig. 14-38). These invade further into the endometrial stroma and disrupt the

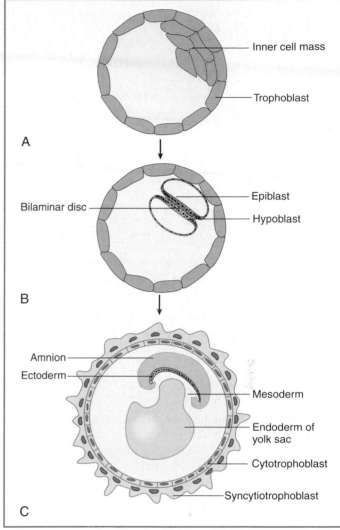

Figure 14-37. Diagram of the development of the blastocyst and placenta. **A,** Embryonic cells have become segregated into an inner cell mass and a trophoblast layer. **B,** At a later time, the inner cell mass has developed cavities that will become the amniotic cavity and the yolk sac, and two cell layers that will form the embryo—the epiblast and hypoblast—have appeared. **C,** At a still later time, the amnion and amniotic cavity have fully formed, the three germ layers of the embryo (ectoderm, mesoderm, and endoderm) have formed, and extraembryonic mesenchyme has filled the interval between the embryo and placenta. The placenta has developed two layers: the outer syncytiotrophoblast and the inner cytotrophoblast.

endothelial lining of maternal blood vessels, so that the surface of the placenta is washed with maternal blood. The stromal cells in contact with the villi themselves differentiate into decidual cells, which have a rounded shape and are filled with glycogen. These cells appear to have a limiting influence on the invasiveness of the placenta and may also suppress immune attacks on the placenta. The most prominent mass of chorionic villi occupies about one fourth of the surface of the blastocyst and eventually expands into a structure called the

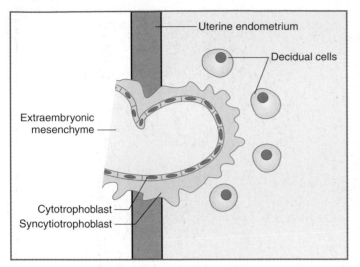

Figure 14-38. Diagram of a chorionic villus within the endometrial stroma. Each villus is covered by syncytiotrophoblast and cytotrophoblast layers that enclose a core of extraembryonic mesenchyme. The invasion of the placenta into the endometrium stimulates the differentiation of stromal cells into large, round decidual cells.

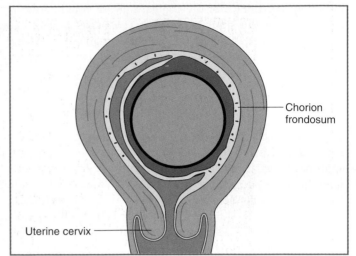

Figure 14-39. Diagram showing the site of implantation of the fetal-placental unit into the uterine endometrium. The basal portion of the placenta, the chorion frondosum, is responsible for most of the exchange of metabolites between baby and mother.

chorion frondosum (Fig. 14-39). The remainder of the trophoblast thins out, becomes adherent to the amnion, and contributes little to the function of the mature placenta.

The cells of the outer syncytiotrophoblast have many unusual features: they secrete hormones such as progesterone, hCG, and human placental somatomammotropin, a hormone with properties similar to GH and prolactin. They also express transporters for molecules such as glucose that allow a transfer of nutrients to the extraembryonic mesenchyme of the fetus through an otherwise impenetrable barrier (Figs. 14-40 and 14-41).

The Placenta and Control of Onset of Labor

When the fetus is fully developed, the uterine myometrium starts contracting and labor ensues. Many hypotheses have been proposed to explain how this critical event is controlled, but no one explanation yet seems to suffice. One crucial step in labor seems to be provoked by a decreased ability of progesterone receptors to suppress uterine contractility. This seems due to a decline in steroid co-activator proteins that enable an activated progesterone receptor to fulfill its function.

Many investigators feel that the signal for labor emanates from the fetus and may involve a release of androgens from the fetal adrenal gland. This increases endometrial levels of labor-inducing molecules such as oxytocin and prostaglandins. Additionally, in human fetuses, lung maturation occurs relatively late in pregnancy and results in an eight-fold increase in levels of lung surfactant proteins in amniotic fluid just before term. These lung proteins cause macrophages to migrate within amniotic fluid, through the extraembryonic mesenchyme, and toward the placenta. These cells appear to then trigger inflammatory processes in the uterus that may

PATHOLOGY

Disorders of Pregnancy

The complex sequence that permits an embryo to implant in the wall of the uterus does not always occur without errors. There are a number of important examples.

Tubal pregnancy

Tubal pregnancy occurs in about 1% of all pregnancies and is due to improper location of blastocyst implantation. Recent results suggest that tubal pregnancies, which can rupture the oviduct and cause serious bleeding, occur when the blastocyst induces the adhesion protein trophinin in the wrong place (the oviduct instead of the endometrium) for reasons that are still uncertain.

Preeclampsia

In preeclampsia, which occurs in as many as 1 in 20 pregnancies, placental blood vessels fail to grow properly, causing hypoxia and starvation of fetal tissues. The fetus, in turn, appears to release uncharacterized molecules that resist this hazardous condition by drastically increasing the blood pressure of the mother and the perfusion by blood of the fetus. These dangerous symptoms make preeclampsia the leading cause of maternal mortality in the United States. The cause of preeclampsia appears to be a circulating molecule that binds growth factors required for placental growth. This molecule, called sFlt-1, is three-fold higher in the blood of preeclamptic mothers than in normal mothers and appears to interfere with the normal growth of placental blood vessels.

Choriocarcinoma

Excessive growth and invasiveness of the placenta—the opposite of preeclampsia—can lead to an excessive growth of the placenta and erosion of the uterus.

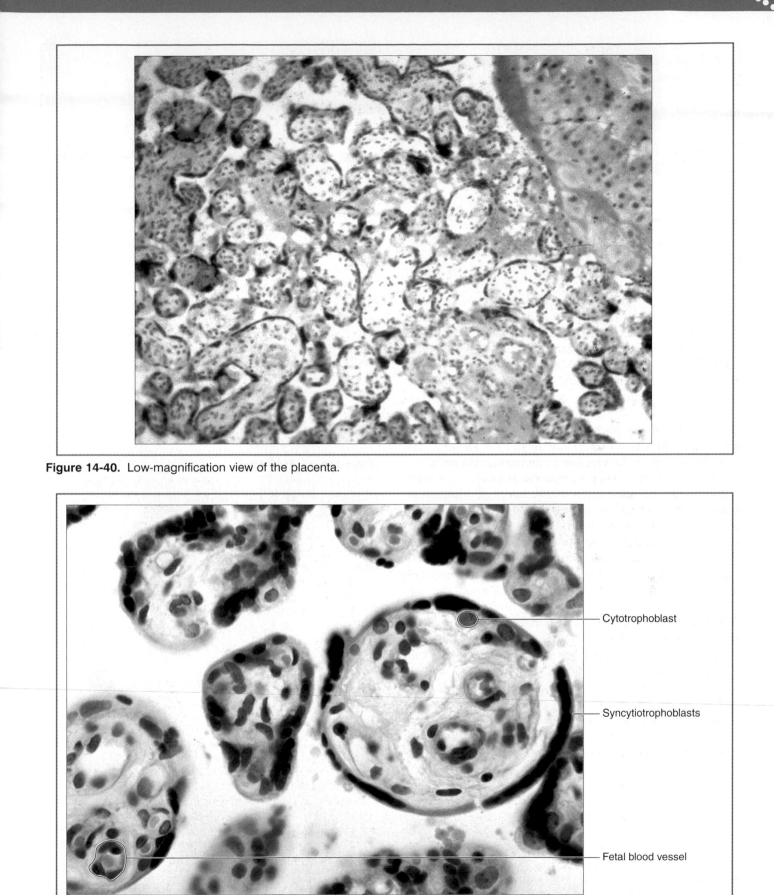

Figure 14-40. Low-magnification view of the placenta.

Figure 14-41. High-magnification view of cross-sections of chorionic villi. The surface of each villus is covered by syncytiotrophoblast. Underlying this outer layer are scattered cells of the cytotrophoblast, plus extraembryonic mesenchyme. Fetal blood vessels are suspended within the extraembryonic mesenchyme.

act as a final signal for labor. This would make sense: a baby is ready to be delivered only when its lungs are prepared for that first breath of air.

One event that facilitates labor is a marked increase in the number of gap junctions connecting smooth muscle cells of the myometrium. This increases the synchronicity of myometrial contractions.

Mammary Glands

In prepubertal women and in adult men, the mammary glands consist of a sparse network of tubules called lactiferous ducts that are surrounded by dense connective tissue and fat and that eventually lead to openings at the nipple. These ducts have a stratified cuboidal epithelium composed of inner secretory cells and outer myoepithelial cells (Fig. 14-42). They are similar in structure to eccrine sweat glands and appear to have derived from these glands during evolution. It would seem that the acquisition of both sweat glands and mammary glands took place as mammals evolved a high metabolic rate and warm bloodedness. This physiologic condition demands structures that (1) cool the body when body temperatures rise too high and (2) provide nourishment for offspring with a high metabolic rate. Sweat glands and their derivatives, mammary glands, accomplish these tasks.

With the onset of puberty, sex steroids stimulate lactiferous ducts to lengthen and grow, and also stimulate a regional enlargement of adipocytes. With the onset of a pregnancy, prolactin and placental hormones stimulate the development of secretory acini (alveoli) at the terminal portions of each duct. The inner secretory cells enlarge, and the lumen of each alveolus becomes distended with milk. The outer layer of myoepithelial cells, in contrast, becomes more attenuated and less noticeable (Fig. 14-43). After the birth of a baby, suckling stimulates the release of oxytocin from the pituitary gland, and oxytocin, by stimulating the contraction of myoepithelial cells, causes a reflex release of milk from the nipple.

Milk produced by mammary epithelial cells contains a complex mixture of nutrients. Milk contains lactose, fats, and a calcium-binding protein called casein. Milk also contains immunoglobulin A, produced by plasma cells of the loose connective tissue surrounding the alveoli. Alveolar epithelial cells bind this secretory form of IgA at their basal surfaces,

PATHOLOGY

Breast Cancer

About 1 in 10 women will develop some form of breast cancer in her lifetime. Most mammary tumors develop from the epithelium of lactiferous ducts and are treated by surgical excision of all or a portion of the breast tissue to prevent the spread of cancer cells (metastasis) via lymphatic vessels to lymph nodes of the axilla or lung. A number of proteins can enhance the risk of developing mammary cancer.

Mutations in a tumor-suppressing protein called BRCA1 or BRCA2 can increase the risk for breast cancer. Approximately 5% to 10% of all forms of breast cancer are due to inherited mutations in these two genes, often characterized by age of onset before 50 years. Genetic screening of women for mutated forms of this protein are useful. Mutations in another protein called HER2, which is a transmembrane protein that controls a number of intracellular signaling pathways and that regulates cellular proliferation, can also predispose to mammary cancer. About 30% of breast cancers show signs of misregulation of this protein. Antibodies to HER2 have been successful in treating this type of cancer.

Breast cancer cells are stimulated to divide by estrogen, so antiestrogen compounds such as tamoxifen have been used to treat breast cancer. Tamoxifen binds to estrogen receptor proteins in a manner similar to estrogen. However, it acts as an antiestrogen for the following reason. When an estrogen receptor protein binds tamoxifen, it undergoes a shape change that is slightly different from that which occurs after binding estrogen. Consequently, the tamoxifen-occupied estrogen receptor is unable to bind to certain steroid co-activator proteins found in mammary epithelium and thus cannot stimulate DNA transcription. However, since various tissues show varying responses to sex steroids and have different steroid co-activator proteins, uterine tissue responds to tamoxifen with an increase rather than a decrease in proliferation. Thus, treatment with tamoxifen is not without potentially hazardous side effects.

move it through the cytoplasm in a process called transcytosis, and secrete it into the alveolar lumen. The milk secreted in the days immediately after the birth of a baby is particularly rich in immunoglobulins and is termed colostrum.

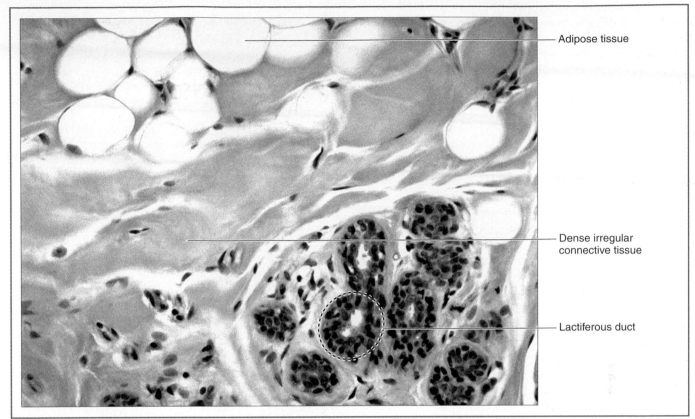

Adipose tissue

Dense irregular
connective tissue

Lactiferous duct

Figure 14-42. Low magnification view of a nonlactating mammary gland showing lactiferous ducts surrounded by loose connective tissue, dense connective tissue, and adipose tissue.

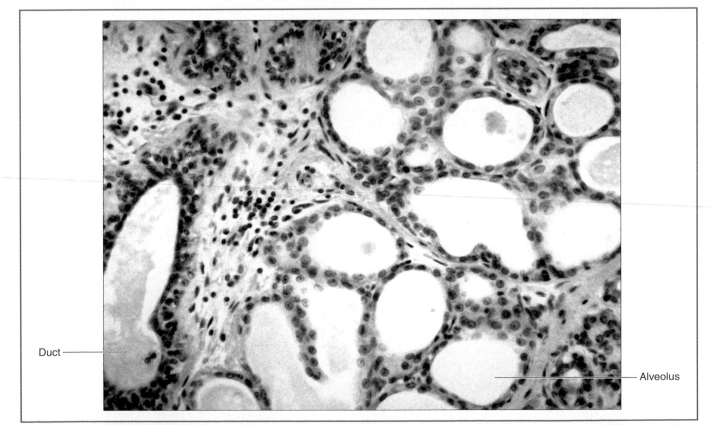

Duct

Alveolus

Figure 14-43. Low-magnification view of a lactating mammary gland. The terminal portions of the ducts have differentiated into secretory alveoli filled with milk.

Case Studies

CASE STUDY 1

A 12-year-old girl visits a new pediatrician with her mother. She has had numerous sinus infections throughout her childhood. Recently, she has developed a chronic cough and feels congested. Her doctor performed a chest radiograph and was surprised to see that the girl's heart was displaced from the left side of the thoracic cavity to the right. Examination of her abdomen with a stethoscope revealed that sounds associated with the stomach were displaced from the right side to the left.

1. **What is most likely to be her medical condition?**

2. **Which organelles have been implicated in this disorder, and why are they particularly critical for respiratory function?**

3. **How would you explain the reverse side placement of her heart and abdominal organs?**

4. **How common is this disorder, and is treatment available?**

CASE STUDY 2

A 57-year-old man has come to his doctor complaining of a number of symptoms. He has developed a persistent cough and sometimes wheezes when he breathes. The wheezing is worse following exertion. He is not a smoker and has never had pneumonia.

1. **What tests should be ordered to evaluate his condition?**

2. **What is the most likely diagnosis for his condition?**

3. **What treatments are available, and what type of prognosis can be expected?**

CASE STUDY 3

A 1-year-old baby girl has developed blisters on her skin that are painful and are particularly prominent on her legs. When she falls or has an injury, large patches of skin exfoliate, heal very poorly, and turn into sores. Since starting on solid food, she has had difficulty eating and has lost weight.

1. **What is most likely to be her medical condition?**

2. **Which molecules or structures have been implicated in this disorder, and why are they particularly critical for skin function?**

3. **Is this disorder common, and is treatment available?**

CASE STUDY 4

A 21-year-old male has always been somewhat overweight (weight, 180 pounds at age 16; height, 5 feel 8 inches), but over the last 2 years, he has gained an additional 20 pounds and his parents have become concerned about his health. When in high school, he usually walked to school, but he now lives on his college campus, and his activity level has declined.

1. **What health problems may be associated with weight gain, and what are the criteria that define the transition from simple overweight to clinically significant obesity?**

2. **To what extent is overweight dependent on changes in lifestyle or environment?**

3. **Which physiologic and biochemical components of the body determine the amount of body fat?**

CASE STUDY 5

A 47-year-old male has come to the doctor with complaints about his right leg. Over the last 4 months, his right thigh has thickened and changed in shape, so that instead of being straight it has acquired a curved, or bowed, profile. These changes have been accompanied by leg pain. In addition, the patient noticed subtle changes in the shape of the back of his head and has had some hearing loss.

1. **What is the most likely explanation of the patient's symptoms? What aspects of his skeletal system are abnormal?**

2. **Is this disorder common, and what is its pathogenesis?**

3. **Are any effective treatments available?**

CASE STUDY 6

A 65-year-old man is beginning to have difficulty with stepping or walking although if someone holds him by the shoulders and moves him from side-to-side as he walks, he can stride along easily. When he sits down to play chess, his hands tremble as he considers the next move. Finally, his facial expressions are beginning to seem more rigid and mask-like.

1. **What is his neurologic condition, and which portion of the brain is most affected?**

2. **What is the pathophysiology of this disorder?**

3. **What explains the apparent connection between this disorder and overall aging?**

CASE STUDY 7

A 25-year-old male arrives at his physician's office complaining of unusual fatigue following clearing his yard of leaves during the fall. Routine blood tests showed that he has a hematocrit of only 30% instead of the normal 45%. Patient history shows that he is of normal weight, is not undernourished, and his intake of iron-containing foods such as meats is normal.

1. **What disorder is affecting the patient? How common is it?**

2. **What is the pathophysiology of this disorder?**

3. **What is the best course of treatment?**

CASE STUDY 8

A 5-month-old male infant is brought to his pediatrician by his father. The child was born with no eyebrows or scalp hair (alopecia) and has fingernails with a slightly concave appearance and longitudinal grooves down the nail. He has had chronic diarrhea for several months and a number of middle ear infections that were difficult to treat. Blood tests show an increased number of circulating eosinophils, and immunocytochemical studies for mature T-cell marker proteins show no detectable mature circulating T lymphocytes.

1. **What disorder does the child have?**

2. **What is the basis for this disease? How common is it?**

3. **How does this disorder relate to the embryologic formation of immune system organs?**

CASE STUDY 9

A 30-year-old male has begun to experience male pattern baldness. The hairs on his scalp have become thinner and sparser, and his hairline has receded noticeably.

1. **Why do some men experience baldness at an earlier age than others?**

2. **Why is hair loss basically confined to the scalp, and why does it not occur in the beard-growing regions of the face?**

3. **Are any effective treatments available?**

CASE STUDY 10

A 51-year-old woman visits her doctor because she has developed a puzzling array of symptoms. She has lost weight, has felt signs of heart palpitations, has become more irritable and nervous, and has difficulty sleeping. She has experienced symptoms of discomfort and burning of her eyes. Her doctor diagnosed an endocrine disorder.

1. **What disorder is the woman suffering from? What is its incidence in the general population and among middle-aged women?**

2. **What is the likely cause of this disorder, and how can it be treated?**

3. **What accounts for the eye abnormalities in this disorder?**

CASE STUDY 11

A 45-year-old man has come to his doctor's office with a variety of complaints. He has begun to experience increased joint pain in his hands, general fatigue, loss of libido, and abdominal pain. Physical examination reveals an enlarged liver. Routine blood work demonstrates a slightly increased level of fasting plasma glucose. He is not a heavy drinker, is not obese, and has no history of diabetes in his family.

1. **The patient is suffering from the most common genetic disorder known. What is it?**

2. **What is the abnormality in this disorder, and what diagnostic tests are most useful in confirming it?**

3. **Are treatments available for this disorder?**

CASE STUDY 12

A woman brings her 1-year-old son to a pediatrician because of a number of symptoms. He is a good eater but has failed to gain weight adequately and is in the 10th percentile for weight for his age. He tends to cough and wheeze and does not digest some foods, like cheese or meat, very well. When the mother kisses her son, his skin has a salty taste.

1. **What disorder is affecting the child, and how common is it?**

2. **What is the main abnormality in this disorder, and how does it explain the symptoms?**

3. **How is this disorder treated?**

CASE STUDY 13

A woman visits her doctor complaining of chronic back pain and frequent urinary tract infections. Her blood pressure is elevated. Suspecting a kidney disorder, her doctor orders ultrasound imaging of her back. The results show substantial renal enlargement and fluid-filled spaces in her kidneys.

1. **What disorder does the woman have? How common is it, and what are its symptoms?**

2. **What is the etiology of the disorder?**

3. **Are any effective treatments available?**

CASE STUDY 14

A 16-year-old girl is brought by her parents to see her pediatrician. Since she was very young, she has been unable to smell any odors. This has not caused any serious problems except for several recent episodes when she was cooking and did not detect the odor of burning. Aside from the safety implications of not being able to smell smoke, her parents have not been concerned for her. Now, however, they have come to the doctor because she has not experienced her first period (menarche) and shows few signs of external sexual differentiation.

1. **What medical condition affects this patient, and how common is it?**

2. **What is the abnormality in this syndrome, and how does it explain the symptoms?**

3. **Is treatment available?**

Case Study Answers

CASE STUDY 1

1. The girl is suffering from Kartagener's syndrome, a disorder first identified in 1933 by a Swiss physician, Manes Kartagener. The syndrome is also known as primary ciliary dyskinesia. Its symptoms include chronic respiratory infections and, in half of the patients, a reversal of the positions of thoracic and abdominal organs to the side opposite from normal (this condition is called situs inversus).

2. and 3. It is likely that these symptoms result from nonmotile cilia. As judged from a comparison between ciliated and nonciliated cells, about 250 genes appear to govern the structure and hence the function of cilia. Several of these have been identified as probable causes of Kartagener's syndrome. These genes are termed DNA genes (from dynein arms) and are called *DNA1*, *DNA5*, and *DNA11*. They code for proteins of the outer dynein arms of ciliary axonemes. Dynein and its associated proteins are ATPases whose main function is to cause cilia to beat and bend. The abnormal ciliary function resulting from mutations in these genes has two major effects:

   a. In embryogenesis, the primary cilia of certain cells of the ventral part of the embryonic node continually sweep fluid toward one side of the embryo. This fluid contains growth factors and possibly some uncharacterized molecules that cause the developing heart to twist toward the left and the stomach and liver to form in their asymmetric positions. In the absence of this fluid movement, these organs are positioned randomly, so that in half of patients with Kartagener's syndrome they form on the "wrong" side.

   b. In both children and adults, cilia play particularly prominent roles in the function of the respiratory epithelium. Without ciliary movement, mucus accumulates in the respiratory tract and sinuses and may provoke repeated infections.

4. This disorder affects approximately 1 in 25,000 persons. Most affected individuals can function relatively normally, even with reversed positioning of organs. Although there is no direct treatment for this syndrome, sinus infections tend to decrease after age 20, perhaps because the air conducting parts of the respiratory system have increased in caliber by adulthood. Males usually have substantially reduced fertility, since flagellar motility is dependent on a functional axoneme.

CASE STUDY 2

1. A chest radiograph and complete blood count are important first diagnostic procedures. Depending on the outcome of these procedures, it may be advisable to perform a CT scan or an MRI. Additionally, intrabronchial lavage with saline can recover cells that can be examined microscopically to determine a specific diagnosis. All these tests can determine whether a cancerous tumor is present in the lung.

2. Lung cancer is a common type of cancer and often is associated with a history of smoking. Nonsmokers also can develop lung cancer, either from second-hand smoke or from other airborne or nonairborne causes. A common form of lung cancer is an adenocarcinoma, derived from epithelial cells of bronchi or bronchioles. A more aggressive, but rarer, form of lung cancer is a mesothelioma, derived from cells that form mesothelial connective tissue and epithelial membrane around the lungs. These two forms of cancer develop from two of the four basic types of tissues. The cancer cells of adenocarcinomas and mesotheliomas look similar under the microscope after conventional staining but often can be distinguished by immunocytochemical stains for specific types of proteins. Mesotheliomas often stain positively for a type of intermediate filament—vimentin—that makes up part of the cytoskeleton of connective tissue cells. These tumors can be provoked by exposure to asbestos, a carcinogen commonly encountered by carpenters who repair old buildings. Adenocarcinomas, in contrast, often stain positively for the epithelial cell protein keratin but are negative for vimentin. There are several other types of lung cancer as well.

3. Current therapies for lung cancer involve the use of irradiation or chemotherapeutic agents (e.g., cisplatin) that damage the DNA of rapidly dividing cancer cells. The 5-year survival rates after treatment for adenocarcinoma are reasonably good, but less so for mesothelioma.

CASE STUDY 3

1. The girl likely has a mild form of epidermolysis bullosa (EB) simplex, a skin disorder in which the

epidermal-dermal attachment has been weakened. In addition to damaging the epidermis, the nonkeratinized stratified squamous epithelium in the esophagus is affected, resulting in damage to the esophagus after contact with solid foods.

2. The molecules affected in this and other skin-blistering diseases are involved in strengthening the skin and attaching the basal layer of the epidermis to the dermis. In EB simplex, a component of the cytoskeleton called an intermediate filament is abnormal. Keratin proteins form the intermediate filaments that are found in epithelial cells. About 30 different types of keratin proteins are known, and each is found in specific types of epithelial cells. In most epithelial cells, keratins account for about 1% of total cell protein, but in basal keratinocytes of the skin, keratins can make up as much as 25% of total cell protein. Basal keratinocytes produce keratin types 5 and 14. Mutations in keratin type 14 result in a disrupted cytoskeleton of the cell and produce cells that rupture in response to mechanical stress. This causes blistering and a very delicate skin. In another blistering skin disorder, bullous pemphigus, patients develop antibodies to a protein found in hemidesmosomes (collagen type XVII), which attach the epidermis to the dermis.

3. EB simplex is a rare genetic disorder and affects approximately 10,000 patients in the United States. Beyond protecting the skin with gauze and soft clothing, there is no effective treatment. Bullous pemphigus is an autoimmune disease that tends to occur more frequently in patients older than 55 years. Like many other autoimmune diseases, bullous pemphigus can be treated with high doses of prednisone. The blisters of bullous pemphigus respond well to treatment and may eventually go away.

CASE STUDY 4

1. In general, obesity increases the risk for type 2 diabetes, high blood pressure, and cardiovascular disease. An individual with a body mass index (BMI) greater than 30 is defined as obese (BMI = weight in kilograms divided by the square of height in meters). At a weight of 200 pounds and a height of 5 feet, 8 inches, his BMI is about 31, putting him in the obese category. Obesity of this type is associated with a statistically significant increase in mortality. However, milder degrees of overweight do not seem to pose a significant risk of increased mortality. Furthermore, consideration of percentage of body fat and muscle mass need to be taken into account in evaluating his obese status.

2. In a nutritionally abundant society like the United States, most people are somewhat at risk for becoming overweight or obese. However, studies of identical twins suggest that as much as 50% to 70% of the variability in body weight is due solely to genetics. Genetic differences in appetite, restlessness, and overall metabolism may play

major roles in the development of obesity. Changes in lifestyle or environment seem to account for the remaining variability in body fat. Any factor that decreases the ratio of calories burned to calories consumed will result in obesity.

3. Studies of genetically obese rodents suggest that a part of the brain called the arcuate nucleus of the hypothalamus plays a major role in determining the amount of body fat, since it contains neurons that regulate appetite and caloric homeostasis. These neurons, in turn, respond to a peptide secreted from fat cells called leptin. When fat stores diminish, blood levels of leptin fall and stimulate the hypothalamus to increase appetite. Increased fat stores provoke increases in circulating levels of leptin, which can diminish appetite. However, if offered tasty foods, animals and humans can override the inhibitory effects of leptin and continue to overconsume calories. This so-called diet-induced hypothalamic resistance to leptin represents a significant problem in reducing body fat. Its cause is uncertain, but it may result from elevations in circulating glucose that are seen in diet-induced obesity. Glucose seems to make the hypothalamus resistant to leptin. Furthermore, studies on the effects of leptin in rodents and in humans indicate that the physiologic role of the hormone is different in rodents and humans.

CASE STUDY 5

1. The patient has Paget's disease, which was first described by the English physician James Paget in 1876. In the first phase of Paget's disease of bone (the osteolytic phase), osteoclasts become abnormally active and large (some can contain as many as 100 nuclei) and degrade bone extensively. In the second phase (the mixed phase), the degraded bone is replaced by osteoblast activity. This results in the formation of excessive amounts of immature (woven) and lamellar bone, which may be found in only a few bones or in many bones. Immature bone is more easily deformed or broken, and the lamellar bone is architecturally abnormal. The skeletal system of adults normally contains very little immature bone. A third phase of the disease (the osteosclerotic phase) is characterized by excessive disorganized deposition of bone. In some cases of Paget's disease, enlargement of skull bones can press upon nerves of the inner ear, which may lead to hearing loss.

2. Paget's disease may be present in as many as 1% of people over 40 years of age, although many affected individuals are unaware of their condition because the symptoms often are not severe. For unknown reasons, this disease is more common in men than in women and is largely confined to individuals from the British Isles and the countries to which they have migrated. The defect seems to be that osteoclasts are excessively responsive to vitamin D and become overactive. This hyperactivity is not due to any abnormalities in the vitamin D receptors, which are similar in structure and function to steroid hormone

receptors. Instead, the osteoclasts overproduce a so-called co-activator protein (TAFII-17), which increases the ability of the vitamin D receptors to activate DNA transcription and promote the synthesis of bone-degrading proteins by the osteoclasts. Evidence indicates that infection with a paramyxovirus (a "slow virus") is the underlying cause of the disease.

3. A common treatment for this disorder is the administration of biphosphonate compounds such as alendronate (Fosamax), which enhance calcium deposition in bone.

CASE STUDY 6

1. The patient suffers from Parkinson's disease (PD). In PD, a specific subset of neurons within the midbrain (substantia nigra) degenerate and die. These neurons utilize dopamine, a neurotransmitter, to communicate with the corpus striatum, a more anterior brain structure that regulates movement. Dopamine is metabolized to form dark-staining intracellular deposits of neuromelanin, which is responsible for the dark appearance of the substantia nigra (Latin, "black substance"). When these dopamine-containing neurons die, a disordered regulation of movement by the striatum results in rest tremor, facial rigidity, and difficulty walking.

2. Most cases of Parkinson's disease do *not* have a genetic basis, and therefore the specific causes of the disorder are uncertain. The incidence of PD is greater among those who work on farms or with agricultural equipment, so many clinicians suspect that exposure to the toxins in pesticides or other farm chemicals may have a damaging effect on dopaminergic neurons. This hypothesis is supported by the discovery of an artificial morphine-type neurotoxin, 1-methyl-4-phenyl-1,2,3,6-tetrahydropyridine (MPTP). Unfortunately, MPTP, which is abused as an ingredient of illicit drugs, can cause the sudden onset of PD. MPTP is taken up into cells in the substantia nigra via dopamine transporters on the cell membrane that normally function in reuptake of dopamine secreted by a neuron. After exposure to MPTP, dopaminergic neurons experience oxidative stress and degenerate in a way similar to the degeneration seen in PD. Some pesticides (e.g., paraquat) have structural similarities to MPTP and may be involved in producing spontaneous PD. Finally, rare cases of inherited PD have shown that neuronal proteins called parkin or synuclein may react to environmental toxins by injuring dopaminergic neurons.

3. About 1% of all people aged 65 or older can be expected to develop PD. The link between aging and PD is probably related to the fact that neurons of the brain have limited regenerative ability. Thus, long-lived neurons gradually accumulate damage from metabolic processes (e.g., oxidation), which take place primarily in mitochondria. As neurons acquire more oxidative stress over a lifetime, they develop mitochondrial abnormalities and become more vulnerable to environmental toxins.

CASE STUDY 7

1. He suffers from a mild form of congenital anemia called thalassemia minor. This genetic disorder is more common in populations from southern Europe or Mediterranean North Africa, where it can be present in as much as 6% of the population.

2. Thalassemia minor results from a defect in the gene coding for the β-chain of hemoglobin, resulting in diminished transcription of the gene and consequent low protein levels. This genetic trait is detectable in patients heterozygous for a mutation on chromosome 11 from one parent. Since these patients have a normal gene on the other chromosome, they still can produce small amounts of the normal β-chain. Low amounts of the β-chain in a red blood cell produce a relative excess of the normal α-chain of hemoglobin, causing insoluble aggregates to form that provoke the premature death of red blood cells. Thus, a mild anemia will be present in thalassemia minor patients that leads to a lowered O_2-carrying capacity of the blood and fatigue upon exercise. If a heterozygous individual marries another heterozygous individual, there is a 25% chance that any offspring will be homozygous for thalassemia and will inherit two damaged genes for hemoglobin (thalassemia major). The homozygous condition is far more serious, producing severe anemia, elevated levels of blood iron due to erythrocyte destruction, and an enlarged spleen.

3. No special treatments are applicable or usually necessary. Excessive supplementation of the diet with iron is not helpful and can even produce symptoms of iron overload.

CASE STUDY 8

1. The child has severe combined immunodeficiency disease (SCID), which results from failure of the thymus to form normally during embryogenesis. As a result, mature T lymphocytes do not form and immune defenses are weakened. This is the human equivalent of a special mutant mouse called the nude mouse. This animal is athymic and lacks hair, hence its name. The nude mouse is widely used by immunologists because it lacks T lymphocytes and cannot reject foreign tissue transplants from other mice. For example, a patch of hairy skin from another mouse can be transplanted onto the back of a nude mouse and will not be rejected.

2. The disorder results from a mutation in a transcription-regulating protein called FOXN1. This protein is selectively expressed in the ectodermal cells of the skin and the thymic portion of the third pharyngeal pouch during embryogenesis. In the skin, this transcription factor is required for the synthesis of calbindin in hair follicles; if it is disrupted, hair will not grow. The formation of nails in the mouse and in the human also is abnormal in the absence of a functioning *FOXN1* gene. The disorder is

uncommon in humans. It has been studied mainly in a small village in Italy, where descendants from an affected ancestor are still living.

3. In the thymus, *FOXN1* appears to be required for the normal function of a subpopulation of thymic epithelial-reticular cells that cause the thymus to become populated with pre-T cells originating in the bone marrow. The requirement of both skin and thymic cells for this transcription factor is just another feature these two cell types have in common in addition to similar histologic morphology and to common production of skin-type keratin.

CASE STUDY 9

1. By about age 50 years, about 50% of men will develop male pattern baldness to some degree. Although not all factors causing male pattern baldness are understood, it is now clear that most (46%) of the variability in baldness between individuals is due to variability in the structure of the androgen receptor. The amino acid sequence of the androgen receptor protein is rather unusual in that the amino terminal portion of the protein contains a variable number of polyglutamine residues. The number of glutamine residues varies between a minimum of 8 to a maximum of 34. As the number of glutamines in the androgen receptor increases, the translation efficiency of the androgen receptor mRNA declines. Cells possessing androgen receptors with 23 or fewer glutamines are synthesized in greater numbers, whereas cells possessing the gene that codes for 24 or more glutamines in the receptor tend to synthesize fewer androgen receptors. Thus, variability in the structure of the androgen receptor promotes an increased sensitivity to androgen in some men and a decreased sensitivity in others.

2. The growth of the epidermis in general and of hair follicles in particular is greatly affected by signaling molecules produced by dermal fibroblasts. Dermal fibroblasts of the skin of the cheeks and chin respond to testosterone by secreting insulin-like growth factor 1, which stimulates hair growth. Dermal fibroblasts of the scalp seem to respond to testosterone by secreting transforming growth factor β, which inhibits hair growth. Why these cells, located in neighboring locations, respond to testosterone so differently is still unknown.

3. One treatment that seems to diminish the rate of hair loss in the scalp is application of minoxidil. This drug activates ATP-sensitive potassium channels in dermal cells and stimulates them to secrete vascular endothelial growth factor, which increases hair growth. However, this treatment works best in younger men and when started shortly after the onset of hair loss.

CASE STUDY 10

1. The woman has Graves' disease (GD), an autoimmune disorder that results in an overproduction of thyroxin. Excess thyroxin stimulates the basal metabolic rate, causing weight loss and tachycardia. Its incidence increases with age; within the general population, less than 0.25% of all people are affected by this disorder. However, in middle-aged women, the incidence is 8-fold higher than in middle-aged men.

2. Graves' disease is caused by production of autoantibodies that bind to the TSH receptor protein in the plasma membrane of thyroid follicular cells. This apparently does not harm the cells but mimics the effects of TSH itself and stimulates increased production of thyroxin. To diminish thyroxin production, a common means of treatment is the systemic administration of a radioactive isotope of iodine. This radioactive iodine is concentrated in the thyroid and causes a partial damage to thyroid follicular cells, diminishing thyroxin production.

3. Ocular symptoms in GD can progress from irritation to exophthalmos, a condition in which the eyeballs protrude forward in their sockets. This is due to an expansion of retro-orbital tissues, including adipose tissue and extraocular muscles. Since rearward expansion of these tissues is blocked by the bones of the orbit, forward expansion is the only route possible. The reasons retro-orbital tissues are particularly affected in GD are uncertain. Recently, it has been demonstrated that retro-orbital fibroblasts appear to possess small numbers of TSH receptors. TSH receptor levels, although 1000-fold lower than those in the thyroid gland, are nevertheless elevated in retro-orbital fibroblasts as compared with fibroblasts elsewhere in the body. Thus, autoantibodies against TSH receptors may stimulate inflammation and adipogenesis within the orbital cavity but not elsewhere.

CASE STUDY 11

1. The patient is suffering from hereditary hemochromatosis (HH). About 10% of people are heterozygotes for the abnormal gene *HFE*, which causes this disorder, and as many as 1 in 400 are homozygous for the gene and exhibit clinical signs of hemochromatosis. The main problem in HH is an overload of iron in a number of organs, primarily the liver, pancreas, and anterior pituitary. Iron deposits in anterior pituitary gonadotropes damage these cells and produce lower secretions of LH and FSH and hence less testosterone, which is responsible for a decrease in the male libido. In the liver, iron overloading causes hepatocyte damage and cirrhosis, leading to an enlarged liver and abnormalities in carbohydrate metabolism.

2. The abnormal protein in HH is called HFE. HFE is a 343-amino-acid protein that shows homology with the major histocompatibility protein MHC-1 on the surface of many cells of the immune system. However, HFE does not seem to assist in recognition or presentation of foreign antigens. HFE is normally expressed at the cell surface and binds to transferrin receptors in the plasma membrane. Transferrin receptors bind the serum iron-carrying protein, transferrin, to the cell surface. People suffering from HH have an abnormal HFE protein (in which a cysteine is replaced by a tyrosine) that becomes misdirected within cells and is not sent to the cell surface. In the absence of HFE, the transferrin receptors deliver too much iron to the interior of cells. If liver damage has progressed significantly, a number of liver enzymes released from damaged hepatocytes will be detectable in the blood. Also, a needle biopsy of the liver may reveal liver cirrhosis. However, the best diagnostic test for HH is elevated transferrin saturation with iron, although measurements of total serum iron and ferritin are also useful. Most patients with this disorder are of northern European ancestry.

3. The body has no normal pathway for iron secretion, so iron overload is difficult to control by homeostatic mechanisms. One means of reducing iron stores is phlebotomy—blood donation or bloodletting. Thus, loss of iron through bleeding is a simple treatment for HH. The fact that symptoms of HH are relatively rare in premenopausal women is explained by blood loss via monthly menstrual periods.

Additionally, ducts of sweat glands, which normally remove chloride from sweat, do not function normally, causing the sweat and the surface of the skin to have a higher salt concentration than normal.

CF patients also suffer from dietary insufficiency since the exocrine ducts of the pancreas become clogged with their own secretions for the same reasons as stated above. The ducts have a cystic and fibrotic appearance, which gives the disease its name. As a result, the pancreatic digestive enzymes are not delivered to the duodenum. CF patients have watery stools and are undernourished. This is treated by oral administration of pancreatic enzymes and careful attention to diet.

3. A number of treatments have become available in the last 10 years that have increased the life expectancy of these patients from the teens to the mid-thirties. Traditional therapy of clapping the back vigorously each day to dislodge mucus from the air passages is an important part of treatment. In addition, administration of antibiotic aerosols that diminish lung infections has been helpful. Experiments in mice suggest that a component present in the spice turmeric, curcumin, may have some protective influence. Curcumin prevents the import of calcium into the endoplasmic reticulum and appears to interfere with the function of quality-control proteases of the rER. This may allow even abnormal CFTR proteins to leave the rER, migrate to the plasma membrane, and carry out a limited amount of Cl^- transport.

CASE STUDY 12

1. The child has cystic fibrosis, one of the most common inheritable diseases (incidence of about 1 in 3500 births).

2. This disease is caused by many different mutations in a protein called the cystic fibrosis transmembrane conductance regulator (CTFR). This protein, normally located at the apical surface of many epithelial cells, is a chloride channel protein and is responsible for the secretion or uptake of chloride into the lumen of airway passages or other ducts. When chloride is secreted, sodium is also pumped out of the cell to maintain the intracellular electrochemical balance, and then water follows passively. CTFR has a similar function in the ducts of exocrine glands such as sweat glands and the pancreas. Mutations in the gene for this protein alter its structure and function. Misfolded CFTR protein is tagged by quality-control protein degradation mechanisms of the endoplasmic reticulum that prevent defective CFTR protein from being transported to the plasma membrane. As a consequence, cells from a patient with cystic fibrosis cannot add sufficient Cl^-, Na^+, or water to the mucus present in the airways, which becomes thick and viscous. Furthermore, dying cells become trapped in the mucus and add to its viscosity by exuding their DNA. The thickened mucus occludes air passages and the ducts of exocrine glands.

CASE STUDY 13

1. The woman is experiencing polycystic kidney disease (PKD). This is a relatively common inheritable disorder, affecting about 1 in 700 persons. The disorder is progressive, so that few symptoms are apparent early in life but are detectable mostly in patients 40 years of age or older. In this disorder, fluid-filled cysts appear in the kidneys and gradually enlarge, slowly replacing the normal parenchyma of the kidney; the kidneys can become very large and heavy—as much as 22 pounds per kidney. The enlarged kidneys are functionally impaired, so that disturbances in fluid balance and blood pressure appear.

2. PKD is a progressive, genetic disorder of the kidneys. It occurs in humans and other animals. PKD is characterized by the presence of multiple cysts (polycystic disease) in both kidneys. The disease can also damage the liver, pancreas, and rarely the heart and brain. There is a more common autosomal dominant form and a less common recessive form of PKD. Two genes called *PKD1* and *PKD2* have been identified as causing this disorder. These genes encode for proteins located on the apical surfaces of epithelial cells of the collecting ducts. They are single, nonmotile cilia called primary cilia that act as chemosensors for these cells. The abnormal proteins present in polycystic kidney disease form transient receptor calcium channels and receptors for epidermal

growth factor. An abnormal activity of these proteins causes an intracellular accumulation of cAMP, which stimulates fluid secretion and an overgrowth of these cells that eventually results in cyst formation.

3. Treatment mainly relies on compounds that reduce blood pressure. These include angiotensin-converting enzyme (ACE) inhibitors, such as losartan, which block the formation of angiotensin II. Since angiotensin II raises blood pressure by constricting arterioles and by causing sodium retention, a decrease in its formation is effective in treating this disease. More recently, the use of vasopressin receptor blockers has been effective as treatment in experimental animals.

CASE STUDY 14

1. This girl's symptoms are a combination of anosmia and hypogonadism, classic signs of Kallmann syndrome, which was recognized in the 1800s and definitively described by Kallmann in 1944. Its incidence is about 1 in 8000 men and 1 in 40,000 women. This sex difference is due to the fact that one of the two abnormal genes, called *KAL1*, is located on the X chromosome. Since women possess two X chromosomes, damage to a gene on one X chromosome can be compensated for by the intact gene on the other X chromosome.

2. The *KAL1* and *KAL2* genes code for a protein called anosmin-1 and for fibroblast growth factor receptor–1, respectively. During embryogenesis, these genes govern the formation of the olfactory placodes that will generate olfactory neurons. In addition, neurons that synthesize GnRH originate in the olfactory bulbs and migrate to the basomedial hypothalamus before initiating their function of regulating the release of pituitary gonadotropins. Defective function of these two genes thus leads to an inability to smell and to a failure to initiate puberty. This comingling of reproductive and olfactory functions of the brain is a reminder of the importance of olfaction in the initiation of mating behavior and reproduction in many mammals.

3. The sexual deficiencies present in Kallmann syndrome can be treated successfully, in women, by administration of sex steroids such as estrogen and progesterone to initiate sexual maturation. To promote ovarian maturation and ovulation, administration of gonadotropins has proved effective.

Index

Page numbers followed by f indicate figures; those followed by t indicate tables; and those followed by b indicate boxed material.

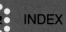